Reference Guide for Essential Oils

Connie and Alan Higley

This book has been designed to provide information to help educate the reader in regard to the subject matter covered. It is sold with the understanding that the publisher and the authors are nc liable for the misconception or misuse of the information provided. It is not provided in order to diagnose, prescribe, or treat any disease, illness, or injured condition of the body. The authors an publisher shall have neither liability nor responsibility to any person or entity with respect to any loss, damage, or injury caused or alleged to be caused directly or indirectly by the information contained in this book. The information presented herein is in no way intended as a substitute for medical counseling. Anyone suffering from any disease, illness, or injury should consult a qualified health care professional.

Library of Congress Cataloging-in-Publication Data.

Higley, Connie.

Reference guide for essential oils / Connie and Alan Higley

p. ill. cm.

Includes bibliographical references.

1. Essences and essential oils–Therapeutic use–Handbooks, manuals, etc.
2. Aromatherapy–Handbooks, manuals, etc.

00-500404

Published and distributed by Abundant Health
PO Box 281, Spanish Fork, UT 84660
Phone: 1-888-718-3068 (toll-free) / 801-798-0642 (local)
Fax: 1-877-568-1988 (toll-free) / 801-798-0644 (local)
Internet: www.abundant-health4u.com
E-Mail: orders@abundant-health4u.com

Printed and bound in the United States of America.

International Standard Book Number: 0-9706583-0-3

Dedication

We, the authors (compilers) of this information, were introduced to Young Living Essential Oils in 1995. At that time, there was no compiled information on the use of these valuable oils, so together with Pat Leatham, we set out to find what we could. We gathered notes from lectures and seminars by D. Gary Young, N.D. and product information from Young Living Essential Oils. Extensive research into the works of other aromatherapy experts have shown us that Dr. Young, through his own research and clinical study, not only supports, but expands their solid foundation of knowledge and expertise. When this book was first made available in 1996, we made a conscious decision to keep the names of D. Gary Young and Young Living Essential Oils out of this book so as to remove all possibility of recrimination or harm to Dr. Young or his company. However, all past, present, and future readers of this work need to understand that all of us, author and reader alike, are deeply indebted to Dr. Young for his brilliant insight, extensive research, and incredible vision of the healing power of essential oils.

We, therefore, dedicate this book to D. Gary Young, N.D. as a tribute to his vision of health for all who will embrace the oils and use them to their fullest potential. Dr. Young is one of the foremost experts on the organic cultivation, distillation, and clinical use of essential oils in North America. His unwavering passion for maintaining the highest quality in his products have produced some astounding healing results. We applaud his heroic and often solitary effort to continue proving, by clinical study, the efficacy of essential oils as indispensable tools for combating disease.

Acknowledgments

To our 5 young children who demonstrate much patience and responsibility with the freedom they are given during the on-going compilation and updating of this book.

To the late Pat Leatham who provided the initial impetus for its creation. Her many hours of research and meticulous note-taking will forever be appreciated.

And to all of you who are discovering, or re-discovering, for yourselves the healing powers of essential oils. May this book provide quick access to the information you need to help yourself, and those you love, progress on the road to better health.

A special thanks goes to our families and to all of our "Essential Oil" friends! Without your love, friendship, suggestions, support, patience, and prodding, we would have crumbled under the strain of compiling a book such as this while trying to raise a family and have a life.

Contents

The section tabs shown on the right, correspond to each individual section listed below. By holding the spine of the book in the left hand and bending the right side back with the right hand, section markings become visible along the right edge. This should allow you quick and easy reference to any applicable section.

The sections on Personal Care Products, Bath Gels and Bar Soaps, Tinctures, Massage Oils, and Supplements and Vitamins list commercially available products that include pure essential oils either for additional therapeutic benefits or to enhance the bio-availability of the other ingredients.

Science and Application
Single Oils
Oil Blends
Personal Care Products
Bath Gels and Bar Soaps
Tinctures
Massage Oils
Supplements
Personal Guide

BASIC FACTS ABOUT ESSENTIAL OILS

How long have essential oils been around?

Essential oils were mankind's first medicine. From Egyptian hieroglyphics and Chinese manuscripts, we know that priests and physicians have been using essential oils for thousands of years. In Egypt, essential oils were used in the embalming process and well preserved oils were found in alabaster jars in King Tut's tomb. Egyptian temples were dedicated to the production and blending of the oils and recipes were recorded on the walls in hieroglyphics. There is even a sacred room in the temple of Isis on the island of Philae where a ritual called "Cleansing the Flesh and Blood of Evil Deities" was practiced. This form of emotional clearing required three days of cleansing using particular essential oils and oil baths.

There are 188 references to essential oils in the Bible. Oils such as frankincense, myrrh, rosemary, hyssop, and spikenard were used for anointing and healing the sick. In Exodus, the Lord gave the following recipe to Moses for "an holy anointing oil":

Myrrh ("five hundred shekels"— approximately 1 gallon)
Sweet Cinnamon ("two hundred and fifty shekels"— approximately ½ gallon)
Sweet Calamus ("two hundred and fifty shekels")
Cassia ("five hundred shekels")
Olive Oil ("an hin"— approximately 1⅓ gallons)

The three wise men presented the Christ child with essential oils of frankincense and myrrh. There are also accounts in the New Testament of the Bible where Jesus was anointed with spikenard oil; "And being in Bethany in the house of Simon the leper, as he sat at meat, there came a woman having an alabaster box of ointment of spikenard very precious; and she brake the box, and poured [it] on his head" (Mark 14:3). "Then took Mary a pound of ointment of spikenard, very costly, and anointed the feet of Jesus, and wiped his feet with her hair: and the house was filled with the odour of the ointment" (John 12:3). Some have even said that essential oils carry the consciousness of Christ.

What are *PURE, THERAPEUTIC-GRADE* essential oils?

Essential oils are the volatile liquids that are distilled from plants (including their respective parts such as seeds, bark, leaves, stems, roots, flowers, fruit, etc.). One of the factors that determine the purity and therapeutic value of an oil is its chemical constituents. These constituents can be affected by a vast number of variables including: the part(s) of the plant from which the oil was produced, soil condition, fertilizer (organic or chemical), geographical region, climate, altitude, harvest season and methods, and distillation process. For example, common thyme, or thyme vulgaris, produces several different chemotypes (biochemical specifics or simple species) depending on the conditions of its growth, climate, and altitude. One will produce high levels of thymol depending on the time of year it is distilled. If distilled during mid-summer or lat fall, there can be higher levels of carvacrol which can cause the oil to be more caustic or irritating to the skin. Low pressure and low temperature are also keys to maintaining the purity, the ultima fragrance, and the therapeutic value of the oil.

As we begin to understand the power of essential oils in the realm of personal, holistic healthcare, we comprehend the absolute necessity for obtaining the purest therapeutic-grade essential oils possible. No matter how costly pure therapeutic-grade essential oils may be, there can be no substitutes. Chemists can replicate some of the known individual constituents, but they have yet to successfully recreate complete essential oils in the laboratory.

The information in this book is based upon the use of pure, therapeutic-grade essential oil Those who are beginning their journey into the realm of aromatherapy and essential oils, must actively seek for the purest quality and highest therapeutic-grade oils available. Anything less tha pure, therapeutic-grade essential oil may not produce the desired results and can, in some cases, b extremely toxic.

Why is it so difficult to find *PURE, THERAPEUTIC-GRADE* essential oils?

Producing the purest of oils can be very costly because it may require several hundred pounds, or even several thousand pounds of plant material to extract one pound of pure essential oil. For example, one pound of pure melissa oil sells for $9,000 - $15,000. Although this sounds quite expensive, one must realize that three tons of plant material are required to produce that single pound of oil. Because the vast majority of all the oils produced in the world today are used by the perfume industry, the oils are being purchased for their aromatic qualities only. High pressure, high temperatures, rapid processing and the use of chemical solvents are often employec during the distillation process so that a greater *quantity* of oil can be produced at a faster rate. These oils may smell just as good and cost much less, but will lack most, if not all, of the chemica constituents necessary to produce the expected therapeutic results.

What benefits do *PURE, THERAPEUTIC-GRADE* essential oils provide?

1. Essential oils are the regenerating, oxygenating, and immune defense properties of plants.
2. Essential oils are so small in molecular size that they can quickly penetrate the tissues of the skin.
3. Essential oils are lipid soluble and are capable of penetrating cell walls, even if they have hardened because of an oxygen deficiency. In fact, essential oils can affect every cell of the body within 20 minutes and are then metabolized like other nutrients.
4. Essential oils contain oxygen molecules which help to transport nutrients to the starving human cells. Because a nutritional deficiency is an oxygen deficiency, disease begins when the cells lack the oxygen for proper nutrient assimilation. By providing the needed oxygen, essential oils also work to stimulate the immune system.
5. Essential oils are very powerful antioxidants. Antioxidants create an unfriendly environment for free radicals. They prevent all mutations, work as free radical scavengers, prevent fungus, and prevent oxidation in the cells.
6. Essential oils are anti-bacterial, anti-cancerous, anti-fungal, anti-infectious, anti-microbial, anti-tumoral, anti-parasitic, anti-viral, and antiseptic. Essential oils have been shown to destroy all tested bacteria and viruses while simultaneously restoring balance to the body.
7. Essential oils may detoxify the cells and blood in the body.
8. Essential oils containing sesquiterpenes have the ability to pass the blood brain barrier, enabling them to be effective in the treatment of Alzheimer's disease, Lou Gehrig's disease, Parkinson's disease, and multiple sclerosis.
9. Essential oils are aromatic. When diffused, they provide air purification by:
   A. Removing metallic particles and toxins from the air;
   B. Increasing atmospheric oxygen;
   C. Increasing ozone and negative ions in the area, which inhibits bacterial growth;
   D. Destroying odors from mold, cigarettes, and animals; and
   E. Filling the air with a fresh, aromatic scent.
10. Essential oils help promote emotional, physical, and spiritual healing.
11. Essential oils have a bio-electrical frequency that is several times greater than the frequency of herbs, food, and even the human body. Clinical research has shown that essential oils can quickly raise the frequency of the human body, restoring it to its normal, healthy level.

What is frequency and how does it pertain to essential oils?

Frequency is a measurable rate of electrical energy that is constant between any two points. Everything has an electrical frequency. Bruce Tainio of Tainio Technology in Cheny, Washington, developed new equipment to measure the bio-frequency of humans and foods. Bruce

Tainio and Dr. D. Gary Young, a North American expert on essential oils, used this bio-frequenc monitor to determine the relationship between frequency and disease. Some of the results of their studies are as follows:

Human Brain	72-90 MHz	Processed/canned food	0 MHz
Human Body (day)	62-68 MHz	Fresh Produce	up to 15 MHz
Cold Symptoms	58 MHz	Dry Herbs	12-22 MHz
Flu Symptoms	57 MHz	Fresh Herbs	20-27 MHz
Candida	55 MHz	Essential Oils	52-320 MHz
Epstein Barr	52 MHz		
Cancer	42 MHz		
Death Begins	25 MHz		

Note: Due to the sensitivity of the instruments, these results are not easily duplicatable. What is important is the relativity of the numbers and the fact that the higher frequency of the essential oils can help raise the frequency of the human body to a more normal level.

Another part of this same study measured the frequency fluctuations within the human body as different substances were introduced. The chart shown below illustrates the frequency reaction of the human body to the introduction of coffee. The subsequent time necessary for the frequency to return to its original measurement was shown to be substantially reduced with the us of essential oils.

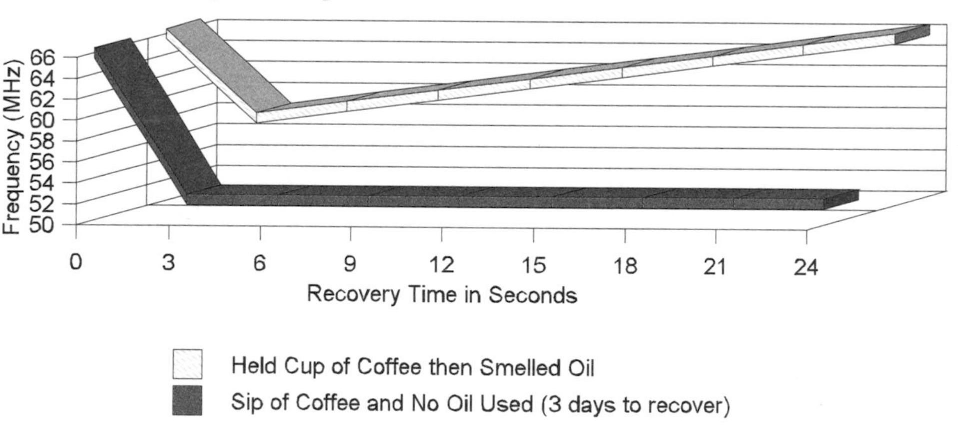

Initially, the frequency of each of two different individuals—the first a 26 yr. old male an the second a 24 yr. old male—was measured at 66 MHz for both. The first individual held a cup of coffee (without drinking any) and his frequency dropped to 58 MHz in 3 seconds. He then removed the coffee and inhaled an aroma of essential oils. Within 21 seconds, his frequency had returned to 66 MHz. The second individual took a sip of coffee and his frequency dropped to 52 MHz in the same 3 seconds. However, no essential oils were used during the recovery time and it took 3 days for his frequency to return to the initial 66 MHz.

Another very interesting result of this study was the influence that thoughts have on our frequency as well. Negative thoughts lowered the measured frequency by 12 MHz and positive thoughts raised the measured frequency by 10 MHz. It was also found that prayer and meditation increased the measured frequency levels by 15 MHz.

How do *PURE, THERAPEUTIC-GRADE* essential oils affect the brain?

The blood-brain barrier is the barrier membrane between the circulating blood and the brain that prevents certain damaging substances from reaching brain tissue and cerebrospinal fluid. The American Medical Association (AMA) determined that if they could find an agent that would pass the blood-brain barrier, they would be able to cure Alzheimer's disease, Lou Gehrig's disease, multiple sclerosis, and Parkinson's disease. In June of 1994, it was documented by the Medical University of Berlin, Germany and Vienna, Austria that sesquiterpenes have the ability to go beyond the blood-brain barrier.

High levels of sesquiterpenes, found in the essential oils of frankincense and sandalwood, help increase the amount oxygen in the limbic system of the brain, particularly around the pineal and pituitary glands. This leads to an increase in secretions of antibodies, endorphins, and neurotransmitters.

Also present in the limbic system of the brain, is a gland called the amygdala. In 1989, it was discovered that the amygdala plays a major role in the storing and releasing of emotional trauma. The only way to stimulate this gland is with fragrance or the sense of smell. Therefore, with Aromatherapy and essential oils, we are now able to release emotional trauma.

What enables *PURE, THERAPEUTIC-GRADE* essential oils to provide such incredible benefits?

Essential oils are chemically very heterogenetic; meaning they are very diverse in their effects and can perform several different functions. Synthetic chemicals are completely opposite in that they have basically one action. This gives essential oils a paradoxical nature which can be difficult to understand. However, they can be compared to another paradoxical group—human beings. For example, a man can play many roles: father, husband, friend, co-worker, accountant, school teacher, church volunteer, scout master, minister. etc. and so it is with essential oils. Lavender can be used for burns, insect bites, headaches, PMS, insomnia, stress and so forth.

The heterogenetic benefits of an oil depend greatly on its chemical constituents; and not only on the existence of specific constituents, but also their amounts in proportion to the other constituents that are present in the same oil. Some individual oils may have anywhere from 200 to

800 different chemical constituents. However, of the possible 800 different constituents, only about 200 of those have so far been identified. Although not everything is known about all the different constituents, most of them can be grouped into a few distinct families, each with some dominant characteristics. The following section provides greater insights into these constituent families.

ESSENTIAL OIL CONSTITUENTS

As was mentioned previously, the chemical constituents of an oil are affected by a vast number of variables. However, most of these variables are controlled by the oil producers. One thing that the student of aromatherapy can do, is to ask questions about the company from which they are purchasing the oils. Some of the most important questions should be, "Does the company utilize gas chromatography (GC) in their quality control process?" "Does their GC equipment utilize a column of at least 50 to 60 meters in length in order to properly identify the hundreds of natural constituents found in an essential oil?" A gas chromatogram shows a pattern of the separated constituents of an oil and helps a trained technician determine its purity and therapeutic quality. The following information can help us understand the functions of some of the main chemical constituents.

In general, *pure* essential oils can be subdivided into two distinct groups of chemical constituents; the **hydrocarbons** which are made up almost exclusively of *terpenes* (monoterpenes, sesquiterpenes, and diterpenes), and the **oxygenated compounds** which are mainly *esters, aldehydes, ketones, alcohols, phenols,* and *oxides.*

Monoterpenes—occur in practically all essential oils and have many different activities. Most tend to inhibit the accumulation of toxins and help discharge existing toxins from the liver and kidneys. Some are antiseptic, anti-bacterial, stimulating, analgesic (weak), and expectorant, while other specific terpenes have anti-fungal, anti-viral, antihistaminic, anti-rheumatic, anti-tumor (antiblastic, anti-carcinogenic), hypotensive, insecticidal, purgative, and pheromonal properties. Most citrus oils (not bergamot) and pine oils, as well as Black pepper, nutmeg, and angelica, contain a high proportion of terpenes. Some common monoterpenes include the following:

Pinenes (α- & β-) have strong antiseptic, anti-bacterial, anti-fungal, and expectorant properties.

Camphene is an insect repellant and according to the Phytochemical Dictionary, it is "used to reduce cholesterol saturation index in the treatment of gallstones".

β-Myrcene is a cancer-preventative.

Limonene is anti-cancerous, anti-bacterial, anti-fungal, antiseptic (5x phenol), and highly anti-viral. It can be found in 90% of the citrus oils.

Sesquiterpenes are found in great abundance in essential oils. They are anti-bacterial, strongly anti-inflammatory, slightly antiseptic and hypotensive, and sedative. Some have analgesic properties while others are highly anti-spasmodic. They also work as liver and gland stimulants. Research from the universities of Berlin and Vienna show increased oxygenation around the pineal and pituitary glands. Further research has shown that sesquiterpenes have the ability to surpass the blood-brain barrier and enter the brain tissue.

β-Caryophyllene is anti-edemic, anti-inflammatory, anti-spasmodic, and an insect and termite repellant. Found in high proportions in plants from the Labiatae family.

Chamazulene is very high in anti-inflammatory and anti-bacterial activity.

Farnesene is anti-viral in action.

Alcohols—are commonly recognized for their anti-bacterial, anti-infectious, and anti-viral activities. They create an uplifting quality and are regarded as safe and effective for young and old alike.

Monoterpene Alcohols (or Monoterpenols) stimulate the immune system, work as a diuretic and a general tonic, and are anti-bacterial and mildly antiseptic as well.

Linalol can help relieve discomfort. It is anti-bacterial, anti-fungal, antiseptic (5x phenol), anti-spasmodic, anti-viral, and sedative.

Citronellol is anti-bacterial, anti-fungal, antiseptic (3.8x phenol), and sedative.

Geraniol is anti-fungal, antiseptic (7x phenol), cancer-preventative, and sedative.

Farnesol is good for the mucous membranes and prevents bacterial growth from perspiration.

Other terpene alcohols include borneol, menthol, nerol, terpineol (which Dr. Gattefosse considered to be a decongestant), vetiverol, and cedrol.

Sesquiterpene Alcohols (Sesquiterpenols) are anti-allergic, anti-bacterial, anti-inflammatory, ulcer-protective (preventative), and a liver and glandular stimulant.

Bisabolol is one of the strongest sesquiterpene alcohols. Others include nerolidol and zingiberol.

Esters—are the compounds resulting from the reaction of an alcohol with an acid (known as esterification). Esters are very common and are found in a large number of essential oils. They are anti-fungal, anti-spasmodic, calming and relaxing. They also have a balancing or regulatory effect, especially on the nervous system. Some examples are **linalyl acetate**, **geranyl acetate** (with strong anti-fungal properties), and **bornyl acetate** (effective on bronchial candida). Other esters include eugenyl acetate and lavendulyl acetate.

Aldehydes—are highly reactive and characterized by the group C-H-O (Carbon, Hydrogen, Oxygen). In general, they are anti-infectious, anti-inflammatory, calming to the central nervous system, fever-reducing, hypotensive, and tonic. They can be quite irritating when applied topically (citrals being an example). However, it has been shown that adding an essential oil with an equal amount of d-limonene can negate the irritant properties of a high citral oil.

Citrals (like neral, geranial, and citronellal) are very common with a distinctive antiseptic action. They also have an anti-viral application as with melissa oil when applied topically on herpes simplex.

Other aldehydes include benzaldehyde, cinnamic aldehyde, cuminic aldehyde, and perillaldehyde.

Ketones—are sometimes mucolytic and neuro-toxic when isolated from other constituents. However, all recorded toxic effects come from laboratory testing on guinea pigs and rats. No documented cases exist where oils with a high concentration of ketones (such as mugwort, tansy, sage, and wormwood) have ever caused a toxic effect on a human being. Also, large amounts of these oils would have to be consumed for them to result in a toxic neurological effect. Ketones stimulate cell regeneration, promote the formation of tissue, and liquefy mucous. They are helpful with such conditions as dry asthma, colds, flu, and dry cough and are largely found in oils used for the upper respiratory system, such as hyssop, Clary sage, and sage.

Thujone is one of the most toxic members of the ketone family. It can be an irritant and upsetting to the central nervous system and may be neuro-toxic when taken internally as in the banned drink *Absinthe*. Although oils containing thujone may be inhaled to relieve respiratory distress and may stimulate the immune system, they should usually be used in dilution (1-2%) and/or for short periods of time.

Jasmone (found in jasmine) and **fenchone** (found in fennel) are both non-toxic.

Other ketones include camphor, carvone, menthone, methyl nonyl ketone, and pinocamphone.

Phenols—are responsible for the fragrance of an oil. They are the most powerful anti-bacterial, anti-infectious, and antiseptic constituents in the plant world. They are also very stimulating to both the nervous and immune systems. They contain high levels of oxygenating molecules and have antioxidant properties. However, they can be quite caustic to the skin and they present some concerns regarding liver toxicity. Essential oils that contain a high proportion of phenols should be diluted and/or used for short periods of time.

Eugenol is analgesic, anesthetic (in dentistry), anticonvulsant, anti-fungal, anti-inflammatory, antioxidant, antiseptic, cancer-preventative, and sedative.

Thymol may not be as caustic as other phenols. It is anti-bacterial, anti-fungal, anti-inflammatory, antioxidant, anti-plaque, anti-rheumatic, antiseptic (20x phenol), anti-spasmodic, deodorant, expectorant.

Carvacrol is a product of auto-oxidation of d-limonene. It is anti-bacterial, anti-fungal, anti-inflammatory, antiseptic (1.5x phenol), anti-spasmodic, and an expectorant. Researchers believe it may possibly contain some anti-cancerous properties.

Others in the phenol family include methyl eugenol, methyl chavicol, anethole, and safrole.

Oxides—According to *The American Heritage® Dictionary of the English Language*, an oxide is "a binary compound of an element or a radical with oxygen."

1,8-Cineol (or eucalyptol) is, by far, the most prevalent member of this family and virtually exists in a class of its own. It is anesthetic, antiseptic, and works as a strong mucolytic as it thins mucus in respiratory tract infections.

Other oxides include linalol oxide, ascaridol, bisabolol oxide, and bisabolone oxide.

All pure essential oils have some anti-bacterial properties. They increase the production of hite blood cells, which help fight infectious illnesses. It is through these properties that aromatic erbs have been esteemed so highly throughout the ages and so widely used during the onsets of alaria, typhoid, and of course, the epidemic plagues during the 16th century. Research has found at people who consistently use pure essential oils have a higher level of **resistance to illnesses**, olds, flues, and diseases than the average person. Further indications show that such individuals, fter contracting a cold, flu, or other illness, will **recover 60-75 percent faster** than those who do ot use essential oils.

THE ART OF BLENDING

Blending essential oils is an art and usually requires a little bit of training and xperimentation. If you choose to create your own blends, it is important to understand that the rder in which the oils are blended is key to maintaining the desired therapeutic properties in a ynergistic blend. An alteration in the sequence of adding selected oils to a blend may change the hemical properties, the fragrance, and thus the desired results. The "Blend Classification", and Blends With" listings under each oil in the Single Oils section of this book should assist one in the lending process. In general, oils that are from the same botanical family, usually blend well ogether. In addition, oils with similar constituents also mix well.

Another method utilizes four blending classifications. The following information explains ne characteristics of each classification, the order in which they should be added to the blend (i.e. ersonifiers first, Enhancers second, Equalizers third, and Modifiers fourth), and the amount of ach type of oil as a percentage of the blend.

st—The **Personifier** (1-5% of blend) oils have very sharp, strong and long-lasting fragrances. They also have dominant properties with strong therapeutic action.

Oils in this classification may include: Angelica, birch, cardamom, cinnamon bark, cistus, Clary sage, clove, coriander, German chamomile, ginger, helichrysum, mandarin, neroli, nutmeg, orange, patchouli, peppermint, petitgrain, rose, spearmint, tangerine, tarragon, wintergreen, ylang ylang.

nd—The **Enhancer** (50-80% of blend) oil should be the predominant oil as it serves to enhance the properties of the other oils in the blend. Its fragrance is not as sharp as the personifiers and is usually of a shorter duration.

Oils in this classification may include: Basil, bergamot, birch, cajeput, cedarwood, cumin, dill, eucalyptus, frankincense, galbanum, geranium, grapefruit, hyssop, jasmine, lavender, lemon, lemongrass, lime, marjoram, melaleuca (Tea Tree), melissa, myrtle, orange, oregano, palmarosa, patchouli, petitgrain, ravensara, roman chamomile, rose, rosemary, sage, spruce, thyme, wintergreen.

3rd—The **Equalizer** (10-15% of blend) oils create balance and synergy among the oils contained i the blend. Their fragrance is also not as sharp as the personifier and is of a shorter duration.

Oils in this classification may include: Basil, bergamot, cedarwood, cypress, fennel, fir frankincense, geranium, ginger, hyssop, jasmine, juniper, lavender, lemongrass, lime, marjoram, melaleuca (Tea Tree), melissa, myrrh, myrtle, neroli, oregano, pine, roman chamomile, rose, rosewood, sandalwood, spruce, tarragon, thyme.

4th—The **Modifier** (5-8% of blend) oils have a mild and short fragrance. These oils add harmony to the blend.

Oils in this classification may include: Angelica, bergamot, cardamom, coriander, eucalyptus, fennel, grapefruit, hyssop, jasmine, lavender, lemon, mandarin, melissa, myrrh, neroli, petitgrain, rose, rosewood, sandalwood, tangerine, ylang ylang.

Depending upon the topical application of your blend, you will want to add some carrier/base oil. When creating a **therapeutic essential oil blend**, you may want to use about **28 drops of essential oil to ½ oz. of V-6 Mixing Oil**. When creating a **body massage blend**, you will want to use a total of about **50 drops of essential oils to 4 oz. of V-6 Mixing Oil**. Remembe to store your fragrant creation in dark-colored glass bottles.

As essential oils can vary in thickness, the following are approximate measurements:

25-30 drops	= 1/4 teaspoon	= 1-2 milliliters	= 5/8 dram
45-50 drops	= 1/2 teaspoon	= 2-3 milliliters	= 1 dram
75-80 drops	= 3/4 teaspoon	= 3-4 milliliters	= 1/8 oz.
100-120 drops	= 1 teaspoon	= 5 milliliters	= 1/6 oz.
160 drops	= 1½ teaspoons	= 6-8 milliliters	= 1/4 oz.
320-400 drops	= 3 teaspoons	= 13-15 milliliters	= 1/2 oz.
600-650 drops	= 6 teaspoons	= 25-30 milliliters	= 1 oz.

Learn to trust your nose as it can help you decide which classification an oil should be in. More detailed information about these methods of blending is beyond the scope of this revision of the book. For additional information on using these classifications in your blending, we highly recommend Marcel Lavabre's Aromatherapy Workbook. Another very simple book about blending, with recipes and easy-to-follow guidelines, is Mindy Green's Natural Perfumes, which uses perfume notes (top, middle, base), odor, and odor intensity to help guide you in making your own fragrant blend creations (refer to the following chart).

Essential Oils Odor Chart

The following chart was compiled from the book Natural Perfumes, by Mindy Green, and various other sources. It lists essential oils by note types in order of odor intensity, 1-lightest to 5-strongest)

ssential Oil	Scent	Intensity
op Notes		(5-20% of the blend)
range	Fresh, citrusy, fruity, sweet, light	1
ergamot	Sweet, lively, citrus, fruity	2
rapefruit	Clean, fresh, bitter, citrusy	2
itronella	Citrusy, slightly fruity, fresh, sweet	3
emon	Sweet, sharp, clear, citrusy	3
ime	Sweet, tart, intense, lively	3
andarin	Very sweet, citrusy, fruity	3
etitgrain	Fresh, floral, citrusy, slightly woody	3
avensara	Slightly medicinal, eucalyptus-like	3
pearmint	Minty, slightly fruity	3
angerine	Fresh, sweet, citrusy	3
uc. Polybrac.	Fresh, woody, earthy	4
emongrass	Grassy, lemony, pungent, earthy	4
uc. Globulus	Fresh, medicinal, woody, earthy	5
albanum	Warm, earthy, green, woody, spicy	5
emon Myrtle	Extremely lemony and crisp	5
op to Middle Notes		(20-80% of the blend)
nise	Licorice-like, rich, sweet	3
aurel	Sweet, fresh, spicy, medicinal	3
avandin	Fresh, sweet, floral, herbaceous	3
lyrtle	Sweet, slightly camphorous, floral hint	3
almarosa	Lemony, fresh, green, hints of rose	3
ngelica	Earthy, peppery, green, spicy	4
asil	Spicy, anise-like, camphorous, lively	4
ennel	Sweet, somewhat spicy, licorice-like	4
Iiddle Notes		(50-80% of the blend)
arrot Seed	Sweet, fruity, warm, earthy	2
ill	Fresh, sweet, herbaceous, slight earthy	2
ir, Balsam	Fresh, clean, green, balsamic, sweet	2
avender	Floral, sweet, balsamic, slightly woody	2
lelissa	Delicate, lemony	2
ajeput	Fresh, camphorous, with fruity note	3
oriander	Woody, spicy, sweet	3
ypress	Fresh, herbaceous, slightly woody	3
lemi	Balsamic, fresh, citrusy, peppery, spicy	3
uc Citriodora	Sweet, lemony, fresh, slightly woody	3
uc. Radiata	Slightly camphorous, sweet, fruity	3
ir	Fresh, woody, earthy, sweet	3
eranium	Sweet, green, citrus-rosy, fresh	3

Essential Oil	Scent	Intensity
Middle Notes (continued)		(50-80% of the blend)
Helichrysum	Rich, sweet, fruity, slightly honey-like	3
Hyssop	Fresh, earthy, woody, fruity	3
Juniper	Sweet, musky, tenacious	3
Marjoram	Herbaceous, green, spicy	3
Melaleuca	Medicinal, fresh, woody, earthy	3
Neroli	Floral, citrusy, semi-sweet, delicate	3
Niaouli	Earthy, musty, harsh	3
Black Pepper	Spicy, peppery, musky, warm	3
Rosemary Cin.	Strong, camphorous, slightly woody	3
Rosewood	Sweet, woody, fruity, floral	3
Spruce	Fresh, woody, earthy, sweet	3
Cardamom	Sweet, spicy, balsamic, slightly floral	4
G. Chamomile	Deep, rich, tenacious, cocoa-like	4
R. Chamomile	Fresh, sweet, fruity, apple-like	4
Ginger	Sweet, spicy-woody, warm, fresh, sharp	4
Nutmeg	Sweet, musky, spicy	4
Pine, Scotch	Fresh, woody, earthy, balsamic	4
Thyme	Fresh, medicinal, herbaceous	4
Yarrow	Sharp, woody, herbaceous, slight floral	4
Oregano	Herbaceous, sharp	5
Peppermint	Minty, sharp, intense	5
Middle to Base Notes		(20-80% of the blend)
Clary Sage	Spicy, hay-like, sharp, fixative	3
Rose	Floral, spicy, rich, deep, sensual, green	3
Clove Bud	Spicy, warming, slightly bitter, woody	5
Ylang Ylang	Sweet, heavy, narcotic, tropical floral	5
Base Notes		(5-20% of the blend)
Onycha	Rich, warm, slightly woody, creamy	1
Cedarwood	Warm, soft, woody	3
Cypress, Blue	Long-lasting, warm, woody, earthy	3
Frankincense	Rich, deep, warm, balsamic, sweet	3
Sandalwood	Soft, woody, sweet, earthy, balsamic	3
Jasmine	Powerful, sweet, tenacious, floral	4
Myrrh	Warm, earthy, woody, balsamic	4
Patchouli	Earthy, sweet-balsamic, rich, wood-like	4
Vanilla	Sweet, balsamic, heavy, warm	4
Spikenard	Heavy, earthy, animal-like	5
Vetiver	Heavy, earthy, balsamic, smoky	5

METHODS OF APPLICATION

TOPICAL APPLICATION

1. **Direct Application.** Apply the oils directly on the area of concern using one to six drops of oil. More oil is not necessarily better since a large amount of oil can trigger a detoxification of the surrounding tissue and blood. Such a quick detoxification can be somewhat uncomfortable. To achieve the desired results, one to three drops of oil is usually adequate. A few guidelines for direct application of the oils are as follows:
   - ✓ The feet are the second fastest area of the body to absorb oils because of the larg pores. Other quick absorbing areas include behind the ears and on the wrists.
   - ✓ To experience a feeling of peace, relaxation, or energy, three to six drops per foo are adequate.
   - ✓ When massaging a large area of the body, always dilute the oils by 15 to 30% with the V-6 Mixing Oil.
   - ✓ When applying oils to infants and small children, dilute with V-6 Mixing Oil. Us one to three drops of an essential oil to one tablespoon (Tbs.) of V-6 Mixing Oil for infants and one to three drops of an essential oil to one teaspoon (tsp.) V-6 Mixing Oil for children from two to five years old.
   - ✓ Do not mix oil blends. Commercially available blends have been specially formulated by someone who understands the chemical constituents of each oil anc which oils blend well. The chemical properties of the oils can be altered when mixed improperly, resulting in some undesirable reactions.
   - ✓ Layering individual oils is preferred over mixing your own blends. Layering refers to the process of applying one oil, rubbing it in, and then applying another oil. There is no need to wait more than a couple of seconds between each oil as absorption occurs quite rapidly. If dilution is necessary, the V-6 Mixing Oil may be applied on top. The layering technique is not only useful in physical healing, but also when doing emotional clearing.
   - ✓ The FDA has approved some essential oils for internal use and given them the designation of GRAS (Generally Regarded As Safe for internal consumption). *This designation is listed in the Single Oil Summary Information chart in the Appendix of this book under Safety Data.* **Oils without this designation should never be used internally.**

1. **Vita Flex Therapy.** A simple method of applying oils to contact points (or nerve endings in the feet or hands. Then a series of hand rotation movements at those control points create a vibrational healing energy that carries the oils along the neuroelectrical pathways. The oils help increase the frequency of this healing energy and serve to either help remove any blockage along the pathways or travel the length of the pathway to benefit the particular organ. Refer to the following pages on Vita Flex Therapy for more details.

Raindrop Technique. A simple application of dropping certain oils like little drops of rain from about six inches above the body along the entire length of the spine. It is also a tremendous boost to the immune system as it releases toxins and kills viruses and bacteria that have accumulated along the spine. See the pages on Raindrop Technique in this section of the reference guide for more details.

Auricular Therapy. A method of applying the oils to the rim of the ears. This technique works extremely well for emotional clearing. Some physical benefits can also be obtained from this technique. See the pages on Auricular Therapy in this section of the reference guide for more details.

Perfume or Cologne. Wearing the oils as a perfume or cologne can provide some wonderful emotional support, and physical support as well; not just a beautiful fragrance. (For some simple, yet exquisite perfume/cologne blends, refer to the book Natural Perfumes, by Mindy Green)

COMPRESSES

Basin. Fill a wash basin with two quarts of hot or cold water and add the desired essential oils. Stir the water vigorously then lay a towel on top of the water. Since the oils will float to the top, the towel will absorb the oils with the water. After the towel is completely saturated, wring out the excess water (leaving much of the oils in the towel) and place over the area needing the compress. For a **hot** compress, cover with a dry towel and a hot water bottle. For a **cold** compress, cover with a piece of plastic or plastic wrap. Finally, put another towel on top and leave for as long as possible (one to two hours is best).

Massage. Apply a hot wet towel and a dry towel on top of an already massaged area. The moist heat will force the oils deeper into the tissues of the body.

INHALATIONS

Diffuser. The easiest and simplest way of putting the oils into the air for inhalation is to use an aromatic diffuser. Diffusers that use a heat source (such as a light bulb ring) will alter the chemical make-up of the oil and its therapeutic qualities. A cold air diffuser uses room-temperature air to blow the oil up against some kind of a nebulizer. This breaks the oils up into a micro-fine mist that is then dispersed into the air, covering hundreds of square feet in seconds. The oils, with their oxygenating molecules, will then remain suspended for several hours to freshen and improve the quality of the air. The anti-viral, anti-bacterial, and antiseptic properties of the oils, kill bacteria and help to reduce fungus and mold. Essential oils, when diffused, have been found to reduce the amount of airbo chemicals and metallics as well as help to create greater spiritual, physical, and emotion harmony. The greatest therapeutic benefit is received by diffusing oils for only 15 minu out of an hour so that the olfactory system has time to recover before receiving more oil

2. **Cloth or Tissue.** Put one to three drops of an essential oil on a paper towel, tissue, cott ball, handkerchief, towel, or pillow case and hold it close to your face and inhale.

3. **Hot Water.** Put one to three drops of an essential oil into hot water and inhale. Again, heat reduces some of the benefits.

4. **Vaporizer or Humidifier.** Put oil in a vaporizer or a humidifier. The cold air types are best since heat reduces some of the benefits.

5. **Fan or Vent.** Put oil on a cotton ball and attach to ceiling fans or air vents. This can a work well in a vehicle as the area is so small.

BATHS

1. **Bath Water.** Begin by adding three to six drops of oil to the bath water while the tub is filling. Because the individual oils will separate as the water calms down, the skin will quickly draw the oils from the top of the water. People have commented that they were unable to endure more than six drops of oil. Such individuals may benefit from adding t oils to a bath and shower gel base first. Soak for 15 minutes.

2. **Bath and Shower Gel.** Begin by adding three to six drops of oil to ½ oz. of a bath and shower gel base and add to the water while the tub is filling. The number of drops can b increased as described above under *Bath Water*. Adding the oils to a bath and shower g base first allows one to obtain the greatest benefit from the oils as they are more evenly dispersed throughout the water and not allowed to immediately separate.

3. **Wash Cloth.** When showering, add three to six drops of oil to a bath and shower gel ba first before applying to a face cloth to effectively cover the entire body.

4. **Body Sprays.** Fill a small spray bottle with distilled water and add 10-15 drops of your favorite oil blend or single oils. Shake well and spray onto the entire body just after taking a bath or shower.

I love to add a drop or 2 of lemon oil to the Joy blend! It's a wonderful perfume. If you want the blend to last longer and cool you off for the summer, fill a small spray bottle with distilled water and 10 drops of Joy, 2 drops of Lemon. I like to spray it on after I shower.

-Submitted by Nancy Dutton (July 2004)

DISHWATER, CLOTHES WASHERS, and DRYERS

The anti-bacterial properties of essential oils can effectively promote greater hygiene. Add :ouple drops of **Melrose** or **lemon** to dishwater for clean dishes and a great smelling kitchen. ;e **lemon** or another citrus oil to take gum out of clothes. A few drops of **Purification** in the ash water will kill bacteria and germs in clothes. Put **Purification**, **Joy**, or other oil on a wet rag d place in dryer, or mist from a spray bottle directly into the dryer.

COOKING

Essential oils can easily be incorporated into your cooking, as long as you remember that ey are very concentrated. Usually only 1 drop is necessary, and sometimes even less. Use a othpick to help control the addition of smaller amounts of oil, by dipping the toothpick into the l (more oil on the toothpick = stronger flavor, etc.) then stirring it into the food. Here are a uple examples of recipes where people have used the essential oils for flavoring.

Lemon Tarragon Dressing

tablespoon fresh tarragon diced, or 1 teaspoon dried tarragon
tablespoon fresh or 1 teaspoon dried basil leaves
cup organic extra virgin cold pressed olive oil
lash of pepper
lash of red pepper
5 drops lemon essential oil

Mix well and drizzle on salad or fish or anything! Keep unused portion in the fridge.

-Submitted by Jill Burk, Saginaw, Michigan (July 2004)

Cream Cheese Icing

8 oz. package of cream cheese
1½ cups of powdered sugar
1 stick of butter
3 drops of tangerine essential oil

Cream together thoroughly the cream cheese, powdered sugar, and butter with electric beater. Stir in the tangerine oil. Enjoy!

-Submitted by Ellie Ayers (July 2004)

CLEANING and DISINFECTING

Put a few drops of **lemon, spruce, or fir** oil on a dust cloth or ten drops in water in a pray bottle to polish furniture and to clean and disinfect bathrooms and kitchens.

PAINTING

To effectively remove paint fumes and after smell, add one 15 ml. bottle of oil to any five allon bucket of paint. The Abundance blend and citrus oils have been favorites. Either a paint prayer or brush and roller may be used to apply the paint after mixing the oils into the paint by irring vigorously. Oils may eventually rise to the top if using a water-based paint. Occasional irring may be necessary to keep the oils mixed.

VITA FLEX THERAPY

Vita Flex Therapy is based on a small part of a complete system which was developed b Stanley Burroughs during a period of more than fifty years of research and application. Vita Fle uses the reflex system of internal body controls to release tensions, congestions, and maladjustments. When properly applied through specific application of hand rotation movements an control points, a vibrational healing energy is released along the neuro-electrical pathways to an exact point. This healing energy is created by the contact between the fingertips and the reflex (contact) points. The resulting spark of energy follows the neuro pathways of the nervous system where there is a break in the electrical circuit. Upon reaching the break, any necessary changes a made automatically. This technique is believed to have originated in Tibet many thousands of years ago, long before acupuncture was ever discovered.

The Vita Flex Technique is a superior form of reflexology. Reflexology, as used today, h a tendency to ground out the electrical charge from constant compression and rotation, which causes cell separation, loss of oxygen to subdermal tissues, and further injury. With the Vita Fle technique people experience less discomfort. Using the thumb and all four fingers, the applicatio is much more efficient. There are more than 5,000 Vita Flex points throughout the body (in the complete system as developed by Stanley Burroughs) in comparison to the 365 acupuncture poin used in reflexology. With Vita Flex, the weakened or injured areas are corrected on reflected points, thereby preventing further injury.

Combining the electrical frequency of the oils and that of the person receiving the application creates rapid and phenomenal results. "Vita Flex" is derived from the term "vitality through the reflexes" and is a complete, workable system which, when combined with the healing properties of essential oils, can release an unlimited healing power.

Stanley Burroughs' book, Healing for the Age of Enlightenment, explains in detail the system that he designed over many years. For step-by-step instruction of the full Vita Flex treatment, refer to the video, Vita Flex Instruction with Tom Woloshyn. This video teaches the proper Vita Flex technique as developed by Stanley Burroughs, including the Atlas Adjustment (a non-chiropractic technique used to quickly and efficiently re-align the spine or any other misalignment in the body). Stanley Burroughs also designed the **Vita Flex roller**, or "Relax-a-Roller" to assist one in doing Vita Flex on themselves. This device is a special type of roller wit staggered, fine-pointed pegs, placed close enough together so as not to dig in too deeply with hea pressure. Yet, they are far enough apart to reach all Vita Flex points as one rolls both feet back and forth. With just a few minutes of use, tensions, drowsiness, weariness, and discomfort disappear. Also, by adding the desired oils to the feet and rolling them back and forth on the rolle one can easily achieve the benefits of Vita Flex Therapy. These rollers are produced in Canada and are available from Abundant Health.

Key Principles

To reduce any discomfort, fingernails should be cut and filed short.

Remove all jewelry and watches to prevent an interference of energy.

Always **DROP** the oils into the palm of your non-dominant hand and use the dominant hand to stir the oils clockwise three times before application. This method will increase the electrical frequency of the oils and significantly improve the results. **To prevent contamination of the oils, do not touch the top of the bottle with any part of your body.**

Put a drop of White Angelica on each of your shoulders to protect yourself against any negative energies from the person you are working on.

Always start on the bottom of the feet. Put three to six drops of Valor on the bottom of each foot. Some may be applied to the brain stem if desired. Hold the bottoms of the feet with your hands; right hand to right foot and left hand to left foot. Continue holding the feet until you feel the body's energy balance. This usually feels like an energy pulse beating in both feet. Another way to balance, which may be preferable to some, is to put one drop of Valor on the wrists and hold the wrists crossed together for a few minutes, until you feel a pulse in the tips of the thumb and index finger.

5. Use the Vita Flex charts (*shown on the next couple of pages*) to determine where the oils should be placed during the therapy. One to three drops of oil may be applied to the specific Vita Flex points of the foot. Vita Flex points on the hand can be used as an alternative to extremely sensitive or sore feet. Apply the oil(s).

Apply the Vita Flex technique as follows: Starting with the fingers on their pads, curl the fingers up and over onto the nails (see photo examples on the next page). Increasing pressure is applied until the fingers are curled almost completely over on the nails. Pressure is then immediately released to create the spark of energy and send it on its way. The curling should be one continuous motion, not jerky, with medium to heavy pressure being placed on the contact point. Never press and hold while performing this technique. This may be done several times on the same spot to obtain the desired results. Some leverage can be achieved by placing the thumb of the same hand around to the other side of the foot or hand on which the Vita Flex is being performed. This allows the hand to operate in a fashion similar to a pipe wrench, which increases pressure on the pipe as it is twisted.

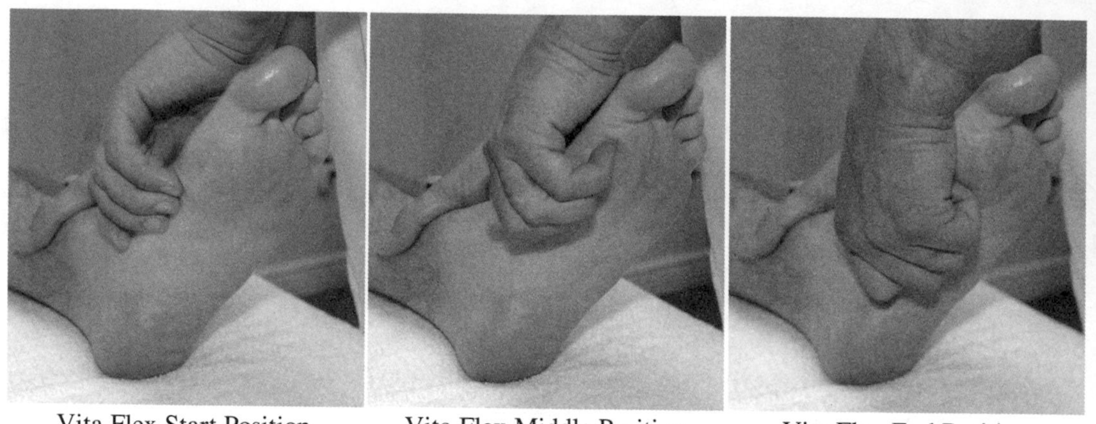

Vita Flex Start Position | Vita Flex Middle Position | Vita Flex End Position

VITA FLEX HAND CHART

Vita Flex points in this hand chart correspond to those in the feet. Occasionally the feet can be too sensitive for typical Vita Flex Therapy. Working with the hands will not only affect th specific body points, but may also help to provide some pain relief to the corresponding points on the feet. (Refer to Stanley Burroughs' book, Healing for the Age of Enlightenment, pg. 78 for a more detailed explanation.)

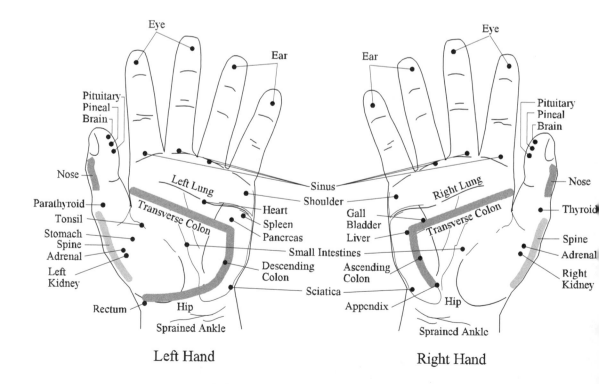

Eye
Ear
Pituitary
Pineal
Brain
Nose
Left Lung
Transverse Colon
Parathyroid
Tonsil
Stomach
Spine
Adrenal
Left Kidney
Rectum
Hip
Sprained Ankle
Heart
Spleen
Pancreas
Descending Colon
Sinus
Shoulder
Small Intestines
Sciatica
Gall Bladder
Liver
Ascending Colon
Appendix
Right Lung
Thyroid
Right Kidney

Left Hand

Right Hand

Science and Application

VITA FLEX FEET CHART

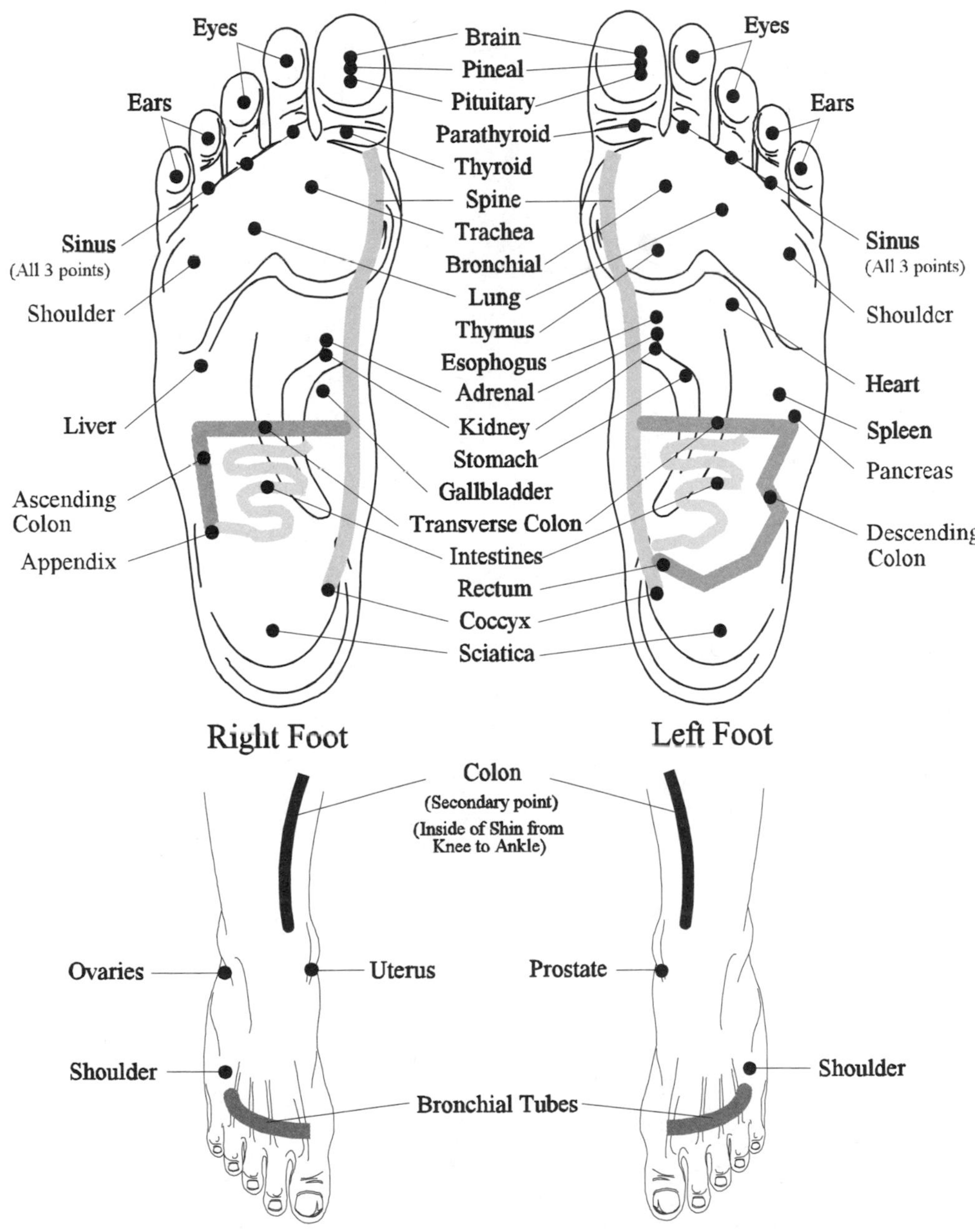

Note:

This chart combines the work of Stanley Burroughs (Vita Flex Charting) and D. Gary Young (Electrical Frequency Tracing). Refer to their respective books, listed in the bibliography, for more detailed information.

AURICULAR INTERNAL BODY POINTS

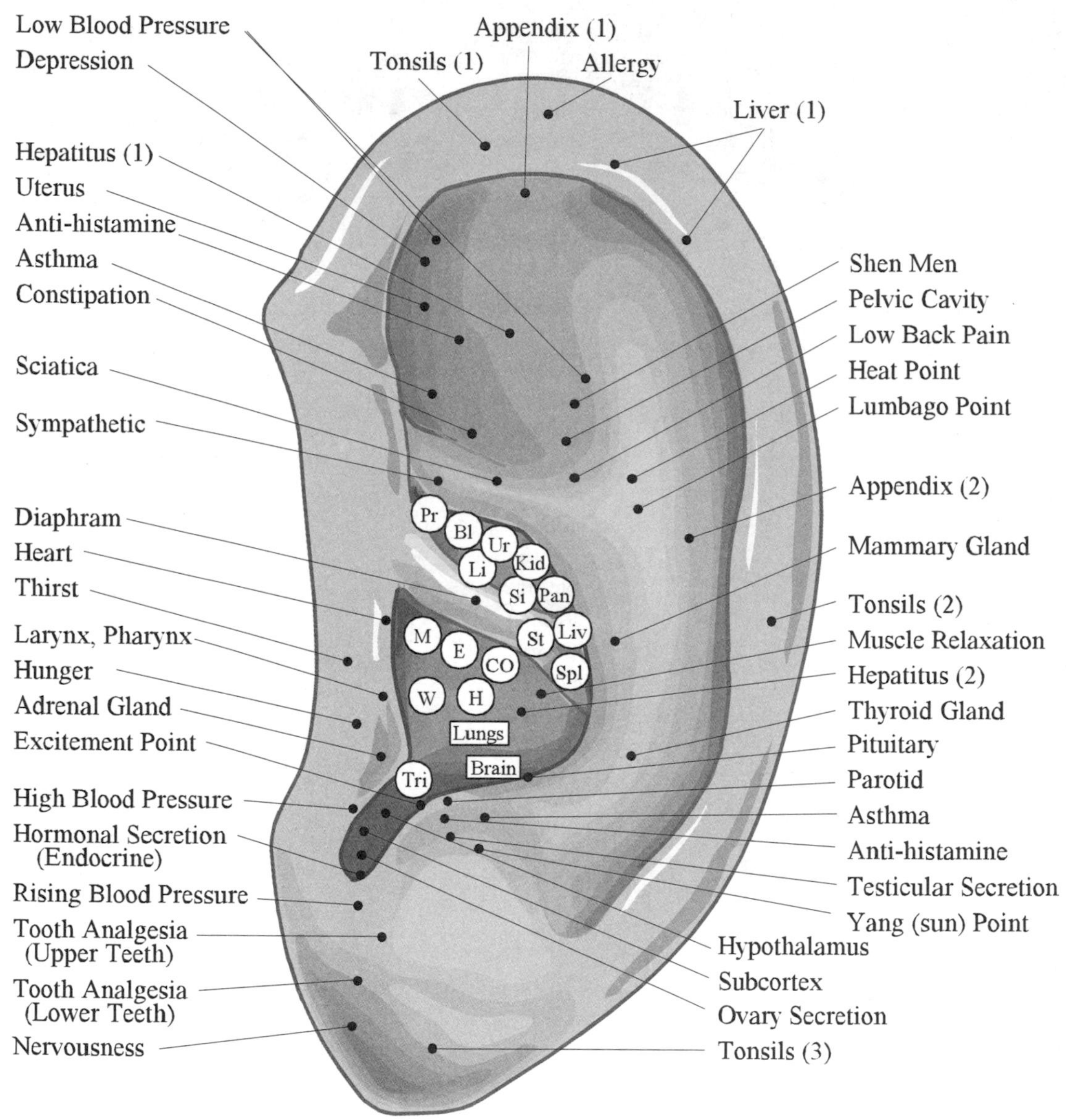

M:	**Mouth**	**Pr:**	**Prostate**	**Liv:**	**Liver**
E:	**Esophagus**	**Bl:**	**Bladder**	**Spl:**	**Spleen**
CO:	**Cardiac Orifice**	**Ur:**	**Ureter**	**H:**	**Heart**
St:	**Stomach**	**Kid:**	**Kidney**	**W:**	**Windpipe, Trachea**
Si:	**Small Intestine**	**Pan:**	**Pancreas, Gall Bladder**	**Tri:**	**Triple Warner**
Li:	**Large Intestine**				

Science and Application

RAINDROP TECHNIQUE

This application technique was developed by Dr. Don Gary Young, N.D. Aromatologist, d one of North America's leading experts on the art and science of aromatherapy. This :hnique involves dropping the oils directly onto the spine from about six inches above the body. ie oils are then worked into the spine using light strokes with the fingers which stimulate energy pulses and disperse the oils along the nervous system throughout the entire body. In this way, body can be brought into balance and the energy centers can be cleared and re-aligned. It will so help to reduce spinal inflammations and kill viruses that hibernate along the spinal column, as ll as help to straighten any spinal curvatures. Although a session lasts for about 45 minutes to hour, the oils will continue to work in the body for a week or more following the treatment. The indrop Technique that is explained below is an abbreviated form. The video entitled Raindrop chnique by D. Gary Young (*available from Abundant Health*) provides step-by-step structions for this technique.

Oils used in the Raindrop Technique

ALOR—is the first and most important oil used in this technique because it helps balance the electrical energies within the body. It also helps create an environment where structural alignment can occur.

HYME—is used for its ability to support the immune system by attacking any bacteria, fungus, infection, or virus that may be present. It may also help one overcome fatigue and physical weakness after an illness.

REGANO—works in conjunction with thyme to strengthen the immune system and to attack bacteria and viruses. It may also act as an antiseptic for the respiratory system, help balance metabolism, and strengthen the vital centers of the body.

YPRESS—is used for its anti-bacterial, anti-infectious, antimicrobial, and diuretic properties. In addition, it may function as a decongestant for the circulatory and lymphatic systems.

IRCH/WINTERGREEN—is great for removing discomfort associated with the inflammation of bones, muscles, and joints. It may also help cleanse the lymphatic system.

ASIL—is relaxing to spastic muscles and is stimulating to the nerves and the adrenal cortex.

EPPERMINT—is used to calm and strengthen the nerves, reduce inflammation, and is highly effective when dealing with conditions related to the respiratory system. It also has a synergistic and enhancing effect on all other oils.

MARJORAM — is used to relax spastic muscles, soothe the nerves, relieve cramps, aches, and pains, and to help calm the respiratory system.

AROMA SIEZ — may help to relax, calm, and relieve the tension of spastic muscles resulting from sports injury, fatigue, or stress.

ORTHO EASE — is the crowning oil to this application. It is used to help relax all the muscles of the back and legs and to help reduce any stress, arthritic pain, or tension that may exist

V-6 MIXING OIL — is used to help dilute any of the oils that may be somewhat caustic to the skin. It should always be used with oregano and thyme and can be used with any of the other oils based upon the person's skin sensitivity.

Note: The oils used in this technique have many more benefits than those listed above. *For mo specific information, please refer to the sections in this book on Singles and Blends.*

Raindrop Technique

1. Remove all jewelry or metal to allow the energy to flow freely. Put a drop of **White Angelica** on each of your shoulders to protect you against any negative energies coming from the person receiving the treatment.

2. Have the person lie face up on a table with their body as straight as possible on the table The person receiving the treatment should be as comfortable as possible, so the arms can be resting along side the body or resting on the top of their hips, whichever they prefer (don't let their hands touch each other as this will tend to short circuit the flow of energy through their body). By covering the person with a sheet, their modesty can be protected as you roll them over and they can be kept warm as you alternate between working on the back and working on the legs and feet.

3. Apply **three** drops of **Valor** on each shoulder as well as six drops on each foot. Hold right foot/shoulder with right hand and left foot/shoulder with left hand (crossing hands if necessary – see the photo illustration entitled, "Valor Balance on Feet") for five to ten minutes or until you can feel an energy pulse in the person's feet. For this part of the application, it works best if there is another person assisting in the treatment. If you are working by yourself, do the feet only. **Valor** is used to balance and it works well on the energy alignment of the body. **This is the most important oil that is used in this application.**

Valor Balance on Feet

First apply 2 drops of **thyme** to the Vita Flex spine points along the inside edge of each foot, working it in three times with the Vita Flex technique (*refer to Vita Flex Technique in this same section, Key Principle #7 and photo illustrations for an explanation of this technique*). Repeat this procedure with each of the following oils, one at a time: **Oregano**, **cypress**, **birch/wintergreen**, **basil**, and **peppermint**. Then, have the person roll over onto their stomach and perform steps 5 through 14 on their spine.

Hold the bottle of **thyme** about six inches from the spine and evenly space **four to five** drops from the sacrum (tailbone) to the neck. Work it in evenly along the curvature of the spine with gentle upward strokes. Apply **five** drops of **oregano** and work it in the same way. Then, apply **ten to fifteen** drops of **V-6 Mixing Oil** to prevent any discomfort since both these oils can be quite caustic.

Using the very tips of the fingers, alternate between left hand and right hand as you very lightly work up the spine from the sacrum to the base of the neck with short, brush-like strokes. Follow the curvature of the spine and repeat two more times.

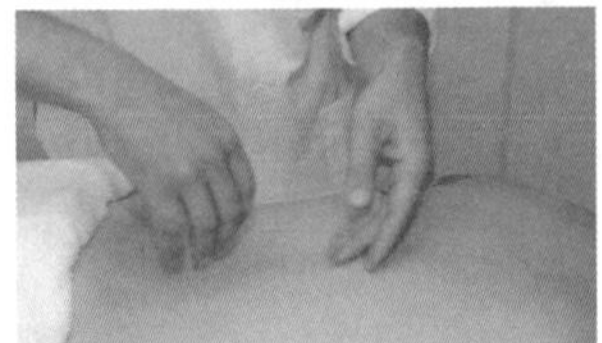 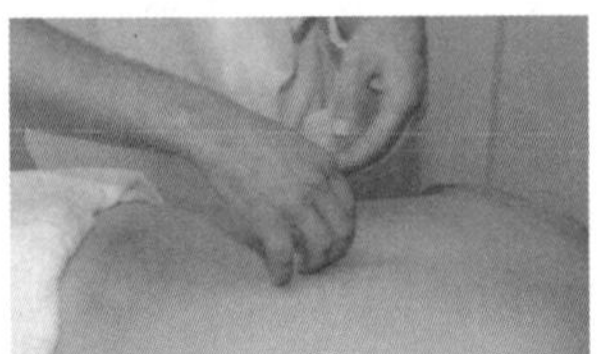 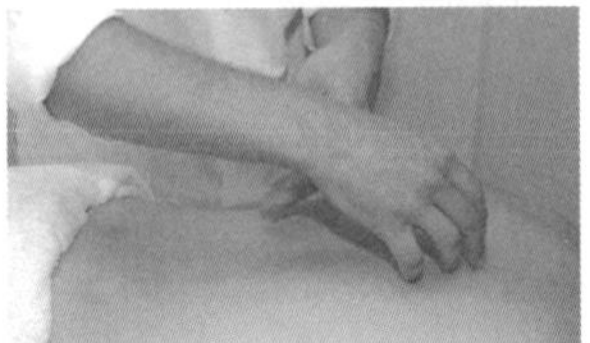

Using your finger tips again, softly brush up a few inches from the sacrum then out to either side of the body; right hand to the right and left hand to the left.

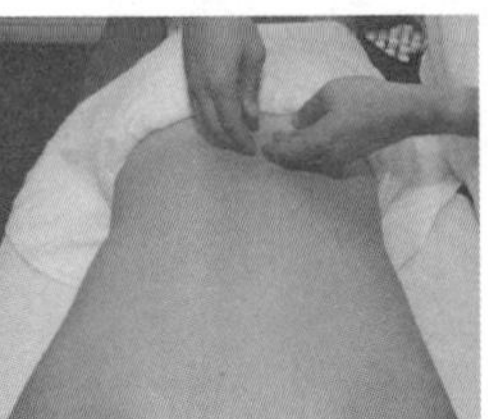 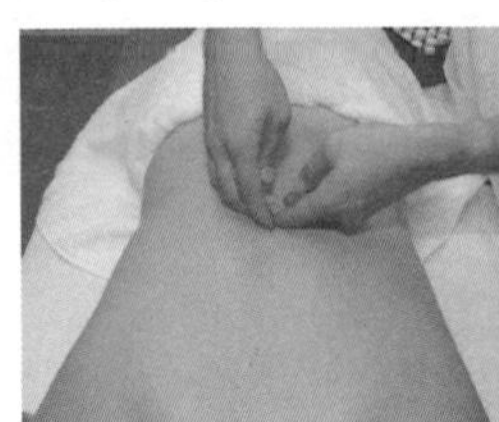 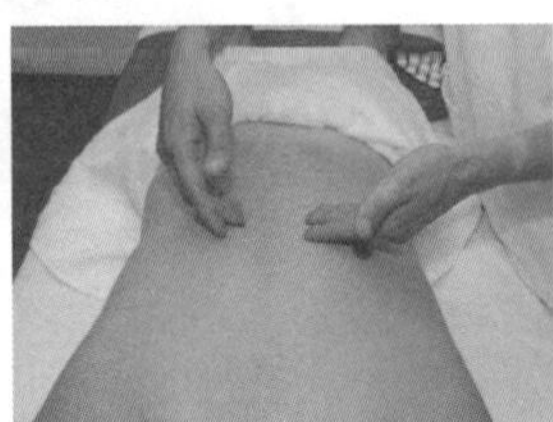 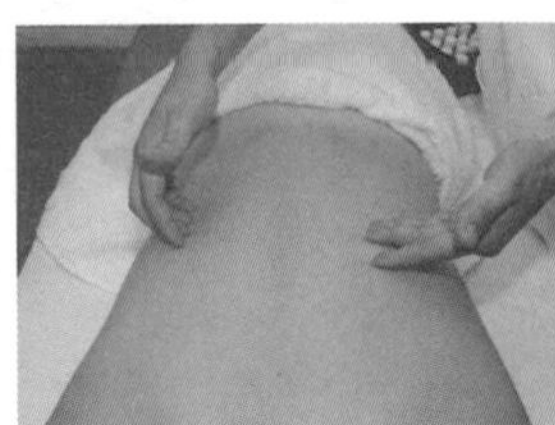

Repeat this step from the sacrum but go a few more inches up the spine then out to the sides. Then again from the sacrum, going up a few more inches then out. Then again, each time going further up the spine until you reach the base of the neck and flare out along the shoulders. This entire step should then be repeated two more times.

Using your finger tips again, start at the sacrum and in full-length strokes, lightly brush all the way up the spine to the base of the neck and then out over the shoulders. Repeat two more times.

9. Evenly space **four to five** drops of **cypress** from the sacrum to the neck. Work it in eve along the curvature of the spine with gentle upward strokes. Then apply the oils of **birch/wintergreen, basil, and peppermint** in the same manner.

10. Place both hands side by side (parallel to the spine) and using the tips of the fingers, massage in a circular, clock-wise motion, just off to one side of the spine, from the sacrum up to the neck. **Remember to never work directly on the spine**. Apply moderate pressure and move a finger's width at a time. This will help to loosen the muscles and allow the spine to straighten itself. After doing one side of the spine, move around the person and work the other side of the spine from the sacrum to the neck in the same manner. Repeat two more times on either side.

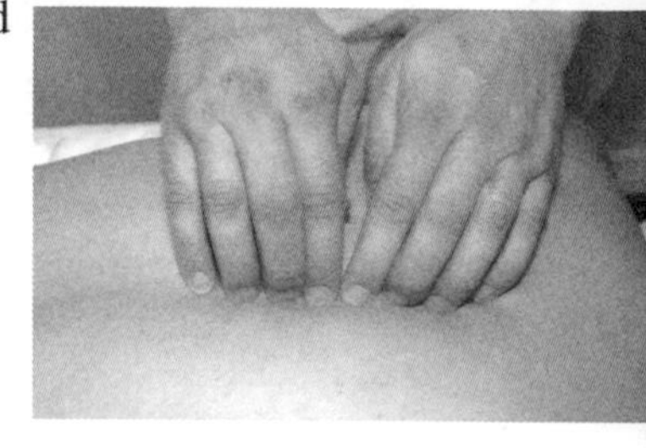

11. Using whichever hand is most comfortable to you, place the index and middle finger on either side of the spine at the sacrum. Place the other hand on top of the first, part way down the two fingers. Apply moderate pressure and with a quick, forward and back continued sawing motion of the hand on top, slide the fingers a little at a time up the spi to the skull. Move the fingers upward slowly during the sawing motion. Once the skull reached, apply gentle but firm pressure to push the skull forward, stretching the spine. Return to the sacrum and repeat two more times.

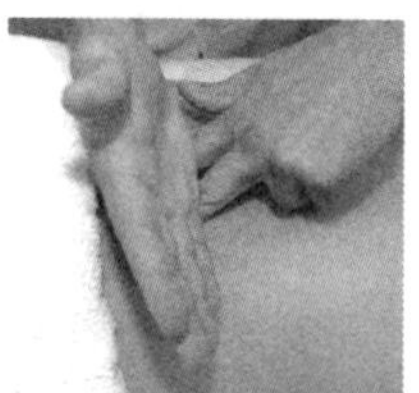

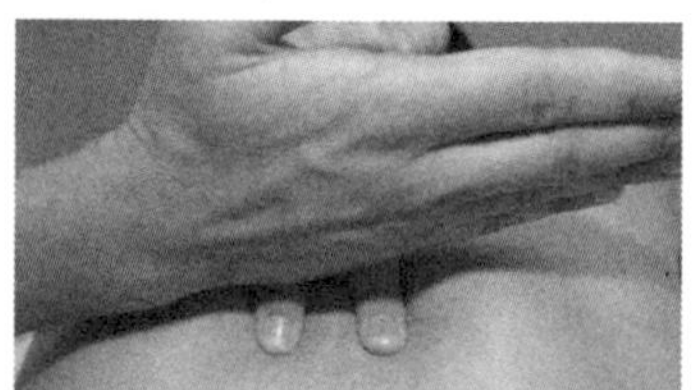

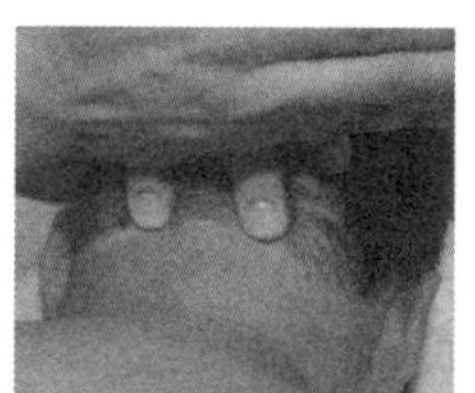

12. Place the thumbs of each hand on either side of the spine at the sacrum and point them towards each other. Next, using the Vita Flex technique, roll the thumbs up and over on the thumbnails, applying some pressure straight down during the roll. Then release and slide the thumbs up an inch or so and repeat the roll with pressure. Continue up to the base of the neck, then return to the sacrum and repeat two more times. This will become easier with practice.

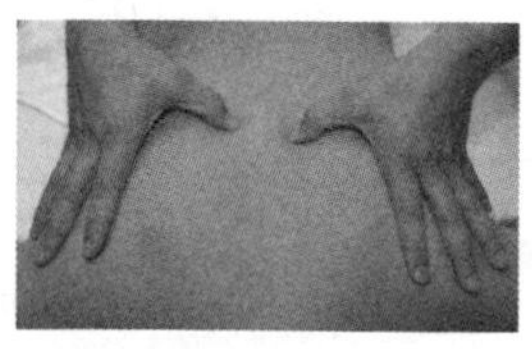

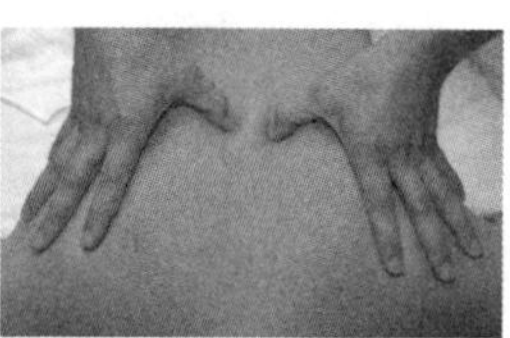

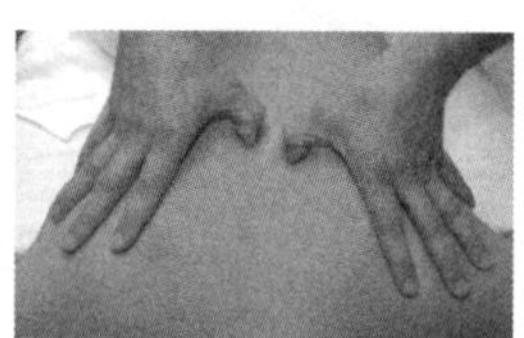

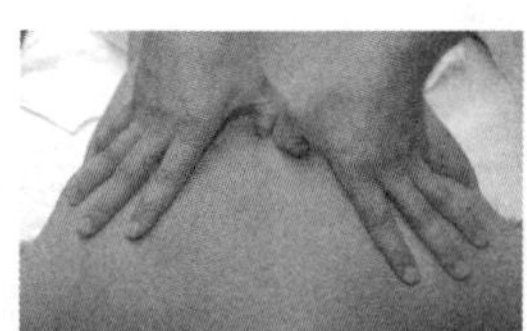

3. Apply five to six drops of **marjoram** up the spine and work it in. Then apply five to six drops of **Aroma Siez** to each side and away from the spine. Gently massage these oils into the muscle tissue all over the back to soothe and relax the patient. After the oils have been massaged in well, you may cover the person with the sheet and rest for approximately five minutes. Apply **Ortho Ease** over the entire area of the back and gently massage it in. Then cover the person to keep them warm and massage **Ortho Ease** into the legs. This will help to relax the muscles that may be pulling on the spine.

4. Fold a hand towel, soak it in hot water, wring it out and lay it along the entire length of the spine. Take a dry bath towel and fold it in half lengthwise and place it over the hot wet towel. Be extremely sensitive to the feelings of the person as the heat may build along the spine. The heat will gradually build for five to eight minutes then cool right down to normal. If the heat becomes too uncomfortable, remove the towels and apply V-6 Mixing Oil. Then replace the towels and continue until the wet towel becomes cold. If the person's back is still hot, cover with a dry towel and allow the back to cool down slowly.

5. After the person's back begins to cool down, gently stretch the spine by crossing hands and straddle the spine with your hands, one pointing towards the top of the spine and the other towards the bottom as shown in the adjacent photo. Starting in the middle, gently press the hands downwards and apart towards opposite ends of the spine. Then move the hands apart more and repeat the stretch. Continue until the ends of the spine are reached.

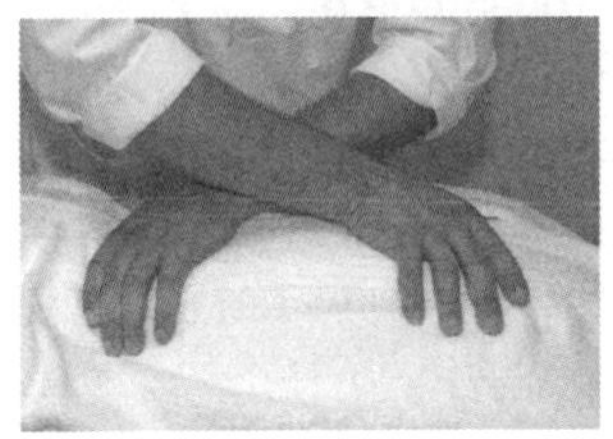

6. Remove the wet towels and have the person roll over onto their back. Apply two to three drops of **birch/wintergreen** along the inside of each leg from the knee to the heel and up the inside of the foot to the big toe. Layer it in and apply the oils of **cypress, basil, and peppermint** in the same fashion. Then work the same area using the Vita Flex technique. The inside of the shin corresponds to the colon. By working this area, you are opening the colon and allowing it to expel any toxins released during the Raindrop Technique.

7. The final step is to perform another gentle stretching of the spine. If you are working alone, put your right hand behind the base of the head and your left hand under the chin. Very gently pull to create a slight tension and release. Do three times then move to the feet. Hold above the ankles and gently pull and release three times. If you have an assistant, one person can hold the head and the other hold the feet. Then together, apply a gentle tension and hold for a few minutes. This is then completed by the person at the head doing a very slight pull and release three times.

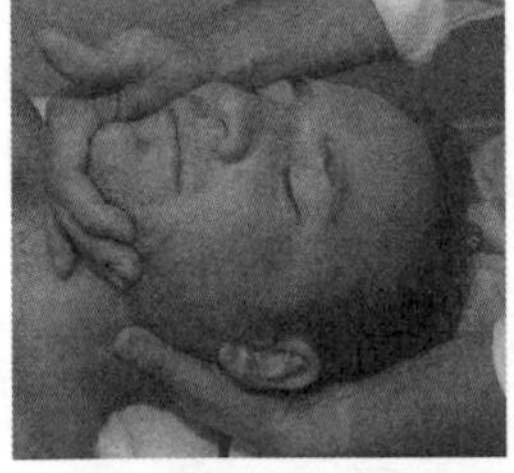

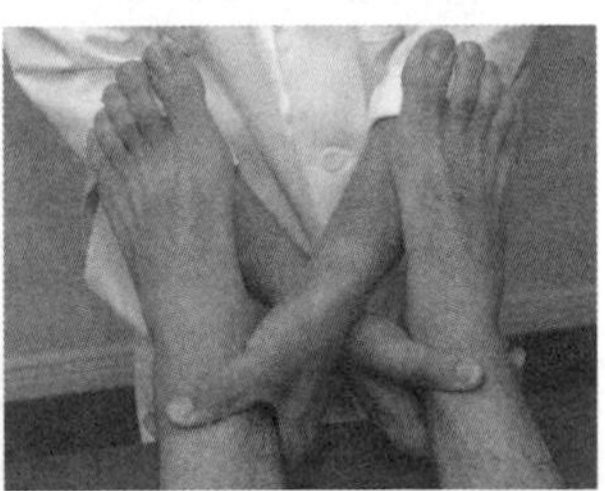

18. If certain systems of the body need work, have the person roll back over onto their stoma and use the applicable blends and/or singles with the Vita Flex Technique on the spine. Refer to the chart of the autonomic nervous system to help with placement of the oils alo the spine.

By stimulating the Central Nervous System, you have just given someone a total treatme affecting every system in the body, including emotional release and support. Even though the oils continue to work in the body for a week or more, one application may last months or it may be necessary to repeat the application every week until the body begins to respond. The object is to develop a new memory in the tissues of the body and train it to hold itself in place. **(For a list of videos that effectively demonstrate this valuable application technique, refer to the *Video Listing* in the Bibliography section of this book.)**

Another aspect to the Raindrop Technique is the ability to **customize it** to the needs of th receiver. Each Raindrop Technique session should begin with the **Valor** essential oil blend, and the single oils of **oregano** (*Origanum compactum* CT carvacrol), and **thyme** (*Thymus vulgaris* C thymol). However, after that, the remaining oils can be replace with others more specific to the condition or body system needing to be affected. To assist with this customization, the following chart is a partial list of single oils and oil blends under the particular body system which they affect. This chart is a condensed excerpt from the Body System Chart shown in the Appendix of this book *(Refer to the full chart in the Appendix for other products that can assist in strengthening a particular body system)*.

Cardiovascular System	**Digestive System**	**Emotional Balance***	**Hormonal System**	**Immune System**	**Nervous System**	**Respiratory System**
anise	anise	angelica	anise	Abundance	angelica	anise
AromaLife	cardamon	Australian Blue	Clary sage	cistus	Brain Power	Aroma Siez
basil	celery seed	chamomile (both)	coriander	Citrus Fresh	carrot	cajeput
cajeput	clove	Chivalry	davana	clove	cedarwood	cedarwood
carrot	coriander	fir, White	Dragon Time	cumin	celery seed	clove
Christmas Spirit	cumin	frankincense	EndoFlex	cypress, Blue	chamomile (both)	eucalyptus (all
clove	cypress, Blue	Gathering	fennel	Exodus II	En-R-Gee	fir (all)
cypress	Di-Tone	geranium	fleabane	frankincense	Idaho Balsam fir	hyssop
fleabane	fennel	jasmine	goldenrod	galbanum	frankincense	laurel
goldenrod	ginger	juniper	jasmine	ImmuPower	hyssop	lavandin
grapefruit	juniper	Lady Sclareol	Mister	laurel	juniper	lemon
helichrysum	JuvaFlex	lavender	myrrh	ledum	lavender	melaleuca (all)
hyssop	Juva Cleanse	onycha	myrtle	lemon	myrrh	Melrose
lavandin	laurel	orange	nutmeg	lemongrass	nutmeg	myrtle
lavender	lemon	palmarosa	sage	lime	PanAway	peppermint
Longevity	mandarin	petitgrain	sage lavender	melaleuca	Peace & Calming	pine
marjoram	myrtle	pine	SclarEssence	Mountain savory	pepper, Black	Raven
onycha	orange	sage lavender	Sensation	myrrh	peppermint	ravensara
palmarosa	peppermint	sandalwood	vetiver	nutmeg	sage lavender	RC
rosemary	Purification	spikenard	yarrow	orange	sandalwood	rosemary verbanc
tsuga	rosemary	spruce	ylang ylang	ravensara	spruce	sage lavender
ylang ylang	SclarEssence	Valor		sage	tansy, Blue	spruce
	spearmint	vetiver		Thieves	valerian	thyme linalol
	tarragon	ylang ylang		yarrow	vetiver	tsuga

**The majority of the essential oil blends in this book deal with emotional balance and are therefore too numerous to list here. Refer to the Body Systems Chart in the Appendix for more possible blends.*

The booklet, entitled A Statistical Validation of Raindrop Technique, by David Stewart, ıD, RA (available from Abundant Health), is the result of research conducted by the distribution ˙ over 3,000 surveys to individuals that have either received a Raindrop Technique session, lministered Raindrop Technique sessions to others, or both. The results of the survey were bulated and the following are excerpts from these results, showing overwhelming evidence that Raindrop is thought by the vast majority of its participants to benefit people in ways both ›jective and subjective, physical and emotional, social and spiritual."

	Perceived Results of Raindrop as Expressed by 416 clients receiving 3,584 Raindrops			Perceived Results of Raindrop as Expressed by Clients to the 265 Facilitators Responding to this Survey for 11,256 Raindrop Procedures Administered		
a.	Positive 97.0%	Neutral 2.5%	Negative 0.5%	Positive 96.3%	Neutral 3.5%	Negative 0.2%
b.	Pleasant 97.9%	Neutral 1.4%	Unpleasant 0.4%	Pleasant 96.4%	Neutral 3.0%	Unpleasant 0.6%
c.	Resulted in Healing 15.9%	No Perceptible Results 83.9%	Resulted in Harm or Injury 0.2%	Resulted in Healing 87.7%	No Perceptible Results 12.0%	Resulted in Harm or Injury 0.3%
d.	Felt Better Afterwards 97.7%	No Change in Feeling 1.4%	Felt Worse Afterwards 0.9%	Felt Better Afterwards 96.0%	No Change in Feeling 3.4%	Felt Worse Afterwards 0.6%
e.	Health Improved 89.1%	No Change in Health 10.9%	Health got Worse 0.0%	Health Improved 90.8%	No Change in Health 9.2%	Health got Worse 0.03%
f.	Emotional State Improved 86.2%	No Change in Emotions 13.4%	Emotional State Worsened 0.4%	Emotional State Improved 91.0%	No Change in Emotions 8.5%	Emotional State Worsened 0.5%
g.	Would Receive It Again 99.9%	Maybe So, Maybe Not 0.1%	Would Never Receive it Again 0.0%	Would Receive It Again 96.7%	Maybe So, Maybe Not 3.2%	Would Never Receive it Again 0.1%

–This information is included here with permission from the author, David Stewart

he following are some personal experiences with Raindrop Technique:

vas in a pitiful state. I had not been able to work for 5 years, lived on disability insurance, and then welfare. I depended on ıarmaceuticals for pain management and depression. My social schedule consisted of doctor appointments and rest periods. I ıd been diagnosed with herniated disks and then fibromyalgia. I was a textbook case with all the symptoms and treatments hich helped temporarily but didn't get rid of anything. Then a wonderful friend talked me into coming to see her to receive the ıindrop Technique. At first, I received the Raindrop Technique once a week for about 6 weeks, then once every other week, en once a month. After the first few sessions, I was feeling so very much better. Then I noticed that I would forget to take my edications and was doing just fine without them. After a while, I did not need to take anything anymore.

—Submitted by Pam Jones, Benton, Arkansas (July 2004)

om had worn a narcotic pain patch for the past two years for her "chronic back pain" due to osteoarthritis, spurring of the ine, and numerous back surgeries. By using PanAway, we were able to discontinue the pain patch. We continued to alternate ınAway with Wintergreen, Peppermint, Clove and V-6 oil to her back and feet with warm compresses once or twice a day as eded for complete relief. Six weeks after she started receiving weekly Raindrop massages, she no longer complained of back ıin. She continues to receive weekly or bi-weekly Raindrop massages, and it's been 6 months since she has complained of ıck pain! Praise God!

—Submitted by E. Pinar (July 2004)

AUTONOMIC NERVOUS SYSTEM

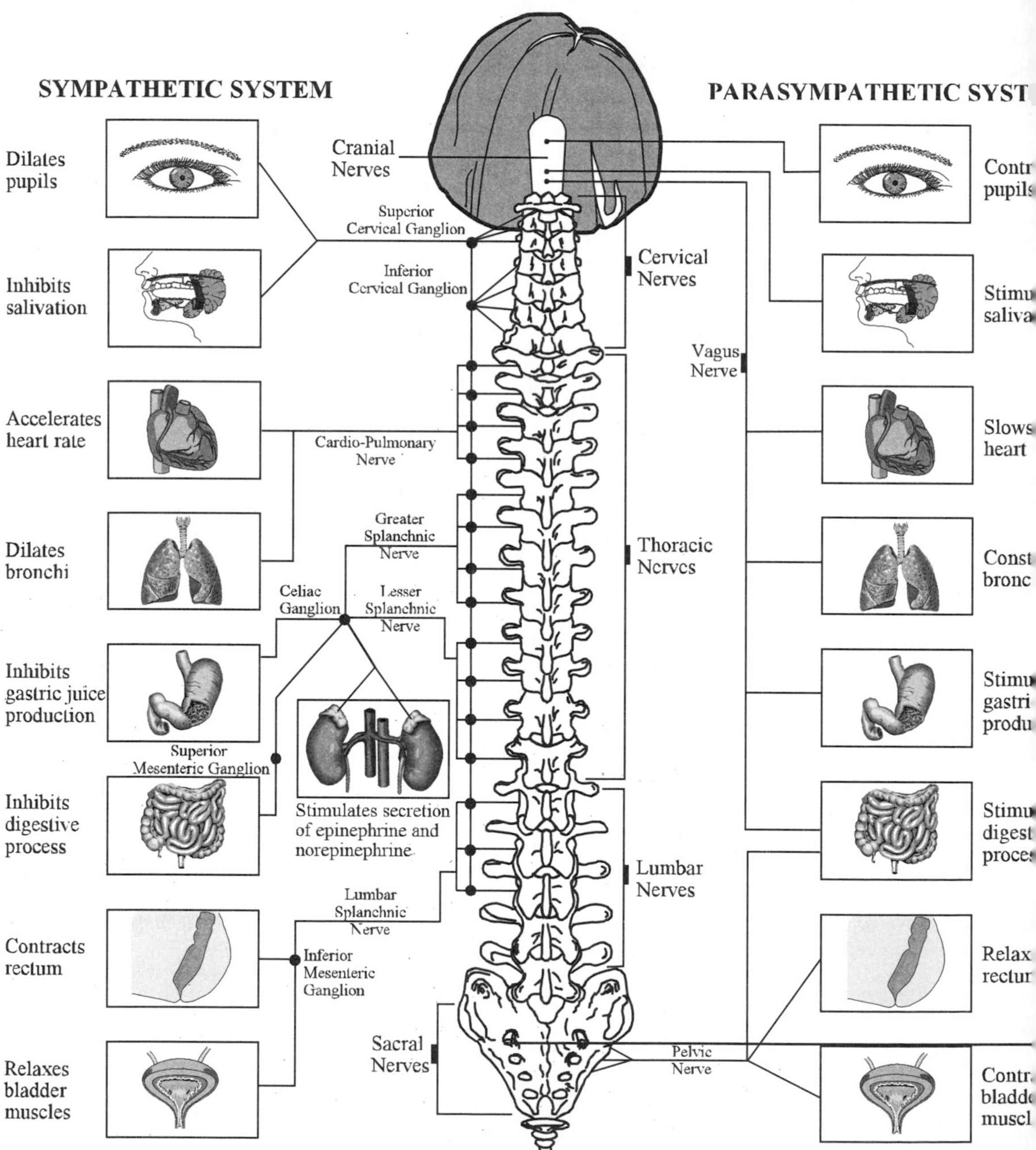
SYMPATHETIC SYSTEM
PARASYMPATHETIC SYST
Dilates pupils
Inhibits salivation
Accelerates heart rate
Dilates bronchi
Inhibits gastric juice production
Inhibits digestive process
Contracts rectum
Relaxes bladder muscles
Cranial Nerves
Superior Cervical Ganglion
Inferior Cervical Ganglion
Cardio-Pulmonary Nerve
Greater Splanchnic Nerve
Celiac Ganglion
Lesser Splanchnic Nerve
Superior Mesenteric Ganglion
Stimulates secretion of epinephrine and norepinephrine
Lumbar Splanchnic Nerve
Inferior Mesenteric Ganglion
Sacral Nerves
Cervical Nerves
Vagus Nerve
Thoracic Nerves
Lumbar Nerves
Pelvic Nerve
Contr pupil
Stimu saliva
Slows heart
Const bronc
Stimu gastri produ
Stimu digest proce
Relax rectur
Contr bladd muscl

DIGESTIVE TRACT

"The gastrointestinal tract is a tube twenty-five to thirty-two feet long, that begins at the iouth and ends at the anus. It comprises the mouth, pharynx, esophagus, stomach, small intestine duodenum, jejunum, and ileum), large intestine (cecum, ascending colon, transverse colon, and escending colon), rectum, and anus. Accessory organs—the liver, pancreas, and gallbladder—all lay an important role in digestion.

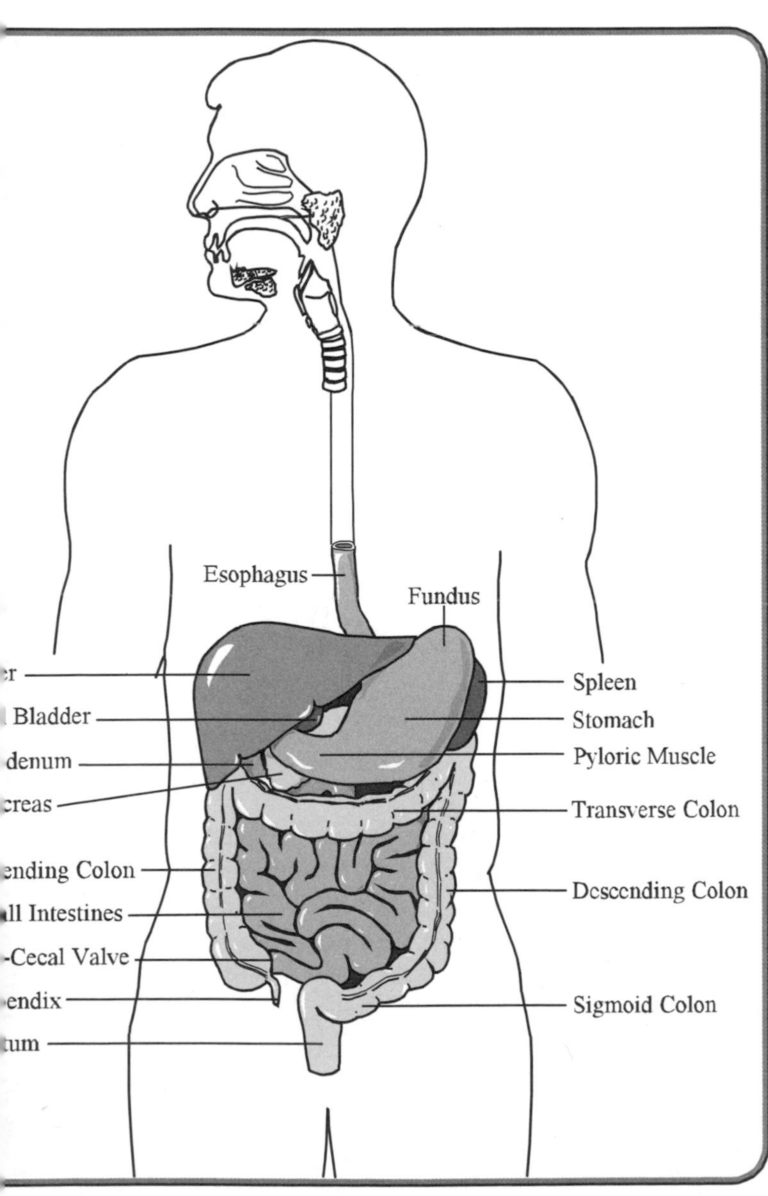

"Digestion begins when food mixes with enzymes in saliva. The process is then carried on in the stomach by hydrochloric acid (HCI) and pepsin. Food is liquified in the stomach and passes into the small intestine, where it is further broken down by digestive enzymes from the pancreas (the enzyme protease digests proteins, the enzyme amylase digests carbohydrates, and the enzyme lipase digests fats). The gallbladder secretes bile, formed by the liver, to aid absorption of fats and fat-soluble vitamins.

"Most food absorption takes place in the small intestine, while water, electrolytes (essential body chemicals), and some of the final products of digestion are absorbed in the large intestine." (Alternative Medicine—The Definitive Guide, p. 680)

NOSE AND OLFACTORY SYSTEM

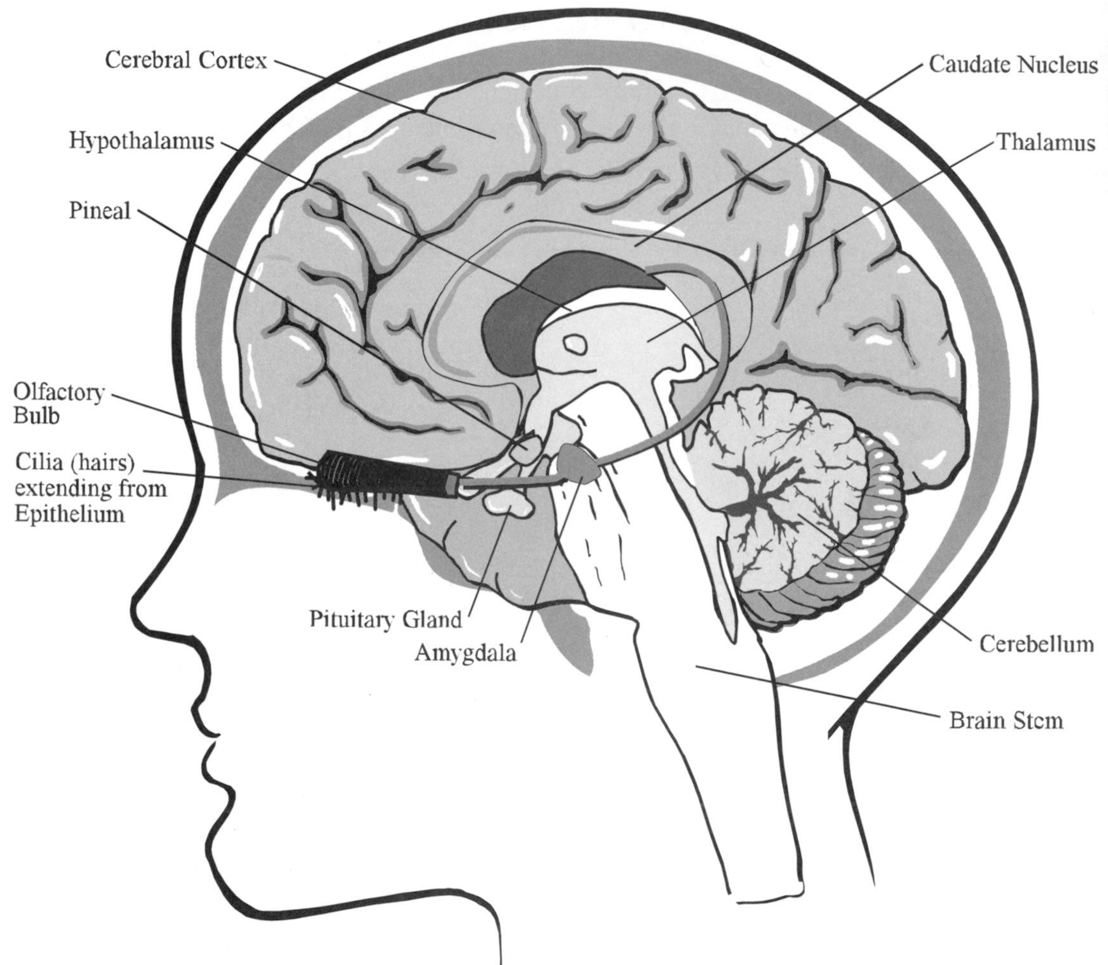

Odor molecules travel to the top of the nasal cavity and fit like little puzzle pieces into specific receptor cells on the cilia. The cilia are little bundles of six to eight tiny hairs which extend from each of about 10 million olfactory nerve cells. These millions of nerve cells (that are replaced every twenty eight days) make up a membrane which is known as the olfactory epithelium. The epithelium serves to transfer electric impulses from the cilia to the olfactory bulb, which it covers. The olfactory bulb, in turn, sends those impulses along to the amygdala (which is responsible for storing and releasing emotional trauma) and further on to the limbic system of the brain. Because the limbic system is directly connected to those parts of the brain that control hear rate, blood pressure, breathing, memory, stress levels, and hormone balance, essential oils can hav some very profound physiological and psychological effects.

AURICULAR EMOTIONAL THERAPY

If more than one oil/blend is indicated, layer them one at a time.

*** When working on the ear, apply Harmony and Forgiveness to the entire ear and apply Valor on the feet.***

10THER: Geranium
:xual Abuse: Geranium, Ylang Ylang
bandonment: Geranium, Forgiveness, Acceptance

'ATHER: Lavender
:xual Abuse: Lavender, Ylang Ylang, Release
lale Abuse: Helichrysum, Lavender

EPRESSION
ny of the following: Valor, Joy, Hope, White Angelica, Peace & Calming, Citrus Fresh, Christmas Spirit, Gentle Baby
se whichever blend(s) work best for you.

)VERWHELMED
se Hope and Acceptance

BEARING BURDENS)F THE WORLD
se Release and Valor

NGER & HATE
se Joy to stimulate the pituitary.
se Valor and Release to release the anger.

ELF EXPRESSION
se Valor and Motivation. Take deep breaths to express oneself.

'EAR
pply Valor, Release, Joy.

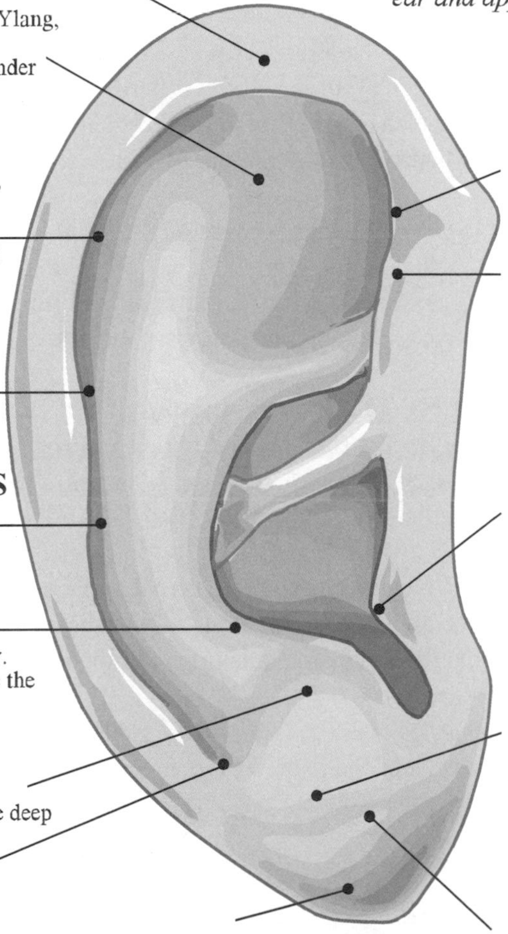

OPEN THE MIND
Apply 3 Wise Men.

SYMPATHY & GUILT
Use Joy and Inspiration.

SELF PITY
Use Acceptance.

REJECTION
Use Forgiveness and Acceptance. Work the rejection points on both ears. For rejection from Mother, use Geranium. For rejection from Father, use Lavender. While applying the oils, say "I choose to accept my Mother/Father for what they have done or not done. It is their life and not mine."

EYES and VISION
To improve eyesight, use 10 Lemongrass, 5 Cypress, 3 Eucalyptus, in ½ oz. of V-6 Mixing Oil.
For Vision of goals, use Dream Catcher, Acceptance, and 3 Wise Men.

HEART
To strengthen the heart and lower blood pressure, use Aroma Life.
For self acceptance, apply Joy, Forgiveness, and Acceptance.

EMOTIONAL RELEASE

Apply each of the following oils in the order suggested. Smell each oil before applying. I you find an oil repulsive, you may choose not to use it in this procedure.

1. Apply three to six drops of **VALOR** to the bottom of the **feet** and balance by holding righ foot in right hand and left foot in left hand. Continue to hold the feet until an energy pulse can be felt in both feet. **VALOR** helps balance electrical energies within the body, helps one overcome fear and opposition, and may give courage, confidence, and increase self esteem. Known as the "Chiropractor in a Bottle", it works best on the bottom of the feet, or on the spine (top and bottom, or entire length—raindrop style).

2. Apply one drop of **HARMONY** either directly on the **energy centers** (chakras), or along the side of the body. **HARMONY** brings about a harmonic balance to the chakras (energy centers), allowing the energy to flow more efficiently through the body. It may reduce stress and create a general overall feeling of well being.

3. Apply one drop of **3 WISE MEN** on the **crown of the head** in a clockwise motion. **3 WISE MEN** opens crown chakra and stimulates the pineal gland to release emotions and deep-seated trauma. It brings a sense of grounding and uplifting through memory recall. It also helps to keep negative energy and negative emotions from reattaching to the body.

4. Apply one drop of **PRESENT TIME** on the **thymus** in a circular motion, close eyes and tap three times with energy fingers (pointer and middle). **PRESENT TIME** helps bring one into the moment. We must forget about the past and stop worrying about the future. We must live in the moment in order to heal.

5. Apply one drop of **INNER CHILD** around the **navel and nose**. **INNER CHILD** may stimulate memory response and help one reconnect with their inner-self or their own identity. This is one of the first steps to achieving emotional balance.

6. Apply one drop of **RELEASE** over the **liver**. **RELEASE** helps to enhance the release of memory trauma from the cells of the liver, where anger and hate emotions are stored. It may also help one let go of negative emotions so that progress is more effective and efficient.

7. Apply one drop of **GROUNDING** to the **brain stem, back of neck and sternum**. **GROUNDING** may help one deal with the reality of their emotions in a peaceful way.

8. Apply one drop of **FORGIVENESS** on the **navel** in a clockwise motion. **FORGIVENESS** may help one move past the barriers in life. It also helps to bring them

into a higher spiritual awareness of their needs and helps raise their frequency to the point where they feel almost compelled to FORGIVE, FORGET, LET GO, and go on with their lives.

Apply one drop of **HOPE** on the **outer edge of the ears**. **HOPE** helps support the body both physically and mentally. It may help one overcome suicidal depression and restore hope for tomorrow. By filling them with a feeling of strength and grounding, it empowers them to go forward with hope and achievement.

0. Apply one drop of **JOY** over the **heart** in a clockwise motion. **JOY** gives one a glorious feeling of self-love, confidence, and creates a frequency around oneself of the energy of love; the true source of all healing.

1. Apply one drop of **SARA** over the **energy centers (chakras), navel, and chest**. **SARA** may enable one to relax into a mental state and allow them to release the memories of traumatic experiences.

2. Apply one drop of **WHITE ANGELICA** on the **crown and shoulders**. **WHITE ANGELICA** strengthens and fortifies one's aura, generating a feeling of protection and an awareness of one's potential. As the final oil in this emotional clearing process, it supports all that has taken place and prepares one to search inward for the strength to proceed with life and to search upward for the true source of love and light.

3. Meditate for 20 minutes.

omments: This procedure has been used successfully by many practitioners.

ote: Energy Centers are commonly known as hakras. For a complete listing of the ppropriate oils for each chakra, refer to the ersonal Guide section of this book under hakras.

Energy Centers

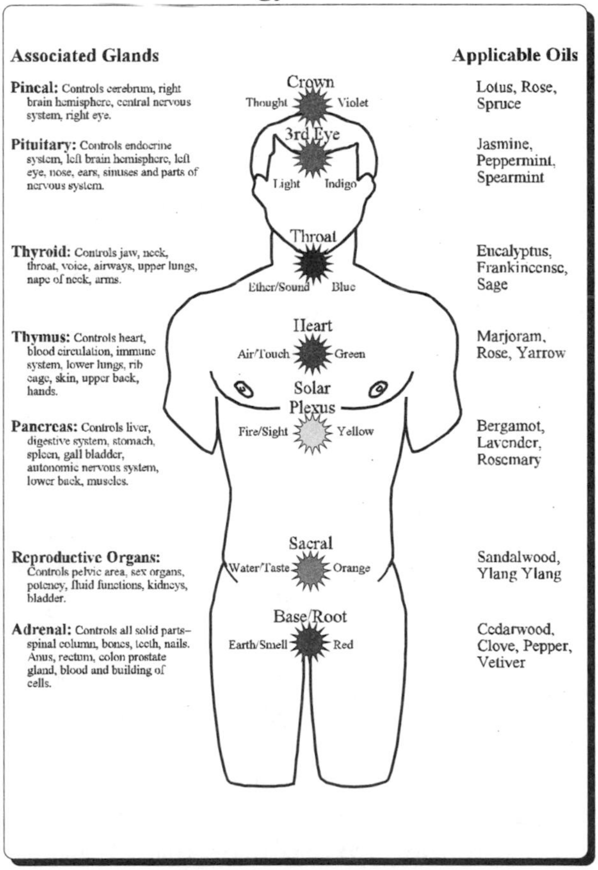

Associated Glands	Energy Center			Applicable Oils
Pineal: Controls cerebrum, right brain hemisphere, central nervous system, right eye.	Crown	Thought	Violet	Lotus, Rose, Spruce
Pituitary: Controls endocrine system, left brain hemisphere, left eye, nose, ears, sinuses and parts of nervous system.	3rd Eye	Light	Indigo	Jasmine, Peppermint, Spearmint
Thyroid: Controls jaw, neck, throat, voice, airways, upper lungs, nape of neck, arms.	Throat	Ether/Sound	Blue	Eucalyptus, Frankincense, Sage
Thymus: Controls heart, blood circulation, immune system, lower lungs, rib cage, skin, upper back, hands.	Heart	Air/Touch	Green	Marjoram, Rose, Yarrow
Pancreas: Controls liver, digestive system, stomach, spleen, gall bladder, autonomic nervous system, lower back, muscles.	Solar Plexus	Fire/Sight	Yellow	Bergamot, Lavender, Rosemary
Reproductive Organs: Controls pelvic area, sex organs, potency, fluid functions, kidneys, bladder.	Sacral	Water/Taste	Orange	Sandalwood, Ylang Ylang
Adrenal: Controls all solid parts–spinal column, bones, teeth, nails. Anus, rectum, colon prostate gland, blood and building of cells.	Base/Root	Earth/Smell	Red	Cedarwood, Clove, Pepper, Vetiver

Music and Aromatherapy

Duets for Peaceful Emotional Healing

by Karyn Grant, Licensed Massage Therapist, Singer, Songwriter

Walking through life is like taking a journey. There are hidden treasures of knowledge along the path. There are precious traveling companions that enlighten our journey and make the way to healing more peaceful, more gentle, more beautiful. Music has become that traveling companion for me. It has never left my side.

I didn't realize it then, but I am aware now that it was as a youth that I learned that musi was healing to the soul. I didn't know why I sang, I just sang. I found that through singing, my spirit was lifted and my mood was brightened. I began writing music by putting scriptures to simple guitar chords (I only knew three). Eventually, my own little handwritten verses became songs too. Just as the poetry of my heart turned to the lyrics of song, the simple everyday sorrow of a teenage girl turned into peaceful happy feelings. I was very happy as a youth. I took voice lessons, wrote songs, sang about everything from a stubbed toe to a broken heart. I didn't know exactly how it worked but I learned that when my heart was making music, I was the happiest. Music became for me, the peaceful way to handle any of life's problems.

I didn't understand then what was happening on a metaphysical level. I did not comprehend that music is a form of "light" and has healing vibrations of its own. I did not yet know what I now know; that music performs a massage on an atomic level in one's body and creates a way for less desirable energies to be transformed into more desirable ones. All I really knew was that when I sang, I got happy. When I wrote out my feelings and expressed them inste of holding them in, I got happy. And when I sang the heartfelt words I wrote, I got twice as happ I had a quote on my wall at age sixteen that read, "I once wrote a poem that no one read, I once sang a song that no one heard, I once drew a picture that no one saw . . . and I was happy."

At nineteen, I was having my preschool class draw pictures as they listened to music blindfolded. I watched amused as they colored slower or scribbled faster to the tempos, rhythms and beats of the songs that I selected for them. I wondered how music could have such a powerfu effect over someone so little? Their feelings and demeanors changed so quickly! Even then, I began learning, by exploring my own emotions and feelings, the mysterious power of music and t effect it had on myself and others.

As I reached my mid-twenties, the songs began coming again in the middle of the night. I learned that the combination of words and music could have a very softening effect on mind, hear body and spirit. As my marriage grew more and more troubled, I realized that the gift of song wa assuaging deep feelings of emotional isolation, spiritual bereavement and loneliness that I could n bear alone. I would arise at 3:00 a.m. every morning to nurse my baby girl back to sleep. Those became my own "feedings" too. That's when I began journeying with song again.

As the isolation grew in my marital relationship, so did the spiritual gift of singing. nging the praises and sorrows of my heart literally took the ache from my heart and transformed ief into comfort, serenity and peace. I was able to focus on spiritual solutions for my less than sirable circumstance. The ability to express the innermost desires and feelings of my heart came easier. Not having developed the talent for writing the melodies, I sung them onto cassettes d hid them away in a drawer never imagining that these treasures would ever serve to bless other uls who were journeying through life carrying hidden wounds that could not be seen, diagnosed solaced.

Not until years later, following my divorce, when I became a massage therapist, did I begin understand the healing effect of music as therapy. I would work with clients during the day and ould help them as best I could. Then, later in the night, I would be awakened with songs of mfort, courage and peace to sing to them at their next appointment. This I would do, and many ept tears of gratitude, saying that they never had anyone take the time to sing to them. N'Shama erling writes:

> When a woman in a certain African tribe knows she is pregnant, she goes out into the wilderness with a few friends and together they pray and meditate until they hear the song of the child. They recognize that every soul has its own vibration that expresses its unique flavor and purpose. When the women attune to the song, they sing it out loud. They then return to the tribe and teach the song of the child to the village.
>
> When the child is born, the community gathers and sings the child's song to him or her. Later, when the child enters education, the village gathers and chants the child's song. When the child passes through the initiation to adulthood, the people would again come together and sing. At the time of marriage, the person hears his or her song. Finally, when the soul is about to pass from this world, the family and friends gather at the person's bed, just as they did at their birth, and they sing the person to the next life.
>
> In this African tribe there is one other occasion upon which the villagers sing to the child. If at any time during his or her life, the person commits a crime or aberrant social act, the individual is called to the center of the village and the people in the community form a circle around them. They sing their song to them. The tribe recognized that the correction for antisocial behavior is not punishment; it is love and the remembrance of your true identity. When you recognize your own song, you have no desire or need to do anything that would hurt another.

A friend is someone who knows your song and sings it to you when you have forgotten it. hose who love you are not fooled by mistakes you have made or dark images you hold about ourself. They remember your beauty when you feel ugly; your wholeness when you are broken; our innocence when you feel guilty; and your purpose when you are confused. You may not have rown up in an African tribe that sings your song to you at crucial life transitions, but life is lways reminding you when you are in tune with yourself and when you are not. When you feel ood, what you are doing matches your song, and when you feel awful, it doesn't. In the end, we hall all recognize our song and sing it well. You may feel your voice is a bit "warbly" at the oment, but so have all the great singers at one time or another. Just keep singing.

I began learning that music was a vibrational soothing balm that could enter into places t physical ointment could not reach. Combining aromatherapy with the music began anchoring in the affirmations and imageries of the songs with scent. I instinctively knew that to reach those hidden wounds that are infected with the energies of loneliness, resentment, anger, despair, sadne fear, doubt and other such emotions that are locked into the cellular memory of the glands, organ tissues, and systems of the body, it would take the healing vibrations of touch, smell, visualizatio and soothing sounds to transform those energies into positive and more joyful emotions.

From The Book of Sound Therapy, we read, "The human being is therefore likened to a very complex, unique, and finely-tuned musical instrument. Every atom, molecule, cell, tissue an organ of the body continually broadcasts the frequencies of physical, emotional, mental and spiritual life. The human voice is an indicator of its body's health on all these levels of existence. It establishes a relationship between the individual and the wondrous network of vibrations that is the cosmos."

In the ancient societies of Egypt, India, Greece, and China, to name a few, music played a vital role in just about everything, from health to architecture to politics. They believed that musi was the bridge linking all things. Physical forms were considered manifestations of music, and it was held that life and health depended upon harmonic balance of rations and relationships. In ancient Greece, for instance, one could not become a physician until he had first become a musician, and prescriptions often included rhythmic singing and chanting from selected sacred melodic sequences.

If we could put a heart, broken and scarred, under a microscope and see the emotional aches manifesting themselves as rips and cuts and then pour the healing balm and vibrations of song and scent into those open and festering sores, I believe that we would watch in amazement as the rips began to mend and the cuts began to close in perfect alignment. For that is what I see in my mind's eye. I see song as living water. I see the vibrations of aromatherapy as more than just scent, but as a healing balm for the soul. I see the wounds being cleansed and mending in perfect closure, having finally been acknowledged, addressed and administered to.

An anonymous quote reads, "Man of himself is an instrument of music; and when the chords of which he is composed are touched as sound salutes the ear, the sound appeals to his spi and the sentiment to his understanding. If the strains are harmonious, he endorses and enjoys the with supreme delight. Whether the tones are from a human voice or from an instrument, they arrest his attention and absorb his whole being."

I have stood at the side of my massage table and beheld as countenances have changed from tearful torment into peaceful, blissful expressions of tranquil gratitude. For the hidden wounds of the heart and the spirit, there are no scalpels, no knives, no needles, no thread, no numbing medications. There is only beauty all around where there are flowers, where there are songs, where there are scents, where there is compassion, where there is pure touch, and where there is hope, but most of all where there is love. We only give the gifts which do the real healing

These are some of Karyn's songs that are currently available from Abundant Health.

Scents of Peace Collection

The Gentle Approach to Wholeness

The music and oils together are excellent for enhancing and anchoring in thoughts and feelings that encourage, inspire, and comfort clients, children, or self. **These CDs can be used with the oils suggested below.**

Vol. 1, The Healer's Touch, Music as Therapy CD &
Vol. 2, The Healer's Touch, Guided Imagery CD
Vocal songs and affirmations to assist in clearing the past.
Suggested oils: *Peace & Calming, Inner Child, Gentle Baby, Forgiveness, Valor, Harmony, Inspiration, Surrender, and White Angelica.*

Vol. 3, Divine Essence, Music as Therapy CD &
Vol. 4, Divine Essence, Guided Imagery CD
Vocal songs, instrumentals and affirmations to bring hope, abundance, restfulness, purpose and rejuvenation to the mind, body, and spirit.
Suggested oils: *Envision, Sacred Mountain, Gentle Baby, Magnify your Purpose, Hope, Abundance, Into the Future, Joy, and Humility.*

Healing Sounds and Scents for Pure Love Collection

Breathe deeply and inhale this collection of songs and oils that simply assist in the mending process of a broken heart. These songs will bring pure comfort to a troubled heart and mind and may assist in lifting one out of despair with the sweet sound of solace. These songs, experienced by many, have been reported to bring comfort and nurture one's soul back to a sense of wholeness.

Vol. 1, Songs for A Broken Heart — Vocal songs that convey love and concern when we are enduring hardship, pain, and suffering.
Suggested oils: Lavender, lemon, peppermint, Joy, PanAway, Peace & Calming, and Purification.

Vol. 2, An Angel's Song — Vocal songs that inspire and give hope to the tender heart that is facing adversity, trials, and hardship.
Suggested oils: Forgiveness, Grounding, Harmony, Hope, Inner Child, Joy, Present Time, Release, SARA, 3 Wise Men, Valor, White Angelica. *and Believe.*

Vol. 3, Angel Lullabies — Vocal songs that will create an atmosphere where love and peace can be felt.
Suggested oils: *Gentle Baby, Dream Catcher, and Inner Child.*

Heaven on Earth Collection

A collection of loving songs to inspire and bless relationship between men and women.

Vol. 1, Angel's Touch — Instrumental music with affirmations for balancing chakras 1-7.
Suggested oils: *Gathering, White Angelica, Humility, Sacred Mountain, Dream Catcher, Awaken, and Inspiration.*

Vol. 2, Heaven on Earth — Instrumental music with affirmations for balancing chakras 8-12.
Suggested oils: *Gratitude, Hope, Present Time, Grounding, Sacred Mountain, Legacy, and Magnify your Purpose.*

Vol. 3, Pure Love Songs — Vocal songs for relationship building and rebuilding.
Suggested oils: *Awaken, Dream Catcher, Gathering, Humility, Inspiration, White Angelica, Inspiration, Gathering, and Sacred Mountain.*

Enlightened Journey Collection

Come take a musical journey that will inspire you to greater heights of faith, hope, love, forgiveness, perseverance, gentleness for yourself, tenderness, creativity, and the joy of overcoming.

Vol. 1, Enlightened Journey — Vocal songs about the journey of life.
Suggested oils: *Magnify your Purpose, Forgiveness, Inner Child, Sacred Mountain, Envision, Sara, Live with Passion, Grounding, Gratitude, Harmony, Valor, Present Time, and Joy.*

Vol. 2, Dancing in the Moment — Vocal songs about moving beyond loss, divorce, and other difficult trials.
Suggested oils: *Humility, Peace & Calming, Purification, SARA, Forgiveness, Gentle Baby, Acceptance, Gratitude, Surrender, Into the Future, Hope, Live with Passion, and Release.*

Vol. 3, Dancing with Joy — Vocal songs about moving along the path into a fullness of joy.
Suggested oils: *Inner Child, Gentle Baby, White Angelica, Envision, Dream Catcher, Harmony, Present Time, Gratitude, Live with Passion, Peace & Calming, Forgiveness, Mister, and Joy.*

Single Oils

This section provides concise information about many of the pure essential oils that are available for use by the general public. The listings of possible uses are meant for external application unless otherwise directed. The included safety data is also based on the external use of the oils and may differ from other published information that is based on oral application.

Other seeming discrepancies between sources of published safety data arise when one does not take into consideration the certain constituents of the oil being reviewed. One glaring example of this is thyme. A linalol type of oil does not have the same caustic/irritant effects that a thymol type would, but the particular application may require the added strength of the thymol type of oil. In this book, care has been taken to differentiate between the different types of essential oil for each application. Since pure essential oils are powerful healing agents, please remember to check the safety data before using an oil. Because there are several different oils that can help the same health condition, it should not be difficult to find one that will work for any particular situation. ***Also, for a listing of products that contain these individual oils, please refer to the Single Oil Summary section in the Appendix.***

Angelica

(*Angelica archangelica*)

BOTANICAL FAMILY: Apiaceae, Umbelliferae (parsley)

EXTRACTION METHOD/ORIGIN: Steam distillation of roots — France, Belgium

CHEMICAL CONSTITUENTS: Monoterpenes (approx. 70%): phellandrene, α and β-pinenes, limonene (13%); Esters: bornyle acetates; Terpene alkaloids; Coumarins: bergapten.

PROPERTIES: ANTI-COAGULANT, ANTI-INFLAMMATORY (intestinal wall), CALMING, EXPECTORANT, SEDATIVE (nervous system), STOMACHIC, and TONIC.

FOLKLORE: One possible source for this oil's unique name comes from an old legend which states that during a terrible plague, an angel revealed this plant to a monk. History also records the use of the plant during the plague of 1660. The stems were chewed to prevent infection, and the seeds and roots were burned to help purify the air. The German people refer to the essence as the "oil of angels".

ESOTERIC USES/ACTIONS: Astrological: *Sun*; Body type: *Mesomorph*; Chakras: *links 7 to*

8 and 7 to 1, also 8; Character: *Yang*; Crystals: *Apophylite, green tourmaline (lifts 7th to 8th chakra), moss agate, bloodstone (links crown to base chakra or 7th to 1st)* ; Element: *Fire*; Oriental: *Cold & damp conditions*

POSSIBLE USES: Angelica may help with ANOREXIA, APPETITE (loss of), BRUISES, COLDS, COLIC, COUGHS, FLATULENCE, INDIGESTION, MENOPAUSE, PRE-MENSTRUAL TENSION, RESPIRATORY INFECTIONS, and RHEUMATIC CONDITIONS.

BODY SYSTEM(S) AFFECTED: EMOTIONAL BALANCE, NERVOUS SYSTEM.

AROMATIC INFLUENCE: It may help one release and let go of negative feelings by bringing one's memory back to a point of origin before TRAUMA or ANGER was experienced.

APPLICATION: Apply to SHOULDERS, VITA FLEX POINTS, bottoms of FEET, and/or directly on AREA of concern; Diffuse.

ORAL USE AS DIETARY SUPPLEMENT: Generally regarded as safe (GRAS) for internal consumption by the FDA. *DILUTE one drop oil in 1 tsp. honey or 4 oz. of beverage (ie. soy/rice milk).* ***Not for children under 6 years old; use with CAUTION and in GREATER DILUTION for children 6 years old and over.***

SAFETY DATA: Avoid if DIABETIC. Use with caution during PREGNANCY. Avoid direct SUNLIGHT for up to 12 hours after use.

BLEND CLASSIFICATION: Personifier, Modifier.

BLENDS WITH: Clary sage, patchouli, vetiver, florals, woods, and most citrus oils.

ODOR: Type: *Top to Middle Notes (20-80% of the blend)*; Scent: *Herbaceous, earthy, peppery, green, spicy*; Intensity: *4*

FREQUENCY: Physical and Emotional; approximately 85 MHz.

Anise

(*Pimpinella anisum*)

BOTANICAL FAMILY: Umbelliferae (dainty, white-flowered annual)

EXTRACTION METHOD/ORIGIN: Steam distillation from seeds (fruit) — Turkey

CHEMICAL CONSTITUENTS: Phenol methyl-ethers: Trans-anethol (75-95%) and Estragole (1-4%); Sesquiterpenes: γ-himachalene.

PROPERTIES: ANTISEPTIC, ANTISPASMODIC, ESTROGEN-LIKE, DIURETIC, STIMULANT (heart), and TONIC (heart).

ESOTERIC USES/ACTIONS: Astrological: *Sun, Mercury, Pluto, and Jupiter*; Body type: *Mesomorph*; Character: *Yang*; Element: *Air*; Oriental: *Cold & damp conditions*

HISTORICAL USES: This oil has been used for dry irritable COUGHS, BRONCHITIS, and WHOOPING COUGH.

OTHER POSSIBLE USES: ALKALOSIS, BLOOD OXYGENATION, BRONCHITIS, COLITIS, CONSTIPATION, DIGESTION (accelerates), DIVERTICULITIS,

ESTROGEN (increases), FERTILITY, FLATULENCE, HORMONAL IMBALANCE, IRRITABLE BOWEL SYNDROME, MENOPAUSE, PARASITES, PMS, PROSTATE CANCER (blend with frankincense), and RESPIRATORY SYSTEM (strengthens).

BODY SYSTEM(S) AFFECTED: CARDIOVASCULAR, DIGESTIVE, HORMONAL, and RESPIRATORY SYSTEMS.

APPLICATION: Apply to VITA FLEX POINTS and directly on AREA of concern; Diffuse.

ORAL USE AS DIETARY SUPPLEMENT: Generally regarded as safe (GRAS) for internal consumption by the FDA. *DILUTE one drop oil in 1 tsp. honey or 4 oz. of beverage (ie soy/rice milk).* ***Not for children under 6 years old; use with CAUTION and in GREATER DILUTION for children 6 years old and over.***

SAFETY DATA: Can irritate sensitive SKIN and has been known to cause DERMATITIS in some individuals. Best if used in moderation.

BLEND CLASSIFICATION: Difficult to use in blending. Use only in very small amounts.

BLENDS WITH: Bergamot, Blue tansy, fennel, ginger, juniper, lemongrass, patchouli, Black pepper, peppermint, tangerine, tarragon, and ylang ylang.

ODOR: Type: *Top to Middle Notes (20-80% of the blend)*

Balsam Fir

(***See Fir, Balsam***)

Basil (or French Basil)

(*Ocimum basilicum*)

BOTANICAL FAMILY: Lamiaceae or Labiatae (mint)

EXTRACTION METHOD/ORIGIN: Steam distillation of leaves, stems, and flowers — Egypt India, Utah, France

CHEMICAL CONSTITUENTS: Alcohols (up to 65%): linalol (>55%), fenchol (>10%); Phenc methyl-ethers (<50%): methyl chavicol (up to 47%), methyl eugenol; Phenols (6%): eugenol; Oxides (6%): 1,8 cineol; Monoterpenes (2%): α & β-pinene, myrcene; Esters (<7%): fenchyl acetate, linalyl acetate; Sesquiterpenes: Isocaryophyllene, β-caryophyllene β-elemene. *NOTE: There are several cultivars and chemotypes of basil, each with widel varying constituencies. The basil described here, French Basil, is the preferred variety for use in aromatherapy due to its higher content of linalol and 1,8 cineol.*

PROPERTIES: ANTI-BACTERIAL, ANTI-INFECTIOUS, ANTI-INFLAMMATORY, ANTISEPTIC (stomach/intestinal), ANTISPASMODIC (powerful), ANTIVIRAL, DECONGESTANT (veins, arteries of the lungs, prostate), STIMULANT (nerves, adrena cortex), and UPLIFTING. Basil may also be anti-catarrhal, anti-depressant, energizing, and restorative.

OLKLORE: Considered by the ancient Greeks as the "king of plants", basil was used to anoint kings. Hindus placed sprigs of basil on the chests of deceased loved ones to protect them from evil and provide safe passage into the next life. Due to its supposed aphrodisiac qualities, Italian women displayed basil to alert possible suitors, and the men would present the women with basil sprigs.

SOTERIC USES/ACTIONS: Astrological: *Mars*; Ayurvedic: *Vata*; Body type: *Endomorph*; Chakras: *2*; Character: *Yang*; Element: *Fire*; Number: *1*

ISTORICAL USES: Basil was used anciently for respiratory problems, digestive and kidney ailments, epilepsy, poisonous insect or snake bites, fevers, epidemics, and malaria.

RENCH MEDICINAL USES: MIGRAINES (especially from liver and gall bladder problems), MENTAL FATIGUE, MENSTRUAL PERIODS (scanty).

THER POSSIBLE USES: This oil may be used for ACHES/PAINS, ANXIETY, BRONCHITIS, CHRONIC COLDS, CONCENTRATION, nervous DEPRESSION, DIGESTION, EARACHE, FAINTING, FATIGUE (mental), FEVER, GOUT, HEADACHES, HEMORRHOIDS, HICCOUGHS, INSECT BITES (soothing), INSECT REPELLANT, INSOMNIA (from nervous tension), INTESTINAL PROBLEMS, poor MEMORY, chronic MUCUS, **MUSCLE SPASMS**, OVARIAN CYSTS, PROSTATE PROBLEMS, RHINITIS (inflammation of nasal mucus membranes), loss of SMELL, SNAKE BITES, VOMITING, WASP STINGS, and WHOOPING COUGH.

ODY SYSTEM(S) AFFECTED: CARDIOVASCULAR SYSTEM, MUSCLES and BONES.

ROMATIC INFLUENCE: Helps one maintain an OPEN MIND and increases CLARITY of thought.

PPLICATION: Apply to TEMPLES, tip of NOSE, VITA FLEX POINTS, and/or directly on AREA of concern; diffuse. May also be added to food or water as a dietary supplement.

RAL USE AS DIETARY SUPPLEMENT: Generally regarded as safe (GRAS) for internal consumption by the FDA. *DILUTE one drop oil in 1 tsp. honey or 4 oz. of beverage (ie. soy/rice milk).* ***Not for children under 6 years old; use with CAUTION and in GREATER DILUTION for children 6 years old and over.***

AFETY DATA: Avoid during PREGNANCY. Not for use by people with EPILEPSY. It may also irritate sensitive skin (test a small area first).

LEND CLASSIFICATION: Enhancer and Equalizer

LENDS WITH: Bergamot, birch, cypress, fir, geranium, helichrysum, lavender, lemongrass, marjoram, peppermint, spruce, wintergreen.

DOR: Type: *Top to Middle Notes (20-80% of the blend)*; Scent: *Herbaceous, spicy, anise-like, camphorous, lively*; Intensity: *4*

REQUENCY: Low (Physical); approximately 52 MHz.

Bergamot

(*Citrus bergamia*)

BOTANICAL FAMILY: Rutaceae (citrus)

EXTRACTION METHOD/ORIGIN: Solvent extraction or vacuum distilled; pressed from rir or peel; rectified and void of terpenes — Italy, Ivory Coast

CHEMICAL CONSTITUENTS: Monoterpenes: d-limonene (30%), γ-terpinene, α & β-pinene Esters: linalyl acetate (usually around 20%); Alcohols: linalol, nerol, geraniol, α-terpinec Aldehydes: citrals; Furocoumarins: bergamotine, bergapten, bergaptol.

PROPERTIES: ANALGESIC, ANTI-BACTERIAL (strep and staph infection), ANTI-INFECTIOUS, ANTI-INFLAMMATORY, ANTI-PARASITIC, ANTISEPTIC, ANTISPASMODIC, DIGESTIVE, SEDATIVE, and UPLIFTING.

FOLKLORE: Christopher Columbus is credited with bringing bergamot to Italy from the Cana Islands.

ESOTERIC USES/ACTIONS: Astrological: *Sun*; Body type: *Endomorph*; Chakras: *3, 4, & 5* Character: *mildly Yang*; Crystals: *Watermelon tourmaline*; Element: *Fire*; Number: *2*; Oriental: *Qi stagnation (pts: Liv-3, GB-34)*

HISTORICAL USES: Bergamot was used by the Italians to cool and relieve fevers, protect against malaria, and expel intestinal worms.

FRENCH MEDICINAL USES: AGITATION, APPETITE (loss of), COLIC, DEPRESSION INDIGESTION, INFECTION, INFLAMMATION, INSECT REPELLENT, INSOMNIA, INTESTINAL PARASITES, RHEUMATISM, STRESS, and VAGINAL CANDIDA.

OTHER POSSIBLE USES: This oil may help ACNE, ANXIETY, regulate APPETITE, BOILS, BRONCHITIS, CARBUNCLES, COLD SORES, oily COMPLEXION, COUGHS, CYSTITIS, DIGESTION, ECZEMA, EMOTIONS, ENDOCRINE SYSTEM, FEVER, GALLSTONES, GONORRHEA, INFECTIOUS DISEASE, INSECT BITES, soothe LUNGS, PSORIASIS, RESPIRATORY INFECTION, SCABIES, SORE THROAT, nervous TENSION, THRUSH, acute TONSILLITIS, ULCERS, URINARY TRACT INFECTION, spot VARICOSE VEINS, and WOUNDS

BODY SYSTEM(S) AFFECTED: DIGESTIVE SYSTEM, EMOTIONAL BALANCE, SKIN

AROMATIC INFLUENCE: It may help to RELIEVE ANXIETY, DEPRESSION, STRESS, and TENSION. It is UPLIFTING and REFRESHING. It helps to expand and open the HEART CHAKRA, and to radiate LOVE ENERGY.

APPLICATION: Apply to FOREHEAD, TEMPLES, VITA FLEX POINTS, and/or directly o AREA of concern; diffuse. May also be applied as a DEODORANT or added to food or water as a dietary supplement.

ORAL USE AS DIETARY SUPPLEMENT: Generally regarded as safe (GRAS) for internal consumption by the FDA. *DILUTE one drop oil in 1 tsp. honey or 4 oz. of beverage (ie soy/rice milk).* ***Not for children under 6 years old; use with CAUTION and in***

GREATER DILUTION for children 6 years old and over.

AFETY DATA: ***Repeated use can result in extreme CONTACT SENSITIZATION. Avoid direct SUNLIGHT or ULTRAVIOLET LIGHT for up to 72 hours after use.***

LEND CLASSIFICATION: Equalizer, Modifier, and Enhancer

LENDS WITH: Chamomile, cypress, eucalyptus, geranium, jasmine, juniper, lavender, lemon, palmarosa, patchouli, and ylang ylang.

DOR: Type: *Top Note (5-20% of the blend)*; Scent: *Sweet, lively, citrusy, fruity*; Intensity: *2*

Birch (Yellow Birch)

(*Betula alleghaniensis*)

OTANICAL FAMILY: Betulaceae

XTRACTION METHOD/ORIGIN: Steam distillation from wood — Canada, Scandinavia

HEMICAL CONSTITUENTS: Esters: methyl salicylate (89%); Salicylic Acid; Sesquiterpenes.

ROPERTIES: ANALGESIC, ANTI-INFLAMMATORY, ANTI-RHEUMATIC, ANTISEPTIC, ANTISPASMODIC, DISINFECTANT, DIURETIC, STIMULANT (bone, liver), and WARMING.

IISTORICAL USES: Birch oil has a strong, penetrating aroma that most people recognize as wintergreen. Although birch (*Betula alleghaniensis* or *Betula lenta*) is completely unrelated to wintergreen (*Gaultheria procumbens*), they are almost identical in chemical constituents. The American Indians and early European settlers enjoyed a tea that was flavored with birch bark or wintergreen. According to Julia Lawless, "...this has been translated into a preference for 'root beer' flavourings [sic]." A synthetic methyl salicylate is now widely used as a flavoring agent, especially in 'root beer', chewing gum, toothpaste, etc.

RENCH MEDICINAL USES: RHEUMATISM, MUSCULAR PAIN, CRAMPS, ARTHRITIS, TENDONITIS, HYPERTENSION, INFLAMMATION.

)THER POSSIBLE USES: This oil may be beneficial for ACNE, BLADDER INFECTION, CYSTITIS, DROPSY, ECZEMA, EDEMA, reducing FEVER, GALLSTONES, GOUT, INFECTION, reducing discomfort in JOINTS, KIDNEY STONES, draining and cleansing the LYMPHATIC SYSTEM, OBESITY, OSTEOPOROSIS, SKIN DISEASES, ULCERS, and URINARY TRACT DISORDERS. It is known for its ability to alleviate **BONE PAIN**. It has a cortisone-like action due to the high content of methyl salicylate. For tissue pain, use Relieve It.

3ODY SYSTEM(S) AFFECTED: MUSCLES and BONES.

AROMATIC INFLUENCE: It influences, elevates, opens, and increases AWARENESS in SENSORY SYSTEM (senses or sensations).

APPLICATION: Apply to VITA FLEX POINTS and/or directly on AREA of concern; diffuse.

Apply topically on location and use only small amounts (dilute with V-6 Mixing Oil for application on larger areas).

ORAL USE AS DIETARY SUPPLEMENT: None.

SAFETY DATA: ***Avoid during PREGNANCY. Not for use by people with EPILEPSY. Son people are very allergic to methyl salicylate. TEST A SMALL AREA OF SKIN FIR FOR ALLERGIES!***

BLEND CLASSIFICATION: Personifier and Enhancer

BLENDS WITH: Basil, bergamot, chamomile, cypress, geranium, juniper, lavender, lemongras marjoram, peppermint, and rosewood.

Black Pepper

(*See Pepper, Black*)

Blue Cypress

(*See Cypress, Blue*)

Cajeput

(*Melaleuca leucadendra*)

BOTANICAL FAMILY: Myrtaceae (myrtle shrubs and trees)

CHEMICAL CONSTITUENTS: Oxides: 1,8 cineol (<50%); Alcohols: α-terpineol (8%), viridiflorol, nerolidol; Monoterpenes: α- & β-pinenes, limonene; Sesquiterpenes: β-caryophyllene; Esters: terpinyl acetate; Aldehydes: benzaldehyde; Acids: acetic, propionic valeric.

PROPERTIES: ANALGESIC (mild), ANTI-CATARRHAL, ANTI-INFECTIOUS, ANTI-INFLAMMATORY, ANTIMICROBIAL, ANTI-NEURALGIC, ANTISEPTIC (pulmonary, urinary, intestinal), ANTISPASMODIC, EXPECTORANT, INSECTICIDAL, and TONIC.

ESOTERIC USES/ACTIONS: Chakra: *6*; Character: *Neutral*

HISTORICAL USES: In Malaysia and other Indonesian islands, cajeput was considered valuable for cholera, colds, flu, headaches, rheumatism, throat infections, toothache, various skin conditions, and sore muscles.

OTHER POSSIBLE USES: Cajeput may help with ACNE, ARTHRITIS, ASTHMA, BRONCHITIS, BURSITIS, CATARRH, COLDS, COUGHS, CYSTITIS, DYSENTERY, ENTERITIS, FLU, HAY FEVER, HEADACHES, INFECTIONS of the URETHRA, INSECT BITES, INTESTINAL PROBLEMS, stiff JOINTS,

LARYNGITIS, PNEUMONIA, PSORIASIS, RESPIRATORY INFECTIONS, RHEUMATISM, SINUSITIS, SKIN (oily and spots), SORE THROAT, TOOTHACHE, URINARY COMPLAINTS, VIRAL INFECTIONS.

)DY SYSTEM(S) AFFECTED: CARDIOVASCULAR and RESPIRATORY SYSTEMS.

'PLICATION: Apply to VITA FLEX POINTS and/or directly on AREA of concern. Diffuse for RESPIRATORY INFECTIONS.

RAL USE AS DIETARY SUPPLEMENT: Approved by the FDA for use as a Food Additive (FA) or Flavoring Agent (FL). *DILUTE one drop oil in 1 tsp. honey or 4 oz. of beverage (ie. soy/rice milk).* ***Not for children under 6 years old; use with CAUTION and in GREATER DILUTION for children 6 years old and over.***

FETY DATA: If not absolutely pure, cajeput could cause further blistering and skin eruptions! Even when pure, it can irritate sensitive SKIN. Use with CAUTION.

.END CLASSIFICATION: Enhancer.

.ENDS WITH: Birch, eucalyptus, juniper, peppermint, and wintergreen.

DOR: Type: *Top Note (5-20% of the blend)*

Single Oils

Canadian Red Cedar

(See Cedar, Canadian Red)

Cardamom

(Elettaria cardamomum)

OTANICAL FAMILY: Zingiberaceae (ginger)

HEMICAL CONSTITUENTS: Esters (>40%): α-terpenyl acetate (30-45%), linalyl acetate (3%); Oxides: 1,8 cineol (up to 45%); Alcohols (7%): linalol, terpinen-4-ol, α-terpineol; Monoterpenes (6%): sabinene, myrcene, limonene, pinene, zingiberene; Aldehyde: geranial.

ROPERTIES: ANTI-BACTERIAL, ANTI-INFECTIOUS, ANTISEPTIC, ANTISPASMODIC, APHRODISIAC, DIGESTIVE, DIURETIC, STOMACHIC, and TONIC.

SOTERIC USES/ACTIONS: Astrological: *Venus & Mercury*; Body type: *Ectomorph*; Chakra: *1*; Character: *Yang*; Crystals: *Carnelian* ; Element: *Water & Air*; Number: *4*; Oriental: *Cold dampness (pts: Sp 9 & 6), Qi deficiency Spleen (pts: Sp-6)*

ISTORICAL USES: Anciently, cardamom was used for epilepsy, spasms, paralysis, rheumatism, cardiac disorders, all intestinal illnesses, pulmonary disease, fever, and digestive and urinary complaints. It is said to be able to neutralize the lingering odor of garlic.

THER POSSIBLE USES: Cardamom may help with APPETITE (loss of), COLIC, COUGHS, DEBILITY, DYSPEPSIA, FLATULENCE, HALITOSIS, HEADACHES,

MENTAL FATIGUE, NAUSEA, PYROSIS (or HEARTBURN), SCIATICA, and VOMITING. It may also help with MENSTRUAL PERIODS, MENOPAUSE, and nervous INDIGESTION. *Note: Cardamom has the same properties as ginger but is l irritant.*

BODY SYSTEM(S) AFFECTED: DIGESTIVE SYSTEM.

AROMATIC INFLUENCE: Cardamom is UPLIFTING, REFRESHING, and INVIGORATING. It may be beneficial for CLEARING CONFUSION.

APPLICATION: Apply to VITA FLEX POINTS and/or directly on AREA of concern. Dilut with a base oil and MASSAGE over the stomach, solar plexus, and thighs. Excellent as BATH oil.

ORAL USE AS DIETARY SUPPLEMENT: Generally regarded as safe (GRAS) for interna consumption by the FDA. *DILUTE one drop oil in 1 tsp. honey or 4 oz. of beverage (i soy/rice milk).* ***Not for children under 6 years old; use with CAUTION and in GREATER DILUTION for children 6 years old and over.***

BLEND CLASSIFICATION: Personifier and Modifier

BLENDS WITH: Bergamot, cedarwood, cinnamon bark, cistus, clove, neroli, orange, rose, an ylang ylang.

ODOR: Type: *Middle Note (50-80% of the blend)*; Scent: *Sweet, spicy, balsamic, with floral undertones*; Intensity: *4*

Carrot

(*Daucus carota*)

BOTANICAL FAMILY: Umbelliferae (parsley)

CHEMICAL CONSTITUENTS: Sesquiterpene alcohols: carotol (up to 50%); Sesquiterpenes: daucene, β-bisabolene (10%), β-caryophyllene (4%); Monoterpenes: limonene, α- & β-pinenes, sabinene; Oxides: epoxy β-caryophyllene; Alcohols: geraniol, linalol, α-terpineo borneol, citronellol; Alcohol-oxide: daucol (up to 5%); Esters: geranyl acetate; Phenol methyl-ether: asarone.

PROPERTIES: CARMINATIVE, HEPATIC (cleanses the liver), STOMACHIC.

HISTORICAL USES: Carrots have been used as a blood cleanser, for liver and skin problems, pulmonary conditions, allergies, inflammation of the intestines, as a tonic for the nervous system, and for eyesight. Carrots where used during the Second World War to help pilot with their night vision.

OTHER POSSIBLE USES: Carrot oil may help with ANEMIA, COLIC (with fennel), CONSTIPATION, DIARRHEA, EYE PROBLEMS, GALLBLADDER PROBLEMS, LIVER PROBLEMS, RHEUMATISM, and SKIN PROBLEMS (AGING SKIN, WRINKLES, SUNBURN, and DRYNESS).

BODY SYSTEM(S) AFFECTED: CARDIOVASCULAR and NERVOUS SYSTEMS, SKIN

PLICATION: Apply to VITA FLEX POINTS and/or directly on AREA of concern. To promote a healthy SUNTAN, apply carrot oil (dilute with Hazelnut oil) for a few days before exposure to the sun.

AL USE AS DIETARY SUPPLEMENT: Generally regarded as safe (GRAS) for internal consumption by the FDA. *DILUTE one drop oil in 1 tsp. honey or 4 oz. of beverage (ie. soy/rice milk).* ***Not for children under 6 years old; use with CAUTION and in GREATER DILUTION for children 6 years old and over.***

END CLASSIFICATION: Considered as more of an active carrier oil (same as Vitamin E Oil and Wheatgerm Oil).

ENDS WITH: Citrus oils, fennel, frankincense, geranium, spice oils.

OR: Type: *Middle Note (50-80% of the blend)*; Scent: *Sweet, fruity, warm, earthy*; Intensity: *2*

Cassia

(*Cinnamomum cassia*)

TANICAL FAMILY: Lauraceae (laurel)

TRACTION METHOD/ORIGIN: Steam distillation from bark — China

IEMICAL CONSTITUENTS: Aldehydes: trans-cinnamaldehyde (up to 85%), benzaldehyde; Phenols (>7%): phenol, 2-vinyl-phenol, isoeugenol, chavicol.

OPERTIES: ANTI-BACTERIAL, ANTI-FUNGAL, ANTIVIRAL.

OTERIC USES/ACTIONS: Astrological: *Mercury & Sun*; Character: *Yang*

ISTORICAL USES: Has been used extensively as a domestic spice. Medicinally, it has been used for colds, colic, flatulent dyspepsia, diarrhea, nausea, rheumatism, and kidney and reproductive complaints.

THER POSSIBLE USES: This oil is best not used individually in aromatherapy as it can be extremely sensitizing to the dermal tissues. Can provide some powerful support to blends when used in very small quantities.

PPLICATION: None.

RAL USE AS DIETARY SUPPLEMENT: Generally regarded as safe (GRAS) for internal consumption by the FDA. *DILUTE one drop oil in 2 tsp. honey or 8 oz. of beverage (ie. soy/rice milk). May need to increase dilution even more due to this oil's potential for irritating mucus membranes.* ***Not for children under 6 years old; use with CAUTION and in GREATER DILUTION for children 6 years old and over.***

AFETY DATA: Repeated use can result in extreme CONTACT SENSITIZATION. Avoid during PREGNANCY. Can cause extreme SKIN IRRITATION. Diffuse with caution; it will irritate the nasal membranes if it is inhaled directly from the diffuser.

LEND CLASSIFICATION: Personifier/Enhancer.

DOR: Type: *Middle Note (50-80% of the blend)*; Scent: *Spicy, warm, sweet*; Intensity: *5*

Cedar, Canadian Red

(*Thuja plicata*)

BOTANICAL FAMILY: Cupressaceae (conifer - cypress)

EXTRACTION METHOD/ORIGIN: Steam distillation from bark and sawdust — Canada

CHEMICAL CONSTITUENTS: Thujyl acid methyl ester; Terpene alcohols: terpinen-4-ol; Sesquiterpenes: β-caryophyllene; Monoterpene esters: lilalyl acetate.

PROPERTIES: ANTI-BACTERIAL, ANTI-FUNGAL, ANTISEPTIC, INSECT REPELLENT, and STIMULANT (follicle stimulator).

HISTORICAL USES: Cedar has been used by the Canadian Native American Indians to enhance their potential for spiritual communication by helping them achieve a higher lev of spiritual being. They would also apply it to the scalp to help stimulate hair growth.

OTHER POSSIBLE USES: This oil may help DANDRUFF and HAIR LOSS. It may also h OPEN the PINEAL GLAND.

BODY SYSTEM(S) AFFECTED: EMOTIONAL BALANCE, RESPIRATORY SYSTEM, SKIN.

AROMATIC INFLUENCE: It may help enhance SPIRITUAL AWARENESS or MEDITATION.

APPLICATION: Apply to VITA FLEX POINTS and/or directly on AREA of concern. DIFFUSE (though it is quite thick and can be somewhat messy in the diffuser) or apply the palms of the hands for DIRECT INHALATION. May also be applied directly to th SKIN or SCALP (dilute slightly to avoid any possible skin irritation). May be applied t the CROWN of the HEAD. Add to BATH WATER. Put a few drops on a cotton ball and place in a mesh bag. Then place the mesh bag in the CLOTHES CLOSET or in bo used for STORING CLOTHES to protect against moths.

ORAL USE AS DIETARY SUPPLEMENT: None.

SAFETY DATA:* *Repeated use can possibly result in CONTACT SENSITIZATION.

Cedar, Western Red

(*Thuja plicata*)

BOTANICAL FAMILY: Cupressaceae (conifer - cypress)

EXTRACTION METHOD/ORIGIN: Steam distillation from leaves — USA

CHEMICAL CONSTITUENTS: Monoterpenes: sabinene, pinene; Ketones: thujone (up to 60%), fenchone, camphor.

PROPERTIES: ANTI-BACTERIAL and ANTISEPTIC.

ESOTERIC USES/ACTIONS: Astrological: *Mercury*; Chakra: *1 & 6*; Character: *Yin*; Elemen *Earth & Ether*

ISTORICAL USES: The Western Red cedar has been referred to as the "Tree of Life". It has been used by ancient civilizations to enhance their potential for spiritual communication during rituals and other ceremonies. It has also been used for coughs, fevers, intestinal parasites, cystitis, and venereal diseases.

THER POSSIBLE USES: This oil may help with HAIR LOSS, SKIN (nourishing), RHEUMATISM, WARTS, and PSORIASIS. It has powerful effects on the SUBCONSCIOUS and UNCONSCIOUS MIND.

ODY SYSTEM(S) AFFECTED: SKIN.

ROMATIC INFLUENCE: It is CALMING and may help enhance SPIRITUAL AWARENESS or MEDITATION.

PPLICATION: Apply to VITA FLEX POINTS and/or directly on AREA of concern. DIFFUSE.

RAL USE AS DIETARY SUPPLEMENT: None.

AFETY DATA: FOR TOPICAL USE ONLY. Due to high Thujone content, use SPARINGLY and DILUTE WELL with V-6 Mixing Oil or Massage Oil.

Cedar Leaf (Thuja)

(*Thuja occidentalis*)

OTANICAL FAMILY: Cupressaceae (conifer - cypress)

XTRACTION METHOD/ORIGIN: Steam distillation from leaves, twigs, and bark — Canada, USA

HEMICAL CONSTITUENTS: Ketones: thujone (up to 60%), isothujone (up to 14%), fenchone (up to 14%), camphor (>3%), piperitone; Esters: bornyl acetate (up to 12%), formlate; Monoterpenols: terpinen-4-ol (>6%); Sesquiterpenols: occidentalol, occidol, α-, β-, & γ-eudesmols; Monoterpenes: limonene, sabinene, α-pinene.

ROPERTIES: ANTI-RHEUMATIC, ASTRINGENT, EXPECTORANT, INSECT REPELLENT, and STIMULANT (nerves, uterus and heart muscles).

SOTERIC USES/ACTIONS: Astrological: *Mercury*; Chakra: *1 & 6*; Character: *Yin*; Element: *Earth & Ether*

IISTORICAL USES: Has been used by ancient civilizations to enhance their potential for spiritual communication during rituals and other ceremonies. It has also been used for coughs, fevers, intestinal parasites, cystitis, and venereal diseases.

THER POSSIBLE USES: May help with RHEUMATISM, WARTS, and PSORIASIS.

ROMATIC INFLUENCE: May help enhance SPIRITUAL AWARENESS or MEDITATION.

PPLICATION: Apply to VITA FLEX POINTS and directly on AREA of concern. DIFFUSE.

RAL USE AS DIETARY SUPPLEMENT: *Has been approved by the FDA for use as a Food Additive (FA) or Flavoring Agent (FL) as long as the finished food is thujone-free. (see 21CFR172.510)* ***Best NOT to use this oil as a dietary supplement.***

SAFETY DATA: FOR TOPICAL USE ONLY. Due to high Thujone content, use SPARINGLY and DILUTE WELL with V-6 Mixing Oil or Massage Oil.

Cedarwood

(*Cedrus atlantica*)

BOTANICAL FAMILY: Pinaceae (conifer)

EXTRACTION METHOD/ORIGIN: Steam distillation from bark — Morocco, USA

CHEMICAL CONSTITUENTS: Sesquiterpenes (50%): cedrene, caryophyllene, cadinene, himachalene; Sesquiterpenols (30%): atlantol, cedrol, cedrenol; Ketones (20%): α- & β-atlantones.

PROPERTIES: ANTI-FUNGAL, ANTI-INFECTIOUS, ANTISEPTIC (urinary and pulmonary), ASTRINGENT, DIURETIC, INSECT REPELLENT, and SEDATIVE.

FOLKLORE: *Cedrus atlantica* is supposed to be the species most closely related to the biblical Cedars of Lebanon.

ESOTERIC USES/ACTIONS: Astrological: *Saturn, Sun, Jupiter, & Uranus*; Body type: *Mesomorph*; Chakra: *1 & 6*; Character: *Yang*; Crystals: *Lepidolite, amethyst, sapphire*; Element: *Fire, Light, & Air*; Number: *6*; Oriental: *Cold, dampness (pts: Sp-9 & 6), Qi deficiency (pts: Kid-3)*

HISTORICAL USES: Cedarwood was used traditionally by the North American Indians to enhance their potential for spiritual communication. It creates the symbolic effect of the umbrella protecting the earth and bringing energy in from the universe. At night the animals in the wild lie down under the tree for the protection, recharging, and rejuvenation the trees bring them.

FRENCH MEDICINAL USES: ANGER (calming effect), ARTERIOSCLEROSIS, BRONCHITIS, CALMING, CELLULITE, DIURETIC, HAIR LOSS, NERVOUS TENSION, TUBERCULOSIS, URINARY INFECTIONS.

OTHER POSSIBLE USES: This oil is recognized for its PURIFYING properties. It may also help ACNE, ANXIETY, ARTHRITIS, CONGESTION, COUGHS, CYSTITIS, DANDRUFF, PSORIASIS, PURIFICATION, SINUSITIS, SKIN DISEASES, and WATER RETENTION. It may help OPEN the PINEAL GLAND. It also helps to reduce OILY SECRETIONS.

BODY SYSTEM(S) AFFECTED: NERVOUS and RESPIRATORY SYSTEMS.

APPLICATION: Apply to VITA FLEX POINTS and/or directly on AREA of concern.

ORAL USE AS DIETARY SUPPLEMENT: None.

SAFETY DATA: Use with caution during PREGNANCY.

BLEND CLASSIFICATION: Enhancer and Equalizer

BLENDS WITH: Bergamot, Clary sage, cypress, eucalyptus, floral oils, juniper, resinous oils, and rosemary.

DOR: Type: *Base Note (5-20% of the blend)*; Scent: *Warm, soft, woody*; Intensity: *3*
BLE: Lev. 14:4, 6, 49, 51, 52

Celery Seed

(*Apium graveolens*)

OTANICAL FAMILY: Umbeliferae

XTRACTION METHOD/ORIGIN: Steam distilled from seed — France

HEMICAL CONSTITUENTS: Monoterpenes (approx. 50%): limonene (up to 50%); Sesquiterpenes (approx. 39%): β-selinene (up to 33%); Phthalides (approx. 15%): sedanolic acid, 3-n-butylphthalide (up to 7%), sedanenolide (>1%), 4-dihydro-phthalide (1%), dihydro-ligustilide (3%); Coumarin ethers: umbelliprenin celerin, apigravin; also apiole, santalol, and others.

ROPERTIES: ANTIOXIDANT, ANTI-RHEUMATIC, ANTISEPTIC (urinary), ANTISPASMODIC, HEPATIC (stimulates drainage), STIMULANT (uterine), TONIC (neuro-muscular).

SOTERIC USES/ACTIONS: Astrological: *Moon, Mercury, Sun*; Character: *Yin?*; Element: *Fire*; Color: *pale yellow*

OSSIBLE USES: Celery seed may help with ARTHRITIS, BLOATING, BRONCHITIS, CONGESTION (respiratory), CYSTITIS, FLATULENCE, GLANDS (swollen), GOUT (reduces uric acid), HEMORRHOIDS, INDIGESTION, JAUNDICE, KIDNEY detoxification (after illness), LACTATION (increases flow of breast milk), LIVER congestion (after infection), LYMPHATIC drainage, MENSTRUATION (induces), NERVOUS disorders, NEURALGIA, RHEUMATISM, SCIATICA, SEXUAL problems (minimizes), SKIN (puffiness, redness, spots, water-logged), URINE flow (increases). It may help to balance the ENDOCRINE SYSTEM to help with glandular problems. It is also a sedative and tonic for the CENTRAL NERVOUS SYSTEM and may help provide a more RESTFUL SLEEP.

ODY SYSTEM(S) AFFECTED: DIGESTIVE SYSTEM, MUSCLE and BONE, NERVOUS SYSTEM.

ROMATIC INFLUENCE: Celery seed has a spicy, warm sweet, tenacious odor. It is fairly strong and long-lasting. The aroma is CALMING and RELAXING to the mind and body.

PPLICATION: Apply to VITA FLEX POINTS of the feet and directly on AREA of concern.

RAL USE AS DIETARY SUPPLEMENT: Generally regarded as safe (GRAS) for internal consumption by the FDA. *DILUTE one drop oil in 1 tsp. honey or 4 oz. of beverage (ie. soy/rice milk).* ***Not for children under 6 years old; use with CAUTION and in GREATER DILUTION for children 6 years old and over.***

AFETY DATA: Repeated use can possibly result in CONTACT SENSITIZATION or SKIN IRRITATION. Avoid during PREGNANCY.

BLEND CLASSIFICATION: Personifier.

ODOR: Type: *Middle Note (50-80% of the blend)*; Scent: *Spicy, warm, sweet, tenacious*; Intensity: *3*

Chamomile, German (Blue)

(*Matricaria recutita*)

BOTANICAL FAMILY: Compositae (daisy)

EXTRACTION METHOD/ORIGIN: Steam distillation from flowers — Egypt, Hungary, Uta

CHEMICAL CONSTITUENTS: Sesquiterpenes: chamazulene, dihydrochamazulene I & II, bisabolenes, trans-β-farnesene; Alcohols: α-bisabolol (8%), spathulenol, fanesol; Oxides: bisabololoxides A (>24%), B, & C; Coumarins: umbelliferone, herniarin.

PROPERTIES: ANALGESIC, ANTI-INFECTIOUS, ANTI-INFLAMMATORY, ANTIOXIDANT, ANTISPASMODIC, DECONGESTANT, DIGESTIVE TONIC, and is HORMONE-LIKE.

ESOTERIC USES/ACTIONS: Astrological: *Venus, Moon, & Mercury*; Body type: *Ectomorp* Chakra: *5*; Character: *Yin*; Crystals: *Blue tourmaline* ; Element: *Ether & Water*; Number *7*; Oriental: *Excess heat (yang), rising heat, internal wind, (pts: Liv-2, He-3)*

HISTORICAL USES: Native to Europe, it is no longer grown in Germany. It has a long histor of use for all symptoms related to or resulting from tension.

FRENCH MEDICINAL USES: ACNE, CYSTITIS, DECONGESTANT, DIGESTIVE TONIC, ECZEMA, GALLBLADDER, HORMONE-LIKE, LIVER, ULCERS.

OTHER POSSIBLE USES: Chamomile neutralizes ALLERGIES and increases the ability of the SKIN to REGENERATE. It is a cleanser of the BLOOD and also helps OPEN the LIVER, INCREASE LIVER FUNCTION and SECRETION, and SUPPORT the PANCREAS. This oil may be used for ABSCESSES, ACNE, BOILS, BURNS, CUTS, CYSTITIS, DERMATITIS, ECZEMA, GALLBLADDER, chronic GASTRITIS, HAIR CARE, INFLAMED JOINTS, INGROWN NAILS (infected), INSOMNIA, LIVER PROBLEMS, MENOPAUSAL PROBLEMS, MIGRAINE HEADACHES, OPEN LEG SORES, RASHES, SKIN DISORDERS, STRESS RELATED COMPLAINTS, TEETHING PAINS, TOOTHACHES, ULCERS, and WOUNDS.

BODY SYSTEM(S) AFFECTED: EMOTIONAL BALANCE, NERVOUS SYSTEM, SKIN.

AROMATIC INFLUENCE: It can dispel ANGER, stabilize the EMOTIONS, and help to release emotions linked to the past. It may also be used to SOOTHE and CLEAR the MIND creating an atmosphere of PEACE and PATIENCE.

APPLICATION: Apply to VITA FLEX POINTS and directly on AREA of concern; diffuse.

ORAL USE AS DIETARY SUPPLEMENT: Generally regarded as safe (GRAS) for internal consumption by the FDA. *DILUTE one drop oil in 1 tsp. honey or 4 oz. of beverage (ie. soy/rice milk).* ***Not for children under 6 years old; use with CAUTION and in GREATER DILUTION for children 6 years old and over.***

FETY DATA: Use with caution during PREGNANCY. Can irritate sensitive SKIN.

.END CLASSIFICATION: Personifier

.ENDS WITH: Birch, fir, geranium, helichrysum, hyssop, lavender, lemongrass, marjoram, sandalwood, spearmint, spruce, melaleuca (Tea Tree), and wintergreen.

)OR: Type: *Middle Note (50-80% of the blend)*; Scent: *Deep, rich, tenacious, cocoa-like, herbaceous*; Intensity: *4*

EQUENCY: Emotional; approximately 105.

Chamomile, Mixta

(*Chamaemelum mixtum*)

)TANICAL FAMILY: Compositae (daisy)

IEMICAL CONSTITUENTS: Alcohols: santolina alcohol (up to 33%), yomoglalcohol, α-terpineol; Monoterpenes: α-pinene; Ketones: camphor; Oxides: 1,8 cineol.

:OPERTIES: ANTI-CONVULSIVE, ANTI-DEPRESSANT, ANTIOXIDANT, ANTISEPTIC, RELAXANT, and TONIC.

;OTERIC USES/ACTIONS: Astrological: *Venus*; Element: *Water*; Color: *Golden yellow*

)SSIBLE USES: This hybrid oil may be beneficial for CONJUNCTIVITIS, DEPRESSION, DIGESTION, GINGIVITIS, INSOMNIA, MENSTRUATION, dry SKIN, SORE THROATS, TOOTHACHES, and TISSUES in general.

'PLICATION: Apply to VITA FLEX POINTS and/or directly on AREA of concern.

:AL USE AS DIETARY SUPPLEMENT: None.

.END CLASSIFICATION: Personifier.

.ENDS WITH: Bergamot, geranium, juniper, lavender, lemon, rosemary, and ylang ylang.

)OR: Type: *Middle Note (50-80% of the blend)*; Scent: *Spicy, fruity;* Intensity: *4*

Chamomile, Roman

(*Chamaemelum nobile* or *Anthemis nobilis*)

)TANICAL FAMILY: Compositae (daisy)

:TRACTION METHOD/ORIGIN: Steam distillation from flowers — Egypt, Utah

IEMICAL CONSTITUENTS: Esters (>80%): δ-isobutyl angelate, angelic and tiglic acids; Ketones: pinocarvone (>14%); Sesquiterpene lactones: 3-deshydronobiline; Alcohols (>7%): trans-pinocarveol, farnesol, nerolidol; Also pinene, chamazulene, and 1,8 cineol.

:OPERTIES: ANTI-INFECTIOUS, ANTI-INFLAMMATORY, ANTI-PARASITIC, ANTISPASMODIC, CALMING, and RELAXING.

;OTERIC USES/ACTIONS: Astrological: *Moon*; Body type: *Ectomorph*; Chakra: *5*;

Character: *Yin/Yang*; Crystals: *Aquamarine, aqua aura, amazonite* ; Element: *Water*; Number: *5*; Oriental: *Excessive Yang (heat) (pts: Liv-2, He-3)*; Color: *Pale blue to clea*

HISTORICAL USES: It was traditionally used by the ancient Romans to give them a CLEAR MIND and to empower them with COURAGE for their battles. According to Roberta Wilson, "...chamomile was nicknamed the "plant's physician" because it supposedly cu any ailing plant placed near it."

FRENCH MEDICINAL USES: INTESTINAL PARASITES, NEURITIS, NEURALGIA, SHOCK (nervous).

OTHER POSSIBLE USES: Chamomile neutralizes ALLERGIES and increases the ability of the SKIN to REGENERATE. It is a cleanser of the BLOOD and also helps the LIVER reject POISONS and to discharge them. This oil may help with ALLERGIES, BRUISE CUTS, DEPRESSION, INSOMNIA, MUSCLE TENSION, NERVES (calming and promoting nerve health), RESTLESS LEGS, and SKIN CONDITIONS like, ACNE, BOILS, DERMATITIS, ECZEMA, RASHES, and SENSITIVE SKIN. Chamomile is mild enough to use on INFANTS and CHILDREN. For centuries, mothers have used chamomile to CALM CRYING CHILDREN, ease EARACHES, fight FEVERS, sooth STOMACHACHES and COLIC, and relieve TOOTHACHES and TEETHING PAIN. can safely and effectively reduce IRRITABILITY and minimize NERVOUSNESS in children, especially HYPERACTIVE CHILDREN.

BODY SYSTEM(S) AFFECTED: EMOTIONAL BALANCE, NERVOUS SYSTEM, SKIN

AROMATIC INFLUENCE: Because it is calming and relaxing it can combat DEPRESSION INSOMNIA, and STRESS. It eliminates some of the emotional charge of ANXIETY, IRRITABILITY, and NERVOUSNESS. It can dispel ANGER, stabilize the EMOTIONS, and help to release emotions that are linked to the past. It may also be us to SOOTHE and CLEAR the MIND creating an atmosphere of PEACE and PATIENC

APPLICATION: Apply to VITA FLEX POINTS and/or directly on AREA of concern; diffus Applied over the THROAT, it can help a person express his or her true feelings.

ORAL USE AS DIETARY SUPPLEMENT: Generally regarded as safe (GRAS) for interna consumption by the FDA. *DILUTE one drop oil in 1 tsp. honey or 4 oz. of beverage (i. soy/rice milk).* ***Not for children under 6 years old; use with CAUTION and in GREATER DILUTION for children 6 years old and over.***

SAFETY DATA: Can irritate sensitive SKIN.

BLEND CLASSIFICATION: Personifier.

BLENDS WITH: Lavender, rose, geranium, or Clary sage.

ODOR: Type: *Middle Note (50-80% of the blend)*; Scent: *Fresh, sweet, fruity-herbaceous, apple-like, no tenacity*; Intensity: *4*

Cinnamon Bark

(*Cinnamomum verum* or *C. zeylanicum*)

)TANICAL FAMILY: Lauraceae (laurel)

{TRACTION METHOD/ORIGIN: Steam distillation from bark — India, Madagascar, Sri Lanka

IEMICAL CONSTITUENTS: Aldehydes: Cinnamaldehyde (<75%), hydroxycinnamaldehyde, benzaldehyde, cuminaldehyde; Phenols (up to 10%): eugenol, isoeugenol, phenol, 2-vinyl-phenol, camphor; Esters: benzyl benzoate, 2-phenyl ethyl benzoate, methyl cinnamate, cinnamyl acetate; Alcohols: 2-phenylethyl, cinnamic, benzyl alcohol, linalol, α-terpineol, borneol; Sesquiterpenes: β-caryophyllene; Monoterpenes: β-phellandrene, limonene, p-cymene.

{OPERTIES: ANTI-BACTERIAL (98% pathogenic bacteria, cocci gr +, bacillus gr -), ANTI-DEPRESSANT, ANTI-FUNGAL, ANTI-INFECTIOUS (intestinal, urinary), ANTI-INFLAMMATORY, ANTIMICROBIAL, ANTIOXIDANT, ANTI-PARASITIC, ANTISEPTIC, ANTISPASMODIC (light), ANTIVIRAL, ASTRINGENT, IMMUNE-STIMULANT, PURIFIER, SEXUAL STIMULANT, and WARMING. It also ENHANCES the action and activity of other oils.

SOTERIC USES/ACTIONS: Astrological: *Sun & Mercury*; Ayurvedic: *Pitta*; Body type: *Endomorph*; Chakra: *1, 2, & 5*; Character: *Yang*; Crystals: *Tourmaline* ; Element: *Fire & Water*; Number: *2*; Oriental: *Yang deficiency (pts: St-36, Dir Ves-6)*

ISTORICAL USES: This most ancient of spices was included in just about every prescription issued in ancient China. It was regarded as a tranquilizer, tonic, and stomachic and as being good for depression and a weak heart.

{RENCH MEDICINAL USES: SEXUAL STIMULANT, TROPICAL INFECTION, TYPHOID, VAGINITIS.

THER POSSIBLE USES: This oil may be beneficial for CIRCULATION, COLDS, COUGHS, DIGESTION, EXHAUSTION, FLU, INFECTIONS, RHEUMATISM, and WARTS. This oil fights VIRAL and INFECTIOUS DISEASES, and testing has yet to find a VIRUS, BACTERIA, or FUNGUS that can survive in its presence.

ODY SYSTEM(S) AFFECTED: IMMUNE SYSTEM.

PPLICATION: Apply to VITA FLEX POINTS and directly on AREA of concern. Best diluted with V-6 Mixing Oil as the high amount of phenols can irritate the skin.

RAL USE AS DIETARY SUPPLEMENT: Generally regarded as safe (GRAS) for internal consumption by the FDA. *DILUTE one drop oil in 2 tsp. honey or 8 oz. of beverage (ie. soy/rice milk). May need to increase dilution even more due to this oil's potential for irritating mucus membranes.* ***Not for children under 6 years old; use with CAUTION and in GREATER DILUTION for children 6 years old and over.***

AFETY DATA: Repeated use can result in extreme CONTACT SENSITIZATION. Avoid during PREGNANCY. Can cause extreme SKIN IRRITATION. Diffuse with caution; it will irritate the nasal membranes if it is inhaled directly from the diffuser.

Use EXTREME CAUTION when DIFFUSING cinnamon bark because it may burn the nostrils if you put your nose directly next to the nebulizer of the diffuser.

BLEND CLASSIFICATION: Personifier

BLENDS WITH: All citrus oils, cypress, frankincense, geranium, juniper, lavender, rosemary, and all spice oils.

ODOR: Type: *Base Note (5-60% of the blend)*; Scent: *Spicy, warm, sweet*; Intensity: *5*

FREQUENCY: Traditionally thought to have a frequency that attracted wealth.

BIBLE: Exod. 30:23, Prov. 7:17, Song. 4:14, Rev. 18:13

Cistus (Labdanum)

(*Cistus ladanifer*)

BOTANICAL FAMILY: Cistaceae

EXTRACTION METHOD/ORIGIN: Steam distillation from branches — France, Spain

CHEMICAL CONSTITUENTS: Monoterpenes: α- & β-pinenes (50%), camphene (4%), sabinene, myrcene, phellandrene, limonene (2%), cymene; Alcohols: borneol & α-terpine (>5%), linalol, terpinen-4-ol, nerol, geraniol; Esters: linalyle acetate, bornyl & geranyl acetate (3%), methyl benzoate, benzyl benzoate, phenyl methyl phenylpropanate; Phenols eugenol (>2%), thymol; Aldehydes: benzaldehyde (>3%), neral; Ketones: 2,2,6-trimethylcyclohexanone (2%), fenchone (1%); Acids (>2%).

PROPERTIES: ANTIMICROBIAL, ANTISEPTIC, ASTRINGENT, DIURETIC, EXPECTORANT, and TONIC.

FOLKLORE: Anciently, cistus was among the first aromatic substances used.

ESOTERIC USES/ACTIONS: Astrological: *Pluto*; Chakra: *7*; Character: *Yang*; Element: *Earth*

HISTORICAL USES: Used for catarrh, diarrhea, dysentery, and promoting menstruation.

OTHER POSSIBLE USES: Cistus may help with BLEEDING (stop), BOILS, BRONCHITIS COLDS, COUGHS, RHINITIS, URINARY INFECTIONS, WOUNDS, and WRINKLES.

BODY SYSTEM(S) AFFECTED: IMMUNE SYSTEM. It may also assist the AUTO-IMMUNE SYSTEM.

AROMATIC INFLUENCE: STIMULATING to the SENSES of touch, feeling, sight, and sound. It affects the upper part of the BRAIN. It may also help quiet the NERVES, calm the INSOMNIAC, and elevate the emotions in MEDITATION.

APPLICATION: Apply to VITA FLEX POINTS and/or directly on AREA of concern; diffuse.

ORAL USE AS DIETARY SUPPLEMENT: Approved by the FDA for use as a Food Additive (FA) or Flavoring Agent (FL). *DILUTE one drop oil in 1 tsp. honey or 4 oz. of beverage (ie. soy/rice milk).* ***Not for children under 6 years old; use with CAUTION and in GREATER DILUTION for children 6 years old and over.***

AFETY DATA: ***Use with caution during PREGNANCY.***

LEND CLASSIFICATION: Personifier.

LENDS WITH: Bergamot, calamus, chamomile, Clary sage, cypress, juniper, lavender, lavandin, patchouli, pine, sandalwood, and vetiver.

Citronella

(*Cymbopogon nardus*)

OTANICAL FAMILY: Gramineae (grasses)

XTRACTION METHOD/ORIGIN: Steam distillation from grass — Egypt, Philippines, Sri lanka

HEMICAL CONSTITUENTS: Terpene alcohols (35%): geraniol (>16%), borneol (6%), citronnellol (8%); Aldehydes: citronnellal (>17%); Esters (>10%); Phenols: isoeugenol (7%).

ROPERTIES: ANTI-BACTERIAL, ANTI-FUNGAL, ANTI-INFLAMMATORY, ANTISEPTIC, ANTISPASMODIC, DEODORANT, and INSECTICIDAL.

SOTERIC USES/ACTIONS: Astrological: *Venus*; Character: *Yang?*

ISTORICAL USES: This oil belongs to the same family of aromatic, oil-rich tropical grasses as lemongrass and palmarosa. It has been used as an insecticide and for rheumatic problems or other aches and pains. The leaves of citronella have been utilized by many diverse cultures for fever, intestinal parasites, digestive and menstrual problems, and as a stimulant. This oil is hardly used alone in therapy, but because of its highly antiseptic and deodorizing properties, it is used a great deal in commercial preparations and some aromatherapy blends.

THER POSSIBLE USES: Citronella may help with COLDS, FATIGUE, FLU, HEADACHES, minor INFECTIONS, MIGRAINE, NEURALGIA, excessive PERSPIRATION, and OILY SKIN. Can be used as an antiseptic to SANITIZE and DEODORIZE SURFACES where food has been prepared. Combined with cedarwood, it makes an excellent insect repellent.

ODY SYSTEM(S) AFFECTED: MUSCLES and BONES, SKIN.

ROMATIC INFLUENCE: May increase the heart rate.

PPLICATION: Dilute and apply directly on AREA of concern.

RAL USE AS DIETARY SUPPLEMENT: Generally regarded as safe (GRAS) for internal consumption by the FDA. *DILUTE one drop oil in 1 tsp. honey or 4 oz. of beverage (ie. soy/rice milk).* ***Not for children under 6 years old; use with CAUTION and in GREATER DILUTION for children 6 years old and over.***

AFETY DATA: ***Repeated use can result in extreme CONTACT SENSITIZATION. Use with caution during PREGNANCY. Can irritate sensitive SKIN. Inhaling citronella can increase the heart rate.***

BLEND CLASSIFICATION: Personifier.

BLENDS WITH: Bergamot, cedarwood, geranium, lemon, orange, and pine.

ODOR: Type: *Top Note (5-20% of the blend)*; Scent: *Citrusy, slightly fruity, fresh, sweet*; Intensity: *3*

Clary Sage

(*Salvia sclarea*)

BOTANICAL FAMILY: Labiatae (mint)

EXTRACTION METHOD/ORIGIN: Steam distillation from flowing plant — France, Utah

CHEMICAL CONSTITUENTS: Terpene esters (75%): linalyl acetate (62-75%); Monoterpene alcohols (20%): linalol (10-20%), terpinene; Monoterpenes: α and β-pinenes, camphene, myrcene, limonene; Sesquiterpenes; Sesquiterpene alcohols; Diterpene alcohols: sclareol (normally 0.5-2.5%, but 5-7% from distillation in Utah); Ethers; Oxides: 1,8 cineol, linalo oxide; Ketones; Aldehydes; Coumarins. *(More than 250 constituents)*

PROPERTIES: ANTI-CONVULSIVE, ANTI-FUNGAL, ANTISEPTIC, ANTISPASMODIC, ASTRINGENT, NERVE TONIC, SEDATIVE, SOOTHING, TONIC, and WARMING

ESOTERIC USES/ACTIONS: Astrological: *Mercury & Saturn*; Body type: *Ectomorph*; Chakras: *2 & 6*; Character: *Yang, with high Yin*; Crystals: *Malachite* ; Element: *Water, Light, & Earth*; Number: *7*

HISTORICAL USES: Nicknamed "clear eyes", it was famous during the Middle Ages for its ability to clear eye problems. During that same time, it was widely used for female complaints, kidney/digestive/skin disorders, inflammation, sore throats, and wounds.

FRENCH MEDICINAL USES: BRONCHITIS, CHOLESTEROL, FRIGIDITY, GENITALIA, HEMORRHOIDS, HORMONAL IMBALANCE, IMPOTENCE, INFECTIONS, INTESTINAL CRAMPS, MENSTRUAL CRAMPS, PMS, PRE-MENOPAUSE, WEAK DIGESTION.

OTHER POSSIBLE USES: This oil may be used for AMENORRHEA, CELL REGULATION, CIRCULATORY PROBLEMS, DEPRESSION, INSECT BITES, INSOMNIA, KIDNEY DISORDERS, dry SKIN, THROAT INFECTION, ULCERS, and WHOOPING COUGH.

BODY SYSTEM(S) AFFECTED: HORMONAL SYSTEM.

AROMATIC INFLUENCE: It may calm and enhance the DREAM STATE, helping to bring about a feeling of EUPHORIA.

APPLICATION: Apply to VITA FLEX POINTS and/or directly on AREA of concern; diffuse.

ORAL USE AS DIETARY SUPPLEMENT: Generally regarded as safe (GRAS) for internal consumption by the FDA. *DILUTE one drop oil in 1 tsp. honey or 4 oz. of beverage (ie. soy/rice milk).* ***Not for children under 6 years old; use with CAUTION and in GREATER DILUTION for children 6 years old and over.***

AFETY DATA: ***Use with caution during PREGNANCY. Not for babies. Avoid during and after consumption of ALCOHOL.***

LEND CLASSIFICATION: Personifier

LENDS WITH: Bergamot, cedarwood, citrus oils, cypress, geranium, juniper, and sandalwood.

DOR: Type: *Middle to Base Notes (5-60% of the blend)*; Scent: *Herbaceous, spicy, hay-like, sharp, fixative*; Intensity: *3*

Clove

(*Syzygium aromaticum*)

OTANICAL FAMILY: Myrtaceae (shrubs and trees)

XTRACTION METHOD/ORIGIN: Steam distillation from bud and stem — Madagascar, Spice Islands

HEMICAL CONSTITUENTS: Phenols: eugenol (up to 85%), chavicol, 4-allylphenol; Esters: eugenyl acetate (22%), styralyl, benzyl, terpenyl, ethyl phenyl acetates, methyl salicylate (tr.); Sesquiterpenes (up to 6%): α- & β-caryophyllene, α- & β-humulene, α-amorphene, α-muurolene, calamenene, calacorene, pinene; Oxides (<3%): caryophyllene oxide, humulene oxide; Also: benzylic acid, vanillin (tr.), furfurol, acetyleugenol.

ROPERTIES: ANALGESIC, ANTI-BACTERIAL, ANTI-FUNGAL, ANTI-INFECTIOUS, ANTI-INFLAMMATORY, ANTI-PARASITIC, strong ANTISEPTIC, ANTI-TUMORAL, ANTIVIRAL, DISINFECTANT, and IMMUNE-STIMULANT.

OLKLORE: Some old tales say that walking near clove trees while wearing a hat would frighten them into no longer bearing fruit. While the trees may have been afraid of hats, they were not afraid of viruses. History has it that the people of Penang (among the "Spice Islands") were free from epidemics until the sixteenth century, when Dutch conquerors destroyed the clove trees that flourished on those islands. Many of the islanders died from the epidemics that followed.

SOTERIC USES/ACTIONS: Astrological: *Mars, Jupiter*; Ayurvedic: *Kapha*; Chakra: *1*; Character: *Yang*; Element: *Fire*

ISTORICAL USES: Cloves were historically used for skin infections, digestive upsets, intestinal parasites, childbirth, and most notably for toothache. The Chinese also used cloves for diarrhea, hernia, bad breath and bronchitis.

RENCH MEDICINAL USES: IMPOTENCE, INTESTINAL PARASITES, MEMORY DEFICIENCY, PAIN, PLAGUE, TOOTHACHE, WOUNDS (infected).

THER POSSIBLE USES: This oil may help AMEBIC DYSENTERY, ARTHRITIS, BACTERIAL COLITIS, BONES, BRONCHITIS, CHOLERA, CYSTITIS, DENTAL INFECTION, DIARRHEA, INFECTIOUS ACNE, FATIGUE, FLATULENCE (gas), FLU, HALITOSIS (bad breath), tension HEADACHES, HYPERTENSION, INFECTION (wounds and more), INSECT BITES AND STINGS, LUPUS, NAUSEA,

NEURITIS, NETTLES and POISON OAK (takes out sting), RHEUMATISM, SINUSITIS, SKIN CANCER, chronic SKIN DISEASE, SMOKING (removes desire), SORES (speeds healing of mouth and skin sores), TUBERCULOSIS, THYROID DYSFUNCTION, leg ULCERS, VIRAL HEPATITIS, VOMITING, and WARTS. *(Se WARTS in the Personal Guide section of this book.)*

BODY SYSTEM(S) AFFECTED: CARDIOVASCULAR, DIGESTIVE, IMMUNE, and RESPIRATORY SYSTEMS.

AROMATIC INFLUENCE: It may influence HEALING, improve MEMORY (mental stimulant), and create a feeling of PROTECTION and COURAGE. Septimas Piesse considered clove scent to VIBRATE in the KEY of B and in the color of VIOLET. It ca also cause a good sleep, generally culminating in stimulating dreams.

APPLICATION: Apply to VITA FLEX POINTS and/or directly on AREA of concern. Rub directly on the GUMS surrounding an infected tooth. Place on TONGUE with finger to remove desire to smoke, or back of tongue for tickling cough. Diffuse.

ORAL USE AS DIETARY SUPPLEMENT: Generally regarded as safe (GRAS) for internal consumption by the FDA. *DILUTE one drop oil in 1 tsp. honey or 4 oz. of beverage (ie soy/rice milk).* ***Not for children under 6 years old; use with CAUTION and in GREATER DILUTION for children 6 years old and over.***

SAFETY DATA: Repeated use can result in extreme CONTACT SENSITIZATION. Use wi caution during PREGNANCY. Can irritate sensitive SKIN.

BLEND CLASSIFICATION: Personifier

BLENDS WITH: Basil, bergamot, cinnamon bark, Clary sage, grapefruit, lavender, lemon, nutmeg, orange, peppermint, rose, rosemary, and ylang ylang.

ODOR: Type: *Middle to Base Notes (20-80% of the blend)*; Scent: *Spicy, warming, slightly bitter, woody, reminiscent of true clove buds, but richer*; Intensity: *5*

Coriander

(*Coriandrum sativum* L.)

BOTANICAL FAMILY: Umbelliferae (parsley)

EXTRACTION METHOD/ORIGIN: Steam distillation from seeds — India, Russia

CHEMICAL CONSTITUENTS: Aldehydes (up to 95%): octanal, decanal, undecanal, 3.6-undecadienal, dodecanal, 7-dodecanal (<20%), tridecanal, tridecenal, 5,8-tridecadienal, 9 tetradecanal (9%); Alcohols: linalol, borneol, geraniol; Ketones: carvone; Phenol methyl-ethers: anethole.

PROPERTIES: ANALGESIC, ANTI-BACTERIAL, ANTI-FUNGAL, ANTIOXIDANT, ANTI-RHEUMATIC, ANTISPASMODIC, and STIMULANT (cardiac, circulatory, nervous systems). It also has ANTI-INFLAMMATORY and SEDATIVE properties.

FOLKLORE: The seeds were found in the ancient Egyptian tomb of Rameses II.

ESOTERIC USES/ACTIONS: Astrological: *Mars*; Body type: *Endomorph*; Chakra: *2*; Character: *Yin?*; Element: *Fire & Water*; Number: *5*

HISTORICAL USES: The Chinese have used coriander for dysentery, piles, measles, nausea, toothache, and painful hernias.

OTHER POSSIBLE USES: Coriander may help with ANOREXIA, ARTHRITIS, COLDS, COLIC, DIARRHEA, DIGESTIVE SPASMS, DYSPEPSIA, FLATULENCE, FLU, GOUT, INFECTIONS (general), MEASLES, MIGRAINE, MUSCULAR ACHES AND PAINS, NAUSEA, NERVOUS EXHAUSTION, NEURALGIA, PILES, POOR CIRCULATION, RHEUMATISM, SKIN (oily skin, blackheads, and other impurities), and STIFFNESS. Current research at Cairo University indicates that coriander lowers GLUCOSE levels by normalizing insulin levels and supporting the PANCREAS FUNCTION. It may also help during CONVALESCENCE and after a difficult childbirth. Because of its estrogen content, it may regulate and help control pain related to MENSTRUATION.

BODY SYSTEM(S) AFFECTED: DIGESTIVE and HORMONAL SYSTEMS.

AROMATIC INFLUENCE: Coriander is a gentle stimulant for those with LOW PHYSICAL ENERGY. It also helps one relax during times of STRESS, IRRITABILITY, AND NERVOUSNESS. It may also provide a CALMING influence to those suffering from SHOCK or FEAR.

APPLICATION: Apply to VITA FLEX POINTS and directly on AREA of concern; diffuse.

ORAL USE AS DIETARY SUPPLEMENT: Generally regarded as safe (GRAS) for internal consumption by the FDA. *DILUTE one drop oil in 1 tsp. honey or 4 oz. of beverage (ie. soy/rice milk).* ***Not for children under 6 years old; use with CAUTION and in GREATER DILUTION for children 6 years old and over.***

SAFETY DATA: Use sparingly as coriander can be STUPIFYING in large doses.

BLEND CLASSIFICATION: Personifier and Modifier

BLENDS WITH: Bergamot, cinnamon bark, citronella, Clary sage, cypress, ginger, jasmine, neroli, petitgrain, pine, sandalwood, and other spice oils.

ODOR: Type: *Middle Note (50-80% of the blend)*; Scent: *Woody, spicy, sweet*; Intensity: *3*

Cumin

(*Cuminum cyminum*)

BOTANICAL FAMILY: Umbelliferae (parsley)

EXTRACTION METHOD/ORIGIN: Steam distillation from seeds — Egypt

CHEMICAL CONSTITUENTS: Aldehydes (up to 60%): cuminaldehyde (up to 32%), dihydrocuminaldehyde, p-mentha-3-en-7-ol, p-mentha-1,3-diene-7-al, p-mentha-1,4-diene-7-al; Monoterpenes (up to 60%): α- & β-pinenes, paracymene, α-terpinene, limonene, γ-terpinene, camphene; Sesquiterpenes: β-caryophyllene; Alcohols: cuminol, terpineol; Ester:

cuminyl ester; Coumarins: scopoletin (tr.).

PROPERTIES: ANTI-BACTERIAL, ANTIOXIDANT, ANTI-PARASITIC, ANTISEPTIC, ANTISPASMODIC, ANTITOXIC, ANTI-VIRAL, APHRODISIAC, DIGESTIVE, STIMULANT (heart, immune and nervous systems), and TONIC.

FOLKLORE: Cumin seeds were found in Egyptian tombs, and used by the Romans as a food preservative.

ESOTERIC USES/ACTIONS: Astrological: *Saturn & Mars*; Body type: *Endomorph*; Character: *Yin, with high Yang?*; Element: *Fire & Water*; Number: *3*; Perfume note: *Top*

HISTORICAL USES: During biblical times it was used by the Hebrews as an antiseptic during their ceremony of circumcision. Traditionally one of the main ingredients in curry, it was also used to help with flatulence, the digestive system, for rheumatic conditions, the heart, and the nervous system.

OTHER POSSIBLE USES: This oil may help with CELLULITE, poor CIRCULATION, COLIC, DEAFNESS following a bad viral FLU infection, DIGESTIVE SPASMS, DYSPEPSIA, FLATULENCE, HEADACHES, INDIGESTION, LYMPHATIC CONGESTION, MIGRAINES, and NERVOUS DEBILITY and EXHAUSTION.

BODY SYSTEM(S) AFFECTED: DIGESTIVE and IMMUNE SYSTEMS.

AROMATIC INFLUENCE: Used by one source to encourage BOWEL MOVEMENTS in thei child. It has also been used at dinner parties to STIMULATE the APPETITE.

APPLICATION: Apply to VITA FLEX POINTS and directly on AREA of concern; diffuse.

ORAL USE AS DIETARY SUPPLEMENT: Generally regarded as safe (GRAS) for internal consumption by the FDA. *DILUTE one drop oil in 1 tsp. honey or 4 oz. of beverage (ie. soy/rice milk).* ***Not for children under 6 years old; use with CAUTION and in GREATER DILUTION for children 6 years old and over.***

SAFETY DATA: Use with caution during PREGNANCY. Avoid direct SUNLIGHT for up to 12 hours after use.

BLEND CLASSIFICATION: Enhancer

BLENDS WITH: Cinnamon bark, jasmine, patchouli, rose, sandalwood, and ylang ylang.

Cypress

(*Cupressus sempervirens*)

BOTANICAL FAMILY: Cupressaceae (conifer - cypress)

EXTRACTION METHOD/ORIGIN: Steam distillation from branches — France, Spain

CHEMICAL CONSTITUENTS: Monoterpenes: α-pinene (>55%), Δ-3-carene (>30%), limonene, terpinolene, sabinene, β-pinene; Sesquiterpenes: α-cedrene, δ-cadinene; Sesquiterpenols: cedrol (7%), cadinol; Monoterpenols: terpinene-4-ol, α-terpineol, borneol Diterpenols (labdanic): manool, sempervirol; Esters: α-terpinyl acetate.

PROPERTIES: ANTI-BACTERIAL, ANTI-INFECTIOUS, ANTIMICROBIAL,

MUCOLYTIC, ANTISEPTIC, ASTRINGENT, DEODORANT, DIURETIC, LYMPHATIC and PROSTATE DECONGESTANT, REFRESHING, RELAXING, and a VASOCONSTRICTOR.

FOLKLORE: According to Roberta Wilson, "The evergreen branches of the cypress tree were considered symbolic of life after death. In fact, *sempervirens* means 'ever-living'."

ESOTERIC USES/ACTIONS: Astrological: *Saturn*; Body type: *Ectomorph*; Chakra: *5*; Character: *Yang*; Element: *Ether & Earth*; Number: *7*; Oriental: *Blood stagnation (pts: Sp-10 & 6)*

HISTORICAL USES: It was used anciently for its benefits on the urinary system and other places where there is excessive loss of fluids, such as perspiration, diarrhea, and menstrual flow. The Chinese valued cypress for its benefits to the liver and respiratory system.

FRENCH MEDICINAL USES: ARTHRITIS, BRONCHITIS, **CIRCULATION**, CRAMPS, HEMORRHOIDS, INSOMNIA, INTESTINAL PARASITES, LYMPHATIC DECONGESTANT, MENOPAUSAL PROBLEMS, MENSTRUAL PAIN, PANCREAS INSUFFICIENCIES, PLEURISY, PROSTATE DECONGESTANT, PULMONARY TUBERCULOSIS, RHEUMATISM, SPASMS, THROAT PROBLEMS, VARICOSE VEINS, WATER RETENTION.

OTHER POSSIBLE USES: This oil may be beneficial for ASTHMA, strengthening BLOOD CAPILLARY WALLS, reducing CELLULITE, **CIRCULATORY SYSTEM**, COLDS, strengthening CONNECTIVE TISSUE, spasmodic COUGHS, DIARRHEA, EDEMA, ENERGY, FEVER, GALLBLADDER, bleeding GUMS, HEMORRHAGING, INFLUENZA, LARYNGITIS, LIVER DISORDERS, LUNG CIRCULATION, MUSCULAR CRAMPS, NERVOUS TENSION, NOSE BLEEDS, OVARIAN CYSTS, increasing PERSPIRATION, SKIN CARE, SCAR TISSUE, WHOOPING COUGH, and WOUNDS.

BODY SYSTEM(S) AFFECTED: CARDIOVASCULAR SYSTEM, MUSCLES and BONES.

AROMATIC INFLUENCE: It influences, strengthens, and helps ease the feeling of LOSS. It creates a feeling of SECURITY, GROUNDING, and it helps to heal EMOTIONS.

APPLICATION: Apply to VITA FLEX POINTS and directly on AREA of concern; diffuse.

ORAL USE AS DIETARY SUPPLEMENT: None.

SAFETY DATA: Use with caution during PREGNANCY.

BLEND CLASSIFICATION: Equalizer

BLENDS WITH: Bergamot, Clary sage, juniper, lavender, lemon, orange, and sandalwood.

ODOR: Type: *Middle Note (50-80% of the blend)*; Scent: *Fresh, herbaceous, slightly woody with evergreen undertones*; Intensity: *3*

Cypress, Blue

(*Callitris intratropica*)

BOTANICAL FAMILY: Cupressaceae

EXTRACTION METHOD/ORIGIN: Steam distillation from the heartwood, which makes up 70% of the tree trunk — Australia

CHEMICAL CONSTITUENTS: Selinenes, gaueenes, guaiol, lactones, eudesmols, elemol, and guaiazulene.

PROPERTIES: ANTI-INFLAMMATORY, ANTI-VIRAL, INSECT REPELLANT, and STIMULANT (to amygdala, pineal gland, pituitary gland, and hypothalamus).

HISTORICAL USES: Blue cypress has been used historically for incense, perfume and embalming. The resin was used for sores, cuts, and upset stomachs. The aboriginal Tiwi people of Australia would throw the wood onto the fire to drive away the mosquitoes and midges. The guaiazulene gives blue cypress oil its azure blue color.

OTHER POSSIBLE USES: Blue cypress may help with ABDOMINAL CRAMPS, ACHES and PAIN (minor), BRAIN function (improves circulation and oxygenates), COLD SORES, HERPES SIMPLEX, HERPES ZOSTER, and the HUMAN PAPILLOMA VIRUS (HPV).

BODY SYSTEM(S) AFFECTED: DIGESTIVE and IMMUNE SYSTEMS.

APPLICATION: Apply to VITA FLEX POINTS and directly on AREA of concern; Diffuse.

ORAL USE AS DIETARY SUPPLEMENT: None.

SAFETY DATA: None available.

BLENDS WITH: Cedarwood, frankincense, helichrysum, lavender, melissa, and sandalwood.

ODOR: Type: *Base Note (5-20% of the blend)*; Scent: *Long-lasting, warm, woody, earthy*; Intensity: *3*

FOUND IN: Brain Power, Australian Blue, AromaGuard Mountain Mint Deodorant.

Davana

(*Artemisia pallens*)

BOTANICAL FAMILY: Compositae (daisy)

CHEMICAL CONSTITUENTS: Ketones: davanone (>52%), isodavanone, nordavanone, artemone; Diethers: davana-ether; Difuranes: davana-furane; Esters; Sesquiterpenes; Also acetoeugenol, γ-cadinene, linalol.

PROPERTIES: ANTI-INFECTIOUS.

POSSIBLE USES: This oil may help stimulate the ENDOCRINE SYSTEM, improve HORMONAL BALANCE, and soothe ROUGH, DRY, and CHAPPED SKIN. It may also help with COUGHING ATTACKS with THICK MUCUS and SPASMODIC

COUGHS, as well as help ease ANXIOUS FEELINGS and NERVOUSNESS.

ODY SYSTEM(S) AFFECTED: HORMONAL SYSTEM.

RAL USE AS DIETARY SUPPLEMENT: Approved by the FDA for use as a Food Additive (FA) or Flavoring Agent (FL). *DILUTE one drop oil in 1 tsp. honey or 4 oz. of beverage (ie. soy/rice milk).* ***Not for children under 6 years old; use with CAUTION and in GREATER DILUTION for children 6 years old and over.***

AFETY DATA: Use with caution during PREGNANCY.

Dill

(*Anethum graveolens*)

OTANICAL FAMILY: Umbelliferae (parsley)

XTRACTION METHOD/ORIGIN: Steam distillation from whole plant — Austria, Hungary

HEMICAL CONSTITUENTS: Ketones: carvone (up to 45%); Monoterpenes: pinene, limonene (up to 25%), α- & β-phellandrenes (up to 35%).

ROPERTIES: ANTISPASMODIC, ANTI-BACTERIAL, EXPECTORANT, and STIMULANT.

OLKLORE: The dill plant is mentioned in the Papyrus of Ebers from Egypt (1550 B.C.). Roman Gladiators would rub it into their skin before a fight.

OSSIBLE USES: This oil may help BRONCHIAL CATARRH, COLIC, CONSTIPATION, DYSPEPSIA, FLATULENCE, HEADACHES, INDIGESTION, LIVER DEFICIENCIES, LOWER GLUCOSE LEVELS, NERVOUSNESS, NORMALIZE INSULIN LEVELS, PROMOTE MILK FLOW in nursing mothers, and SUPPORT the PANCREAS FUNCTION.

ODY SYSTEM(S) AFFECTED: DIGESTIVE SYSTEM.

ROMATIC INFLUENCE: It calms the autonomic nervous system and, when diffused with Roman chamomile, may help fidgety children

PPLICATION: Apply to VITA FLEX POINTS and/or directly on AREA of concern; diffuse. A drop or two on the WRISTS can help remove ADDICTIONS to SWEETS.

RAL USE AS DIETARY SUPPLEMENT: Generally regarded as safe (GRAS) for internal consumption by the FDA. *DILUTE one drop oil in 1 tsp. honey or 4 oz. of beverage (ie. soy/rice milk).* ***Not for children under 6 years old; use with CAUTION and in GREATER DILUTION for children 6 years old and over.***

AFETY DATA: Use with caution if susceptible to EPILEPSY.

LEND CLASSIFICATION: Enhancer

LENDS WITH: Nutmeg and citrus oils.

DOR: Type: *Middle Note (50-80% of the blend)*; Scent: *Fresh, sweet, herbaceous, slightly earthy*; Intensity: *2*

Douglas Fir

(*See Fir, Douglas*)

Elemi

(*Canarium luzonicum*)

BOTANICAL FAMILY: Burseraceae

EXTRACTION METHOD/ORIGIN: Steam distillation from the gum of the tree — Philippin

CHEMICAL CONSTITUENTS: Monoterpenes: α- phellandrene (15%), β-phellandrene (7%) limonene (up to 70%), terpinolene, pinene, dipentene; Sesquiterpenes: elemenes; Alcohol elemol (up to 25%), terpineol; Ketones: carvone. Also elemicin.

PROPERTIES: ANTI-CATARRHAL, ANTI-DEPRESSANT, ANTI-INFECTIOUS, ANTISEPTIC, EXPECTORANT, and SEDATIVE.

FOLKLORE: The name, elemi, comes from an Arabic phrase meaning "As above, so below". This helps us understand its action on both the emotional and spiritual planes. Because the similar properties and uses, it has come to be known as the "poor man's frankincense

ESOTERIC USES/ACTIONS: Astrological: *Sun*; Chakras: 7; Crystals: *Elestial, skeleton quartz* ; Color: *Yellow pale*

HISTORICAL USES: Native to the Philippine Islands and the Moluccas, it is used locally for skin conditions and respiratory problems. Anciently, the Egyptians used the oil that was distilled from the resin in part of the embalming process.

OTHER POSSIBLE USES: This oil may help with BRONCHITIS (chronic), CHEST INFECTIONS, CHILDBIRTH, COUGHS (unproductive), CUTS (infected), GANGRENE, INFLAMMATION (breast and uterus), PREGNANCY, RASHES (allergic), REJUVENATION, SKIN (chapped), THYMUS GLAND, TISSUE (builds), ULCERS, WOUNDS (infected), and WRINKLES. ***See frankincense and myrrh for other possible uses.***

BODY SYSTEM(S) AFFECTED: SKIN.

AROMATIC INFLUENCE: When diffused, this oil may help with NERVOUS EXHAUSTION, STRESS, SINUSITIS, and other BRONCHIAL INFECTIONS. Duri MEDITATION, it may help to CALM and CENTER the individual. It may also help to bring the MIND, BODY, and SPIRIT into alignment with each other. It is psychologica BALANCING and STRENGTHENING as well as FORTIFYING to the PSYCHIC CENTERS.

APPLICATION: Apply to VITA FLEX POINTS and/or directly on AREA of concern. May b used as a COMPRESS for infected WOUNDS and ABSCESSES. May also be diluted for use during a MASSAGE, or added to a BATH.

ORAL USE AS DIETARY SUPPLEMENT: Approved by the FDA for use as a Food Additi (FA) or Flavoring Agent (FL). *DILUTE one drop oil in 1 tsp. honey or 4 oz. of bevera*

(ie. soy/rice milk). ***Not for children under 6 years old; use with CAUTION and in GREATER DILUTION for children 6 years old and over.***

LEND CLASSIFICATION: Enhancer; the hint of lemon gives it more of a middle note.

LENDS WITH: Cinnamon bark & other spices, frankincense, lavender, myrrh, rosemary, sage.

DOR: Type: *Middle Note (50-80% of the blend)*; Scent: *Balsamic, fresh, citrusy, peppery, spicy*; Intensity: *3*

Eucalyptus

(*Eucalyptus globulus*)

OTANICAL FAMILY: Myrtaceae (Myrtle shrubs and trees)

XTRACTION METHOD/ORIGIN: Steam distillation from leaves — Australia, Brazil

HEMICAL CONSTITUENTS: Oxides: 1,8 cineol (up to 78%); Monoterpenes (>20%): α- & β-pinenes, limonene, ρ-cymene, α-terpinene; Sesquiterpenes: aromadendrene (>7%), allo-aromadendrene (>2%), δ-guaiazulene, α-humulene; Alcohols: trans-pinocarveol, linalol, terpinen-4-ol, globulol (>7%), ledol (>2%), eudesmol; Esters: terpenyl acetate; Aldehydes: butyraldehyde, valeraldehyde, caproaldehyde, myrtenol.

ROPERTIES: ANALGESIC, ANTI-BACTERIAL, ANTI-CATARRHAL, ANTI-INFECTIOUS, ANTI-INFLAMMATORY, ANTISEPTIC, ANTIVIRAL, DIURETIC, EXPECTORANT, INSECT REPELLENT, and STIMULANT.

SOTERIC USES/ACTIONS: Astrological: *Saturn & Mercury*; Ayurvedic: *Kapha*; Chakra: *4, 5, & 6*; Character: *Yang*; Crystals: *Aquamarine* ; Element: *Air & Earth*; Oriental: *Cold phlegm (pts: St-40, Sp-6)*

ISTORICAL USES: Australian aborigines used the eucalyptus leaves to bind up serious wounds. This would not only prevent infection but also expedite healing.

RENCH MEDICINAL USES: ASTHMA, CANDIDA, COUGHS, DIABETES, FEVER, HYPOGLYCEMIA, LUNGS, MEASLES, MIGRAINES, RESPIRATORY STIMULANT, SINUSITIS, TUBERCULOSIS, URINARY STIMULANT.

THER POSSIBLE USES: This oil may be used for ACHES/PAINS, ACNE, ALLERGIES, BRONCHITIS, BURNS, COLDS, CYSTITIS, DIARRHEA, ENDOMETRIOSIS, increasing ENERGY, FLU, GALLSTONES, GONORRHEA, HAY FEVER, HERPES, INFLAMMATION of the EAR, INFLAMMATION of the IRIS, INFLAMMATION of the NASAL MUCOUS MEMBRANE, MALARIA, NASOPHARYNX, RHEUMATISM, SKIN INFECTION/SORES, SORE THROAT, ULCERS, VAGINITIS, VIRUSES, and WOUNDS.

ODY SYSTEM(S) AFFECTED: MUSCLES and BONES, RESPIRATORY SYSTEM.

ROMATIC INFLUENCE: It promotes HEALTH, WELL BEING, PURIFICATION, and HEALING.

PPLICATION: Apply to VITA FLEX POINTS and/or directly on AREA of concern; *diffuse.*

Apply under the nose and on each side of the nose for quick SINUS RELIEF.

ORAL USE AS DIETARY SUPPLEMENT: Approved by the FDA for use as a Food Additi (FA) or Flavoring Agent (FL). *DILUTE one drop oil in 1 tsp. honey or 4 oz. of beverag (ie. soy/rice milk).* ***Not for children under 6 years old; use with CAUTION and in GREATER DILUTION for children 6 years old and over.***

BLEND CLASSIFICATION: Enhancer

BLENDS WITH: Geranium, lavender, lemon, sandalwood, juniper, lemongrass, melissa, pine, and thyme.

ODOR: Type: *Top Note (5-20% of the blend)*; Scent: *Fresh, medicinal, woody, earthy*; Intensity: *5*

Eucalyptus Citriodora

(or Lemon Eucalyptus)

(*Eucalyptus citriodora*)

BOTANICAL FAMILY: Myrtaceae (Myrtle shrubs and trees)

EXTRACTION METHOD/ORIGIN: Steam distillation from leaves — China

CHEMICAL CONSTITUENTS: Aldehydes: citronellal (>80%); Alcohols: citronellol (>20%), trans-pinocarveol, geraniol, cis- & trans-p-menthane-3,8-diols; Esters: citronellyl citronellate & butyrate.

PROPERTIES: ANTI-BACTERIAL, ANTI-FUNGAL, ANTI-INFECTIOUS, ANTI-INFLAMMATORY, ANTI-RHEUMATIC, ANTISEPTIC, ANTIVIRAL, DEODORANT, EXPECTORANT, and INSECTICIDAL.

ESOTERIC USES/ACTIONS: Astrological: *Mercury & Saturn*; Character: *Yin*; Element: *Air*; Oriental: *Hot wind, phlegm (pts: St-40, Sp-6)*

HISTORICAL USES: *Eucalyptus citriodora* has been used to perfume the linen closet, and as an insect repellent, especially for cockroaches and silverfish.

OTHER POSSIBLE USES: *Eucalyptus citriodora* may help with ASTHMA, ATHLETE'S FOOT and other FUNGAL INFECTIONS, COLDS, CUTS, DANDRUFF, FEVERS, HERPES, INFECTIOUS SKIN CONDITIONS such as CHICKENPOX, INFECTIOUS DISEASES, INSECT REPELLENT, LARYNGITIS, SCABS, SORE THROAT, SORES, WOUNDS.

BODY SYSTEM(S) AFFECTED: RESPIRATORY SYSTEM.

APPLICATION: Apply to VITA FLEX POINTS and/or directly on AREA of concern.

ORAL USE AS DIETARY SUPPLEMENT: None.

SAFETY DATA: Repeated use can possibly result in CONTACT SENSITIZATION.

ODOR: Type: *Middle Note (50-80% of the blend)*; Scent: *Sweet, lemony, fresh, with a woody hint*; Intensity: *3*

Eucalyptus Dives

(*Eucalyptus dives var. piperitone*)

BOTANICAL FAMILY: Myrtaceae (Myrtle shrubs and trees)

EXTRACTION METHOD/ORIGIN: Steam distillation from leaves — Australia, Brazil

CHEMICAL CONSTITUENTS: Ketones: piperitone (up to 50%); Monoterpenes: α-phellandrene (>30%), β-phellandrene, camphene, cymene, terpinene, thujene; Sesquiterpenes: α-cubebene, β-caryophyllene, longifolene, γ-elemene, δ-cadinene; Monoterpenols: linalol, terpinen-4-ol, α-terpineol, piperitol;.

PROPERTIES: ANTI-BACTERIAL (more specific than other varieties of eucalyptus oil)

ESOTERIC USES/ACTIONS: Astrological: *Mercury & Saturn*; Chakras: *4 & 6*; Character: *slightly Yang*; Element: *Air & Earth*

POSSIBLE USES: See other varieties of eucalyptus for possible uses.

BODY SYSTEM(S) AFFECTED: RESPIRATORY SYSTEM.

APPLICATION: Diffuse; Apply to VITA FLEX POINTS and directly on AREA of concern.

ORAL USE AS DIETARY SUPPLEMENT: None.

Eucalyptus Polybractea

(*Eucalyptus polybractea*)

BOTANICAL FAMILY: Myrtaceae (Myrtle shrubs and trees)

EXTRACTION METHOD/ORIGIN: Steam distillation from leaves — Australia, Brazil

CHEMICAL CONSTITUENTS: Oxides: 1,8 cineol (up to 80%); Monoterpenes: limonene, paracymene, α-pinene.

PROPERTIES: ANTI-BACTERIAL, ANTI-INFECTIOUS, ANTI-INFLAMMATORY, ANTIVIRAL, EXPECTORANT, MUCOLYTIC, and INSECTICIDAL.

ESOTERIC USES/ACTIONS: Astrological: *Mercury & Saturn*; Character: *Neutral?*; Element: *Air & Earth*

POSSIBLE USES: ACNE, CYSTITIS. See other varieties of eucalyptus for possible uses.

BODY SYSTEM(S) AFFECTED: RESPIRATORY SYSTEM.

APPLICATION: Diffuse; Apply to VITA FLEX POINTS and directly on AREA of concern.

ORAL USE AS DIETARY SUPPLEMENT: None.

ODOR: Type: *Top Note (5-20% of the blend)*; Scent: *Fresh, woody, earthy*; Intensity: *4*

Eucalyptus Radiata

(*Eucalyptus radiata*)

BOTANICAL FAMILY: Myrtaceae (Myrtle shrubs and trees)

EXTRACTION METHOD/ORIGIN: Steam distillation from leaves — Australia

CHEMICAL CONSTITUENTS: Oxides: 1,8 cineol (62-72%), caryophyllene oxide; Monoterpenols (20%): linalol, borneol, geraniol α-terpinol (14%); Monoterpenes (8%): α- & β-pinenes, myrene; Aldehydes (8%): myrtenal, citronellal, geranial, neral.

PROPERTIES: ANTI-BACTERIAL, ANTI-CATARRHAL, ANTI-INFECTIOUS, ANTI-INFLAMMATORY, ANTIVIRAL, and EXPECTORANT.

ESOTERIC USES/ACTIONS: Astrological: *Saturn & Mercury*; Chakra: *6*; Character: *Yang*; Element: *Air & Earth*; Oriental: *Cools and quiets fire element of lungs - massage over chest, back, ribs, & over spleen/pancreas & lung meridians*

OTHER POSSIBLE USES: This oil, when combined with bergamot, has been used effectively on HERPES SIMPLEX. It may also help with ACNE, BRONCHITIS, EAR (inflammation), ENDOMETRIOSIS, FLU, HAY FEVER, IRIS (inflammation), NASAL MUCOUS MEMBRANE (inflammation), SINUSITIS, and VAGINITIS.

BODY SYSTEM(S) AFFECTED: RESPIRATORY SYSTEM, SKIN.

APPLICATION: Apply to VITA FLEX points and/or directly on AREA of concern; diffuse.

ODOR: Type: *Middle Note (50-80% of the blend)*; Scent: *Slightly camphorous, sweet, fruity*; Intensity: *3*

Fennel

(*Foeniculum vulgare*)

BOTANICAL FAMILY: Umbelliferae (parsley)

EXTRACTION METHOD/ORIGIN: Steam distillation from the crushed seeds — Australia, Spain

CHEMICAL CONSTITUENTS: Phenyl methyl-ethers: trans-anethole (70%), methyl chavicol (>3%); Ketones: fenchone (12%), phellandrene; Monoterpenes: α- & β-pinenes, limonene (18-29%), camphene, trans-ocimene

PROPERTIES: ANTI-PARASITIC, ANTISEPTIC, ANTISPASMODIC, ANTI-TOXIN, DIURETIC, and EXPECTORANT.

FOLKLORE: During Medieval times, fennel was believed to ward off evil spirits and block spells cast by witches.

ESOTERIC USES/ACTIONS: Astrological: *Mercury*; Body type: *Lymphatic*; Chakra: *1*; Character: *Yang, Yin*; Element: *Air*; Oriental: *Cold damp (pts: Sp-9 & 6)*

HISTORICAL USES: The ancient Egyptians and Romans awarded garlands of fennel as praise to victorious warriors because fennel was believed to bestow strength, courage, and longevity. It has been used for thousands of years for snakebite, to stave off hunger pains, to tone the female reproductive system, for earaches, eye problems, insect bites, kidney complaints, lung infections, and to expel worms.

FRENCH MEDICINAL USES: CYSTITIS, sluggish DIGESTION, FLATULENCE, GOUT, INTESTINAL PARASITES, INTESTINAL SPASMS, increases LACTATION, MENOPAUSE PROBLEMS, PRE-MENOPAUSE, URINARY STONES, VOMITING.

OTHER POSSIBLE USES: Fennel oil may be used for COLIC, stimulating the CARDIOVASCULAR SYSTEM, CONSTIPATION, DIGESTION (supports the LIVER), balancing HORMONES, KIDNEY STONES, NAUSEA, OBESITY, supporting PANCREATIC FUNCTION, and PMS. It may break up FLUIDS and TOXINS, and CLEANSE the TISSUES.

BODY SYSTEM(S) AFFECTED: DIGESTIVE and HORMONAL SYSTEMS.

AROMATIC INFLUENCE: It influences and increases LONGEVITY, COURAGE and PURIFICATION.

APPLICATION: Apply to VITA FLEX POINTS and directly on AREA of concern; diffuse.

ORAL USE AS DIETARY SUPPLEMENT: Generally regarded as safe (GRAS) for internal consumption by the FDA. *DILUTE one drop oil in 1 tsp. honey or 4 oz. of beverage (ie. soy/rice milk).* ***Not for children under 6 years old; use with CAUTION and in GREATER DILUTION for children 6 years old and over.***

SAFETY DATA: Repeated use can possibly result in CONTACT SENSITIZATION. Use with caution if susceptible to EPILEPSY. Use with caution during PREGNANCY.

BLEND CLASSIFICATION: Equalizer and Modifier

BLENDS WITH: Basil, geranium, lavender, lemon, rosemary, and sandalwood.

ODOR: Type: *Top to Middle Notes (20-80% of the blend)*; Scent: *Sweet, somewhat spicy, licorice-like*; Intensity: *4*

Fir (Silver Fir or Fir Needle)

(*Abies alba*)

BOTANICAL FAMILY: Pinaceae (conifer)

EXTRACTION METHOD/ORIGIN: Steam distillation from needles — Balkans

CHEMICAL CONSTITUENTS: Monoterpenes (75-95%): α-pinenes (24%), camphene (21%), limonene (34%), santene, Δ-3-carene; Esters: bornyle acetate (up to 10%).

PROPERTIES: ANALGESIC, ANTI-ARTHRITIC, ANTI-CATARRHAL, ANTISEPTIC (pulmonary), EXPECTORANT, and STIMULANT.

ESOTERIC USES/ACTIONS: Astrological: *Jupiter*; Character: *Yang*

HISTORICAL USES: The fir tree is the classic Christmas tree (short with the perfect pyramidal shape and silvery white bark). Though highly regarded for its fragrant scent, the fir tree has been prized through the ages for its medicinal virtues in regards to respiratory complaints, fever, muscular and rheumatic pain.

FRENCH MEDICINAL USES: BRONCHITIS, RESPIRATORY CONGESTION, ENERGY

OTHER POSSIBLE USES: Fir creates the symbolic effect of the umbrella protecting the earth and bringing energy in from the universe. At night the animals in the wild lie down under the tree for the protection, recharging, and rejuvenation the trees bring them. It may be beneficial for reducing ACHES/PAINS from COLDS and the FLU, fighting AIRBORNE GERMS/BACTERIA, ARTHRITIS, ASTHMA, supporting the BLOOD, BRONCHIAL obstructions, COUGHS, FEVERS, OXYGENATING the cells, RHEUMATISM, SINUSITIS, and URINARY TRACT INFECTIONS.

BODY SYSTEM(S) AFFECTED: RESPIRATORY SYSTEM.

AROMATIC INFLUENCE: It creates a feeling of GROUNDING, ANCHORING, and EMPOWERMENT. It can STIMULATE the MIND while allowing the body to relax.

APPLICATION: Apply to VITA FLEX POINTS and/or directly on AREA of concern; diffuse.

ORAL USE AS DIETARY SUPPLEMENT: Approved by the FDA for use as a Food Additive (FA) and Flavoring Agent (FL). *DILUTE one drop oil in 1 tsp. honey or 4 oz. of beverage (ie. soy/rice milk).* ***Not for children under 6 years old; use with CAUTION and in GREATER DILUTION for children 6 years old and over.***

SAFETY DATA: Can irritate sensitive SKIN.

BLEND CLASSIFICATION: Equalizer

BLENDS WITH: German chamomile, cedarwood, frankincense, lavender, myrtle, and rosewood

ODOR: Type: *Middle Notes (50-80% of the blend)*; Scent: *Fresh, woody, earthy, sweet*; Intensity: *3*

Fir, Balsam (Canadian Balsam)

(Abies balsamea)

BOTANICAL FAMILY: Pinaceae (conifer)

EXTRACTION METHOD/ORIGIN: Steam distillation from branches — Canada, USA

CHEMICAL CONSTITUENTS: Monoterpenes (approx. 90%): limonene, pinene, camphene, phellandrene, bisabolene, dipentene,; Esters (approx. 25%): bornyl acetate, terpinyl acetate.

PROPERTIES: ANTISEPTIC (genito-urinary, pulmonary), ASTRINGENT, DIURETIC, EXPECTORANT, SEDATIVE (nerves), and TONIC.

ESOTERIC USES/ACTIONS: Astrological: *Jupiter, Saturn*; Character: *Yang*; Element: *Air*

HISTORICAL USES: This fir tree is tall and graceful with a perfect conical shape. Though highly regarded for its fragrant scent, the fir tree has been prized through the ages for its medicinal virtues in regards to respiratory complaints, fever, muscular and rheumatic pain. The oleoresin from the balsam fir tree has been used extensively for ritual purposes and for the external treatment of burns, sores, cuts, heart and chest pains, and for coughs.

THER POSSIBLE USES: This oil may be beneficial for ASTHMA, BRONCHITIS, BURNS, CATARRH, CHRONIC COUGHS, CUTS, CYSTITIS, DEPRESSION, HEMORRHOIDS, STRESS-RELATED CONDITIONS, SORE THROAT, TENSION (nervous), URINARY INFECTIONS, WOUNDS. This oil may help with ANXIETY, COLDS, FLU, INFECTIONS, and PAIN (reduces). It may help enhance the production of hGH (human Growth Hormone) and reduce the levels of cortisol. It has been found to be very effective for soothing **OVERWORKED** or **TIRED MUSCLES, LIGAMENTS, TENDONS,** and **JOINTS**. It may also help with back pain.

ODY SYSTEM(S) AFFECTED: EMOTIONAL BALANCE, MUSCLES and BONES, NERVOUS SYSTEM, RESPIRATORY SYSTEM.

ROMATIC INFLUENCE: It creates a feeling of GROUNDING, ANCHORING, and EMPOWERMENT. It can STIMULATE the MIND while allowing the BODY to RELAX. It has been described as APPEASING, ELEVATING, and OPENING. It is also very emotionally balancing.

PPLICATION: Diffuse; Apply to VITA FLEX POINTS and directly on AREA of concern.

RAL USE AS DIETARY SUPPLEMENT: Approved by the FDA for use as a Food Additive (FA) and Flavoring Agent (FL). *DILUTE one drop oil in 1 tsp. honey or 4 oz. of beverage (ie. soy/rice milk).* ***Not for children under 6 years old; use with CAUTION and in GREATER DILUTION for children 6 years old and over.***

AFETY DATA: Can irritate sensitive SKIN. Avoid direct SUNLIGHT for 3 to 6 hours after use.

LEND CLASSIFICATION: Equalizer

LENDS WITH: German chamomile, cedarwood, cypress, frankincense, juniper, lavender, lemon, myrtle, pine, sandalwood, and rosewood.

DOR: Type: *Middle Note (50-80% of the blend)*; Scent: *Fresh, clean, green, balsamic, coniferous, sweet*; Intensity: 2

Fir, Douglas

(*Pseudotsuga menziesii*)

OTANICAL FAMILY: Pinaceae (conifer)

XTRACTION METHOD/ORIGIN: Steam distillation of leaves and twigs — Canada, USA

HEMICAL CONSTITUENTS: Monoterpenes (approx. 75%): α- & β-pinenes, limonene (up to 18%), Δ-3-carene, camphene, terpinolene; Alcohols (approx. 10%): borneol, geraniol; Esters (approx. 8%): geranyl, bornyl & citronellyl acetates & caproates; Aldehydes: citrals (tr.), benzoic aldehyde; Ketones: camphor; Oxides: 1,8 cineol.

ROPERTIES: ANTISEPTIC, ASTRINGENT, DIURETIC, EXPECTORANT, SEDATIVE (joints, muscles, nerves), and TONIC.

HISTORICAL USES: Though highly regarded for its fragrant scent, the fir tree has been prize through the ages for its medicinal virtues in regards to respiratory complaints, fever, muscular and rheumatic pain.

OTHER POSSIBLE USES: This oil may help with ANXIETY, ASTHMA, BRONCHITIS, CATARRH, COLDS, COUGHS, FLU, INFECTIONS, RESPIRATORY WEAKNESS RHEUMATISM, TENSION (nervous), and WOUNDS. It is very soothing for SORE MUSCLES and has been found to be very effective for calming OVERWORKED or TIRED MUSCLES and JOINTS.

BODY SYSTEM(S) AFFECTED: RESPIRATORY SYSTEM, MUSCLES and BONES.

AROMATIC INFLUENCE: It creates a feeling of GROUNDING, ANCHORING, and EMPOWERMENT. It can STIMULATE the MIND while allowing the BODY to RELAX.

APPLICATION: Diffuse; Apply to VITA FLEX POINTS and directly on AREA of concern.

ORAL USE AS DIETARY SUPPLEMENT: None.

SAFETY DATA: Can irritate sensitive SKIN.

BLEND CLASSIFICATION: Equalizer

BLENDS WITH: German chamomile, cedarwood, cypress, frankincense, juniper, lavender, lemon, myrtle, pine, sandalwood, and rosewood.

Fir, Idaho Balsam

(See Fir, Balsam)

Fir, White (or Giant Fir)

(*Abies grandis*)

BOTANICAL FAMILY: Pinaceae (conifer)

EXTRACTION METHOD/ORIGIN: Steam distillation of leaves/twigs—Canada, France, USA

CHEMICAL CONSTITUENTS: Monoterpenes: pinenes, phellandrene; Esters; Alcohols.

PROPERTIES: ANALGESIC, ANTISEPTIC, ASTRINGENT, DIURETIC, EXPECTORANT SEDATIVE (joints, muscles, nerves), and TONIC.

HISTORICAL USES: Though highly regarded for its fragrant scent, the fir tree has been prized through the ages for its medicinal virtues in regards to respiratory complaints, fever, muscular and rheumatic pain.

OTHER POSSIBLE USES: This oil may help with ANXIETY, ASTHMA, BRONCHITIS, CATARRH, COLDS, COUGHS, FLU, INFECTIONS, RESPIRATORY WEAKNESS, RHEUMATISM, TENSION (nervous), and WOUNDS. It has been found to be very effective for calming OVERWORKED or TIRED MUSCLES and JOINTS and for relieving **PAIN** resulting **FROM INFLAMMATION**.

ODY SYSTEM(S) AFFECTED: EMOTIONAL BALANCE, MUSCLES and BONES, RESPIRATORY SYSTEM.

ROMATIC INFLUENCE: It creates a feeling of GROUNDING, ANCHORING, and EMPOWERMENT. It can STIMULATE the MIND while allowing the BODY to RELAX.

PPLICATION: DIFFUSE; Apply to VITA FLEX POINTS and/or directly on AREA of concern.

RAL USE AS DIETARY SUPPLEMENT: None.

AFETY DATA: Can irritate sensitive SKIN.

LEND CLASSIFICATION: Equalizer

LENDS WITH: German chamomile, cedarwood, cypress, frankincense, juniper, lavender, lemon, myrtle, pine, sandalwood, and rosewood.

Fleabane

(*Conyza canadensis*)

OTANICAL FAMILY: Compositae (daisy)

XTRACTION METHOD/ORIGIN: Steam distillation from stems, leaves, and flowers — Canada

HEMICAL CONSTITUENTS: Monoterpenes: limonene (up to 75%); Sesquiterpenes; Terpene alcohols; Esters: methyl esters (up to 30%), lactones.

ROPERTIES: ANTI-RHEUMATIC, ANTISPASMODIC, CARDIOVASCULAR DILATOR, HORMONE-LIKE.

RENCH MEDICINAL USES: Used by Daniel Pénoël, M.D. to treat children with RETARDED PUBERTY.

THER POSSIBLE USES: May help stimulate the LIVER and PANCREAS. It is a MOOD ENHANCER and promoter of hGH.

ODY SYSTEM(S) AFFECTED: CARDIOVASCULAR and HORMONAL SYSTEMS.

PPLICATION: Apply to VITA FLEX POINTS and directly on AREA of concern; diffuse.

RAL USE AS DIETARY SUPPLEMENT: None.

AFETY DATA: This oil is still under study. Best to DILUTE with V-6 Mixing Oil or Massage Oil.

Frankincense (Olibanum)

(*Boswellia carterii*)

BOTANICAL FAMILY: Burseraceae (resinous trees and shrubs)

EXTRACTION METHOD/ORIGIN: Steam distillation from gum/resin — Somalia

CHEMICAL CONSTITUENTS: Monoterpenes (up to 49%): α-pinene (43%), α-thujene (<8% limonene (<16%), sabinene, myrcene, phellandrene, cymene; Sesquiterpenes: α-gurjunene α-guaiene; Alcohols: borneol, trans-pinocarveol, farnesol; Ketone alcohol: olibanol; Alcohol oxide: incensoloxide.

PROPERTIES: ANTI-CATARRHAL, ANTI-DEPRESSANT, ANTI-INFECTIOUS, ANTISEPTIC, ANTI-TUMORAL, EXPECTORANT, IMMUNE-STIMULANT, and SEDATIVE.

FOLKLORE: One of the gifts given to Christ at His birth. There are over 52 references to frankincense in the Bible (considering that "incense" is translated from the Hebrew/Greek "frankincense" and either refers to the same oil or to a mixture, of which frankincense wa one of the ingredients).

ESOTERIC USES/ACTIONS: Astrological: *Sun & Saturn*; Body type: *Ectomorph*; Chakras: *Links 1 to 7, also 4, 5, & 6*; Character: *Yang-Hot 2nd degree*; Crystals: *Tiger's eye (links 1st to 7th chakra), Amber, Topaz*; Element: *Air, Ether, Light, & Fire*; Number: *3*

HISTORICAL USES: Frankincense is a HOLY OIL in the Middle East. As an ingredient in th holy incense, it was used anciently during sacrificial ceremonies to help improve communication with the CREATOR.

FRENCH MEDICINAL USES: ASTHMA, DEPRESSION, ULCERS.

OTHER POSSIBLE USES: This oil may help with AGING, ALLERGIES, BITES (insect and snake), BRONCHITIS, CANCER, CARBUNCLES, CATARRH, COLDS, COUGHS, DIARRHEA, DIPHTHERIA, GONORRHEA, HEADACHES, HEALING, HEMORRHAGING, HERPES, HIGH BLOOD PRESSURE, INFLAMMATION, JAUNDICE, LARYNGITIS, MENINGITIS, NERVOUS conditions, PROSTATE problems, PNEUMONIA, RESPIRATORY PROBLEMS, preventing SCARRING, SCIATIC PAIN, SORES, SPIRITUAL AWARENESS, STAPH, STREP, STRESS, SYPHILIS, T.B., TENSION, TONSILLITIS, TYPHOID, WOUNDS, and WARTS. It contains sesquiterpenes, enabling it to go beyond the blood-brain barrier. It may also help OXYGENATE the PINEAL and PITUITARY GLANDS. It increases the activity of LEUKOCYTES in defense of the body against infection. Frankincense may also help one have a better attitude, which may help to strengthen the IMMUNE SYSTEM.

BODY SYSTEM(S) AFFECTED: EMOTIONAL BALANCE, IMMUNE and NERVOUS SYSTEMS, SKIN.

AROMATIC INFLUENCE: It increases SPIRITUAL AWARENESS and MEDITATION.

APPLICATION: Apply to VITA FLEX POINTS and/or directly on AREA of concern; diffuse.

ORAL USE AS DIETARY SUPPLEMENT: Approved by the FDA for use as a Food Additive

(FA) and Flavoring Agent (FL). *DILUTE one drop oil in 1 tsp. honey or 4 oz. of beverage (ie. soy/rice milk).* ***Not for children under 6 years old; use with CAUTION and in GREATER DILUTION for children 6 years old and over.***

.END CLASSIFICATION: Enhancer and Equalizer

.ENDS WITH: All oils.

)OR: Type: *Base Note (5-20% of the blend)*; Scent: *Rich, deep, warm, balsamic, sweet, with incense-like overtones*; Intensity: *3*

{EQUENCY: High (Spiritual)

BLE: Exod. 30:34, Lev. 2:1, 2, 15, 16; 5:11; 6:15; 24:7, Num. 5:15, Matt 2:11, Rev. 18:13

Galbanum

(*Ferula gummosa* or *F. galbaniflua*)

)TANICAL FAMILY: Umbelliferae (parsley)

{TRACTION METHOD/ORIGIN: Steam distillation from resin derived from stems and branches — Iran, Turkey, Afghanistan, Lebanon

HEMICAL CONSTITUENTS: Monoterpernes (>84%), α-pinene (>12%), β-pinene (>40%), Δ-3-carene (10-20%), tricyclene, camphene, limonene, myrcene, sabinene, terpinolene, β-phellandrene; Sesquiterpenes: cadinene, myrcene; Sesquiterpenols: guaiol, bulsenol, α-, β-, & γ-eudesmols (=galbanol), 10-γ-epi-junenol, α-cadinol; Ketones: carvone; Esters: fenchyl acetate, linalyl acetate, terpenyl acetate, bornyl acetate; Coumarins: umbelliferone.

{OPERTIES: ANALGESIC, ANTI-INFECTIOUS, ANTI-INFLAMMATORY, ANTIMICROBIAL, ANTISEPTIC, ANTISPASMODIC, ANTIVIRAL, DIURETIC, EXPECTORANT, RESTORATIVE, and TONIC.

SOTERIC USES/ACTIONS: Astrological: *Saturn & Venus*; Character: *Drying, preserving*; Color: *Green*; Odor: *Warm, earthy, green*

ISTORICAL USES: Galbanum was used anciently as an incense and for embalming. It was also combined with frankincense as a holy incense (Exodus 30:34-38) and was only used in the tabernacle during sacrifices. It has also been used for treating wounds, inflammation, and skin disorders.

THER POSSIBLE USES: Galbanum is similar to hyssop, oregano, and frankincense and is recognized for its ANTIVIRAL, body STRENGTHENING and SUPPORTING properties. It may also help with ABSCESSES, ACNE, ASTHMA, BOILS, BRONCHITIS, CATARRH, CHRONIC COUGHS, CRAMPS, CUTS, FLATULENCE, INDIGESTION, INFLAMMATION, MUSCULAR ACHES and PAINS, NERVOUS TENSION, the PINEAL GLAND, POOR CIRCULATION, RHEUMATISM, SCAR TISSUE, SKIN (tones), STRESS RELATED COMPLAINTS, SWOLLEN GLANDS, WRINKLES, and WOUNDS. Some very interesting research is being done with galbanum. It has a low frequency, but when combined with other oils, such as frankincense or sandalwood, the frequency changes drastically. This oil is more than ju medicinal oil.

BODY SYSTEM(S) AFFECTED: IMMUNE SYSTEM.

AROMATIC INFLUENCE: It may help increase SPIRITUAL AWARENESS and MEDITATION and may have a HARMONIZING and BALANCING effect on the psyche.

APPLICATION: Apply to VITA FLEX POINTS and directly on AREA of concern; diffuse.

ORAL USE AS DIETARY SUPPLEMENT: Approved by the FDA for use as a Food Additi (FA) and Flavoring Agent (FL). *DILUTE one drop oil in 1 tsp. honey or 4 oz. of beverage (ie. soy/rice milk).* ***Not for children under 6 years old; use with CAUTION and in GREATER DILUTION for children 6 years old and over.***

BLEND CLASSIFICATION: Enhancer and Equalizer

BLENDS WITH: All oils.

ODOR: Type: *Top Note (5-20% of the blend)*; Scent: *Warm, earthy, green, woody, spicy*; Intensity: *5*

FREQUENCY: Low (Physical); approximately 56.

BIBLE: Exodus 30:34

Geranium

(*Pelargonium graveolens*)

BOTANICAL FAMILY: Geraniaceae

EXTRACTION METHOD/ORIGIN: Steam distillation from leaves — Egypt, India

CHEMICAL CONSTITUENTS: Monoterpenes: α- & β-phellandrene; Sesquiterpenes: 4-guaiadiene-6,9, α-copaene, d- & γ-cadinenes, α- & β-bourbonenes, guaiazulene; Monoterpenols (approx. 65%): geraniol (<23%), citronellol (>32%), linalol, α-terpineol, nerol, menthol; Esters (approx. 35%): citronellyl formiate (>14%), geranyl linalyl formiates, citronellyl & geranyl acetate, citronellyl, geranyl, phenylethyl tiglates; Ketone isomenthone (>8%), methylheptenone, menthone, piperitone; Oxides: 1,8 cineol, cis- & trans-linalol oxide; Aldehydes: neral, geranial (9%), citronellal.

PROPERTIES: ANTI-DEPRESSANT, ANTISEPTIC, ASTRINGENT, DIURETIC, INSECT REPELLENT, REFRESHING, RELAXING, SEDATIVE, and TONIC.

FOLKLORE: During the 1600's, European gardeners would plant geraniums around their hous to keep the evil spirits out. However, this oil is not produced from the same geranium as the house plants.

ESOTERIC USES/ACTIONS: Astrological: *Venus*; Body type: *Endomorph*; Chakra: *2 & 5*; Character: *Yin*; Crystal: *Red Tourmaline*; Element: *Water & Ether*; Number: *4*; Oriental: *Yin deficiencies (pts: Kid-6,Sp-6)*

HISTORICAL USES: Geranium oil has been used for dysentery, hemorrhoids, inflammations, heavy menstrual flow, and possibly even cancer (if the folk tale is correct). It has also been said to be a remedy for bone fractures, tumors, and wounds.

RENCH MEDICINAL USES: DIABETES, DIARRHEA, GALLBLADDER, GASTRIC ULCER, JAUNDICE, LIVER, STERILITY, URINARY STONES.

THER POSSIBLE USES: This oil may be used for ACNE, BLEEDING (increases to eliminate toxins, then stops), BURNS, CIRCULATORY PROBLEMS (improves blood flow), DEPRESSION, DIGESTION, ECZEMA, HORMONAL IMBALANCE, INSOMNIA, KIDNEY STONES, dilating biliary ducts for LIVER DETOXIFICATION, MENSTRUAL PROBLEMS, NEURALGIA (severe pain along the nerve), regenerating TISSUE and NERVES, PANCREAS (balances), RINGWORM, SHINGLES, SKIN (may balance the sebum which is the fatty secretion in the sebaceous glands of the skin that keep the skin supple. Good for expectant mothers, oily skin - as a cleanser, and may even liven up pale skin), SORES, SORE THROATS, and WOUNDS. Geranium opens the LIVER CHAKRA and discharges toxins from the liver that prevent us from having balance.

ODY SYSTEM(S) AFFECTED: EMOTIONAL BALANCE, SKIN.

ROMATIC INFLUENCE: It may help to release NEGATIVE MEMORIES and take us back to PEACEFUL, JOYFUL MOMENTS. It may also help EASE NERVOUS TENSION and STRESS, BALANCE the EMOTIONS, LIFT the SPIRIT, and foster PEACE, WELL BEING, and HOPE.

PPLICATION: Apply to VITA FLEX POINTS and directly on AREA of concern; diffuse.

RAL USE AS DIETARY SUPPLEMENT: Generally regarded as safe (GRAS) for internal consumption by the FDA. *DILUTE one drop oil in 1 tsp. honey or 4 oz. of beverage (ie. soy/rice milk).* ***Not for children under 6 years old; use with CAUTION and in GREATER DILUTION for children 6 years old and over.***

AFETY DATA: Repeated use can possibly result in some CONTACT SENSITIZATION.

LEND CLASSIFICATION: Enhancer and Equalizer

LENDS WITH: All oils.

DOR: Type: *Middle Note (50-80% of the blend)*; Scent: *Sweet, green, citrus-rosy, fresh*; Intensity: *3*

German Chamomile

(See Chamomile, German)

Ginger

(*Zingiber officinale*)

OTANICAL FAMILY: Zingiberaceae (ginger)

EXTRACTION METHOD/ORIGIN: Steam distillation from rhizomes — China, West Indie and many others.

CHEMICAL CONSTITUENTS: Monoterpenes: α and β-pinenes, camphene (8%), myrcene, limonene, β-phellandrene; Sesquiterpenes: zingiberene (up to 30%), cis-γ-bisabolene (>8%), β-sesquiphellandrene (>90%), ar-curcumene (>8%); Monoterpenols: linalol (>1% citronellol (2%); Sesquiterpenols: nerolidol, elemol; Aldehydes: butanal, pentanal, citronellal, geranial; Ketones: acetone, 2-hexanone (>1%), gingerone; Oxide: cineol.

PROPERTIES: ANTISEPTIC, LAXATIVE, STIMULANT, TONIC, and WARMING.

ESOTERIC USES/ACTIONS: Astrological: *Mars*; Body type: *Endomorph*; Chakra: *3 or 1, balances all*; Character: *Yang*; Crystal: *Rhodochrosite*; Element: *Fire*; Number: *8*; Oriental: *Yang deficiencies (pts: St-3, Dir Ves-6)*

HISTORICAL USES: Anciently esteemed as a spice and recognized for its affinity for the digestive system, it has been used in gingerbread (up to 4,000 years ago in Greece), in Egyptian cuisine to ward off epidemics, in Roman wine (for its aphrodisiac powers), in Indian tea (to soothe upset stomachs), and in Chinese tonics (to strengthen the heart and relieve head congestion). It has also been used in Hawaii to scent the clothing, cook with and cure indigestion. They also added it to their shampoos and massage oils.

FRENCH MEDICINAL USES: ANGINA, prevention of CONTAGIOUS DISEASES, COOKING, DIARRHEA, FLATULENCE, IMPOTENCE, RHEUMATIC PAIN, SCURVY, and TONSILLITIS.

OTHER POSSIBLE USES: Ginger may be used for ALCOHOLISM, loss of APPETITE, ARTHRITIS, BROKEN BONES, CATARRH (mucus), CHILLS, COLDS, COLIC, CONGESTION, COUGHS, CRAMPS, DIGESTIVE disorders, FEVERS, FLU, IMPOTENCE, INDIGESTION, INFECTIOUS DISEASES, MEMORY, MOTION SICKNESS, MUSCULAR ACHES/PAINS, NAUSEA, RHEUMATISM, SINUSITIS, SORE THROATS, and SPRAINS. It may also be used in COOKING.

BODY SYSTEM(S) AFFECTED: DIGESTIVE and NERVOUS SYSTEMS.

AROMATIC INFLUENCE: The aroma may help influence physical energy, sex, love, money, and courage.

APPLICATION: Apply to VITA FLEX POINTS and directly on AREA of concern; diffuse.

ORAL USE AS DIETARY SUPPLEMENT: Generally regarded as safe (GRAS) for internal consumption by the FDA. *DILUTE one drop oil in 1 tsp. honey or 4 oz. of beverage (ie soy/rice milk).* ***Not for children under 6 years old; use with CAUTION and in GREATER DILUTION for children 6 years old and over.***

SAFETY DATA: Repeated use can possibly result in CONTACT SENSITIZATION. Avoid direct SUNLIGHT for 3 to 6 hours after use.

BLEND CLASSIFICATION: Personifier and Equalizer

BLENDS WITH: All spice oils, all citrus oils, eucalyptus, frankincense, geranium, myrtle, rosemary, and spearmint.

ODOR: Type: *Middle Note (50-80% of the blend)*; Scent: *Sweet, spicy-woody, warm, tenacious fresh, sharp*; Intensity: *4*

Goldenrod

(*Solidago canadensis*)

OTANICAL FAMILY: Asteraceae or Compositae (daisy)

XTRACTION METHOD/ORIGIN: Steam distillation from stems, leaves, and flowers — Eastern Canada

HEMICAL CONSTITUENTS: Monoterpenes: α-pinene, myrcene, α-phellandrene, limonene; Sesquiterpenes: isolongifolene, germacrene-D; Esters: bornyl acetate, benzoates; Also: methyl chavicol, borneol.

ROPERTIES: RELAXING and CALMING.

SOTERIC USES/ACTIONS: Astrological: *Venus*; Element: *Air*

RADITIONAL USES: DIPHTHERIA, DYSPEPSIA, HYPERTENSION, INFLUENZA, NERVOUSNESS, RESPIRATORY MUCUS, TONSILLITIS and PHARYNGITIS (these uses have not been substantiated by modern clinical research).

THER POSSIBLE USES: According to Franchomme (1990) and as mentioned in the Swiss Pharmacopia, *faltrank*, goldenrod supports the CIRCULATORY SYSTEM including CARDIOVASCULAR PROBLEMS (like tachycardia and arrhythmia), URINARY TRACT, and LIVER FUNCTION. According to the University of Montreal in Canada, goldenrod shows great potential for help with IMPOTENCE.

ODY SYSTEM(S) AFFECTED: CARDIOVASCULAR SYSTEM, HORMONAL SYSTEM.

PPLICATION: Apply to VITA FLEX POINTS and/or directly on AREA of concern; diffuse. According to literature from Young Living Essential Oils, may also be used as a dietary supplement by diluting one drop in 4 oz. of liquid (ie. soy/rice milk or honey).

RAL USE AS DIETARY SUPPLEMENT: None. *Although Young Living Essential Oils recommends the use of this oil as a dietary supplement, the FDA has* ***not yet*** *approved it for use as a food additive (FA) or flavoring agent (FL) (as of 07/01/2004 - see 21CFR172.510 and 21CFR182.20).*

OMPANION OILS: <u>JuvaFlex</u>

OMPANION PRODUCTS: CardiaCare, HRT tincture, JuvaTone, K&B tincture

Grapefruit

(*Citrus x paradisi*)

BOTANICAL FAMILY: Rutaceae (hybrid between *Citrus maxima* and *Citrus sinensis*)

EXTRACTION METHOD/ORIGIN: Cold pressed from rind — California

HEMICAL CONSTITUENTS: Monoterpenes: d-limonene (up to 95%), myrcene, α-pinene, sabinene, β-phellandrene; Ketones: nootketone (very small % but used to detremine harvest time); Terpenols: octonol; Aldehydes (>2%): nonanal, decanal, citrals, citronellal, and others; Coumarins; Furocoumarins.

PROPERTIES: ANTI-DEPRESSANT, ANTISEPTIC, DISINFECTANT, DIURETIC, STIMULANT, and TONIC.

ESOTERIC USES/ACTIONS: Astrological: *Sun*; Body type: *Ectomorph*; Chakra: *1*; Character: *Yang*; Number: *5*; Oriental: *Hot dampness (pts: Sp-9 & 6)*

FRENCH MEDICINAL USES: CELLULITE, DIGESTION, DYSPEPSIA, LYMPHATIC DECONGESTANT, WATER RETENTION.

OTHER POSSIBLE USES: Grapefruit oil may help with DEPRESSION, DRUG WITHDRAWAL, EATING disorders, FATIGUE, GALLSTONES, JET LAG, LIVER disorders, MIGRAINE HEADACHES, OBESITY, PRE-MENSTRUAL TENSION, and STRESS. It may also have a cleansing effect on the KIDNEYS, the LYMPHATIC SYSTEM, and the VASCULAR SYSTEM.

BODY SYSTEM(S) AFFECTED: CARDIOVASCULAR SYSTEM.

AROMATIC INFLUENCE: It may help prevent one from drowning in their own negativity. It is BALANCING and UPLIFTING to the mind, and may help to RELIEVE ANXIETY.

APPLICATION: Apply to VITA FLEX POINTS and/or directly on AREA of concern; diffuse. Because grapefruit oil has many of the same uses as other citrus oils, it can be used in the place when immediate exposure to the sun is unavoidable. This is because grapefruit oil does not have the photosensitivity that the other citrus oils have.

ORAL USE AS DIETARY SUPPLEMENT: Generally regarded as safe (GRAS) for internal consumption by the FDA. *DILUTE one drop oil in 1 tsp. honey or 4 oz. of beverage (ie. soy/rice milk).* ***Not for children under 6 years old; use with CAUTION and in GREATER DILUTION for children 6 years old and over.***

COMPANION OILS: Citrus oils.

BLEND CLASSIFICATION: Modifier and Enhancer.

BLENDS WITH: Basil, bergamot, cedarwood, chamomile, cypress, frankincense, geranium, juniper, lavender, peppermint, rosemary, rosewood, and ylang ylang.

ODOR: Type: *Top Note (5-20% of the blend)*; Scent: *Clean, fresh, bitter, citrusy*; Intensity: *2*

Helichrysum

(*Helichrysum angustifolia var. italicum*)

BOTANICAL FAMILY: Compositae

EXTRACTION METHOD/ORIGIN: Steam distilled from flowers — Yugoslavia, France, Italy *(Note: Since the supply of pure, therapeutic grade helichrysum can be somewhat erratic at times, similar therapeutic results have been achieved by using a blend of 3 oils as follows: 5 drops elemi, 5 drops Idaho tansy, 1 drop birch or wintergreen)*

CHEMICAL CONSTITUENTS: Monoterpenes: limonene (<13%), α-pinene (<8%), γ-curcumene (<15%); Sesquiterpenes: β-caryophyllene; Monoterpenols: nerol (<5%), geraniol, linalol (<4%); Phenol: eugenol; Terpene esters: neryl acetate (up to 35%); Ketones.

ROPERTIES: ANTI-CATARRHAL, ANTI-COAGULANT, ANTIOXIDANT, ANTISPASMODIC, EXPECTORANT, and MUCOLYTIC.

OLKLORE: Helichrysum, as an ornamental dried flower, retains its fragrance, color, and shape almost forever. Hence the other names, "Everlasting" or "Immortelle", by which it is commonly known.

SOTERIC USES/ACTIONS: Astrological: *Jupiter*; Chakra: *6*; Character: *Yin*

IISTORICAL USES: Helichrysum has been used for asthma, bronchitis, whooping cough, headaches, liver ailments, and skin disorders.

RENCH MEDICINAL USES: BLOOD CLEANSING, CHELATING AGENT for METALLICS, CHEMICALS, and TOXINS, viral COLITIS, DETOXIFICATION, GALLBLADDER INFECTION, HEMATOMA, HYPO-CHOLESTEROL, LIVER CELL FUNCTION STIMULANT, LYMPH DRAINAGE, reduces PAIN, PANCREAS STIMULANT, PHLEBITIS, SCIATICA, SINUS INFECTION, SKIN CONDITIONS (Eczema, Dermatitis, Psoriasis), STOMACH CRAMPS, SUN SCREEN.

THER POSSIBLE USES: This oil may help ANGER, stop BLEEDING, CIRCULATORY functions, GALLBLADDER INFECTION, improve **HEARING**, HEMATOMA (swelling or tumor full of diffused blood), detoxify and stimulate the LIVER cell function, LYMPH DRAINAGE, PAIN (acute), relieve RESPIRATORY conditions, reduce SCARRING, SCAR TISSUE, reduce TISSUE PAIN, regenerate TISSUE, and VARICOSE VEINS.

ODY SYSTEM(S) AFFECTED: CARDIOVASCULAR SYSTEM, MUSCLES and BONES.

ROMATIC INFLUENCE: It is UPLIFTING to the subconscious and may possess the ability to cut through BARRIERS of anger, allowing one to forgive trespasses against them and move forward in life.

PPLICATION: Apply to VITA FLEX POINTS and directly on AREA of concern; diffuse.

RAL USE AS DIETARY SUPPLEMENT: Generally regarded as safe (GRAS) for internal consumption by the FDA. *DILUTE one drop oil in 1 tsp. honey or 4 oz. of beverage (ie. soy/rice milk).* ***Not for children under 6 years old; use with CAUTION and in GREATER DILUTION for children 6 years old and over.***

LEND CLASSIFICATION: Personifier

LENDS WITH: Geranium, Clary sage, rose, lavender, spice oils and citrus oils.

DOR: Type: *Middle Note (50-80% of the blend)*; Scent: *Rich, sweet, fruity, with tea and honey undertones*; Intensity: *3*

REQUENCY: High (Spiritual); approximately 181 MHz.

Hyssop

(*Hyssopus officinalis*)

BOTANICAL FAMILY: Labiatae (mint)

EXTRACTION METHOD/ORIGIN: Steam distilled from stems/leaves — France, Hungary

CHEMICAL CONSTITUENTS: Monoterpenes (< 25%); β-pinenes (15-22%), limonene, camphene, cadinene; Sesquiterpenes (12%): β-caryophyllene, germacrene-D, phellandrene Phenol methyl-ethers (4%): myrtenol, chavicol; Ketones (up to 58%): α and β-thujones, camphor, isopinocamphone (up to 31%), pinocamphone (up to 12%); Alcohols: nerolidol linalol, geraniol, borneol; Oxide: 1,8 cineol.

PROPERTIES: ANTI-ASTHMATIC, ANTI-CATARRHAL, ANTI-INFECTIOUS, ANTI-INFLAMMATORY, ANTIOXIDANT, ANTI-PARASITIC, ANTISEPTIC, ANTISPASMODIC, ANTIVIRAL, ASTRINGENT, DECONGESTANT, DIURETIC, MUCOLYTIC, and SEDATIVE.

ESOTERIC USES/ACTIONS: Astrological: *Jupiter*; Chakra: *4, 3*; Character: *Yang*; Crystals: *Lapis lazuli, Amethyst*; Element: *Fire*

HISTORICAL USES: Hyssop is mentioned in Exodus Chapter 12 as the oil in lamb's blood. I was used to prevent the Plague, which may be similar to AIDS today.

OTHER POSSIBLE USES: This oil may be beneficial for ANXIETY, restoring APPETITE, ARTHRITIS, ASTHMA, BRUISES, CLEANSING and purifying, COLDS, CONCENTRATION (alertness - stimulating and clearing the mind), COUGHS, CUTS, DERMATITIS, DIGESTION, FATIGUE (strengthens and enlivens the body), FEVER, expelling GAS from intestines, GOUT, GRIEF, regulating LIPID METABOLISM, raising LOW BLOOD PRESSURE, clearing LUNGS, promoting and regulating MENSTRUAL FLOW, discharging MUCUS, NERVOUS TENSION, PARASITES (expelling worms), increasing PERSPIRATION, RHEUMATISM, preventing SCARRING, SCAR TISSUE, SORE THROATS, STRESS related conditions, TONSILLITIS, discharging TOXINS, VIRAL INFECTIONS, and WOUNDS.

BODY SYSTEM(S) AFFECTED: CARDIOVASCULAR, NERVOUS, and RESPIRATORY SYSTEMS.

AROMATIC INFLUENCE: It may help stimulate CREATIVITY and MEDITATION and promote CENTERING.

APPLICATION: Apply to VITA FLEX POINTS and directly on AREA of concern; *diffuse*.

ORAL USE AS DIETARY SUPPLEMENT: Generally regarded as safe (GRAS) for internal consumption by the FDA. *DILUTE one drop oil in 1 tsp. honey or 4 oz. of beverage (ie. soy/rice milk). However, due to high ketone content, extreme caution should be taken.* ***Best AVOIDED by children of any age.***

SAFETY DATA: According to some sources, the pinocamphone can cause toxic effects. Avoid during PREGNANCY. Avoid if dealing with HIGH BLOOD PRESSURE. Not for use by people with EPILEPSY. Use extreme caution and DILUTE WELL when unsure!

OMPANION OILS: All citrus oils, Clary sage, sage, myrtle, geranium, and fennel.

LEND CLASSIFICATION: Enhancer, Equalizer, and Modifier

DOR: Type: *Middle Note (50-80% of the blend)*; Scent: *Fresh, earthy, woody, fruity, slightly sweet*; Intensity: *3*

IBLE: According to the Bible, hyssop ***purges*** and ***cleanses***. See the following: Exodus 12:22; Lev. 14:4, 6, 49,51,52; Num. 19:6,18; 1Kings 4:33; Psalms 51:7

Idaho Balsam Fir

(***See Fir, Balsam***)

Idaho Tansy

(***See Tansy, Idaho***)

Jasmine

(*Jasminum officinale*)

OTANICAL FAMILY: Oleaceae (olive)

XTRACTION METHOD/ORIGIN: Absolute extraction from flowers (jasmine is actually an "essence" not an essential oil. The flowers must be picked at night to maximize the fragrance) — India

HEMICAL CONSTITUENTS: Esters: benzyl acetate (<28%), benzyl benzoate (<21%), methyl anthralilate, methyl jasmonate; Alcohols: linalol (<8%), phytol (<12%), benzyl alcohol, farnesol; Ketone: cis-jasmone.

ROPERTIES: ANTI-CATARRHAL, ANTI-DEPRESSANT, and ANTISPASMODIC.

SOTERIC USES/ACTIONS: Astrological: *Moon & Jupiter*; Ayurvedic: *Pitta*; Body type: *Mesomorph*; Chakra: *2*; Character: *Yang (flowers-Yin, oil-Yang, Yin when diluted)*; Crystals: *Ruby, Red Jasper, Quartz, Moonstone, Sapphire*; Element: *Water & Fire*; Number: *9*; Oriental: *Cold & Dry*

ISTORICAL USES: Known in India as the "queen of the night" and "moonlight of the grove", women have treasured it for centuries for its beautiful, aphrodisiac-like fragrance. According to Roberta Wilson, "In many religious traditions, the jasmine flower symbolizes hope, happiness, and love." Jasmine has been used for hepatitis, cirrhosis of the liver, dysentery, depression, nervousness, coughs, respiratory congestion, reproductive problems, and "to stimulate uterine contractions in pregnant women as childbirth approached." It was also used in teas, perfumes, and incense.

OTHER POSSIBLE USES: This oil may help with CATARRH (mucus), CONJUNCTIVITIS, COUGHS, DYSENTERY, ECZEMA (when caused by emotions), FRIGIDITY, HEPATITIS (cirrhosis of the liver), HOARSENESS, LABOR PAINS, LARYNGITIS, LETHARGY (abnormal drowsiness), MENSTRUAL PAIN and PROBLEMS, MUSCLE SPASMS, NERVOUS EXHAUSTION and TENSION, PAIN RELIEF, RESPIRATORY conditions, SEX, SKIN CARE (dry, greasy, irritated, and sensitive), SPRAINS, and UTERINE disorders. Jasmine is an oil that affects the EMOTIONS; it penetrates the deepest layers of the soul, opening doors to our emotions. It produces a feeling of CONFIDENCE, ENERGY, EUPHORIA, and OPTIMISM. It helps to reduce ANXIETY, APATHY, DEPRESSION, DILEMMAS that deal with RELATIONSHIPS, INDIFFERENCE, and LISTLESSNESS. When worn as a cologne, it increases feelings of ATTRACTIVENESS.

BODY SYSTEM(S) AFFECTED: EMOTIONAL BALANCE, HORMONAL SYSTEM.

AROMATIC INFLUENCE: It is very UPLIFTING to the EMOTIONS and may help increase INTUITIVE powers and WISDOM. It may also help to promote powerful, inspirational RELATIONSHIPS.

APPLICATION: Apply to VITA FLEX POINTS and directly on AREA of concern; diffuse.

ORAL USE AS DIETARY SUPPLEMENT: Generally regarded as safe (GRAS) for internal consumption by the FDA. *DILUTE one drop oil in 1 tsp. honey or 4 oz. of beverage (ie soy/rice milk).* ***Not for children under 6 years old; use with CAUTION and in GREATER DILUTION for children 6 years old and over.***

BLEND CLASSIFICATION: Equalizer, Modifier, and Enhancer

BLENDS WITH: Bergamot, frankincense, geranium, helichrysum, lemongrass, mandarin, melissa, orange, palmarosa, rose, rosewood, sandalwood, spearmint.

ODOR: Type: *Base Note (5-20% of the blend)*; Scent: *Powerful, sweet, tenacious, floral with fruity-herbaceous undertones*; Intensity: *4*

NOTE: *One pound of jasmine oil requires about 1,000 pounds of jasmine or 3.6 million fresh picked blossoms. The blossoms must be collected before sunrise, or much of the fragrance will have evaporated. The quality of the blossoms can also be compromised they are squashed. A single 1 lb. can of pure jasmine oil can cost from $1,200 to $4,500. In contrast, synthetic jasmine oils can be obtained for $3.50 per pound, but th obviously do not possess the same therapeutic qualities as pure jasmine oil. The above mentioned properties and possible uses are based on pure jasmine oil, not synthetic oil*

Juniper (or Rocky Mountain Juniper)

(*Juniperus osteosperma* and/or *J. scopulorum*)

BOTANICAL FAMILY: Cupressaceae (conifer - cypress)

EXTRACTION METHOD/ORIGIN: Steam distilled from berries and twigs — Utah

IEMICAL CONSTITUENTS: Monoterpenes (>50%): α-pinene (up to 40%), sabinene (<18%), myrcene (<6%), limonene (<8%); Sesquiterpenes; Esters: bornyl acetate (up to 20%); Alcohols (up to 18%): camphor, terpinen-4-ol (<8%); Aldyhydes; Ketones: pinocamphone.

ROPERTIES: ANTISEPTIC, ANTISPASMODIC, ASTRINGENT, CLEANSER, DETOXIFIER, DIURETIC, STIMULANT, and TONIC.

)LKLORE: According to Roberta Wilson, "During biblical times, juniper was often used to banish evil spirits." Also, during Medieval times, "Bundles of juniper berries were hung over doors to ward off witches, and burning juniper wood supposedly deterred demons."

SOTERIC USES/ACTIONS: Astrological: *Sun & Jupiter*; Ayurvedic: *Kapha*; Chakra: *3 & 6*; Character: *Yin*; Crystal: *Red Jasper*; Element: *Fire*

ISTORICAL USES: Over the centuries, juniper has been used for embalming, for physical and spiritual purification, to cleanse infections and heal wounds, for liver complaints, to relieve arthritis and urinary tract infections, to ward off plagues, epidemics, and contagious diseases, for headaches, kidney and bladder problems, pulmonary infections, and fevers.

RENCH MEDICINAL USES: ACNE, DERMATITIS, ECZEMA.

THER POSSIBLE USES: This oil may work as a DETOXIFIER and a CLEANSER which may reduce ACNE, DERMATITIS, and ECZEMA. It may also help COUGHS, DEPRESSION, ENERGY, INFECTION, increase circulation through KIDNEYS, KIDNEY STONES, LIVER PROBLEMS, aching MUSCLES, NERVE FUNCTION and REGENERATION, OBESITY, RHEUMATISM (promotes excretion of uric acid and toxins), ULCERS, URINARY INFECTIONS, WATER RETENTION, and WOUNDS.

ODY SYSTEM(S) AFFECTED: DIGESTIVE SYSTEM, EMOTIONAL BALANCE (aromatic), NERVOUS SYSTEM, SKIN.

ROMATIC INFLUENCE: Juniper evokes feelings of HEALTH, LOVE, and PEACE and may help to ELEVATE one's SPIRITUAL AWARENESS.

PPLICATION: Apply to VITA FLEX POINTS and/or directly on AREA of concern; diffuse. Juniper may also be applied to the FOREHEAD to enhance feelings of OPTIMISM, or on the CHEEKS for CONFIDENCE and EUPHORIA.

RAL USE AS DIETARY SUPPLEMENT: *As of July 1, 2004, the FDA has NOT given this variety of juniper the designation of GRAS (Generally Regarded As Safe for internal consumption) (see 21CFR182.20).* ***Not recommended for internal consumption.***

LEND CLASSIFICATION: Equalizer

LENDS WITH: Bergamot, all citrus oils, cypress, geranium, lavender, melaleuca (tea-tree), Melrose, and rosemary.

DOR: Type: *Middle Note (50-80% of the blend)*; Scent: *Sweet, musky, tenacious*; Intensity: *3*

REQUENCY: Emotional; approximately 98 MHz.

IBLE: Job 30:4

Laurel (Bay or Sweet Bay)

(*Laurus nobilis*)

BOTANICAL FAMILY: Lauraceae

EXTRACTION METHOD/ORIGIN: Steam distilled from leaves — France

CHEMICAL CONSTITUENTS: Monoterpenes: α and β-pinenes, sabinene (> 10%), limonen Sesquiterpenes: β-elemene, β-caryophyllene, α-humulene, phellandrene; Alcohols: linalo (>15%), geraniol, α-terpineol, terpinen-4-ol, cis-thujanol-4; Esters: terpinyl acetate (up t 10%), bornyl, geranyl & linalyl acetates; Phenol methyl-ethers: eugenol (<2%); Oxides: 1,8 cineol (up to 50%); Sesquiterpene lactones.

PROPERTIES: ANTISEPTIC, DIGESTIVE, DIURETIC, ANTI-FUNGAL.

FOLKLORE: Ancient Greek and Roman generals would wear crowns of laurel leaves when victorious in battle. Both the Greeks and the Romans believed that the laurel tree had great powers of divination and prophecy, and that all one had to do to avoid thunder and lightning or evil spirits was to run under a laurel tree.

ESOTERIC USES/ACTIONS: Astrological: *Sun*; Body type: *Ectomorph*; Chakras: *2, 3, & 4*; Character: *Yin (medium)*; Element: *Fire*; Number: *1*

HISTORICAL USES: Both the leaves and the black berries were also used to alleviate colic, indigestion, and loss of appetite. During the Middle Ages, it was used for angina pectori asthma, fever, gout, migraine, palpitations, and liver and spleen complaints. Laurel has also been used as a fragrance component in cosmetics and perfumes.

OTHER POSSIBLE USES: Laurel oil is primarily produced in the country formerly known as Yugoslavia. Laurel may help with loss of APPETITE, ASTHMATIC CONDITIONS, CHRONIC BRONCHITIS, DYSPEPSIA, FLATULENCE, FLU, HAIR LOSS (after a infection), PEDICULOSIS, SCABIES, VIRAL INFECTIONS.

BODY SYSTEM(S) AFFECTED: DIGESTIVE, IMMUNE, and RESPIRATORY SYSTEM

AROMATIC INFLUENCE: It has a spicy, medicinal odor.

APPLICATION: Apply to VITA FLEX POINTS and/or directly on AREA of concern.

ORAL USE AS DIETARY SUPPLEMENT: Generally regarded as safe (GRAS) for internal consumption by the FDA. *DILUTE one drop oil in 1 tsp. honey or 4 oz. of beverage (i soy/rice milk).* ***Not for children under 6 years old; use with CAUTION and in GREATER DILUTION for children 6 years old and over.***

SAFETY DATA: Repeated use can possibly result in CONTACT SENSITIZATION. Moderate use is recommended. Avoid during PREGNANCY.

ODOR: Type: *Top to Middle Notes (20-80% of the blend)*; Scent: *Sweet, fresh, spicy, camphorous, medicinal*; Intensity: *3*

Lavandin

(*Lavandula x hybrida*)

BOTANICAL FAMILY: Labiatae

CHEMICAL CONSTITUENTS: Monoterpenes: limonene, cis- & trans-ocimenes; Esters (<45%): linalyl acetate, bornyl acetate, lavandulyl acetate, geranyl acetate; Alcohols: linalol (> 40%), borneol, lavendulol, terpineol, terpinen-4-ol; Ketones: camphor (>5%); Oxides: 1,8 cineol.

PROPERTIES: ANTI-BACTERIAL, ANTI-FUNGAL, and strong ANTISEPTIC. (See LAVENDER for additional properties.)

ESOTERIC USES/ACTIONS: Astrological: *Mercury*; Body type: *Endomorph*; Chakra: *4*; Character: *Almost neutral (leans Yang)*; Crystals: *Flourite, Amethyst*; Element: *Air*; Number: *7*

HISTORICAL USES: Also known as *Lavandula x intermedia*, lavandin is a hybrid plant developed by crossing true lavender with spike lavender or aspic (*Lavandula Latifolia*). It has been used to sterilize the animal cages in veterinary clinics and hospitals throughout Europe. There is not a long history of the therapeutic use of lavandin as it was most often used to adulterate true lavender oils.

OTHER POSSIBLE USES: Lavandin can be used in the same way as true lavender (see LAVENDER) ***except NOT for burns***. It is more penetrating and has a much sharper scent.

BODY SYSTEM(S) AFFECTED: CARDIOVASCULAR SYSTEM, MUSCLES and BONES, RESPIRATORY SYSTEM.

AROMATIC INFLUENCE: It has the same calming effects as lavender.

APPLICATION: Apply to VITA FLEX POINTS and/or directly on AREA of concern; diffuse.

ORAL USE AS DIETARY SUPPLEMENT: Generally regarded as safe (GRAS) for internal consumption by the FDA. *DILUTE one drop oil in 1 tsp. honey or 4 oz. of beverage (ie. soy/rice milk).* ***Not for children under 6 years old; use with CAUTION and in GREATER DILUTION for children 6 years old and over.***

SAFETY DATA: Use with caution if susceptible to EPILEPSY. Avoid during PREGNANCY. DO NOT USE FOR BURNS!

BLENDS WITH: Bergamot, cinnamon bark, citronella, clove, cypress, Clary sage, geranium, lime, patchouli, pine, rosemary, and thyme.

ODOR: Type: *Top to Middle Notes (20-80% of the blend)*; Scent: *Fresh, sweet, floral, more herbaceous than Lavender*; Intensity: *3*

Lavender

(*Lavandula angustifolia*)

BOTANICAL FAMILY: Labiatae (mint)

EXTRACTION METHOD/ORIGIN: Steam distilled from flowering top — France, Idaho, Utah

CHEMICAL CONSTITUENTS: Monoterpenes (>5%): α-pinene, camphene, Δ-3-carene, limonene; Sesquiterpenes: β-caryophyllene, β-farnesene; Alcohols (45%): linalol (>41%), geraniol, borneol, lavendulol, nerol; Esters (approx. 50%): linalyl acetate (up to 45%), terpenyl acetate, geranyl & lavendulyl acetate; Oxides: 1,8 cineol, linaloxide, caryophyllene oxide; Ketones: camphor; Aldehydes; Lactones; Coumarins.

PROPERTIES: ANALGESIC, ANTI-COAGULANT, ANTI-CONVULSIVE, ANTI-DEPRESSANT, ANTI-FUNGAL, ANTIHISTAMINE, ANTI-INFECTIOUS, ANTI-INFLAMMATORY, ANTISEPTIC, ANTISPASMODIC, ANTITOXIC, CARDIO-TONIC, REGENERATIVE, and SEDATIVE.

ESOTERIC USES/ACTIONS: Astrological: *Mercury*; Body type: *Ectomorph*; Chakras: *4 & 7* Character: *Neutral, Yin but leans Yang*; Crystals: *Flourite, Amethyst*; Element: *Air & Ether*; Number: *7*; Oriental: *Excess Yang (pts: Liv-2, He-3)*

HISTORICAL USES: During Medieval times, people were obviously divided on the properties of lavender regarding love. Some would claim that it could keep the wearer chaste, while others claimed just the opposite–touting its aphrodisiac qualities. The list of historical uses for lavender is quite long as it was used for just about everything.

FRENCH MEDICINAL USES: ACNE, ALLERGIES, BURNS (cell renewal), CRAMPS (leg) DANDRUFF, DIAPER RASH, FLATULENCE, HAIR LOSS, HERPES, INDIGESTION, INSOMNIA, LOWER BLOOD PRESSURE, LYMPHATIC SYSTEM DRAINAGE, MENOPAUSAL CONDITIONS, MOUTH ABSCESS, NAUSEA, PHLEBITIS, PRE-MENSTRUAL CONDITIONS, SCARRING (minimizes), STRETCH MARKS, TACHYCARDIA, THRUSH, WATER RETENTION.

OTHER POSSIBLE USES: Lavender is a universal oil that has traditionally been known to balance the body and to work wherever there is a need. If in doubt, use lavender. It may help ARTHRITIS, ASTHMA, BALANCING BODY SYSTEMS, BOILS, BRONCHITIS, BRUISES, CARBUNCLES, COLD SORES, CONVULSIONS, DEPRESSION, EARACHES, FAINTING, GALLSTONES, HAY FEVER, relieve HEADACHES, HEART (irregularity), reduce HIGH BLOOD PRESSURE, HIVES (urticaria), HYSTERIA, INSECT BITES and BEE STINGS, INFECTION, INFLUENZA, INJURIES, LARYNGITIS, MIGRAINE HEADACHES, MOUTH ABSCESS, reduce MUCUS, NERVOUS TENSION, PINEAL GLAND (activates), RESPIRATORY FUNCTION, RHEUMATISM, SKIN CONDITIONS (eczema, psoriasis, rashes), SPRAINS, STRESS, SUNBURNS (including lips), SUNSTROKE, TENSION, THROAT INFECTIONS, TUBERCULOSIS, TYPHOID FEVER, WHOOPING COUGH, AND WOUNDS. One of our readers suggested putting a drop of lavender in the mascara bottle to thin it out and get more shine from eye lashes.

ODY SYSTEM(S) AFFECTED: CARDIOVASCULAR SYSTEM, EMOTIONAL BALANCE, NERVOUS SYSTEM, SKIN.

ROMATIC INFLUENCE: It promotes CONSCIOUSNESS, HEALTH, LOVE, PEACE and a general sense of WELL BEING.

PPLICATION: Apply to VITA FLEX POINTS and directly on AREA of concern; diffuse.

RAL USE AS DIETARY SUPPLEMENT: *As of July 1, 2004, the FDA has NOT given this variety of lavender the designation of GRAS (Generally Regarded As Safe for internal consumption) (see 21CFR182.20).* ***Not recommended for internal consumption.***

LEND CLASSIFICATION: Enhancer and Modifier and Equalizer

LENDS WITH: Most oils especially citrus oils, chamomile, Clary sage, and geranium.

DOR: Type: *Middle Note (50-80% of the blend)*; Scent: *Floral, sweet, herbaceous, balsamic, woody undertones*; Intensity: *2*

REQUENCY: Emotional and Spiritual; approximately 118.

Ledum (or Labrador Tea)

(*Ledum groenlandicum*)

OTANICAL FAMILY: Ericaceae (heather)

XTRACTION METHOD/ORIGIN: Steam distilled from leaves — Canada

HEMICAL CONSTITUENTS: Monoterpenes (mostly): limonene (up to 35%), α and β-terpenes, sabinene, γ-terpinenes; Sesquiterpenes: α-selinene, selinadiene; Alcohols: α-terpineol, terpinen-4-ol, ledol; Aldehydes: myrtenal; Ketones: germacrone; Esters: bornyl acetate & butyrate.

ROPERTIES: ANTI-CANCEROUS, ANTI-TUMORAL, ANTIVIRAL, NERVE-STIMULANT, and TONIC.

ISTORICAL USES: Ledum tea has been used for all types of skin problems, kidney-related problems, coughs, and hoarseness. Some sources say it was used by the eskimos of the arctic region to fight cancer. Other natives of North America have used ledum tea to fight scurvy for thousands of years. According to Laurie Lacey, "The Cree named this plant **muskeko-pukwan**, and used it to treat fevers, colds, and other conditions."

THER POSSIBLE USES: This oil may be beneficial for ADD, ALLERGIES, BRONCHITIS, COLDS, EDEMA, FEVER, HEPATITIS (viral), INFLUENZA, LARYNGITIS, LYMPH NODES (inflamed), SKIN PROBLEMS (all kinds), and THYROID REGULATION. It may also be a wonderful support to the URINARY TRACT, RESPIRATORY SYSTEM, and IMMUNE SYSTEM, as well as a powerful LIVER support and detoxifier (best when combined with JuvaTone). Research has indicated that this oil may contain more anti-cancerous and anti-tumoral properties than frankincense.

BODY SYSTEM(S) AFFECTED: DIGESTIVE and IMMUNE SYSTEMS, SKIN.

APPLICATION: DIFFUSE or apply to VITA FLEX POINTS and/or directly on AREA of concern. Best DILUTED in one teaspoon of V-6 Mixing Oil or Massage Oil for topical application. According to literature from Young Living Essential Oils, may also be used as a dietary supplement by diluting one drop of oil in 4 oz. of liquid (ie. soy/rice milk or honey).

ORAL USE AS DIETARY SUPPLEMENT: None. *Although Young Living Essential Oils recommends the use of this oil as a dietary supplement, the FDA has **not yet** approved for use as a food additive (FA) or flavoring agent (FL) (as of 07/01/2004 - see 21CFR172.510 and 21CFR182.20).*

COMPANION OILS: JuvaFlex, Raven, R.C..

COMPANION PRODUCTS: JuvaTone, K&B Tincture, Super C, Thyromin.

Lemon

(*Citrus limon*)

BOTANICAL FAMILY: Rutaceae (citrus)

EXTRACTION METHOD/ORIGIN: Cold pressed from rind (requires 3,000 lemons to produ a kilo of oil) — California, Italy

CHEMICAL CONSTITUENTS: Monoterpenes: d-limonene (up to 72%), α- & γ-terpinenes (14%), paracymene, α- & β-phellandrene, terpinolene, sabinene; Sesquiterpenes: β-bisabolene; Alcohols: Hexanol, octanol, nonanol, decanol, linalol, geraniol; Aldehydes (> 3%): heptanal, octanal, geranial, neral; Coumarins and Furocoumarins (>5%): umberlliferone, bergamotene, bergaptol, bergaptene. Also contains flavonoids, carotenoids, steroids.

PROPERTIES: ANTISEPTIC, ANTIVIRAL, ASTRINGENT, INVIGORATING, REFRESHING, and TONIC.

ESOTERIC USES/ACTIONS: Astrological: *Saturn & Moon*; Body type: *Mesomorph*; Chakra *3*; Character: *Yang*; Element: *Water & Fire*; Number: *7*; Oriental: *Blood stagnation (pts Sp-10 & 6), Hot phlegm (pts: St-40, S-6)*

HISTORICAL USES: Lemon has been used to fight food poisoning, malaria and typhoid epidemics, and scurvy (in fact, sources say that Christopher Columbus carried lemon see to America–probably just the left overs from the fruit that was eaten during the trip). Lemon has also been used to lower blood pressure and to help with liver problems, arthritis, and muscular aches and pains.

FRENCH MEDICINAL USES: AIR DISINFECTANT, ANEMIA, ASTHMA, COLD, FEVER (reduces), GERMICIDE, GOUT, HEARTBURN, INTESTINAL PARASITES RED BLOOD CELL FORMATION, RHEUMATISM, THROAT INFECTION, URETER INFECTIONS, VARICOSE VEINS, WATER PURIFICATION, WHITE

BLOOD CELL FORMATION.

OTHER POSSIBLE USES: This oil may be beneficial for ANXIETY, BLOOD PRESSURE, soothing broken CAPILLARIES, dissolving CELLULITE, CLARITY of thought, DEBILITY, DIGESTIVE PROBLEMS, ENERGY, GALLSTONES, HAIR (cleansing), promoting LEUKOCYTE FORMATION, LIVER deficiencies in children, LYMPHATIC SYSTEM CLEANSING, MEMORY IMPROVEMENT, NAILS (strengthening and hardening), NERVOUS CONDITIONS, RESPIRATORY PROBLEMS, cleaning the SKIN of dirty kids, SORE THROATS, and promoting a sense of WELL BEING. It works extremely well in REMOVING GUM, WOOD STAIN, OIL, and GREASE SPOTS. It may also brighten a pale, dull COMPLEXION by removing dead skin cells.

BODY SYSTEM(S) AFFECTED: DIGESTIVE, IMMUNE, and RESPIRATORY SYSTEMS.

AROMATIC INFLUENCE: It promotes HEALTH, HEALING, PHYSICAL ENERGY, and PURIFICATION. Its fragrance is INVIGORATING, ENHANCING, and WARMING.

APPLICATION: Apply to VITA FLEX POINTS and directly on AREA of concern; Diffuse.

ORAL USE AS DIETARY SUPPLEMENT: Generally regarded as safe (GRAS) for internal consumption by the FDA. *DILUTE one drop oil in 1 tsp. honey or 4 oz. of beverage (ie. soy/rice milk).* ***Not for children under 6 years old; use with CAUTION and in GREATER DILUTION for children 6 years old and over.***

SAFETY DATA: Avoid direct SUNLIGHT for up to 12 hours after use. Can cause extreme SKIN IRRITATION.

BLEND CLASSIFICATION: Modifier and Enhancer

BLENDS WITH: Chamomile, eucalyptus, fennel, frankincense, geranium, juniper, peppermint, sandalwood, and ylang ylang.

ODOR: Type: *Top Note (5-20% of the blend)*; Scent: *Sweet, sharp, clear, citrusy*; Intensity: *3*

Lemongrass

(*Cymbopogon flexuosus*)

BOTANICAL FAMILY: Gramineae (grasses)

EXTRACTION METHOD/ORIGIN: Steam distilled from leaves — India, Guatemala

CHEMICAL CONSTITUENTS: Aldehydes: citrals (up to 85%): neral, geranial, farnesal; Alcohols: α-terpenol, borneol, geraniol, nerol, linalol, citronellol; Sesquiterpene alcohols: farnesol (> 13%).

PROPERTIES: ANALGESIC, ANTI-INFLAMMATORY, ANTISEPTIC, INSECT REPELLENT, REVITALIZER, SEDATIVE, TONIC, and VASODILATOR.

HISTORICAL USES: Lemongrass has been used for infectious illnesses and fever, an insecticide, and as a sedative to the central nervous system.

FRENCH MEDICINAL USES: BLADDER INFECTION (cystitis), CONNECTIVE TISSUE (regenerates), DIGESTIVE SYSTEM, EDEMA, FLUID RETENTION, KIDNEY

DISORDERS, LYMPHATIC DRAINAGE, PARASYMPATHETIC NERVOUS SYSTEM (regulates), VARICOSE VEINS, VASCULAR WALLS (strengthens).

OTHER POSSIBLE USES: This oil may help improve CIRCULATION, improve DIGESTION, improve EYESIGHT, FEVERS, FLATULENCE, HEADACHES, clear INFECTIONS, repair **LIGAMENTS**, wake up the LYMPHATIC SYSTEM, get the OXYGEN flowing, PURIFICATION, RESPIRATORY PROBLEMS, SORE THROATS, TISSUE REGENERATION, and WATER RETENTION.

BODY SYSTEM(S) AFFECTED: IMMUNE SYSTEM, MUSCLES and BONES.

AROMATIC INFLUENCE: It promotes PSYCHIC AWARENESS and PURIFICATION.

APPLICATION: Apply to VITA FLEX POINTS or directly on AREA of concern; diffuse.

ORAL USE AS DIETARY SUPPLEMENT: Generally regarded as safe (GRAS) for internal consumption by the FDA. *DILUTE one drop oil in 1 tsp. honey or 4 oz. of beverage (ie. soy/rice milk).* ***Not for children under 6 years old; use with CAUTION and in GREATER DILUTION for children 6 years old and over.***

SAFETY DATA: ***Can cause extreme SKIN IRRITATION.***

BLEND CLASSIFICATION: Enhancer and Equalizer

BLENDS WITH: Basil, cedarwood, Clary sage, eucalyptus, geranium, jasmine, lavender, melaleuca (tea-tree), and rosemary.

ODOR: Type: *Top Note (5-20% of the blend)*; Scent: *Grassy, lemony, pungent, earthy, slightly bitter*; Intensity: *4*

Lime

(*Citrus aurantifolia*)

BOTANICAL FAMILY: Rutaceae (citrus)

EXTRACTION METHOD/ORIGIN: Cold expressed from peel — India, Guatemala

CHEMICAL CONSTITUENTS: Terpenes: d-limonene (>65%), pinenes, camphene, sabinene, myrcene, bisabolene, dipentene, phellandrene, cadinene; Alcohols (4%): linalol, α-terpineol; Esters: terpenyl, geranyl, neryl, & bornyl acetate; Aldehydes (12%): furfural, octanal, nonanal, decanal, lauric aldehyde, neral, geranial, citronellal; Coumarins & Furanocoumarins; Nitrogen: N-methylanthranilate.

PROPERTIES: ANTI-BACTERIAL, ANTISEPTIC, ANTIVIRAL, RESTORATIVE, and TONIC.

ESOTERIC USES/ACTIONS: Astrological: *Saturn, Mercury, & Sun*; Body type: *Endomorph*; Character: *Yang*; Element: *Fire*; Number: *1*

HISTORICAL USES: For some time, lime was used as a remedy for dyspepsia with glycerin of pepsin. Was often used in place of lemon for fevers, infections, sore throats, colds, etc.

OTHER POSSIBLE USES: This oil may be beneficial for ANXIETY, BLOOD PRESSURE, soothing broken CAPILLARIES, dissolving CELLULITE, CLARITY of thought,

DEBILITY, ENERGY, FEVERS, GALLSTONES, HAIR (cleansing), promoting LEUKOCYTE FORMATION, LIVER deficiencies in children, LYMPHATIC SYSTEM CLEANSING, MEMORY IMPROVEMENT, NAILS (strengthening), NERVOUS CONDITIONS, cleaning the SKIN of dirty kids, SORE THROATS, WATER and AIR PURIFICATION, and promoting a sense of WELL BEING. It works extremely well in REMOVING GUM, WOOD STAIN, OIL, and GREASE SPOTS. It may also help brighten a pale, dull COMPLEXION by removing the dead skin cells. Lime oil is capable of TIGHTENING SKIN and CONNECTIVE TISSUE.

BODY SYSTEM(S) AFFECTED: DIGESTIVE, IMMUNE, and RESPIRATORY SYSTEMS.

AROMATIC INFLUENCE: Lime oil has a fresh, lively fragrance that is STIMULATING and REFRESHING. It helps one overcome EXHAUSTION, DEPRESSION, and LISTLESSNESS. Although unverifiable, some sources claim that inhaling the oil may stimulate the muscles around the eyes.

APPLICATION: Apply to VITA FLEX POINTS and/or directly on AREA of concern; diffuse. Excellent addition to BATH and SHOWER GELS, BODY LOTIONS, and DEODORANTS.

ORAL USE AS DIETARY SUPPLEMENT: Generally regarded as safe (GRAS) for internal consumption by the FDA. *DILUTE one drop oil in 1 tsp. honey or 4 oz. of beverage (ie. soy/rice milk).* ***Not for children under 6 years old; use with CAUTION and in GREATER DILUTION for children 6 years old and over.***

SAFETY DATA: Avoid direct SUNLIGHT for up to 12 hours after use.

BLEND CLASSIFICATION: Enhancer and Equalizer

BLENDS WITH: Citronella, Clary sage, lavandin, lavender, neroli, rosemary, other citrus oils.

ODOR: Type: *Top Note (5-20% of the blend)*; Scent: *Sweet, tart, intense, lively*; Intensity: *3*

Mandarin

(*Citrus reticulata*)

BOTANICAL FAMILY: Rutaceae (citrus)

EXTRACTION METHOD/ORIGIN: Cold pressed from peel. — China, Italy, Madagascar

CHEMICAL CONSTITUENTS: Monoterpenes: d-limonene (up to 75%), γ-terpinen, α-pinene, myrcene; Alcohols: nonanol, octanol, geraniol; Monoterpenols: citronellol, linalol; Esters: benzyl acetate; Aldehydes: decanal, citral, citronellal; Coumarins; Nitrogen compounds: methyl-N-methyl anthranilate (>1%), N-methylanthranilate. Also contains flavonoids, carotenoids, steroids.

PROPERTIES: ANTI-FUNGAL, ANTISEPTIC, ANTISPASMODIC, DIGESTIVE, SEDATIVE (nervous system), STIMULANT (digestive, lymphatic), TONIC.

FOLKLORE: The name of the fruit is said to have originated from a group of Imperial Chinese officials called the mandarins. The fruit was a traditional gift given to these officials.

ESOTERIC USES/ACTIONS: Astrological: *Saturn & Sun*; Body type: *Ectomorph*; Chakra: *2*; Character: *Yang/Yin?*; Crystals: *Pink and Gold Topaz*; Element: *Fire*; Number: *3*

HISTORICAL USES: Mandarin has been used in children's remedies for indigestion, hiccoughs etc. Also for the elderly to strengthen the digestive function and the liver.

OTHER POSSIBLE USES: This oil may help ACNE, DIGESTIVE PROBLEMS, DYSPEPSIA, FLUID RETENTION, HEPATIC DUCT FUNCTION, HICCOUGHS, INSOMNIA, INTESTINAL PROBLEMS, SKIN PROBLEMS (congested and oily skin, SCARS, SPOTS, tones the skin), STRETCH MARKS (when combined with either jasmine, lavender, sandalwood, and/or frankincense), NERVOUS TENSION, OBESITY, RESTLESSNESS. Recommended for CHILDREN and PREGNANT WOMEN because it is very gentle.

BODY SYSTEM(S) AFFECTED: DIGESTIVE SYSTEM, SKIN.

AROMATIC INFLUENCE: It is APPEASING, GENTLE, and promotes HAPPINESS. It is also REFRESHING, UPLIFTING, and REVITALIZING. Because of its sedative and slightly hypnotic properties, it is very good for STRESS and IRRITABILITY.

APPLICATION: Apply to VITA FLEX POINTS and/or directly on AREA of concern; diffuse. During pregnancy, combine with Olive oil or Wheat Germ oil and MASSAGE on the ABDOMEN.

ORAL USE AS DIETARY SUPPLEMENT: Generally regarded as safe (GRAS) for internal consumption by the FDA. *DILUTE one drop oil in 1 tsp. honey or 4 oz. of beverage (ie. soy/rice milk).* ***Not for children under 6 years old; use with CAUTION and in GREATER DILUTION for children 6 years old and over.***

SAFETY DATA: Avoid direct SUNLIGHT for 3 to 6 hours after use.

BLEND CLASSIFICATION: Personifier and Modifier

BLENDS WITH: Lavender; neroli and other citrus oils; cinnamon bark, clove, nutmeg, and othe spice oils.

ODOR: Type: *Top Note (5-20% of the blend)*; Scent: *Very sweet, citrusy, fruity*; Intensity: *3*

Marjoram

(*Origanum majorana*)

BOTANICAL FAMILY: Labiatae (mint)

EXTRACTION METHOD/ORIGIN: Steam distilled from leaves — France

CHEMICAL CONSTITUENTS: Monoterpenes (40%) α and β-pinenes, sabinene, myrcene, α- & γ-terpinenes, paracymene, terpinolene, α- & β- phellandrenes; Sesquiterpenes: β-caryophyllene, α-humulene; Alcohols (approx. 50%): linalol, terpinen-4-ol (>21%), terpinene-1-ol-3, α-terpineol, cis- & trans-thujanol-4; Esters: terpenyl acetates, linalyl acetate, geranyl acetates; Phenol methyl-ethers: trans-anethole (tr).

PROPERTIES: ANTI-BACTERIAL, ANTI-INFECTIOUS, ANTISEPTIC, ANTI-SEXUAL,

ANTISPASMODIC, ARTERIAL VASODILATOR, DIGESTIVE STIMULANT, DIURETIC, EXPECTORANT, SEDATIVE, and TONIC.

)LKLORE: Known as the "herb of happiness" to the Romans and "joy of the mountains" to the Greeks, marjoram was used to decorate at both weddings and funerals. Not only would it warm both the body and the emotions, but many believed it would increase longevity. It was also grown on grave sites to comfort the departed soul.

SOTERIC USES/ACTIONS: Astrological: *Mercury & Venus*; Ayurvedic: *Kapha*; Body type: *Mesomorph*; Chakra: *4*; Character: *Yang*; Element: *Air & Water*; Number: *9*

ISTORICAL USES: Marjoram was used for poisoning, fluid retention, muscle spasms, rheumatism, sprains, stiff joints, bruises, obstructions of the liver and spleen, and respiratory congestions. According to Roberta Wilson, "Those curious about their futures anointed themselves with marjoram at bedtime so that they might dream of their future mates."

RENCH MEDICINAL USES: ACHES, ARTHRITIS, ASTHMA, BRONCHITIS, COLIC, CONSTIPATION, CRAMPS, INSOMNIA, INTESTINAL PERISTALSIS, MIGRAINE HEADACHE, MUSCLES, NEURALGIA, PAINS, PARASYMPATHETIC NERVOUS SYSTEM (tones), BLOOD PRESSURE (regulates), RHEUMATISM, SPRAINS.

THER POSSIBLE USES: It may be RELAXING and CALMING to the **MUSCLES** that constrict and sometimes contribute to HEADACHES. It may help ANXIETY, BOILS, BRUISES, BURNS, CARBUNCLES, CELIBACY (vow not to marry), COLDS, COLD SORES, CUTS, FUNGUS and VIRAL INFECTIONS, HYSTERIA, MENSTRUAL PROBLEMS, calm RESPIRATORY SYSTEM, RINGWORM, SHINGLES, SHOCK, SORES, relieve SPASMS, SUNBURNS, TENSION, and WATER RETENTION.

ODY SYSTEM(S) AFFECTED: CARDIOVASCULAR SYSTEM, MUSCLES and BONES.

ROMATIC INFLUENCE: It promotes PEACE and SLEEP.

PPLICATION: Apply to VITA FLEX POINTS and directly on AREA of concern; Diffuse.

RAL USE AS DIETARY SUPPLEMENT: Generally regarded as safe (GRAS) for internal consumption by the FDA. *DILUTE one drop oil in 1 tsp. honey or 4 oz. of beverage (ie. soy/rice milk).* ***Not for children under 6 years old; use with CAUTION and in GREATER DILUTION for children 6 years old and over.***

AFETY DATA: Use with caution during PREGNANCY.

LEND CLASSIFICATION: Enhancer and Equalizer

LENDS WITH: Bergamot, cedarwood, chamomile, cypress, lavender, orange, nutmeg, rosemary, rosewood, ylang ylang.

DOR: Type: *Middle Note (50-80% of the blend)*; Scent: *Herbaceous, green, spicy*; Intensity: *3*

Melaleuca (Tea Tree)

(Melaleuca alternifolia)

BOTANICAL FAMILY: Myrtaceae (Myrtle - shrubs and trees)

EXTRACTION METHOD/ORIGIN: Steam distilled from leaves — Australia

CHEMICAL CONSTITUENTS: Monoterpenes (up to 20%): α and β-pinene, myrcene, α- & terpinenes, paracymene, limonene, terpinolene; Sesquiterpenes: β-caryophyllene, aromadendrene, allo-aromadendrene, viridiflorene, α- & δ-cadinene; Alcohols (approx. 50%): terpinen-4-ol (>59%), α- & β-terpineols, globulol, viridiflorol; Oxides: 1,4-cineol, 1,8-cineol (>18%), epoxycaryophyllene II.

PROPERTIES: ANALGESIC, ANTI-BACTERIAL, ANTI-FUNGAL, ANTI-INFECTIOUS, ANTI-INFLAMMATORY, ANTIOXIDANT, ANTI-PARASITIC, a strong ANTISEPTIC, ANTIVIRAL, DECONGESTANT, DIGESTIVE, EXPECTORANT, IMMUNE-STIMULANT, INSECTICIDAL, NEURO TONIC, STIMULANT, and TISSUE REGENERATOR.

ESOTERIC USES/ACTIONS: Character: *Yang*

HISTORICAL USES: The leaves of the Melaleuca tree (or Tea Tree) have been used for centuries by the aborigines to heal cuts, wounds, and skin infections. With twelve times the antiseptic power of phenol, it has some strong immune building properties.

FRENCH MEDICINAL USES: ATHLETE'S FOOT, BRONCHITIS, COLDS, COUGHS, DIARRHEA, FLU, PERIODONTAL (GUM) DISEASE, RASH, SKIN HEALING, SORE THROAT, SUNBURN, TONSILLITIS, VAGINAL THRUSH.

OTHER POSSIBLE USES: This oil may help ACNE, BURNS, CANDIDA, COLD SORES, DIGESTION, FUNGAL INFECTIONS, HYSTERIA, INFECTIOUS DISEASES, INFLAMMATION, SHOCK, VIRAL INFECTIONS, WARTS, and WOUNDS (promotes healing).

BODY SYSTEM(S) AFFECTED: IMMUNE and RESPIRATORY SYSTEMS, MUSCLES and BONES, SKIN.

AROMATIC INFLUENCE: It promotes CLEANSING and PURITY.

APPLICATION: Apply to VITA FLEX POINTS and/or directly on AREA of concern; diffuse

ORAL USE AS DIETARY SUPPLEMENT: Approved by the FDA for use as a Food Additi (FA) or Flavoring Agent (FL). *DILUTE one drop oil in 1 tsp. honey or 4 oz. of bevera (ie. soy/rice milk).* ***Not for children under 6 years old; use with CAUTION and in GREATER DILUTION for children 6 years old and over.***

SAFETY DATA: Repeated use can possibly result in CONTACT SENSITIZATION.

BLEND CLASSIFICATION: Enhancer and Equalizer

BLENDS WITH: All citrus oils, cypress, eucalyptus, lavender, rosemary, and thyme.

ODOR: Type: *Middle Note (50-80% of the blend)*; Scent: *Medicinal, fresh, woody, earthy, herbaceous*; Intensity: *3*

Melaleuca Ericifolia (or Rosalina)

(Melaleuca ericifolia)

OTANICAL FAMILY: Myrtaceae (Myrtle - shrubs and trees)

RIGIN: Australia

HEMICAL CONSTITUENTS: Terpene alcohols (up to 62%): linalol (up to 45%), α-terpineol (<5%), terpinen-4-ol; Oxides: 1,8-cineol; Monoterpenes: β-phellandrene (<22%), α-pinene (<10%), limonene, γ-terpinene, ρ-cymene (<6%); Sesquiterpenes: aromandrene (<6%), viridiflorene.

ROPERTIES: ANTI-BACTERIAL, ANTI-FUNGAL, ANTI-INFECTIOUS, powerful ANTIMICROBIAL, CALMING, and SEDATIVE.

THER POSSIBLE USES: Because this variety of melaleuca oil is VERY GENTLE and NON-IRRITATING to the skin, it is well suited for YOUTH and others who may be more sensitive to the oils. Research by Dr. Daniel Pénoël, M.D. has shown this oil to help with BRONCHITIS, DERMATITIS, EAR INFECTIONS, ECZEMA, INFLUENZA, INSOMNIA, NERVOUS TENSION, PNEUMONIA, and SINUSITIS.

ODY SYSTEM(S) AFFECTED: RESPIRATORY SYSTEM, SKIN.

PPLICATION: Apply to VITA FLEX POINTS and/or directly on AREA of concern. May also be applied to the CHEST, FACE, TEMPLES, THROAT, or WRISTS. For a FULL BODY MASSAGE, dilute 4-8 drops of *Melaleuca ericifolia* oil in 30 ml. of a pure vegetable oil. May also be diffused or added to bath water. *Caution: Heating or burning this oil can cause it to lose all therapeutic value.*

RAL USE AS DIETARY SUPPLEMENT: Approved by the FDA for use as a Food Additive (FA) or Flavoring Agent (FL). *DILUTE one drop oil in 1 tsp. honey or 4 oz. of beverage (ie. soy/rice milk).* ***Not for children under 6 years old; use with CAUTION and in GREATER DILUTION for children 6 years old and over.***

LEND CLASSIFICATION: Personifier, Enhancer, Equalizer, and Modifier.

Melaleuca Leucadendron

*(**See Cajeput**)*

Melaleuca Quinquenervia (or Niaouli)

(Melaleuca quinquenervia)

OTANICAL FAMILY: Myrtaceae (Myrtle - shrubs and trees)

XTRACTION METHOD/ORIGIN: Steam distilled from leaves and limbs — Australia

HEMICAL CONSTITUENTS: Oxides: 1,8-cineol (>60%); Alcohols: linalol, terpinen-4-ol

(2%), α-terpineol (>20%), viridiflorol (>14%), nerolidol (<6%); Monoterpenes (17%): α & β-pinenes, β-phellandrene, α- & γ-terpinenes, limonene; Sesquiterpenes: β-caryophyllene, aromadendrene, viridiflorene, δ-cadinene; Aldehydes: isovaleraldehyde, benzaldehyde (tr.)

PROPERTIES: ANTI-BACTERIAL, ANTI-FUNGAL (very strong and powerful), ANTI-INFLAMMATORY, ANTISEPTIC, ANTIVIRAL, DIGESTIVE TONIC, PROTECTC AGAINST RADIATION, and a strong TISSUE REGENERATOR.

ESOTERIC USES/ACTIONS: Astrological: *Mercury*; Character: *Neutral?*; Element: *Air*

OTHER POSSIBLE USES: This oil may help with RESPIRATORY ALLERGIES, INFECTIONS, HEMORRHOIDS, and others as listed under MELALEUCA.

BODY SYSTEM(S) AFFECTED: MUSCLES and BONES, RESPIRATORY SYSTEM.

AROMATIC INFLUENCE: Some people may prefer this oil to melaleuca (*M. alternifolia*) because of its sweet, delicate scent. It aids in CONCENTRATION, is REVIVING, and helps CLEAR the HEAD.

APPLICATION: Apply to VITA FLEX POINTS and/or directly on AREA of concern; diffuse DIFFUSE for respiratory problems.

ORAL USE AS DIETARY SUPPLEMENT: Approved by the FDA for use as a Food Additi (FA) or Flavoring Agent (FL). *DILUTE one drop oil in 1 tsp. honey or 4 oz. of beverag (ie. soy/rice milk).* ***Not for children under 6 years old; use with CAUTION and in GREATER DILUTION for children 6 years old and over.***

SAFETY DATA: Repeated use can possibly result in CONTACT SENSITIZATION.

ODOR: Type: *Middle Note (50-80% of the blend)*; Scent: *Earthy, musty, harsh*; Intensity: *3*

Melissa (Lemon Balm)

(*Melissa officinalis*)

BOTANICAL FAMILY: Labiatae (mint)

EXTRACTION METHOD/ORIGIN: Steam distilled from leaves and flowers — France, Idaho, Utah

CHEMICAL CONSTITUENTS: Monoterpenes: cis- & trans-ocimenes; Sesquiterpenes: α-cubebene, α-copaene, β-bourbonene, β-caryophyllene (>7%), α-humulene, germacrene-D (>5%); Alcohols: linalol, nerol, geraniol, citronnellol, α-terpineol, terpinen-4-ol, caryophyllenol, farnesol; Esters: geranyl, neryl, linalyl, & citronellyl acetates; Oxides: 1,8 cineol, caryophyllene oxide; Aldehydes: citrals: neral (>16%), geranial (>15%), citronella Coumarins: aesculetine; Also: eugenol.

PROPERTIES: ANTI-BACTERIAL, ANTI-DEPRESSANT, ANTIHISTAMINE, ANTIMICROBIAL, ANTISPASMODIC, ANTIVIRAL, HYPERTENSIVE, NERVINE SEDATIVE, TONIC, and UTERINE.

FOLKLORE: Melissa, the "Elixir of Life", is one of the earliest known medicinal herbs.

ESOTERIC USES/ACTIONS: Astrological: *Jupiter*; Body type: *Endomorph*; Chakras: *4 & 3*; Character: *Yang with high Yin*; Element: *Fire*; Number: *1*

HISTORICAL USES: Anciently, melissa was used for nervous disorders and many different ailments dealing with the heart or the emotions. It was also used to promote fertility. Melissa was the main ingredient in Carmelite water, distilled in France since 1611 by the Carmelite monks.

OTHER POSSIBLE USES: ALLERGIES, ANXIETY, ASTHMA, BRONCHITIS, CHRONIC COUGHS, COLDS, COLD-SORE BLISTERS (apply directly three times per day), COLIC, DEPRESSION, DYSENTERY, ECZEMA, ERYSIPELAS, FEVERS, HEART CONDITIONS (where there is overstimulation or heat), HYPERTENSION, INDIGESTION, INSECT BITES, INSOMNIA, MENSTRUAL PROBLEMS, MIGRAINE, NAUSEA, NERVOUS TENSION, PALPITATIONS, SHOCK, STERILITY (in women), THROAT INFECTIONS, VERTIGO, and VOMITING. Dr. Dietrich Wabner, a professor at the Technical University of Munich, reported that a one-time application of true melissa oil led to complete remission of HERPES SIMPLEX LESIONS. According to Robert Tisserand, "... melissa is the nearest one can find to a rejuvenator – not something which will make us young again, but which helps to cushion, the effect of our mind and the world outside, on our body."

BODY SYSTEM(S) AFFECTED: EMOTIONAL BALANCE, SKIN.

AROMATIC INFLUENCE: Melissa has a delicate, delightful, lemony scent that is unique among essential oils, providing a wonderful support to both body and mind. It has been known to bring out GENTLE characteristics within people. It is CALMING and UPLIFTING and may help to BALANCE the EMOTIONS. It may also help to remove EMOTIONAL BLOCKS and INSTILL a POSITIVE OUTLOOK on LIFE.

APPLICATION: Apply to VITA FLEX POINTS and/or directly on AREA of concern.

ORAL USE AS DIETARY SUPPLEMENT: Generally regarded as safe (GRAS) for internal consumption by the FDA. *DILUTE one drop oil in 1 tsp. honey or 4 oz. of beverage (ie. soy/rice milk).* ***Not for children under 6 years old; use with CAUTION and in GREATER DILUTION for children 6 years old and over.***

BLEND CLASSIFICATION: Enhancer, Equalizer, and Modifier

BLENDS WITH: Geranium, lavender, and other floral and citrus oils.

ODOR: Type: *Middle Note (50-80% of the blend)*; Scent: *Delicate, lemony*; Intensity: *2*

FREQUENCY: Emotional and Spiritual; approximately 102 MHz.

Mountain Savory (or Winter Savory)

(*Satureja montana*)

BOTANICAL FAMILY: Labiatae (mint)

EXTRACTION METHOD/ORIGIN: Steam distilled from flowering plant — France

CHEMICAL CONSTITUENTS: Monoterpenes: α-thujene, α and β-pinenes, camphene, sabinene, myrcene, Δ-3-carene, Δ-4-carene, α-phellandrene, α- & γ-terpinenes (20%), paracymene (up to 20%), limonene, terpinolene; Sesquiterpenes: β-caryophyllene, calamene, α-humulene, aromadendrene, β-bisabolene, α- & γ-cadinenes, calacornene; Alcohols: linalol, cis- & trans-thujanol-4, terpinen-4-ol, α-terpineol, geraniol, myrtenol, borneol; Esters: bornyl, linalyl, terpenyl, terpinenyl, & geranyl acetates; Phenols: thymol (tr.), carvacrol (up to 50%), eugenol; Phenol methyl-ethers: methyl carvacrol; Oxides: 1,8 cineol (<1%); Ketones: camphor.

PROPERTIES: ANTI-BACTERIAL, ANTI-FUNGAL, strong ANTI-INFECTIOUS (genito-urinary & gastro-intestinal - superior to thyme, rosemary, and lavender), ANTI-PARASITIC, ANTIVIRAL, IMMUNE-STIMULANT, and a general TONIC for the body.

HISTORICAL USES: This oil has been used as a digestive remedy for colic and diarrhea.

OTHER POSSIBLE USES: Due to its high phenol content, Mountain savory is a very strong antiseptic and has been used to hasten the FORMATION of SCAR TISSUE, and to help with ABSCESSES, BURNS, and CUTS. It is also known to stimulate the ADRENAL GLAND.

BODY SYSTEM(S) AFFECTED: IMMUNE SYSTEM.

AROMATIC INFLUENCE: It may produce STRONG PSYCHOLOGICAL EFFECTS and can help revitalize and stimulate the nervous system. It is a powerful ENERGIZER and MOTIVATOR.

APPLICATION: Apply diluted to VITA FLEX POINTS and on AREA of concern; diffuse.

ORAL USE AS DIETARY SUPPLEMENT: Generally regarded as safe (GRAS) for internal consumption by the FDA. *DILUTE one drop oil in 2 tsp. honey or 8 oz. of beverage (ie. soy/rice milk). May need to increase dilution even more due to this oil's potential for irritating mucus membranes.* ***Not for children under 6 years old; use with CAUTION and in GREATER DILUTION for children 6 years old and over.***

SAFETY DATA: Robert Tisserand has classified Mountain savory as a dermal toxin, dermal irritant, and mucous membrane irritant. He recommends it never be used on the skin. However, other sources recommend its use but emphasize that it must always be used in dilution. Can cause extreme SKIN IRRITATION. Avoid during PREGNANCY and use with EXTREME CAUTION. Also, best if used for short duration, may be toxic to the liver during long term use.

Mugwort

(*Artemisia vulgaris*)

BOTANICAL FAMILY: Asteraceae or Compositae (daisy)

EXTRACTION METHOD/ORIGIN: Steam distillation from the leaves and root — Europe

CHEMICAL CONSTITUENTS: Ketones: α- & β-thujones (up to 12%); Oxide: cineol; Monoterpenes: α- & β-pinenes, camphene, sabinene (<14%), myrcene (up to 25%), ρ-cymene, γ-cadinene, limonene, β-phellandrene; Alcohols: α-terpineol, borneol; Also: camphor, germacrene-D.

PROPERTIES: ANTISEPTIC, ANTISPASMODIC, CALMING, DIURETIC, EXPECTORANT.

HISTORICAL USES: Having been associated with superstition and witchcraft, mugwort was seen as a protective charm against danger and evil. It has been used for painful or delayed menstruation, amenorrhea and dysmenorrhea, for hysteria and epilepsy, to expel worms, and control fever. According to some sources, mugwort was used by the Jews as one of the bitter herbs eaten during passover.

OTHER POSSIBLE USES: MUCUS (expels), NERVES (calms), PARASITES (blend with thyme)

BODY SYSTEM(S) AFFECTED: HORMONAL and NERVOUS SYSTEMS.

AROMATIC INFLUENCE: This strongly aromatic oil was anciently believed to increase psychic powers.

APPLICATION: Apply to VITA FLEX POINTS and/or directly on AREA of concern.

ORAL USE AS DIETARY SUPPLEMENT: *Has been approved by the FDA for use as a Food Additive (FA) or Flavoring Agent (FL) as long as the finished food is thujone-free. (see 21CFR172.510)* ***Best NOT to use this oil as a dietary supplement.***

SAFETY DATA: FOR TOPICAL USE ONLY. Due to high Thujone content, use SPARINGLY and DILUTE WELL with V-6 Mixing Oil or Massage Oil. Avoid during PREGNANCY as it may contribute to a miscarriage.

BLENDS WITH: Anise, German chamomile, ginger, peppermint, rosemary, tangerine, and tarragon.

FOUND IN: ComforTone

Myrrh

(*Commiphora myrrha*)

BOTANICAL FAMILY: Burseraceae (resinous trees and shrubs)

EXTRACTION METHOD/ORIGIN: Steam distilled from gum/resin — Somalia

CHEMICAL CONSTITUENTS: Mono/Sesquiterpenes: curzerene (up to 25%), lindestrene (up to 45%), β- & γ-elemenes (<6%), furano-eudesmene, heerabolene, limonene, dipentene, pinenes, cadinene; Phenols: eugenol; Aldehydes: cinnamaldehyde, cuminaldehyde.

PROPERTIES: ANTI-INFECTIOUS, ANTI-INFLAMMATORY, ANTISEPTIC, ASTRINGENT, and TONIC.

FOLKLORE: Well over 2,000 years before the baby Jesus received myrrh as a gift, it was one of the most desired and most expensive items in the world. According to Roberta Wilson, "In

Greek mythology, Aphrodite forced the goddess Myrrha into an incestuous relationship with her father, Cinyras. Cinyras avenged the act by turning his daughter into a myrrh tree. When the tree sprouted its blooms, their child Adonis was born. The resinous drops that exude from cuts in the tree's bark were said to be Myrrha's tears."

ESOTERIC USES/ACTIONS: Astrological: *Saturn, Jupiter, & Sun*; Body type: *Ectomorph*; Chakras: *1 & 2*; Character: *Yang - Hot and Drying*; Crystals: *Hematite, Red Garnet, Pearl*; Element: *Water*; Number: *5*

HISTORICAL USES: Myrrh was used as incense in religious rituals, in embalming, as a cure for cancer, leprosy, and syphilis. Myrrh, mixed with coriander and honey, was used to treat herpes.

FRENCH MEDICINAL USES: BRONCHITIS, DIARRHEA, DYSENTERY, HYPERTHYROIDISM, STRETCH MARKS, THRUSH, ULCERS, VAGINAL THRUSH, VIRAL HEPATITIS.

OTHER POSSIBLE USES: This oil may help increase APPETITE, ASTHMA, ATHLETE'S FOOT, CANDIDA, CATARRH (mucus), COUGHS, ECZEMA, DIGESTION, DYSPEPSIA (impaired digestion), FLATULENCE (gas), FUNGAL INFECTION, GINGIVITIS, GUM INFECTION, HEMORRHOIDS, MOUTH ULCERS, decongest PROSTATE GLAND, RINGWORM, SORE THROATS, SKIN CONDITIONS (chapped, cracked, and inflammation), WOUNDS, and WRINKLES.

BODY SYSTEM(S) AFFECTED: HORMONAL, IMMUNE, and NERVOUS SYSTEMS, SKIN.

AROMATIC INFLUENCE: It promotes SPIRITUAL AWARENESS and is UPLIFTING.

APPLICATION: Apply to VITA FLEX POINTS and/or directly on AREA of concern.

ORAL USE AS DIETARY SUPPLEMENT: Approved by the FDA for use as a Food Additive (FA) and Flavoring Agent (FL). *DILUTE one drop oil in 1 tsp. honey or 4 oz. of beverage (ie. soy/rice milk).* ***Not for children under 6 years old; use with CAUTION and in GREATER DILUTION for children 6 years old and over.***

SAFETY DATA: Use with caution during PREGNANCY.

BLEND CLASSIFICATION: Modifier and Equalizer

BLENDS WITH: Frankincense, lavender, patchouli, sandalwood, and all spice oils.

ODOR: Type: *Base Note (5-20% of the blend)*; Scent: *Warm, earthy, woody, balsamic*; Intensity: *4*

FREQUENCY: Emotional and Spiritual; approximately 105 MHz.

COMMENTS: Myrrh is a true gift. When we open our HEARTS and MINDS to receive the gifts, they will be given.

Myrtle

(*Myrtus communis ssp. red*)

OTANICAL FAMILY: Myrtaceae (Myrtle - shrubs and trees)

XTRACTION METHOD/ORIGIN: Steam distilled from leaves — Morocco, Tunisia

HEMICAL CONSTITUENTS: Monoterpenes: α-pinene (up to 24%), β-pinene, camphene; Sesquiterpenes: β-caryophyllene, α-humulene, dihydroazulenes; Alcohols: linalol, myrtenol (>1%), α-terpineol, terpinen-4-ol, nerol, geraniol; Esters: linalyl, myrtenyl, terpenyl, neryl, geranyl, bornyl, & trans-carvyl acetates; Oxides: 1,8 cineol (up to 45%); Aldehydes.

ROPERTIES: ANTI-BACTERIAL, ANTI-INFLAMMATORY, ANTI-PARASITIC, ANTISEPTIC, ASTRINGENT, EXPECTORANT, DECONGESTANT, and DEODORIZER.

OLKLORE: According to Susanne Fischer-Rizzi, "...myrtle, considered the sacred plant of the goddess Aphrodite, was worshiped as a plant of mystery. Aphrodite, goddess of beauty and love, and born as a beautiful adult woman from sea foam, sought refuge in her new-born nakedness in a myrtle bush. That's why myrtle also stands for chaste beauty. Many brides today still wear myrtle as a symbol for innocence."

SOTERIC USES/ACTIONS: Astrological: *Venus & Mercury*; Character: *Yang (with strong Yin)*; Element: *Water*

ISTORICAL USES: Myrtle was used for diarrhea, dysentery, catarrhal conditions (asthma, bronchitis, chronic coughs, tuberculosis), lung and bladder infections, sinus infections, and skin care.

RENCH MEDICINAL USES: BRONCHITIS, COUGHS, FLU, HYPOTHYROIDISM, INSOMNIA, OVARIES (hormone-like effects), PROSTATE DECONGESTANT, SINUS INFECTION, TUBERCULOSIS, URETER INFECTIONS.

THER POSSIBLE USES: This oil may help ANGER, ASTHMA, CATARRH, CHILDREN (see comment), COLDS, CYSTITIS, DIARRHEA, DYSENTERY, DYSPEPSIA (impaired digestion), FLATULENCE (gas), HEMORRHOIDS, support IMMUNE SYSTEM, INFECTIONS, INFECTIOUS DISEASES, PULMONARY DISORDERS, SKIN CONDITIONS (acne, blemishes, bruises, oily skin, psoriasis, etc.), and SINUSITIS. Useful on CHILDREN for CHEST complaints and COUGHS.

ODY SYSTEM(S) AFFECTED: DIGESTIVE, HORMONAL, and RESPIRATORY SYSTEMS, MUSCLES and BONES.

ROMATIC INFLUENCE: It is ELEVATING and EUPHORIC. It also soothes ANGER.

PPLICATION: Apply to VITA FLEX POINTS or directly on AREA of concern; diffuse.

RAL USE AS DIETARY SUPPLEMENT: Approved by the FDA for use as a Food Additive (FA) and Flavoring Agent (FL). *DILUTE one drop oil in 1 tsp. honey or 4 oz. of beverage (ie. soy/rice milk).* ***Not for children under 6 years old; use with CAUTION and in GREATER DILUTION for children 6 years old and over.***

LEND CLASSIFICATION: Equalizer and Enhancer

BLENDS WITH: Bergamot, lavender, lemon, lemongrass, rosewood, rosemary, spearmint, thyme, and melaleuca (Tea Tree).

ODOR: Type: *Top to Middle Notes (20-80% of the blend)*; Scent: *Sweet, slightly camphorous, with a floral hint*; Intensity: *3*

Myrtle, Lemon

(*Backhousia citriodora*)

BOTANICAL FAMILY: Myrtaceae (Myrtle - shrubs and trees)

EXTRACTION METHOD/ORIGIN: Steam distilled from leaves — Australia

CHEMICAL CONSTITUENTS: Aldehydes: Citrals (up to 90%): neral and geranial. Other trace elements include myrcene, linalol, citronellal, cyclocitral, and methyl-heptenone..

PROPERTIES: ANTI-BACTERIAL, ANTIFUNGAL, ANTIMICROBIAL, ANTISEPTIC, ANTIVIRAL, CALMING, CORRECTIVE, and SEDATIVE.

HISTORICAL USES: The leaves from the Lemon Myrtle trees have been dried and used as foo flavoring for poultry and seafood as well as for air fresheners in wardrobes, shoe cabinets and vehicles. Lemon myrtle is said to smell more "lemony than lemon". Research is showing that lemon myrtle oil has very good antibacterial activity and excellent antifunga activity, maybe even more so than *Melaleuca alternifolia.* Other tests have shown lemon myrtle to possess strong germicidal powers, twice that of *Eucalyptus citriodora* and even 19.5 times that of citral alone.

OTHER POSSIBLE USES: This oil may help with VIRAL, BACTERIAL, and FUNGAL INFECTIONS. It has also been reported to help with sprained or torn LIGAMENTS and TENDONS. Due to its anti-bacterial, antifungal, and antimicrobial actions, it would wor well as an additive to any natural cleaning product. And what a better way to clean than with the strong lemon scent from the oil.

BODY SYSTEM(S) AFFECTED: IMMUNE SYSTEM, RESPIRATORY SYSTEM MUSCLES and BONES.

AROMATIC INFLUENCE: It is ELEVATING and REFRESHING.

APPLICATION: Apply to VITA FLEX POINTS or directly on AREA of concern; diffuse.

ODOR: Type: *Top Note (5-20% of the blend)*; Scent: *Extremely lemony and crisp, more "lemony" than true lemon oil*; Intensity: *5*

Neroli (or Orange Blossom)

(*Citrus aurantium bigaradia*)

BOTANICAL FAMILY: Rutaceae (citrus)

XTRACTION METHOD/ORIGIN: Absolute extraction from flowers of the orange tree — Morocco, Tunisia

HEMICAL CONSTITUENTS: Monoterpenes (35%); α-pinene, β-pinene (17%), d-limonene (11%), camphene; Terpene alcohols (40%): linalol (30-32%), α-terpineol, geraniol, nerol; Esters (>21%): linalyl acetate (5-7%), neryl & geranyl acetates; Sesquiterpene alcohols (6%): trans-nerolidol, farnesols; Aldehydes: decanal, benzaldehyde; Ketones: jasmone (tr.).

ROPERTIES: ANTI-BACTERIAL, ANTI-DEPRESSANT, ANTI-INFECTIOUS, ANTI-PARASITIC, ANTISEPTIC, ANTISPASMODIC, ANTIVIRAL, APHRODISIAC, DEODORANT, SEDATIVE, and TONIC.

OLKLORE: The name of this oil is said to originate from a beloved princess of Nerola, Italy, who lavished it on everything. Brides adorned themselves and their bouquets with the orange blossoms, to signify their purity and beauty.

SOTERIC USES/ACTIONS: Astrological: *Sun*; Body type: *Ectomorph*; Chakras: *4, 8 & HIGHER*; Character: *Yin with high Yang*; Crystals: *Selenite (best), Herkemer Diamond, Fluorite, Rutilated quartz, Diamond, &Chrysoprase, Chalcedony*; Element: *Air & Ether*; Number: *1*

ISTORICAL USES: Neroli has been regarded traditionally by the Egyptian people for its great attributes for healing the MIND, BODY, and SPIRIT. It brings everything into the focus of one and at the moment.

THER POSSIBLE USES: It may support the DIGESTIVE SYSTEM and fight BACTERIA, INFECTIONS, PARASITES, and VIRUSES. It may also help with ANXIETY, CHRONIC DIARRHEA, COLIC, DEPRESSION, DIGESTIVE SPASMS, FEAR, FLATULENCE, HEADACHES, HEART (regulates rhythm), HYSTERIA, INSOMNIA, MATURE and SENSITIVE SKIN, NERVOUS DYSPEPSIA, NERVOUS TENSION, PALPITATIONS, PMS, POOR CIRCULATION, SCARS, SHOCK, STRESS RELATED CONDITIONS, STRETCH MARKS, TACHYCARDIA, THREAD VEINS, and WRINKLES. In support of the skin, it works at the cell level to help shed the old skin cells and STIMULATE NEW CELL GROWTH.

ODY SYSTEM(S) AFFECTED: DIGESTIVE SYSTEM, SKIN.

ROMATIC INFLUENCE: As a NATURAL TRANQUILIZER, neroli has some POWERFUL PSYCHOLOGICAL EFFECTS. It has been used successfully to treat DEPRESSION, ANXIETY, and SHOCK. It is CALMING and RELAXING to body and spirit. It may also help to STRENGTHEN and STABILIZE the emotions, and BRING RELIEF to seemingly hopeless situations. It encourages CONFIDENCE, COURAGE, JOY, PEACE, and SENSUALITY. Neroli is said to vibrate in the 2nd and 4th chakra. In the words of one author, "Neroli offers the gift of strength and courage that helps us see life's beauty."

PPLICATION: Apply to VITA FLEX POINTS and directly on AREA of concern; diffuse.

RAL USE AS DIETARY SUPPLEMENT: Generally regarded as safe (GRAS) for internal consumption by the FDA. *DILUTE one drop oil in 1 tsp. honey or 4 oz. of beverage (ie. soy/rice milk).* ***Not for children under 6 years old; use with CAUTION and in***

GREATER DILUTION for children 6 years old and over.

BLEND CLASSIFICATION: Equalizer, Modifier, and Personifier

BLENDS WITH: Rose, lavender, sandalwood, jasmine, cedarwood, geranium, lemon.

ODOR: Type: *Middle Note (50-80% of the blend)*; Scent: *Floral, citrusy, sweet, delicate, slightly bitter*; Intensity: *3*

Niaouli

(*See Melaleuca quinquenervia*)

Nutmeg

(*Myristica fragrans*)

BOTANICAL FAMILY: Myristicaceae

EXTRACTION METHOD/ORIGIN: Steam distilled from fruits and seeds — Indonesia, Tunisia

CHEMICAL CONSTITUENTS: Monoterpenes: α-pinene (25%) and β-pinenes (10%), sabinene (>19%), limonene (4%), α- & γ-terpinenes, camphene; Alcohols: terpinen-4-ol (>10%), linalol, terpineol, geraniol, borneol; Phenols: eugenol, isoeugenol; Phenol methyl-ethers: myristicin (<6%), elemicin (>1.5%); Ether-oxides: safrole (up to 2%), 1,8-cineol (>2%); Acids.

PROPERTIES: ANTI-INFLAMMATORY, ANTI-PARASITIC, ANTISEPTIC, STIMULANT (cerebral, circulatory), LAXATIVE, and TONIC.

ESOTERIC USES/ACTIONS: Astrological: *Jupiter*; Body type: *Ectomorph*; Chakra: *1*; Element: *Fire*; Number: *4*

HISTORICAL USES: Nutmeg has been used for centuries as a remedy for digestive and kidney problems.

FRENCH MEDICINAL USES: APPETITE (loss of), CHRONIC DIARRHEA, DEBILITY, DIGESTION (helps with starchy foods and fats), GALLSTONES, HALITOSIS (bad breath), RHEUMATISM.

OTHER POSSIBLE USES: This oil has adrenal cortex-like activity, which helps support the ADRENAL GLANDS for INCREASED ENERGY. It may also help loss of ARTHRITIS, BACTERIAL INFECTION, CIRCULATION, revive FAINTING, FLATULENCE (gas), FRIGIDITY, GOUT, IMPOTENCE, IMMUNE FUNCTION (support), JOINTS, MENSTRUATION (regulates scanty periods and soothes pains), MUSCLES (also muscle aches and pains), NAUSEA, NERVOUS FATIGUE, NEURALGIA (severe pain along nerve), support NERVOUS SYSTEM, and VOMITING.

)DY SYSTEM(S) AFFECTED: HORMONAL, IMMUNE, and NERVOUS SYSTEMS.

'PLICATION: Apply to VITA FLEX POINTS and/or directly on AREA of Concern.

ʀAL USE AS DIETARY SUPPLEMENT: Generally regarded as safe (GRAS) for internal consumption by the FDA. *DILUTE one drop oil in 1 tsp. honey or 4 oz. of beverage (ie. soy/rice milk).* ***Not for children under 6 years old; use with CAUTION and in GREATER DILUTION for children 6 years old and over.***

.FETY DATA: Not for use by people with EPILEPSY. Use with caution during PREGNANCY. If over used (several undiluted drops at once), it may cause mental discomfort or delirium, and convulsions and could overstimulate the heart. Dilute well or use a single undiluted drop then wait for a period of time.

.END CLASSIFICATION: Personifier

.ENDS WITH: Cinnamon bark, clove, cypress, frankincense, lemon, orange, patchouli, rosemary, melaleuca, melissa.

DOR: Type: *Middle Note (50-80% of the blend)*; Scent: *Sweet, musky, spicy*; Intensity: *4*

Single Oils

Onycha (Benzoin)

(Styrax benzoin)

)TANICAL FAMILY: Styracaceae

KTRACTION METHOD/ORIGIN: Absolute extraction from the resin (Onycha is actually an "essence" not an essential oil) — India, China, Laos, Thailand, or Vietnam.

HEMICAL CONSTITUENTS: Volatile Fraction: Acids: benzoic (up to 20%), cinnamic; Esters: benzyl cinnamate (tr.); **Non Volatile Fraction:** Esters (<70%): coniferyl benzoate.

ROPERTIES: ANTI-INFLAMMATORY, ANTISEPTIC, ANTIOXIDANT, ASTRINGENT, DEODORANT, DIURETIC, EXPECTORANT, and SEDATIVE.

OTERIC USES/ACTIONS: Astrological: *Mercury & Sun*; Chakra: *1*; Character: *Yang*; Element: *Air*; Oriental: *Cold dampness (pts. Sp-9 & 6)*

ISTORICAL USES: Onycha (or benzoin), as either a resin or an absolute, has been used for thousands of years in the east for rituals and ceremonies as either incense or for anointings. It is mentioned in the Bible as one of the ingredients for an "Holy Anointing Oil" (Exodus 30:34). The Chinese used it for its heating and drying qualities and in the west it was used for respiratory complaints.

)SSIBLE USES: This oil may help ARTHRITIS, ASTHMA, BLEEDING (slow or stop), BRONCHITIS, CHILLS, CIRCULATION (poor), COLIC, CUTS, FLATULENCE (gas), FLU, GOUT, LARYNGITIS, MUCUS (helps remove), NERVOUS TENSION, RHEUMATISM, SKIN (lesions; chapped, inflamed, and irritated conditions), STOMACH (gripping pains), STRESS related conditions, URINARY TRACT INFECTION, and WOUNDS. It is very WARMING which makes it good for COLDS, COUGHS, and SORE THROATS.

BODY SYSTEM(S) AFFECTED: CARDIOVASCULAR SYSTEM, EMOTIONAL BALANCE, SKIN.

AROMATIC INFLUENCE: Onycha is WARMING and SOOTHING to the HEART. According to Marguerite Maury, "This essence creates a kind of euphoria; it interposes padded zone between us and events." It may also help overcome SADNESS, LONELINESS, DEPRESSION, and ANXIETY. When combined with rose, it can be very COMFORTING and UPLIFTING.

APPLICATION: Apply to VITA FLEX POINTS and/or directly on AREA of concern; MASSAGE (combine with rose and add to a massage oil base). Because of its thick, resinous nature, thin heavily with lavender or peppermint oils for diffusion.

ORAL USE AS DIETARY SUPPLEMENT: Approved by the FDA for use as a Food Additi (FA) and Flavoring Agent (FL). *DILUTE one drop oil in 1 tsp. honey or 4 oz. of beverage (ie. soy/rice milk).* ***Not for children under 6 years old; use with CAUTION and in GREATER DILUTION for children 6 years old and over.***

BLEND CLASSIFICATION: Enhancer and Equalizer

BLENDS WITH: Coriander, cypress, frankincense, jasmine, juniper, lemon, myrrh, rose, sandalwood, and other spice oils.

ODOR: Type: *Base Note (5-20% of the blend)*; Scent: *Rich, warm, slightly woody, creamy, vanilla-like*; Intensity: *1*

Orange

(*Citrus sinensis*)

BOTANICAL FAMILY: Rutaceae (citrus)

EXTRACTION METHOD/ORIGIN: Cold pressed from rind. — USA, South Africa, Italy, China

CHEMICAL CONSTITUENTS: Monoterpenes (> 89%): d-limonene (90%), α-pinene, myrcene; Alcohols (>6%): linalol, α-terpineol, cis- & trans-carveol, geraniol; Aldehydes: n-octanal, n-decanal, citronellal; Ketones: carvone, α-ionone; Coumarins. Also contains flavonoids, β-carotene, steroids, and acids.

PROPERTIES: ANTI-DEPRESSANT, ANTISEPTIC, ANTISPASMODIC, DIGESTIVE, SEDATIVE, and TONIC.

FOLKLORE: According to Robert Wilson, "From early times, oranges have been associated with generosity and gratitude. Once called "golden apples", oranges symbolized innocen and fertility."

ESOTERIC USES/ACTIONS: Astrological: *Sun*; Ayurvedic: *Vatta*; Body type: *Endomorph*; Chakra: *2*; Character: *Yin*; Element: *Fire*; Number: *1*

HISTORICAL USES: Oranges, particularly the bitter orange, has been used for palpitation, scurvy, jaundice, bleeding, heartburn, relaxed throat, prolapse of the uterus and the anus, diarrhea, and blood in the feces.

RENCH MEDICINAL USES: ANGINA (false), CARDIAC SPASM, CONSTIPATION, DIARRHEA (chronic), DYSPEPSIA (nervous), INSOMNIA, MENOPAUSE, PALPITATION.

THER POSSIBLE USES: This oil may help APPETITE, BONES (rickety), BRONCHITIS, COLDS, COLIC (dilute for infants; helps them sleep), COMPLEXION (dull and oily), DERMATITIS, DIGESTIVE SYSTEM, FEVER, FLU, lowers HIGH CHOLESTEROL, MOUTH ULCERS, MUSCLE SORENESS, OBESITY, SEDATION, TISSUE REPAIR, WATER RETENTION, and WRINKLES.

ODY SYSTEM(S) AFFECTED: DIGESTIVE and IMMUNE SYSTEMS, EMOTIONAL BALANCE, SKIN.

ROMATIC INFLUENCE: Orange brings PEACE and HAPPINESS to the MIND and BODY and JOY to the HEART, which provide EMOTIONAL support to help one overcome depression.

PPLICATION: Apply to VITA FLEX POINTS and directly on AREA of concern; diffuse.

RAL USE AS DIETARY SUPPLEMENT: Generally regarded as safe (GRAS) for internal consumption by the FDA. *DILUTE one drop oil in 1 tsp. honey or 4 oz. of beverage (ie. soy/rice milk).* ***Not for children under 6 years old; use with CAUTION and in GREATER DILUTION for children 6 years old and over.***

AFETY DATA: Avoid direct SUNLIGHT for up to 12 hours after use.

LEND CLASSIFICATION: Enhancer and Personifier

LENDS WITH: Cinnamon bark, clove, cypress, frankincense, geranium, juniper, lavender, nutmeg, rosewood.

DOR: Type: *Top Note (5-20% of the blend)*; Scent: *Fresh, citrusy, fruity, sweet, light*; Intensity: *1*

Oregano

(*Origanum compactum*, CT Carvacrol)

OTANICAL FAMILY: Labiatae

XTRACTION METHOD/ORIGIN: Steam distilled from leaves — Morocco, France

HEMICAL CONSTITUENTS: Monoterpenes (25%): α and β-pinenes, myrcene, γ-terpinene, paracymene; Sesquiterpenes: β-caryophyllene; Alcohols (<10%): linalol, terpinen-4-ol, α-terpineol; Phenols (approx. 65%): carvacrol (majority), thymol; Phenol methyl-ethers: methyl carvacrol; Ketones: camphor.

ROPERTIES: ANTI-BACTERIAL, ANTI-FUNGAL, ANTI-PARASITIC, ANTISEPTIC to the respiratory system, ANTIVIRAL, and IMMUNE-STIMULANT.

SOTERIC USES/ACTIONS: Astrological: *Mercury*; Chakra: *4*; Character: *Yang*; Element: *Air*; Number: *9*

FRENCH MEDICINAL USES: ASTHMA, BRONCHITIS (chronic), MENTAL DISEASE, PULMONARY TUBERCULOSIS, RHEUMATISM (chronic), WHOOPING COUGH

OTHER POSSIBLE USES: This oil may help COLDS, DIGESTION PROBLEMS, balance METABOLISM, viral and bacterial PNEUMONIA, and strengthen VITAL CENTERS

BODY SYSTEM(S) AFFECTED: IMMUNE and RESPIRATORY SYSTEMS, MUSCLES and BONES.

AROMATIC INFLUENCE: Strengthens one's feeling of SECURITY.

APPLICATION: Apply to VITA FLEX POINTS and directly on AREA of concern; Diffuse.

ORAL USE AS DIETARY SUPPLEMENT: Generally regarded as safe (GRAS) for internal consumption by the FDA. *DILUTE one drop oil in 1 tsp. honey or 4 oz. of beverage (i. soy/rice milk).* ***Not for children under 6 years old; use with CAUTION and in GREATER DILUTION for children 6 years old and over.***

SAFETY DATA: Can cause extreme SKIN IRRITATION.

BLEND CLASSIFICATION: Enhancer and Equalizer

BLENDS WITH: Basil, fennel, geranium, lemongrass, myrtle, pine, thyme, rosemary.

ODOR: Type: *Middle Note (50-80% of the blend)*; Scent: *Herbaceous, sharp*; Intensity: *5*

Palmarosa

(*Cymbopogon martinii*)

BOTANICAL FAMILY: Graminaceae

EXTRACTION METHOD/ORIGIN: Steam distilled from leaves — India, Conoros

CHEMICAL CONSTITUENTS: Alcohols (>90%): linalol, geraniol (up to 95%), nerol, citronellol (tr.), farnesol (tr.); Sesquiterpenols: elemol; Esters: geranyl & neryl formates, geranyl acetate, geranyl butyrate, and others.

PROPERTIES: ANTI-BACTERIAL, ANTI-FUNGAL, ANTIMICROBIAL, ANTISEPTIC, ANTIVIRAL, HYDRATING, STIMULANT (digestive and circulatory), and TONIC.

FOLKLORE: Once known as Turkish Geranium oil or Indian Geranium oil, palmarosa was us for centuries by the Turks to adulterate the more costly Turkish Rose oil.

ESOTERIC USES/ACTIONS: Astrological: *Venus*; Body type: *Mesomorph*; Character: *Yang with high Yin*; Crystals: *Lapis Lazuli*; Element: *Water & Air*; Number: *2*

HISTORICAL USES: Used to prevent infections and fight fever, palmarosa was also added to many culinary dishes to kill bacteria and aid digestion.

OTHER POSSIBLE USES: This oil may be beneficial for CANDIDA, CIRCULATION, DIGESTION, FEVER, INFECTION, NERVOUS SYSTEM, and RASHES. It is valuable for all types of SKIN problems because it stimulates new cell growth, regulates oil production, moisturizes and speeds healing.

BODY SYSTEM(S) AFFECTED: CARDIOVASCULAR SYSTEM, EMOTIONAL BALANCE, SKIN.

ROMATIC INFLUENCE: Strengthens one's feeling of SECURITY. It also helps to reduce STRESS and TENSION, and promotes recovery from NERVOUS EXHAUSTION. If uplifts the EMOTIONS, refreshes the MIND, and clarifies THOUGHTS. Inhaling palmarosa may also have a normalizing effect on the THYROID GLAND.

PPLICATION: Apply to VITA FLEX POINTS and directly on AREA of concern; diffuse.

RAL USE AS DIETARY SUPPLEMENT: Generally regarded as safe (GRAS) for internal consumption by the FDA. *DILUTE one drop oil in 1 tsp. honey or 4 oz. of beverage (ie. soy/rice milk).* ***Not for children under 6 years old; use with CAUTION and in GREATER DILUTION for children 6 years old and over.***

LEND CLASSIFICATION: Enhancer and Equalizer

LENDS WITH: Basil, fennel, geranium, lemongrass, myrtle, pine, thyme, rosemary.

DOR: Type: *Top to Middle Notes (20-80% of the blend)*; Scent: *Lemony, fresh, green, with hints of rose and geranium*; Intensity: *3*

Single Oils

Patchouli (or Patchouly)

(*Pogostemon cablin*)

OTANICAL FAMILY: Labiatae (mint)

XTRACTION METHOD/ORIGIN: Steam distilled from leaves and flowers — Sumatra, Java, Malaysia, China, Brazil, Indonesia

HEMICAL CONSTITUENTS: Monoterpenes: α-pinenes; Sesquiterpenes (up to 45%): α-gaiene (>12%), β-gaiene, α-bulnesene (>12%), β-bulnesene (>15%), α-, β- & γ-patchoulenes, β-elemene, saychellene (6%), β-caryophyllene, α-humulene, d-cadinene; Ketones: patchoulenone (>1%); Alcohols: patchoulol (up to 35%), pogostol, bulnesol, guaiol, & others; Epoxysesquiterpenes; Acids; Sesquiterpene alkaloids; Aldehydes.

ROPERTIES: ANTI-INFECTIOUS, ANTI-INFLAMMATORY, ANTI-FUNGAL, ANTISEPTIC, ANTITOXIC, ASTRINGENT, DECONGESTANT, DEODORANT, DIURETIC, INSECTICIDAL, STIMULANT (digestive), and TONIC.

SOTERIC USES/ACTIONS: Astrological: *Sun*; Body type: *Endomorph*; Chakras: *1 & 2*; Character: *Yang*; Crystals: *Green tourmaline, Black obsidian*; Element: *Fire & Earth*; Number: *1*

HISTORICAL USES: For centuries, the Asian people used patchouli to fight infection, cool fevers, tone the skin (and entire body), and as an antidote for insect and snake bites. It was also used to treat colds, headaches, nausea, vomiting, diarrhea, abdominal pain, and halitosis (bad breath).

RENCH MEDICINAL USES: ALLERGIES, DERMATITIS, ECZEMA, HEMORRHOIDS, TISSUE REGENERATION.

OTHER POSSIBLE USES: This oil is a DIGESTER of TOXIC MATERIAL in the body. It may also help ACNE, APPETITE (curbs), BITES (INSECT and SNAKE), CELLULITE,

CONGESTION, DANDRUFF, DEPRESSION, DIGESTIVE SYSTEM, relieve itching from HIVES, SKIN CONDITIONS (chapped and tightens loose skin), UV RADIATION (protects against), WATER RETENTION, WEEPING WOUNDS, WEIGHT REDUCTION, and prevent WRINKLES.

BODY SYSTEM(S) AFFECTED: SKIN.

AROMATIC INFLUENCE: It is SEDATING, CALMING, and RELAXING allowing it to reduce ANXIETY. It may have some particular influence on SEX, PHYSICAL ENERGY, and MONEY.

APPLICATION: Apply to VITA FLEX POINTS and directly on AREA of concern; diffuse.

ORAL USE AS DIETARY SUPPLEMENT: Approved by the FDA for use as a Food Additiv (FA) and Flavoring Agent (FL). *DILUTE one drop oil in 1 tsp. honey or 4 oz. of beverage (ie. soy/rice milk).* ***Not for children under 6 years old; use with CAUTION and in GREATER DILUTION for children 6 years old and over.***

BLEND CLASSIFICATION: Enhancer

BLENDS WITH: Bergamot, Clary sage, frankincense, geranium, ginger, lavender, lemongrass, myrrh, pine, rosewood, sandalwood.

ODOR: Type: *Base Note (5-20% of the blend)*; Scent: *Earthy, herbaceous, sweet-balsamic, rich, with woody undertones*; Intensity: *4*

Pepper, Black

(*Piper nigrum*)

BOTANICAL FAMILY: Piperaceae

EXTRACTION METHOD/ORIGIN: Steam distilled from berries — Egypt, India, Madagascar

CHEMICAL CONSTITUENTS: Monoterpenes: α and β-pinenes (<15%), thujene, camphene, sabinene (<10%), carene, limonene (<12%), phellandrene; Sesquiterpenes (approx. 89%): β-caryophyllene (up to 35%), α-humulene, α-guaiene, α- & β-selinenes, α- & β-cubebenes δ- & β-elemenes, β-bisabolene, calamemene; Alcohols: terpinen-4-ol, α-terpineol, linalol, trans-pinocarveol, trans-carveol; Phenol methyl-ethers: paracymene-8-ol, methyl carvacro Ketones: dihydrocarvone; Acetophenones: m- & p-methylacetophenones; Aldehydes: piperonal; Sulfur; Acids.

PROPERTIES: ANALGESIC, ANTI-CATARRHAL, ANTI-INFLAMMATORY, ANTISEPTIC, ANTISPASMODIC, ANTITOXIC, APHRODISIAC, EXPECTORANT, LAXATIVE, RUBEFACIENT, and STIMULANT (nervous, circulatory, digestive),.

FOLKLORE: Pepper was used by the Egyptians in mummification as evidenced by the discover of Black pepper in the nostrils and abdomen of Ramses II. Indian monks ate several Black pepper corns a day to maintain their incredible stamina and energy.

ESOTERIC USES/ACTIONS: Astrological: *Mars*; Body type: *Mesomorph*; Chakras: *3, 4, & 1*

Character: *Yang*; Crystals: *Malachite, Bloodstone*; Element: *Fire*; Number: *2*

HISTORICAL USES: Pepper has been used for thousands of years for malaria, cholera, and several digestive problems.

OTHER POSSIBLE USES: This oil may increase CELLULAR OXYGENATION, support DIGESTIVE GLANDS, stimulate ENDOCRINE SYSTEM, increase ENERGY, and help RHEUMATOID ARTHRITIS. It may also help with loss of APPETITE, CATARRH, CHILLS, CHOLERA, COLDS, COLIC, CONSTIPATION, COUGHS, DIARRHEA, DYSENTERY, DYSPEPSIA, DYSURIA, FLATULENCE (combine with fennel), FLU, HEARTBURN, INFLUENZA, NAUSEA, NEURALGIA, POOR CIRCULATION, POOR MUSCLE TONE, QUINSY, SPRAINS, TOOTHACHE, VERTIGO, VIRUSES, and VOMITING.

BODY SYSTEM(S) AFFECTED: DIGESTIVE and NERVOUS SYSTEMS.

AROMATIC INFLUENCE: Pepper is considered to be good for the 1st CHAKRA. It is COMFORTING and STIMULATING.

APPLICATION: Apply to VITA FLEX POINTS and/or directly on AREA of concern; diffuse. Mix very sparingly with juniper and lavender in a BATH to help with CHILLS or warm one up in the winter.

ORAL USE AS DIETARY SUPPLEMENT: Generally regarded as safe (GRAS) for internal consumption by the FDA. *DILUTE one drop oil in 1 tsp. honey or 4 oz. of beverage (ie. soy/rice milk).* ***Not for children under 6 years old; use with CAUTION and in GREATER DILUTION for children 6 years old and over.***

SAFETY DATA: Can cause extreme SKIN IRRITATION.

BLENDS WITH: Cumin, fennel, frankincense, lavender, marjoram, rosemary, sandalwood, and other spice oils.

ODOR: Type: *Middle Note (50-80% of the blend)*; Scent: *Spicy, peppery, musky, warm, with herbaceous undertones*; Intensity: *3*

Peppermint

(*Mentha piperita*)

BOTANICAL FAMILY: Labiatae (mint)

EXTRACTION METHOD/ORIGIN: Steam distilled from leaves, stems, and flower buds — North America

CHEMICAL CONSTITUENTS: Monoterpenes (< 16%): α and β-pinene, limonene phellandrene, camphene; Sesquiterpenes: β-caryophyllene, z-bulgarene, germacrene-D; Alcohols: menthol (up to 48%), piperitols; Ketones: menthone (20-30% and up to 65% if distilled in September when flowering), piperitone, pulegone, carvone, jasmone; Oxides: 1,8 cineol (5%); Esters: menthyl acetate, also menthyl butyrate & isovalerate; Coumarins; Sulfurs: di-menthylsulfide, mintsulfide.

PROPERTIES: ANALGESIC, ANTICARCINOGENIC, ANTI-INFLAMMATORY (prostate and nerves), ANTISEPTIC, ANTISPASMODIC, and INVIGORATING.

FOLKLORE: According to Roberta Wilson, "In Roman mythology, when Pluto professed his love for the nymph Mentha, his wife Persephone, afire with jealousy, crushed Mentha into dust on the ground. Pluto, unable to change her back, transformed her into a peppermint plant and gave her a fresh fragrance so she would smell sweet whenever stepped upon."

ESOTERIC USES/ACTIONS: Astrological: *Mercury & Venus*; Ayurvedic: *Pitta*; Chakras: *7, 2, & 6*; Character: *Yang*; Crystals: *Topaz, Chalcedony*; Element: *Air*

HISTORICAL USES: For centuries, peppermint has been used to soothe digestive difficulties, freshen breath, and relieve colic, gas, headaches, heartburn, and indigestion.

FRENCH MEDICINAL USES: ASTHMA, BRONCHITIS, CANDIDA, DIARRHEA, DIGESTIVE AID, FEVER (reduces), FLU, HALITOSIS, HEARTBURN, HEMORRHOIDS, HOT FLASHES, INDIGESTION, MENSTRUAL IRREGULARITY, MIGRAINE HEADACHE, MOTION SICKNESS, NAUSEA, RESPIRATORY FUNCTION (aids), SHOCK, SKIN (itchy), THROAT INFECTION, VARICOSE VEINS, VOMITING.

OTHER POSSIBLE USES: This oil may help ANGER, ARTHRITIS, COLIC, DEPRESSION, FATIGUE, FOOD POISONING, HEADACHES, HIVES, HYSTERIA, INFLAMMATION, LIVER PROBLEMS, MORNING SICKNESS, **NERVES** (regenerate and support), RHEUMATISM, elevate and open SENSORY SYSTEM, soothe and cool SKIN (may help keep body cooler on hot days), TOOTHACHES, TUBERCULOSIS, and add flavor to WATER.

BODY SYSTEM(S) AFFECTED: DIGESTIVE SYSTEM, MUSCLES and BONES, NERVOUS and RESPIRATORY SYSTEMS, SKIN.

AROMATIC INFLUENCE: It is PURIFYING and STIMULATING to the CONSCIOUS MIND. Reduces FEVERS. Dr. Dembar of the University of Cincinnati discovered in a research study that inhaling peppermint oil INCREASED the MENTAL ACCURACY of the students tested by up to 28%.

APPLICATION: Apply to VITA FLEX POINTS and/or directly on AREA of concern.

ORAL USE AS DIETARY SUPPLEMENT: Generally regarded as safe (GRAS) for internal consumption by the FDA. *DILUTE one drop oil in 1 tsp. honey or 4 oz. of beverage (ie. soy/rice milk).* ***Not for children under 6 years old; use with CAUTION and in GREATER DILUTION for children 6 years old and over.***

SAFETY DATA: Repeated use can possibly result in CONTACT SENSITIZATION. Use with caution if dealing with HIGH BLOOD PRESSURE. Use with caution during PREGNANCY.

BLEND CLASSIFICATION: Personifier

ODOR: Type: *Middle Note (50-80% of the blend)*; Scent: *Minty, sharp, intense*; Intensity: *5*

FREQUENCY: Physical; approximately 78.

Single Oils

Petitgrain

(*Citrus aurantium*)

OTANICAL FAMILY: Rutaceae (citrus)

XTRACTION METHOD/ORIGIN: Steam distilled from bitter orange tree leaves — Italy

IEMICAL CONSTITUENTS: Monoterpenes (10%): β-myrcene, cis- & trans-β-ocimene, paracymene, d-limonene, camphene, α-terpinene, β-pinene; Alcohols (40%): linalol (20%), α-terpineol (<8%), nerol, geraniol (<5%); Esters (5-80%): linalyl acetate (up to 55%), neryl & terpenyl acetate, geranyl acetate (<5%); Nitrogen compounds; Aldehydes.

ROPERTIES: ANTI-BACTERIAL, ANTI-INFECTIOUS, ANTI-INFLAMMATORY, ANTISEPTIC, ANTISPASMODIC, DEODORANT, NERVINE, and STIMULANT (digestive, nervous).

OLKLORE: Petitgrain derives its name from the extraction of the oil, which at one time was from the green unripe oranges when they were still about the size of a cherry.

SOTERIC USES/ACTIONS: Astrological: *Jupiter, Mars & Sun*; Body type: *Mesomorph*; Chakras: *2 & 4*; Character: *Yin?*; Element: *Fire*; Number: *1*

ISTORICAL USES: Because of its very pleasing scent, petitgrain has been used extensively in high-quality perfumes and cosmetics.

THER POSSIBLE USES: This oil may help re-establish NERVE EQUILIBRIUM. It may also help with ACNE, DYSPEPSIA, FATIGUE, FLATULENCE, GREASY HAIR, INSOMNIA, and excessive PERSPIRATION.

ODY SYSTEM(S) AFFECTED: EMOTIONAL BALANCE.

ROMATIC INFLUENCE: It is UPLIFTING and REFRESHING and helps to refresh the SENSES, clear CONFUSION, reduce MENTAL FATIGUE, and reduce DEPRESSION. It may also stimulate the MIND, support MEMORY, and gladden the HEART.

PPLICATION: Apply to VITA FLEX POINTS and directly on AREA of concern; Diffuse.

RAL USE AS DIETARY SUPPLEMENT: Generally regarded as safe (GRAS) for internal consumption by the FDA. *DILUTE one drop oil in 1 tsp. honey or 4 oz. of beverage (ie. soy/rice milk).* ***Not for children under 6 years old; use with CAUTION and in GREATER DILUTION for children 6 years old and over.***

LEND CLASSIFICATION: Enhancer, Modifier, and Personifier

LENDS WITH: Bergamot, cistus, Clary sage, clove, geranium, jasmine, lavender, neroli, orange, palmarosa, and rosemary.

DOR: Type: *Top Note (5-20% of the blend)*; Scent: *Fresh, floral, citrusy, lighter in fragrance than neroli and slightly woody*; Intensity: *3*

Pine (or Scotch Pine)

(*Pinus sylvestris*)

BOTANICAL FAMILY: Pinaceae (conifer)

EXTRACTION METHOD/ORIGIN: Steam distilled from needles — Austria, Canada, Russ

CHEMICAL CONSTITUENTS: Monoterpenes (50-90%): α-pinene (>41%) and β-pinene (<12%), limonene (up to 30%), Δ-3-carene (<12%); Sesquiterpenes: longifolene; Alcoho borneol (2%); Esters: bornyl acetate (up to 10%).

PROPERTIES: ANTI-BACTERIAL, ANTIMICROBIAL, ANTI-NEURALGIC, ANTISEPT (pulmonary, urinary, hepatic), ANTIVIRAL, EXPECTORANT, and STIMULANT (adrenal cortex, circulatory, nervous).

FOLKLORE: In some cultures, pine branches were placed on coffins to signify immortality.

ESOTERIC USES/ACTIONS: Astrological: *Mars*; Body type: *Ectomorph*; Chakra: *6*; Character: *Yang*; Crystal: *Malachite*; Element: *Air & Light*; Number: *3*

HISTORICAL USES: Pine was used by the American Indians to prevent scurvy. They also stuffed mattresses with pine to repel lice and fleas. It was used to treat pneumonia and lung infections and was even added to baths to revitalize people suffering from mental or emotional fatigue and nervous exhaustion.

FRENCH MEDICINAL USES: ASTHMA, BRONCHITIS, DIABETES, INFECTIONS (severe), RHEUMATOID ARTHRITIS, SINUSITIS.

OTHER POSSIBLE USES: This oil may help dilate and open the RESPIRATORY SYSTEM particularly the BRONCHIAL TRACT. It may also help with COLDS, COUGHS, CUTS, CYSTITIS, FATIGUE, FEET (excessive sweating), FLU, GOUT, LICE, NERVOUS EXHAUSTION, SCABIES, SKIN PARASITES, SORES, STRESS, and URINARY INFECTION. Pine oil may also help increase BLOOD PRESSURE and STIMULATE the ADRENAL GLANDS and the CIRCULATORY SYSTEM. Pine is a good recommendation for any First Aid kit.

BODY SYSTEM(S) AFFECTED: EMOTIONAL BALANCE, RESPIRATORY SYSTEM.

AROMATIC INFLUENCE: It helps soothe MENTAL STRESS, relieve ANXIETY, FRESHEN and DEODORIZE a room, and REVITALIZE the entire body.

APPLICATION: Apply to VITA FLEX POINTS and/or directly on AREA of concern; diffuse Pine is an excellent tonic when added to water and sprinkled on hot rocks in the SAUNA

ORAL USE AS DIETARY SUPPLEMENT: Approved by the FDA for use as a Food Additi (FA) and Flavoring Agent (FL). *DILUTE one drop oil in 1 tsp. honey or 4 oz. of beverage (ie. soy/rice milk).* ***Not for children under 6 years old; use with CAUTION and in GREATER DILUTION for children 6 years old and over.***

SAFETY DATA: Repeated use can possibly result in SKIN IRRITATION.

BLENDS WITH: Cedarwood, eucalyptus, juniper, lemon, marjoram, melaleuca, and rosemary

ODOR: Type: *Middle Note (50-80% of the blend)*; Scent: *Fresh, woody, earthly, balsamic*; Intensity: *4*

Ravensara

(Ravensara aromatica)

)TANICAL FAMILY: Lauraceae

{TRACTION METHOD/ORIGIN: Steam distilled from leaves and branches — Madagascar

HEMICAL CONSTITUENTS: Monoterpenes: α and β-pinenes (< 10%), sabinene (12%); Sesquiterpenes: β-caryophyllene, α-humulene; Alcohols: α-terpineol (<12%), terpinen-4-ol; Esters: terpenyl acetate; Oxides: 1,8-cineol (up to 49%); Phenols: eugenol (5%), isoeugenol (2%); Phenol methyl-ether: methyl eugenol (>3%).

ROPERTIES: ANTI-BACTERIAL, ANTI-FUNGAL, ANTI-INFECTIOUS, ANTISEPTIC, powerful ANTIVIRAL, and EXPECTORANT.

RENCH MEDICINAL USES: BRONCHITIS, CHOLERA, HERPES, INFECTIOUS MONONUCLEOSIS, INSOMNIA, MUSCLE FATIGUE, RHINO PHARYNGITIS, SHINGLES, SINUSITIS, VIRAL HEPATITIS.

THER POSSIBLE USES: Ravensara is part of the Laurel family (akin to *Laurus nobilis*) and is another universal oil like lavender. It may help ASTHMA, BLADDER, BUNIONS, BURNS (healing), CANCER, COLDS, CUTS, EARS, FLU, LIVER, LUNGS, support the NERVES, PNEUMONIA, SCRAPES, VIRAL INFECTIONS, and WOUNDS. As a cross between clove and nutmeg, it may be very supportive to the ADRENAL GLANDS.

ODY SYSTEM(S) AFFECTED: IMMUNE and RESPIRATORY SYSTEMS.

PPLICATION: Apply to VITA FLEX POINTS and/or directly on AREA of concern; Diffuse.

LEND CLASSIFICATION: Enhancer

DOR: Type: *Top Note (5-20% of the blend)*; Scent: *Slightly medicinal, eucalyptus-like, slightly sweet with a fruity hint*; Intensity: *3*

REQUENCY: High (Spiritual); approximately 134 MHz.

Roman Chamomile

(See Chamomile, Roman)

Rosalina

(See Melaleuca Ericifolia)

Rose (or Bulgarian Rose)

(*Rosa damascena*)

BOTANICAL FAMILY: Rosaceae

EXTRACTION METHOD/ORIGIN: Steam distilled from flowers (a two-part process) — Bulgaria, Turkey

CHEMICAL CONSTITUENTS: Monoterpenols: geraniol (up to 28%), citronellol (up to 45% nerol (5%), linalol; Alcohols: phenyl ethyl alcohol (up to 3%), farnesol (>2%); Esters (>5%); Phenols & Methyl Ethers: eugenol (1%), methyl eugenol (<1%); Oxides: rose oxide (<10%); Ketones: α- & β-damascenone, β-ionone (>1%); Nitrogen Compounds: rosefuran (>1%); Many other trace elements.

PROPERTIES: ANTI-HEMORRHAGING, ANTI-INFECTIOUS, and APHRODISIAC.

ESOTERIC USES/ACTIONS: Astrological: *Venus*; Ayurvedic: *Pitta*; Body type: *Mesomorp* Chakras: *2, 4, 6, & 7 (balances all)*; Character: *Yin; Cold and Dry in 2nd Degree*; Crystals: *Ruby (Chakra-2), Rose Quartz, Emerald (Chakra-4), Kunzite, Pink Calcite, Watermelon Tourmaline (Chakra-7)*; Element: *Water, Air, Light, & Ether*; Number: *6*; Oriental: *Yin deficiency (pts. Kid-6, Sp-6); Excess Yang (heat), (pts. Liv-2, He-3)*

HISTORICAL USES: The healing properties of the rose have been utilized in medicine throughout the ages and still plays an important role in the East. It has been used for digestive and menstrual problems, headaches and nervous tension, liver congestion, poor circulation, fever (plague), eye infections, and skin complaints.

OTHER POSSIBLE USES: This oil may help ASTHMA, chronic BRONCHITIS, FRIGIDITY, GINGIVITIS, HEMORRHAGING, HERPES SIMPLEX, IMPOTENCE, INFECTIONS, prevent SCARRING, SEXUAL DEBILITIES, SKIN DISEASE, SPRAINS, THRUSH, TUBERCULOSIS, ULCERS, WOUNDS, and WRINKLES.

BODY SYSTEM(S) AFFECTED: EMOTIONAL BALANCE, SKIN.

AROMATIC INFLUENCE: It is STIMULATING and ELEVATING to the MIND, creating sense of WELL BEING. Its beautiful fragrance is almost intoxicating and APHRODISIAC-LIKE.

APPLICATION: Apply to VITA FLEX POINTS and/or directly on AREA of concern; diffuse

ORAL USE AS DIETARY SUPPLEMENT: Generally regarded as safe (GRAS) for internal consumption by the FDA. *DILUTE one drop oil in 1 tsp. honey or 4 oz. of beverage (i soy/rice milk).* ***Not for children under 6 years old; use with CAUTION and in GREATER DILUTION for children 6 years old and over.***

SAFETY DATA: Use with caution during PREGNANCY.

BLEND CLASSIFICATION: Personifier, Enhancer, Equalizer, and Modifier.

ODOR: Type: *Middle to Base Notes (20-80% of the blend)*; Scent: *Floral, spicy, rich, deep, sensual, green, honey-like*; Intensity: *3*

FREQUENCY: Highest of all the oils (Spiritual); approximately 320 MHz. It enhances the frequency of every cell, bringing balance and harmony to the body.

Rosehip

(*Rosa canina*)

OTANICAL FAMILY: Rosaceae

ROPERTIES: REGENERATIVE

OSSIBLE USES: Rosehip oil has been used effectively in the treatment of SKIN CONDITIONS. It promotes TISSUE REGENERATION, and may help heal BURNS, reduce SCARRING, retard PREMATURE AGING, and soften SCAR TISSUE.

PPLICATION: Apply directly on AREA of concern.

RAL USE AS DIETARY SUPPLEMENT: Generally regarded as safe (GRAS) for internal consumption by the FDA. *DILUTE one drop oil in 1 tsp. honey or 4 oz. of beverage (ie. soy/rice milk).* ***Not for children under 6 years old; use with CAUTION and in GREATER DILUTION for children 6 years old and over.***

Rosemary Camphor

(*Rosmarinus officinalis*, CT Camphor)

OTANICAL FAMILY: Labiatae (mint)

XTRACTION METHOD/ORIGIN: Steam distilled from flowering plant — France, Spain, Tunisia

HEMICAL CONSTITUENTS: Monoterpenes: α-pinene (>12%), β-pinene, camphene (up to 22%), myrcene (1.5%), α and β-phellandrene, limonene (0.5-2%), α and γ-terpinenes, paracymene (2%); Sesquiterpenes: β-caryophyllene (3%); Alcohols: linalol (<1%), terpinen-4-ol, α-terpineol (>1%), borneol (>4%), isoborneol, cis-thujanol-4, trans-thujanol-4, paracymene-8-ol; Esters: bornyl acetate (<1%), α-fenchyl acetate; Oxides: 1,8 cineol (up to 30%), caryophyllene oxide, humulene epoxides I & II; Ketones: 3-hexanone, methyl-heptanone, camphor (up to 30%), verbenon, carvone.

ROPERTIES: ANALGESIC, ANTI-BACTERIAL, ANTISEPTIC, ANTISPASMODIC, ENDOCRINE EQUILIBRATE, EXPECTORANT, MUCOLYTIC, and STIMULANT.

SOTERIC USES/ACTIONS: Astrological: *Sun*; Body type: *Mesomorph*; Chakras: *3 & 6*; Character: *Yang*; Crystals: *Quartz Crystal, Sugalite*; Element: *Fire & Light*; Number: *6*

IISTORICAL USES: The rosemary plant was regarded as sacred by many civilizations. It was used as a fumigant to help drive away evil spirits, and to protect against plague and infectious illness.

RENCH MEDICINAL USES: ARTHRITIS, BLOOD PRESSURE (low), BRONCHITIS, CELLULITE, CHOLERA, COLDS, DANDRUFF, DEPRESSION (nervous), DIABETES, FATIGUE (nervous/mental), FLU, FLUID RETENTION, HAIR LOSS, HEADACHE, HEPATITIS (viral), MENSTRUAL PERIODS (irregular), SINUSITIS, TACHYCARDIA, VAGINITIS.

OTHER POSSIBLE USES: This oil may help ASTHMA, BALDNESS, CANDIDA, CHOLESTEROL, CIRCULATION, GOUT, balance HEART FUNCTION, INJURIES, MUSCULAR ACHES/PAINS, stimulate NERVES, OBESITY, RESPIRATORY FUNCTIONS, RHEUMATISM, SKIN CONDITIONS, SPRAINS, and WOUNDS. ***Note: This chemotype is said to be best for CRAMPS, FATIGUE, HEART (tonic - a a venous decongestant), INFECTIONS, LIVER (aids production of bile), and as a powerful MUCOLYTIC and a non-hormonal EMMENAGOGUE (promotes MENSTRUATION).***

BODY SYSTEM(S) AFFECTED: CARDIOVASCULAR and DIGESTIVE SYSTEMS, MUSCLES and BONES.

AROMATIC INFLUENCE: It is great for the morning, as it is highly STIMULATING. It help to enliven the BRAIN, clears and aids MEMORY, and opens the CONSCIOUS MIND.

APPLICATION: Apply to VITA FLEX POINTS and/or directly on AREA of concern; Diffuse

ORAL USE AS DIETARY SUPPLEMENT: Generally regarded as safe (GRAS) for internal consumption by the FDA. *DILUTE one drop oil in 1 tsp. honey or 4 oz. of beverage (ie soy/rice milk).* ***Not for children under 6 years old; use with CAUTION and in GREATER DILUTION for children 6 years old and over.***

SAFETY DATA: Avoid during PREGNANCY. Not for use by people with EPILEPSY. Avoi if dealing with HIGH BLOOD PRESSURE. Highly stimulating in small doses, avoic if sleep is needed.

BLEND CLASSIFICATION: Enhancer.

BLENDS WITH: Basil, cedarwood, frankincense, lavender, peppermint, rosewood, eucalyptus.

Rosemary Cineol

(*Rosmarinus officinalis*, CT 1,8 Cineol)

BOTANICAL FAMILY: Labiatae (mint)

EXTRACTION METHOD/ORIGIN: Steam distilled from flowering plant — France, Tunisia USA

CHEMICAL CONSTITUENTS: Monoterpenes: α-pinene (<14%), β-pinene (<9%), camphene (<6%), myrcene, α and β-phellandrene, limonene, α and γ-terpinenes, paracymene; Sesquiterpenes: β-caryophyllene; Monoterpene alcohols: borneol; Esters: bornyl acetate; Oxides: 1,8 cineol (up to 55%); Ketones: camphor (<15%).

PROPERTIES: ANTI-BACTERIAL, ANTI-CATARRHAL, ANTI-INFECTIOUS, and EXPECTORANT.

ESOTERIC USES/ACTIONS: (See Rosemary Camphor)

HISTORICAL USES: (See Rosemary Camphor)

FRENCH MEDICINAL USES: (See Rosemary Camphor)

OTHER POSSIBLE USES: This oil may help ARTERIOSCLEROSIS, BRONCHITIS,

CHILLS, COLDS, COLITIS, CYSTITIS, DYSPEPSIA, nervous EXHAUSTION, FLU, oily HAIR, IMMUNE SYSTEM (stimulate), OTITIS, PALPITATIONS, prevent RESPIRATORY INFECTIONS, SINUSITIS, sour STOMACH, STRESS-RELATED ILLNESS. ***Note: This chemotype is said to be best used for PULMONARY CONGESTION, slow ELIMINATION, CANDIDA, chronic FATIGUE, and INFECTIONS (especially staph and strep).***

ODY SYSTEM(S) AFFECTED: IMMUNE, RESPIRATORY, and NERVOUS SYSTEMS.

ROMATIC INFLUENCE: Stimulates MEMORY and opens the CONSCIOUS MIND.

PPLICATION: Apply to VITA FLEX POINTS and/or directly on AREA of concern; Diffuse.

RAL USE AS DIETARY SUPPLEMENT: Generally regarded as safe (GRAS) for internal consumption by the FDA. *DILUTE one drop oil in 1 tsp. honey or 4 oz. of beverage (ie. soy/rice milk).* ***Not for children under 6 years old; use with CAUTION and in GREATER DILUTION for children 6 years old and over.***

AFETY DATA: Avoid during PREGNANCY. Not for use by people with EPILEPSY. Avoid if dealing with HIGH BLOOD PRESSURE.

LEND CLASSIFICATION: Enhancer.

LENDS WITH: Basil, cedarwood, frankincense, lavender, peppermint, rosewood, eucalyptus, marjoram, pine.

DOR: Type: *Middle Note (50-80% of the blend)*; Scent: *Herbaceous, strong, camphorous, with woody-balsamic and evergreen undertones*; Intensity: *3*

Rosemary Verbenon

(*Rosmarinus officinalis*, CT Verbenon)

OTANICAL FAMILY: Labiatae (mint)

XTRACTION METHOD/ORIGIN: Steam distilled from flowering plant — Corsica

HEMICAL CONSTITUENTS: Monoterpenes: α-pinene (22%), β-pinene, camphene, myrcene, limonene, α-terpinene, terpinolene; Sesquiterpenes: β-caryophyllene; Alcohols: borneol (up to 7%), α-terpineol, terpinen-4-ol; Esters: bornyl acetate; Oxides: 1,8 cineol (> 19%); Ketones: verbenon (up to 37%), camphor (1-15%).

ROPERTIES: ANTI-BACTERIAL, ANTI-CATARRHAL, ANTI-INFECTIOUS, ANTISPASMODIC, CARDIAC regulator, ENDOCRINE regulator (pituitary - regulates ovaries and testicles), EXPECTORANT, MUCOLYTIC, and NERVOUS regulator.

SOTERIC USES/ACTIONS: (See Rosemary Camphor)

ISTORICAL USES: (See Rosemary Camphor)

RENCH MEDICINAL USES: (See Rosemary Camphor)

THER POSSIBLE USES: This oil may help ASTHMA, BALDNESS, CANDIDA, CHOLESTEROL, CIRCULATION, GOUT, balance HEART FUNCTION, support IMMUNE SYSTEM, INJURIES, decongest the LIVER, MUSCULAR ACHES/PAINS, stimulate NERVES, OBESITY, regulate OVARY function, RESPIRATORY FUNCTIONS, RHEUMATISM, SKIN CONDITIONS, energize SOLAR PLEXUS, SPINAL, SPRAINS, regulate TESTICULAR function, VIRUSES, and WOUNDS. ***Note: This chemotype is said to be best used for LIVER and GALL BLADDER support, rejuvenation of SKIN (especially chronic DRY SKIN), middle EAR INFECTIONS, and ENDOCRINE problems (regulates hypothalamic / pituitary / sexual glands).***

BODY SYSTEM(S) AFFECTED: DIGESTIVE and HORMONAL SYSTEMS, SKIN and HAIR.

AROMATIC INFLUENCE: Stimulates MEMORY and opens the CONSCIOUS MIND.

APPLICATION: Apply to VITA FLEX POINTS and directly on AREA of concern; Diffuse.

ORAL USE AS DIETARY SUPPLEMENT: Generally regarded as safe (GRAS) for internal consumption by the FDA. *DILUTE one drop oil in 1 tsp. honey or 4 oz. of beverage (ie soy/rice milk).* ***Not for children under 6 years old; use with CAUTION and in GREATER DILUTION for children 6 years old and over.***

SAFETY DATA: Avoid during PREGNANCY. Not for use by people with EPILEPSY. Avo if dealing with HIGH BLOOD PRESSURE.

BLEND CLASSIFICATION: Enhancer.

BLENDS WITH: Basil, eucalyptus, lavender, marjoram, peppermint, pine.

Rosewood

(*Aniba rosaeodora*)

BOTANICAL FAMILY: Lauraceae

EXTRACTION METHOD/ORIGIN: Steam distilled from wood — Brazil

CHEMICAL CONSTITUENTS: Monoterpene alcohols: linalol (up to 90%), α-terpineol, geraniol; Monoterpenes: limonene, pinene; Oxides: 1,8-cineol; Aldehydes: citronellal.

PROPERTIES: ANTI-BACTERIAL, ANTI-FUNGAL, ANTI-INFECTIOUS, ANTI-PARASITIC, and ANTIVIRAL.

ESOTERIC USES/ACTIONS: Astrological: *Sun, Venus*; Body type: *Mesomorph*; Chakras: *links 7 to 1; also 4*; Character: *Yang*; Crystals: *Rutilated smoky quartz, Apophylite (link 1st to 7th chakra)*; Element: *Earth*; Number: *3*

HISTORICAL USES: According to Roberta Wilson, "The original site of production of *bois de rose*, as the French called rosewood, was French Guiana, on the northern coast of South America. So great was the demand among the French for rosewood oil, . . . that they depleted the colony's rosewood forests." Even now, this tropical, evergreen tree is one of the trees that is being extensively felled in the clearing of the South America rainforests.

FRENCH MEDICINAL USES: ACNE, CANDIDA, DEPRESSION, ECZEMA, ORAL INFECTIONS, SKIN (dry), VAGINITIS.

OTHER POSSIBLE USES: This oil may create SKIN ELASTICITY and is SOOTHING to the SKIN. It is recognized for its ability to get rid of CANDIDA of the SKIN and slow the AGING process. It may also be beneficial for CUTS, NAUSEA, TISSUE REGENERATION, and WOUNDS. It helps to create a synergism with all other oils.

BODY SYSTEM(S) AFFECTED: SKIN.

AROMATIC INFLUENCE: It is APPEASING to the MIND, RELAXING to the BODY, and creates a feeling of PEACE and GENTLENESS.

APPLICATION: Apply to VITA FLEX POINTS and/or directly on AREA of concern; diffuse.

ORAL USE AS DIETARY SUPPLEMENT: Generally regarded as safe (GRAS) for internal consumption by the FDA. *DILUTE one drop oil in 1 tsp. honey or 4 oz. of beverage (ie. soy/rice milk).* ***Not for children under 6 years old; use with CAUTION and in GREATER DILUTION for children 6 years old and over.***

BLEND CLASSIFICATION: Modifier and Equalizer.

ODOR: Type: *Middle Note (50-80% of the blend)*; Scent: *Sweet, woody, fruity, floral aroma*; Intensity: *3*

Sage

(*Salvia officinalis*)

BOTANICAL FAMILY: Labiatae (mint)

EXTRACTION METHOD/ORIGIN: Steam distilled from leaves and flowers — Croatia, France, Spain

CHEMICAL CONSTITUENTS: Monoterpenes: α-thujene, α- & β-pinenes, camphene, myrcene, α-terpinene, limonene; Sesquiterpenes: β-caryophyllene, aromadendrene, α-humulene-4, d-cadinenes; Alcohols: linalol (>11%), terpinen-4-ol (4%), α-terpineol (5%), borneol; Sesquiterpenol: viridiflorol; Esters: methyl isovalerate, bornyl, linalyl, & sabinyl acetates; Phenols: thymol (tr.); Oxides: 1,8 cineol (up to 14%); Ketones (approx. 60%): α-thujone (12-33%), β-thujone (2-14%), camphor (1-26%); Coumarins.

PROPERTIES: ANTI-BACTERIAL, ANTI-CANCEROUS, ANTISEPTIC, ANTISPASMODIC, DECONGESTANT, DIURETIC, and DISINFECTANT. It contains estriol and has ESTROGEN-LIKE PROPERTY.

FOLKLORE: Sage is recognized by the Lakota Indians as a purifier and as the master healer, and was called *herba sacra* or 'sacred herb' by the Romans.

ESOTERIC USES/ACTIONS: Astrological: *Jupiter*; Body type: *Ectomorph*; Chakras: *4, 2, & 3*; Character: *Yang*; Crystal: *Malachite*; Element: *Air*; Number: *7*; Perfume note: *Top*

HISTORICAL USES: Sage has been used for respiratory infections, menstrual difficulties, digestive complaints, inflammations of the mouth, tongue, and throat, and to strengthen the senses and the memory.

FRENCH MEDICINAL USES: ASTHMA, BRONCHITIS (chronic), DIGESTION (sluggish),

GINGIVITIS, GLANDULAR DISORDERS, LYMPHATIC SYSTEM, MENOPAUSE, MENSTRUAL IRREGULARITY, NIGHT SWEATS.

OTHER POSSIBLE USES: This oil may help improve ESTROGEN and PROGESTERONE-TESTOSTERONE BALANCE. It is believed to contain elements that contribute to the SECRETION of PROGESTERONE-TESTOSTERONE. It activates the NERVOUS SYSTEM and ADRENAL CORTEX and may help with illness that is related to DIGESTION and LIVER PROBLEMS. It may also be beneficial for ACNE, ARTHRITIS, BACTERIAL INFECTIONS, CATARRH (mucus), DANDRUFF, DEPRESSION, ECZEMA, FIBROSITIS, HAIR LOSS, LOW BLOOD PRESSURE, MENTAL FATIGUE, METABOLISM, RESPIRATORY PROBLEMS, RHEUMATISM, SKIN CONDITIONS, SORES, SPRAINS, TISSUE (firms), and strengthening the VITAL CENTERS of the body. It may also BALANCE the PELVIC CHAKRA where negative emotions from denial and sexual abuse are stored.

BODY SYSTEM(S) AFFECTED: HORMONAL and IMMUNE SYSTEMS.

AROMATIC INFLUENCE: Helps to relieve DEPRESSION, MENTAL FATIGUE, and STRAIN.

APPLICATION: Apply to VITA FLEX POINTS and/or directly on AREA of concern; diffuse.

ORAL USE AS DIETARY SUPPLEMENT: Generally regarded as safe (GRAS) for internal consumption by the FDA. *DILUTE one drop oil in 2 tsp. honey or 8 oz. of beverage (ie. soy/rice milk). However, due to thujone content, more dilution may be necessary.* ***Best AVOIDED by children of all ages.***

SAFETY DATA: Classified by Robert Tisserand as an ORAL TOXIN due to thujone content However, other sources indicate that for thujone to be toxic, undiluted oil in excess of 30 ml must be ingested in a short period of time. Therefore, use with caution. Best kept away from children. Avoid during PREGNANCY. Not for use by people with EPILEPSY. Avoid if dealing with HIGH BLOOD PRESSURE.

BLEND CLASSIFICATION: Enhancer.

BLENDS WITH: Bergamot, lemon, lavender, peppermint, rosemary, lemongrass, pine.

Sage Lavender (or Spanish Sage)

(Salvia lavandulafolia)

BOTANICAL FAMILY: Labiatae

EXTRACTION METHOD/ORIGIN: Steam distilled from flowering plant — Spain

CHEMICAL CONSTITUENTS: Alcohols (approx. 35%): linalool (>28%), terpinen-4-ol, α- & δ-terpineol, trans-thujanol-4, sabinol, borneol, nerol, geraniol, sesquiterpenols; Oxides: 1,8-cineole (up to 35%); Ketones: camphor (up to 34%); Monoterpenes: α-thujene, α- & β-pinenes (up to 20%), camphene (>20%), sabinene, myrcene, limonene (>20%), cis- & trans-ocimene, allocimene; Sesquiterpenes: α-cubenene, α-coaene, α-gurjunene, cis- &

trans-α-bergamotene, β-caryophyllene, α-humulene; Hydrocarbons: α-p-dimethylstyrene; Esters: linalyl acetate, bornyl acetate, sabinyl acetate, terpenyl acetate

PROPERTIES: ANTI-CATARRHAL, ANTI-DEPRESSANT, ANTI-INFLAMMATORY, ANTIMICROBIAL, ANTISEPTIC, ANTI-INFECTIOUS, ANTISPASMODIC, ASTRINGENT, ANALGESIC, REGULATOR (seborrhea), STIMULANT (liver, adrenal, and circulatory), TONIC.

ESOTERIC USES/ACTIONS: Astrological: *Jupiter*; Body type: *Ectomorph*; Chakras: *4, 2, & 3*; Character: *Yang*; Crystal: *Malachite*; Element: *Air*; Number: *7*; Perfume note: *Top*

POSSIBLE USES: Sage lavender may be beneficial for Alzheimer's Disease. It has been shown to inhibit cholinesterase activity and mimic HORMONES (increasing both estradiol and testosterone levels). It may also be beneficial for ACHES/PAINS (muscle), ACNE, ARTHRITIS, ASTHENIA, ASTHMA, BRONCHITIS, CHILLS, CIRCULATION (poor), COLDS, COUGHS, CUTS, DANDRUFF, DEBILITY, DERMATITIS, ECZEMA, EXHAUSTION (nervous), FEVER, FLU, GUM infections, HAIR loss, HEADACHES, JAUNDICE, LARYNGITIS, LIVER congestion, MENSTRUATION (induces), NEURALGIA, PERIODS (painful and difficult), RHEUMATISM, RHINITIS, SINUSITIS, STERILITY, SWEATING (excessive).

BODY SYSTEM(S) AFFECTED: EMOTIONAL BALANCE, HORMONAL SYSTEM, MUSCLE and BONE, NERVOUS SYSTEM, RESPIRATORY SYSTEM, SKIN.

AROMATIC INFLUENCE: Sage lavender helps improve MOOD and MEMORY. It may also help HARMONIZE and BALANCE the EMOTIONS and reduce STRESS-RELATED conditions.

APPLICATION: Apply to VITA FLEX POINTS of the feet and/or directly on AREA of concern; DIFFUSE.

ORAL USE AS DIETARY SUPPLEMENT: Generally regarded as safe (GRAS) for internal consumption by the FDA. *DILUTE one drop oil in 1 tsp. honey or 4 oz. of beverage (ie. soy/rice milk).* ***Not for children under 6 years old; use with CAUTION and in GREATER DILUTION for children 6 years old and over.***

BLEND CLASSIFICATION: Personifier and Equalizer.

BLENDS WITH: Clary sage, fennel, frankincense, geranium, sandalwood, ylang ylang.

Sandalwood

(*Santalum album*)

BOTANICAL FAMILY: Santalaceae (sandalwood)

EXTRACTION METHOD/ORIGIN: Steam distilled from wood — India, Indonesia

CHEMICAL CONSTITUENTS: Sesquiterpenes: α- & β-santalenes, epi-β-santalene; Sesquiterpene alcohols: α and β-santalols (<65%), epi-β-santalol (>5%); Aldehydes: tersantalal; Carboxylic acid (<2%): nor-tricyclo-eka-santalic acid; Also: borneol

PROPERTIES: ANTI-DEPRESSANT, ANTISEPTIC, APHRODISIAC, ASTRINGENT, CALMING, SEDATIVE, and TONIC.

FOLKLORE: Sandalwood purportedly awakens the latent life force energy during meditation, and frees the souls of the deceased at funerals. Many cultures still consider sandalwood to be sacred.

ESOTERIC USES/ACTIONS: Astrological: *Saturn, Moon, Jupiter & Uranus*; Ayurvedic: *Pitta*; Body type: *Mesomorph*; Chakras: *links 1 & 7, also 4, 5, & 1*; Character: *mildly Yang - Cold & Dry 2nd Degree*; Crystals: *Clear Calcite, Emerald, Turquoise, Citrine (links 2nd & 7th chakras)*; Element: *Water, Fire, & Air*; Number: *6*; Oriental: *Hot dampness (pts: Sp-9 & 6)*

HISTORICAL USES: Sandalwood was traditionally used as an incense during ritual work for enhancing meditation. The Egyptians also used sandalwood for embalming.

FRENCH MEDICINAL USES: BRONCHITIS (chronic), DIARRHEA (obstinate), HEMORRHOIDS, IMPOTENCE.

OTHER POSSIBLE USES: Sandalwood is very similar to frankincense in action. It may support the CARDIOVASCULAR SYSTEM, remove NEGATIVE PROGRAMMING from CELLS, and relieve symptoms associated with LUMBAGO and the SCIATIC NERVES. It may also be beneficial for ACNE, regenerating BONE CARTILAGE, CATARRH, CIRCULATION (similar in action to frankincense), COUGHS, CYSTITIS, DEPRESSION, HICCOUGHS, LYMPHATIC SYSTEM, MEDITATION, MENSTRUAL PROBLEMS, NERVES (similar in action to frankincense), NERVOUS TENSION, increasing OXYGEN around the PINEAL and PITUITARY GLANDS, SKIN INFECTION and REGENERATION, TUBERCULOSIS, and YOGA.

BODY SYSTEM(S) AFFECTED: EMOTIONAL BALANCE, MUSCLE and BONE, NERVOUS SYSTEM, SKIN.

AROMATIC INFLUENCE: Slowly and powerfully CALMS, HARMONIZES, and BALANCES the EMOTIONS. It helps one accept others with an open heart while diminishing one's own egocentricity. It may help ENHANCE MEDITATION by opening the third eye. It can also be stimulating as well as grounding as it is said to vibrate between the 7th and 1st chakra.

APPLICATION: Apply to VITA FLEX POINTS of the feet and/or directly on AREA of concern; diffuse.

ORAL USE AS DIETARY SUPPLEMENT: Approved by the FDA for use as a Food Additive (FA) and Flavoring Agent (FL). *DILUTE one drop oil in 1 tsp. honey or 4 oz. of beverage (ie. soy/rice milk).* ***Not for children under 6 years old; use with CAUTION and in GREATER DILUTION for children 6 years old and over.***

BLEND CLASSIFICATION: Modifier and Equalizer.

BLENDS WITH: Cypress, frankincense, lemon, myrrh, ylang ylang, patchouli, spruce.

ODOR: Type: *Base Note (5-20% of the blend)*; Scent: *Soft, woody, sweet, earthy, balsamic, tenacious*; Intensity: *3*

FREQUENCY: Physical and Emotional; approximately 96 MHz.

Spearmint

(*Mentha spicata*, CT Carvone)

OTANICAL FAMILY: Labiatae (mint)

XTRACTION METHOD/ORIGIN: Steam distilled from leaves — Utah, USA

HEMICAL CONSTITUENTS: Monoterpenes: α and β-pinenes, camphene, myrcene, limonene (> 18%), α-phellandrene; Sesquiterpenes: β-caryophyllene, α-elemene, farnesene, β-bourbonene; Alcohols: menthol, linalol, borneol, trans-thujanol-4 (>20%), farnesol, elemol, cadinol; Esters: dihydrocarvyl acetate, cis- & trans-carvyl acetate; Oxides: 1,8 cineol (>3%); Ketones: carvone (50-60%), dihydrocarvone (<1%), menthone (>1%).

ROPERTIES: ANTI-BACTERIAL, ANTI-CATARRHAL, ANTI-FUNGAL, ANTI-INFLAMMATORY, ANTISEPTIC, ANTISPASMODIC, HORMONE-LIKE, INSECTICIDAL, and STIMULANT.

SOTERIC USES/ACTIONS: Astrological: *Mercury & Venus*; Character: *Yang*; Element: *Air & Water*

ISTORICAL USES: Spearmint has been used to relieve hiccough, colic, nausea, indigestion, flatulence, headaches, sores, and scabs.

RENCH MEDICINAL USES: BRONCHITIS, CANDIDA, CYSTITIS, HYPERTENSION.

THER POSSIBLE USES: This oil may balance and increase METABOLISM, which may help BURN UP FATS and TOXINS in the body. It may aid the GLANDULAR, NERVOUS, and RESPIRATORY SYSTEMS. It may also help with ACNE, APPETITE (stimulates), BAD BREATH, BALANCE, CHILDBIRTH (promotes easier labor), CONSTIPATION, DEPRESSION, DIARRHEA, DIGESTION, DRY SKIN, ECZEMA, FEVERS, HEADACHES, INTESTINES (soothes), KIDNEY STONES, MENSTRUATION (slow, heavy periods), MIGRAINES, NAUSEA, SORE GUMS, STOMACH (relaxes muscles), URINE RETENTION, VAGINITIS, WEIGHT (reduces), and bring about a feeling of WELL BEING.

DY SYSTEM(S) AFFECTED: DIGESTIVE SYSTEM, EMOTIONAL BALANCE.

ROMATIC INFLUENCE: Its HORMONE-LIKE activity may help open and release emotional blocks to bring about a feeling of balance. It acts as an anti-depressant by relieving mental strain and fatigue, and by lifting one's spirits.

PPLICATION: Apply to VITA FLEX POINTS and directly on AREA of concern; Diffuse.

RAL USE AS DIETARY SUPPLEMENT: Generally regarded as safe (GRAS) for internal consumption by the FDA. *DILUTE one drop oil in 1 tsp. honey or 4 oz. of beverage (ie. soy/rice milk).* ***Not for children under 6 years old; use with CAUTION and in GREATER DILUTION for children 6 years old and over.***

AFETY DATA: Use with caution during PREGNANCY. Not for use on babies.

LEND CLASSIFICATION: Personifier.

LENDS WITH: Basil, lavender, peppermint, rosemary.

DOR: Type: *Top Note (5-20% of the blend)*; Scent: *Minty, slightly fruity, less bright than peppermint*; Intensity: *3*

Spikenard

(*Nardostachys jatamansi*)

BOTANICAL FAMILY: Valerianaceae

EXTRACTION METHOD/ORIGIN: Steam distilled from roots — India

CHEMICAL CONSTITUENTS: Sesquiterpenes (93%): calarene (up to 35%), aristolene, dihydroazulenes, β-ionene, β-maaliene; Aldehydes: valerenal; Ketones: valeranone (=jatamansone), nardostachone; Acids: jatamanshinic acid; Coumarins.

PROPERTIES: ANTI-BACTERIAL, ANTI-FUNGAL, ANTI-INFLAMMATORY, DEODORANT, RELAXING, and SKIN TONIC.

FOLKLORE: Spikenard has also been known as "nard" and "'false' Indian valerian root" oil. Prized in early Egypt, it was used in a preparation, called *kyphi*, with other oils like saffron, juniper, myrrh, cassia, and cinnamon. According to Roberta Wilson, "The Egyptians believed that in addition to appeasing the gods, Kyphi incense quelled fear and anxiety, improved meditation, and induced restful sleep with pleasant dreams."

ESOTERIC USES/ACTIONS: Astrological: *Saturn & Sun*; Chakras: *4 & 7*; Character: *Yin*; Element: *Fire & Ether*

HISTORICAL USES: In India, spikenard was notably regarded as a perfume, medicinal herb, and as a skin tonic. Highly prized in the Middle East during the time of Christ, there are several passages in the Bible referring to spikenard. Spikenard was also used in the preparation of *nardinum*, a scented oil of great renown during ancient times.

OTHER POSSIBLE USES: The oil is known for helping in the treatment of ALLERGIC SKI REACTIONS, and according to Victoria Edwards, "The oil redresses the skin's physiological balance and causes permanent regeneration." Spikenard may also help wit ALLERGIES, CANDIDA, FLATULENT INDIGESTION, INSOMNIA, MENSTRUA DIFFICULTIES, MIGRAINE, NAUSEA, RASHES, STAPH INFECTIONS, STRESS TACHYCARDIA, TENSION, and WOUNDS that will not heal.

BODY SYSTEM(S) AFFECTED: EMOTIONAL BALANCE, SKIN.

AROMATIC INFLUENCE: Spikenard has a peaty, earthy, animal-like fragrance, reminiscent of goats. It is BALANCING, SOOTHING, and HARMONIZING.

APPLICATION: Apply to VITA FLEX POINTS and/or directly on AREA of concern.

ORAL USE AS DIETARY SUPPLEMENT: None.

BLENDS WITH: Cistus, lavender, patchouli, pine, and vetiver.

ODOR: Type: *Base Note (5-20% of the blend)*; Scent: *Heavy, earthy, animal-like, similar to valerian*; Intensity: *5*

BIBLE: Song of Solomon 1:12, 4:13-14; Mark 14:3; John 12:3

Spruce (or Black Spruce)

(*Picea mariana*)

OTANICAL FAMILY: Pinaceae (conifer)

XTRACTION METHOD/ORIGIN: Steam distilled from needles — Canada

HEMICAL CONSTITUENTS: Monoterpenes (bi- & tri-cyclic approx. 55%): camphene (13%), tricyclene, α-pinene (up to 16%), Δ-3-carene (up to 15%); Sesquiterpenes: longifolene, longicyclene; Alcohols: borneol (2%); Esters: bornyl acetate (> 35%); Sesquiterpenols: longiborneol.

ROPERTIES: ANTI-INFECTIOUS, ANTI-INFLAMMATORY, ANTISPASMODIC, CORTISONE-LIKE, DISINFECTANT, and TONIC.

SOTERIC USES/ACTIONS: Chakras: *5, 6, & 3*; Character: *Yang*; Element: *Ether & Light*

ISTORICAL USES: It was used by the Lakota Indians to enhance their communication with the Great Spirit.

RENCH MEDICINAL USES: ARTHRITIS, CANDIDA, HYPERTHYROIDISM, IMMUNE-DEPRESSION, PROSTATITIS, RHEUMATISM, SOLAR PLEXUS.

THER POSSIBLE USES: Spruce oil creates the symbolic effect of the umbrella which protects the earth and brings energy in from the universe. At night the animals in the wild lie down under a tree for the protection, recharging, and rejuvenation the trees bring them. It may be beneficial for BONE PAIN, GLANDULAR SYSTEM, aching JOINTS, opening the PINEAL GLAND, SCIATICA PAIN, and stimulating the THYMUS and ADRENAL glands.

ODY SYSTEM(S) AFFECTED: EMOTIONAL BALANCE, NERVOUS and RESPIRATORY SYSTEMS.

ROMATIC INFLUENCE: Spruce oil GROUNDS the body, creating the feeling of BALANCE necessary to receive and to give. Helps release EMOTIONAL BLOCKS.

PPLICATION: Apply to VITA FLEX POINTS and/or directly on AREA of concern.

RAL USE AS DIETARY SUPPLEMENT: Approved by the FDA for use as a Food Additive (FA) and Flavoring Agent (FL). *DILUTE one drop oil in 1 tsp. honey or 4 oz. of beverage (ie. soy/rice milk).* ***Not for children under 6 years old; use with CAUTION and in GREATER DILUTION for children 6 years old and over.***

LEND CLASSIFICATION: Equalizer and Enhancer

LENDS WITH: Birch, eucalyptus, frankincense, helichrysum, ravensara, wintergreen.

DOR: Type: *Middle Note (50-80% of the blend)*; Scent: *Fresh, woody, earthy, sweet, with a hint of a fruity note*; Intensity: *3*

Tamanu

(*Calophyllum inophyllum*)

NOTE: *This is a vegetal oil, not an essential oil. Listed here because of its value as a fixed oil in formulations.*

BOTANICAL FAMILY: Gutiferae or Hypericaceae

EXTRACTION METHOD/ORIGIN: Cold pressed from the nut of the Polynesian Tamanu tree. — Tahiti

CHEMICAL CONSTITUENTS: Terpenic essences, benzoic & oxibenzoic acids, vitamin F, lipids, glycerides, saturated fatty acids, calophyllolide (3,4-dihydro-5-methoxyl-22-dimethyl-6), calophyllic acid, coumarin derivatives, and phosphor-amino acids.

PROPERTIES: ANTIBACTERIAL, ANTI-INFECTIOUS, ANTI-INFLAMMATORY, ANT RHEUMATIC.

HISTORICAL USES: The natives of Tahiti believe that tamanu oil is a "sacred" gift of nature The women use the oil as a natural moisturizing cosmetic on their faces and bodies. It w also used for protection against sunburns.

OTHER POSSIBLE USES: BURNS and WOUNDS (when mixed with helichrysum), HAIR (creates healthy), and NATURAL SUN SCREEN.

BODY SYSTEM(S) AFFECTED: SKIN

AROMATIC INFLUENCE: GROUNDING and SOOTHING. It has an earthly, musky smel with a slight nutty odor.

APPLICATION: Apply directly on area of concern.

ORAL USE AS DIETARY SUPPLEMENT: None.

SAFETY DATA: AVOID if allergic to any kind of nuts.

BLENDS WITH: Helichrysum (burns and wounds), Rosemary camphor for hair growth

Tangerine

(*Citrus nobilis* or *Citrus reticulata* var. tangerine)

BOTANICAL FAMILY: Rutaceae (citrus)

EXTRACTION METHOD/ORIGIN: Cold pressed from rind — USA, Mexico, Brazil, South Africa

CHEMICAL CONSTITUENTS: Monoterpenes: d-limonene (up to 92%), α-pinene, myrcene (<4%), cadinene, γ-terpinene; Alcohols: linalol, citronellol; Aldehydes: citrals.

PROPERTIES: ANTI-COAGULANT, ANTI-INFLAMMATORY, LAXATIVE, and SEDATIVE.

ESOTERIC USES/ACTIONS: Astrological: *Sun*; Body type: *Nervous*; Chakra: *2*; Character: *Yang (some Yin)?*; Element: *Water*

POSSIBLE USES: It may help dissolve CELLULITE, CIRCULATION, CONSTIPATION, DIARRHEA, DIGESTIVE SYSTEM DISORDERS, FAT DIGESTION, DIZZINESS, FEAR, FLATULENCE, GALLBLADDER, INSOMNIA, INTESTINAL SPASMS, IRRITABILITY, LIMBS (tired and aching), LIVER PROBLEMS, decongest LYMPHATIC SYSTEM (helps to stimulate draining), OBESITY, PARASITES, SADNESS, STOMACH tonic, STRETCH MARKS (smooths when blended with lavender), STRESS, **SWELLING**, and alleviate **WATER RETENTION (EDEMA)**.

BODY SYSTEM(S) AFFECTED: EMOTIONAL BALANCE, IMMUNE SYSTEM, SKIN.

AROMATIC INFLUENCE: Tangerine oil contains esters and aldehydes which are SEDATING and CALMING to the NERVOUS SYSTEM. When diffused together with marjoram, it can soothe emotions such as grief, anger, and shock.

APPLICATION: Apply to VITA FLEX POINTS and directly on AREA of concern; diffuse.

ORAL USE AS DIETARY SUPPLEMENT: Generally regarded as safe (GRAS) for internal consumption by the FDA. *DILUTE one drop oil in 1 tsp. honey or 4 oz. of beverage (ie. soy/rice milk).* ***Not for children under 6 years old; use with CAUTION and in GREATER DILUTION for children 6 years old and over.***

BLEND CLASSIFICATION: Modifier and Personifier

BLENDS WITH: Basil, bergamot, chamomile, Clary sage, frankincense, geranium, grapefruit, lavender, lemon, orange.

ODOR: Type: *Top Note (5-20% of the blend)*; Scent: *Fresh, sweet, citrusy*; Intensity: *3*

Tansy, Blue

(*Tanacetum annum*)

BOTANICAL FAMILY: Compositae (daisy)

EXTRACTION METHOD/ORIGIN: Steam distilled from leaves and flowers — France, Morocco

CHEMICAL CONSTITUENTS: Monoterpenes: limonene, sabinene (<17%), β-pinene (<10%), myrcene (<13%), α-phellandrene (<10%), paracymene (<8%); Sesquiterpenes: chamazulene (<29%); Ketones: camphor (<17%).

PROPERTIES: ANALGESIC, ANTI-BACTERIAL, ANTI-INFLAMMATORY, ANTIHISTAMINE, HYPOTENSIVE, HORMONE-LIKE, and NERVINE.

OTHER POSSIBLE USES: May help with LOW BLOOD PRESSURE, relieve ITCHING, reduce PAIN, and sedate the NERVES.

BODY SYSTEM(S) AFFECTED: NERVOUS SYSTEM.

APPLICATION: Apply to VITA FLEX POINTS and/or directly on AREA of concern.

ORAL USE AS DIETARY SUPPLEMENT: None.

SAFETY DATA: This oil should only be used EXTERNALLY and with CAUTION.

Tansy, Idaho

(*Tanacetum vulgare*)

BOTANICAL FAMILY: Compositae (daisy)

EXTRACTION METHOD/ORIGIN: Steam distilled from leaves — Idaho, Washington

CHEMICAL CONSTITUENTS: Ketones: β-thujone (approx. 65%, can be as high as 81%), isothujone, isopinocamphone, umbellulone, piperitone; Oxides: 1,8-cineol, camphor (<8%); Monoterpenes: sabinene (<4%), germacrene-D (<7%), camphene; Alcohols: borneol, thujyl alcohol; Esters: bornyl acetate, cis-chrysanthenyl acetate.

PROPERTIES: ANTI-BACTERIAL, ANTI-FUNGAL, ANTI-INFECTIOUS, ANTI-INFLAMMATORY, ANTISPASMODIC, ANTIVIRAL, NERVINE, and STIMULANT

CARRIER OILS: Some commercial companies will dilute this oil with almond oil.

HISTORICAL USES: Wild tansy (similar in chemical make-up to Idaho tansy) was used historically among the gypsies as a sort of "cure all". It has been used for worms, colds, fever, miscarriage, dyspepsia, cramping pains, scabies, bruises, sprains, nervous disorders and to keep flies and vermin away.

OTHER POSSIBLE USES: Idaho tansy may be supportive to the IMMUNE SYSTEM in helping to FIGHT COLDS, FLU, and INFECTIONS. It may also be beneficial for STOMACH conditions, ARTHRITIS symptoms, and possibly TUMORS. It has been shown to soothe the BOWELS and tone the entire system,. The properties in this oil suggest that it may help with ANEURISMS, BRUISES, DIARRHEA, DYSPEPSIA, FRECKLES, GOUT, HEART DISORDERS, INFLAMED EYES, IRRITABLE BOWEL SYNDROME, JAUNDICE, KIDNEYS, LIVER SPOTS, MENSTRUATION (promotes), PALPITATIONS, RESPIRATORY INFECTIONS, RHEUMATISM, SCIATICA, SPRAINS, SUNBURN, TOOTHACHES, TUBERCULOSIS, and VOMITING.

BODY SYSTEM(S) AFFECTED: IMMUNE SYSTEM.

AROMATIC INFLUENCE: It encourages an UPLIFTING FEELING, a POSITIVE ATTITUDE and a general feeling of WELL BEING.

APPLICATION: Apply to VITA FLEX POINTS and/or directly on AREA of concern.

ORAL USE AS DIETARY SUPPLEMENT: None.

***SAFETY DATA:** Because Idaho tansy contains a high concentration of thujone, this oil has been classified (along with Wild tansy) as an Oral Toxin by Robert Tisserand. However, other sources indicate that for thujone to be toxic, undiluted oil in excess of 30 ml must be ingested in a short period of time. Best for this oil to only be used EXTERNALLY and with CAUTION. Avoid during PREGNANCY. Not for use by people with EPILEPSY.*

BLENDS WITH: Most oils; perfumers in France have found that Wild tansy (similar in chemical make-up to Idaho tansy) has a greater fixative capability than any other oil.

FREQUENCY: Emotional; approximately 105 MHz.

Tarragon

(*Artemisia dracunculus*)

BOTANICAL FAMILY: Compositae

EXTRACTION METHOD/ORIGIN: Steam distilled from leaves — France, Slovenia

CHEMICAL CONSTITUENTS: Phenol methyl-ethers: methyl chavicol (up to 75%), anethole; Coumarins: esculetin; Mono- & Sesquiterpenes: capillene, cis- & trans-β-ocimenes (<12%), phellandrene, cymene; Also: nerol, thujone, cineol, linalyl acetate.

PROPERTIES: ANTI-BACTERIAL, ANTI-CANCEROUS, ANTI-INFECTIOUS, ANTI-INFLAMMATORY, ANTISEPTIC, ANTISPASMODIC, ANTI-PARASITIC, ANTIVIRAL, DIURETIC, LAXATIVE, NEUROMUSCULAR, and STIMULANT.

FOLKLORE: The name is said to come from an ancient use as a remedy for bites from venomous creatures.

ESOTERIC USES/ACTIONS: Astrological: *Mars*; Character: *Yang, Yin*; Perfume note: *Top*

HISTORICAL USES: Tarragon was used to induce appetite, for digestive and menstrual irregularities, and as a remedy for toothache.

FRENCH MEDICINAL USES: COLITIS, HICCOUGHS, INTESTINAL SPASMS, PARASITES, RHEUMATIC PAIN, SCIATICA.

OTHER POSSIBLE USES: It may be beneficial for ABDOMINAL DISCOMFORT and SPASMS, ARTHRITIS, DYSPEPSIA (impaired digestion), preventing FERMENTATION, GENITAL URINARY TRACT INFECTION, KIDNEYS, NAUSEA, NERVOUS and SLUGGISH DIGESTION, PRE-MENSTRUAL discomfort, and WEEPING WOUNDS.

BODY SYSTEM(S) AFFECTED: DIGESTIVE SYSTEM. It may also help balance the AUTONOMIC NERVOUS SYSTEM.

APPLICATION: Apply to VITA FLEX POINTS and/or directly on AREA of concern. Best to DILUTE with V-6 Mixing Oil or Massage Oil.

ORAL USE AS DIETARY SUPPLEMENT: Generally regarded as safe (GRAS) for internal consumption by the FDA. *DILUTE one drop oil in 1 tsp. honey or 4 oz. of beverage (ie. soy/rice milk).* ***Not for children under 6 years old; use with CAUTION and in GREATER DILUTION for children 6 years old and over.***

SAFETY DATA: Avoid during PREGNANCY. Not for use by people with EPILEPSY.

BLEND CLASSIFICATION: Equalizer

BLENDS WITH: Chamomile, Clary sage, fir, juniper, lavender, pine, rosewood, orange, and tangerine.

Thyme

(*Thymus vulgaris*, CT Thymol)

BOTANICAL FAMILY: Labiatae (mint)

EXTRACTION METHOD/ORIGIN: Steam distilled from leaves, stems, and flowers — Utah, Idaho, France

CHEMICAL CONSTITUENTS: Phenols: thymol (up to 55%), carvacrol (<6%); Monoterpenes: paracymene (up to 28%), γ-terpinene (<11%), pinene, camphene, β-caryophyllene; Alcohols: terpinen-4-ol, borneol, linalol (<7%), thujanol, geraniol; Esters: linalyl & bornyl acetate; Ethers: methyl thymol (tr.), methyl carvacrol (tr.); Oxide: cineol (tr.); Ketone: camphor; Also: menthone, triterpenic acids.

PROPERTIES: Highly ANTIMICROBIAL, ANTIFUNGAL, ANTIVIRAL, ANTISEPTIC.

ESOTERIC USES/ACTIONS: Astrological: *Venus*; Chakras: *6 & 3*; Character: *Yang*; Crystal *Pearl, Sodalite*; Element: *Fire & Water*; Oriental: *Cold phlegm (pts: St-40, Sp-6); Qi deficiencies (pts: Lu-9, St-36, Dir Ves-6); Hot phlegm (pts: St-40, Sp-6)*

HISTORICAL USES: It was used by the Egyptians for embalming and by the ancient Greeks against infectious illnesses. It has also been used for respiratory problems, digestive complaints, the prevention and treatment of infection, dyspepsia, chronic gastritis, bronchitis, pertussis, asthma, laryngitis, tonsillitis, and enuresis in children.

FRENCH MEDICINAL USES: ANTHRAX, ASTHMA, BRONCHITIS, COLITIS (infectious), CYSTITIS, DERMATITIS, DYSPEPSIA, FATIGUE (general), PLEURISY PSORIASIS, SCIATICA, TUBERCULOSIS, VAGINAL CANDIDA.

OTHER POSSIBLE USES: This oil is a general TONIC for the NERVES and STOMACH. It may also help with BACTERIAL INFECTIONS, COLDS, CIRCULATION, DEPRESSION, DIGESTION, PHYSICAL WEAKNESS after ILLNESS, FLU, HEADACHES, IMMUNOLOGICAL functions, INSOMNIA, RHEUMATISM, URINARY INFECTIONS, VIRUSES along the SPINE, and WOUNDS.

BODY SYSTEM(S) AFFECTED: IMMUNE SYSTEM, MUSCLES and BONES.

AROMATIC INFLUENCE: It helps SUPPLY ENERGY in times of PHYSICAL WEAKNESS and STRESS. It has also been thought to increase INTELLIGENCE and aid CONCENTRATION. It is UPLIFTING and helps to relieve DEPRESSION.

APPLICATION: Apply to VITA FLEX POINTS and/or directly on AREA of concern.

ORAL USE AS DIETARY SUPPLEMENT: Generally regarded as safe (GRAS) for internal consumption by the FDA. *DILUTE one drop oil in 2 tsp. honey or 8 oz. of beverage (ie. soy/rice milk). However, more dilution may be necessary due to this oil's potential for irritating mucus membranes.* ***Not for children under 6 years old; use with CAUTION and in GREATER DILUTION for children 6 years old and over.***

SAFETY DATA: This type of thyme oil may be somewhat irritating to the mucous membrane and dermal tissues (skin). This type of thyme should be avoided during PREGNANCY. Use this type with caution when dealing with HIGH BLOOD PRESSURE.

LEND CLASSIFICATION: Equalizer and Enhancer
LENDS WITH: Bergamot, cedarwood, juniper, melaleuca, oregano, and rosemary.
DOR: Type: *Middle Note (50-80% of the blend)*; Scent: *Fresh, medicinal, herbaceous*; Intensity: *4*

Thyme Linalol

(*Thymus vulgaris*, CT Linalol)

OTANICAL FAMILY: Labiatae (mint)
XTRACTION METHOD/ORIGIN: Steam distilled from leaves, stems, and flowers — France
HEMICAL CONSTITUENTS: Monoterpenes (small %): β-myrcene, p-cymene; Sesquiterpenes (small %): β-caryophyllene, α-humulene; Monoterpenols: linalol (up to 78%), terpinen-4-ol, α-terpineol, geraniol; Esters: linalyl acetate (5-30% varies with uv light); Phenols (<1%): thymol, carvacrol; Also: 1,8-cineol, camphor.
ROPERTIES: ANTI-BACTERIAL, ANTI-FUNGAL, ANTI-INFECTIOUS, ANTI-INFLAMMATORY, ANTIMICROBIAL, ANTI-PARASITIC, ANTISEPTIC, ANTIVIRAL, CARDIO-TONIC, NEURO-TONIC, and UTERO-TONIC.
SOTERIC USES/ACTIONS: Astrological: *Venus*; Chakras: *3 & 6*; Character: *Yang*; Element: *Fire & Water*; Perfume note: *Top to Mid*
ISTORICAL USES: It was used by the Egyptians for embalming and by the ancient Greeks against infectious illnesses. It has also been used for respiratory problems, digestive complaints, the prevention and treatment of infection, dyspepsia, chronic gastritis, bronchitis, pertussis, asthma, laryngitis, tonsillitis, and enuresis in children.
RENCH MEDICINAL USES: ANTHRAX, ASTHMA, BRONCHITIS, COLITIS (infectious), CYSTITIS, DERMATITIS, DYSPEPSIA, FATIGUE (general), PLEURISY, PSORIASIS, SCIATICA, TUBERCULOSIS, VAGINAL CANDIDA.
THER POSSIBLE USES: This oil is a general TONIC for the NERVES and STOMACH. It may also help with BACTERIAL INFECTIONS, COLDS, CIRCULATION, DEPRESSION, DIGESTION, PHYSICAL WEAKNESS after ILLNESS, FLU, HEADACHES, IMMUNOLOGICAL functions, INSOMNIA, RHEUMATISM, URINARY INFECTIONS, VIRUSES along the SPINE, and WOUNDS. ***Note: This chemotype is said to be the best suited to kill BACTERIA, relieve discomfort in stomach or gut (CANDIDA, PARASITES), and nervous FATIGUE. It is non-irritating, especially for children, elderly, and the infirm.***
ODY SYSTEM(S) AFFECTED: RESPIRATORY SYSTEM, SKIN.
ROMATIC INFLUENCE: It helps SUPPLY ENERGY in times of PHYSICAL WEAKNESS and STRESS. It has also been thought to increase INTELLIGENCE and aid CONCENTRATION. It is UPLIFTING and helps to relieve DEPRESSION.
PPLICATION: Apply to VITA FLEX POINTS and/or directly on AREA of concern.

ORAL USE AS DIETARY SUPPLEMENT: Generally regarded as safe (GRAS) for internal consumption by the FDA. *DILUTE one drop oil in 1 tsp. honey or 4 oz. of beverage (ie soy/rice milk).* ***Not for children under 6 years old; use with CAUTION and in GREATER DILUTION for children 6 years old and over.***

SAFETY DATA: Because this type of thyme oil is a 'linalol type', it is safe for use on the sk and with children. Other varieties of thyme oil can contain large amounts of thymol and carvacrol, making them somewhat toxic, irritating to the mucous membranes, an dermal (skin) irritants. While this type of thyme may be used during pregnancy, the other types should be avoided! Use this type with caution when dealing with HIGH BLOOD PRESSURE.

BLEND CLASSIFICATION: Equalizer and Enhancer

BLENDS WITH: Bergamot, citrus oil, cedarwood, juniper, melaleuca, oregano, and rosemary.

Tsuga (or Hemlock Spruce)

(*Tsuga canadensis*)

BOTANICAL FAMILY: Pinaceae (pine)

EXTRACTION METHOD/ORIGIN: Steam distilled from leaves and twigs — Idaho, Canada ***This oil is not to be confused with hemlock (Conium maculatum), which contains tox alkaloids, and is not a source of essential oil.***

CHEMICAL CONSTITUENTS: Monoterpenes: α- & β-pinenes (up to 25%), camphene (up t 18%), limonene (<5%), tricyclene (<8%), β-phellandrene (<5%), myrcene (<3%), dipentene, cadinene; Esters: bornyl acetate (up to 38%); Ketones: thujone.

PROPERTIES: ANTIMICROBIAL, ANTISEPTIC, ASTRINGENT, DIURETIC, EXPECTORANT, NERVINE, TONIC.

ESOTERIC USES/ACTIONS: Astrological: *Saturn*; Chakra: *6*; Element: *Light*; Perfume note *Base*

HISTORICAL USES: It has been used for diarrhea, cystitis, mucous colitis, leucorrhea, uterin prolapse, pharyngitis, stomatitis, gingivitis, wounds, sores, digestive disorders, diseases c the mouth and throat and scurvy.

OTHER POSSIBLE USES: This oil may help with ANXIETY, ASTHMA, BRONCHITIS, poor CIRCULATION, COLDS, COUGHS, FLU, INFECTIONS, MUSCULAR ACHE and PAINS, PERIODONTAL (GUM) DISEASE, RESPIRATORY WEAKNESS (open and dilates for better oxygen exchange), RHEUMATISM, STRESS-RELATED CONDITIONS, and WOUNDS. It can also be used in VETERINARY LINIMENTS.

BODY SYSTEM(S) AFFECTED: CARDIOVASCULAR and RESPIRATORY SYSTEMS.

AROMATIC INFLUENCE: It is UPLIFTING to the EMOTIONS as it OPENS and ELEVATES while GROUNDING at the same time. Some have found it excellent for us during YOGA and MEDITATION.

PPLICATION: DIFFUSE. Apply to VITA FLEX POINTS and/or directly on AREA of concern. For topical use, DILUTE in one teaspoon V-6 Mixing Oil or Massage Oil.

RAL USE AS DIETARY SUPPLEMENT: Approved by the FDA for use as a Food Additive (FA) or Flavoring Agent (FL) (see 21CFR172.510). *DILUTE one drop oil in 1 tsp. honey or 4 oz. of beverage (ie. soy/rice milk).* ***Not for children under 6 years old; use with CAUTION and in GREATER DILUTION for children 6 years old and over.***

AFETY DATA: Repeated use can possibly result in SKIN IRRITATION.

OMPANION PRODUCTS: Di-Tone, Essentialzyme, Fresh Essence Mouthwash, K&B Tincture, Rose Ointment.

LENDS WITH: Pine, cedarwood, galbanum, lavender, lavandin, and rosemary.

Valerian

(*Valeriana officinalis*)

OTANICAL FAMILY: Valerianaceae

XTRACTION METHOD/ORIGIN: Steam distilled from roots — Belgium, Croatia, France

HEMICAL CONSTITUENTS: Monoterpenes: α-pinene (<8%), β-pinene (<6%), camphene, vitivene, cadinene; Sesquiterpenes: β-caryophyllene, azulene, α-fenchene (up to 30%); Alcohols: geraniol, α-terpineol, borneol, patchouli alcohol, valerianol; Esters: bornyl acetate (up to 44%), bornyl formiate & butyrate, and bornyl isovalerate (responsible for odor & therapeutic effects), eugenyl isovalerate; Aldehydes: valerenal; Ketones: valerone, ionone; Acids: valerenic acid, isovaleric and acetoxyvaleric acid.

ROPERTIES: ANTI-BACTERIAL, ANTI-DANDRUFF, ANTISPASMODIC, DEPRESSANT (central nervous system), DIURETIC, HYPNOTIC, REGULATOR, SEDATIVE.

OLKLORE: Once called "all heal", valerian has been treasured since medieval times.

SOTERIC USES/ACTIONS: Astrological: *Venus*; Element: *Water*; Perfume note: *Base*

IISTORICAL USES: Down through the centuries, valerian has been used for insomnia, migraine, dysmenorrhea, intestinal colic, rheumatism, cholera, epilepsy, skin complaints, backache, colds, menstrual problems, and sores. During that last few decades, it has been studied for its tranquilizing properties.

THER POSSIBLE USES: Because of its effect on the nervous system, it may help with INSOMNIA, NERVOUS INDIGESTION, MIGRAINE, RESTLESSNESS, SLEEP DISTURBANCES, and TENSION.

ODY SYSTEM(S) AFFECTED: NERVOUS SYSTEM.

ROMATIC INFLUENCE: It may be useful in meditation as it helps cut through the tension and stress of our everyday lives to help us focus on our inner self, where true peace and calm can be found. It is profoundly CALMING, RELAXING, GROUNDING, and BALANCING.

APPLICATION: Apply to VITA FLEX POINTS and/or directly on AREA of concern. May also be applied to the WRISTS or bottom of the FEET. Is actually more effective when taken internally as a dietary supplement.

ORAL USE AS DIETARY SUPPLEMENT: Approved by the FDA for use as a Food Additi (FA) and Flavoring Agent (FL). *DILUTE one drop oil in 1 tsp. honey or 4 oz. of beverage (ie. soy/rice milk).* ***Not for children under 6 years old; use with CAUTION and in GREATER DILUTION for children 6 years old and over.***

SAFETY DATA: Repeated use can possibly result in CONTACT SENSITIZATION.

BLENDS WITH: Cedarwood, lavender, mandarin, patchouli, petitgrain, pine, and rosemary.

Vetiver

(*Vetiveria zizanoides*)

BOTANICAL FAMILY: Gramineae (grasses)

EXTRACTION METHOD/ORIGIN: Steam distilled from roots — India, Haiti (best)

CHEMICAL CONSTITUENTS: Sesquiterpenes: vitivene, tricyclovetivene, vetivazulene; Alcohols: isovalencenol (up to 15%), khusenol (up to 11%), vetiverol, tricyclovetivenol, zizanol, furfurol; Ketones: α- & β-vitiverones (<12%), khusimone (<6%), nootkatone (<5%); Esters: vetivenyl acetate; Also: benzoic acid.

PROPERTIES: ANTISEPTIC, ANTISPASMODIC, CALMING, GROUNDING, IMMUNE-STIMULANT, RUBEFACIENT (locally warming), SEDATIVE (nervous system), STIMULANT (circulatory, production of red corpuscles).

FOLKLORE: Known in India as "oil of tranquility", vetiver is distilled from the root of a scente grass native to India that is botanically related to citronella and lemongrass

ESOTERIC USES/ACTIONS: Astrological: *Venus & Saturn*; Body type: *Mesomorph*; Chakras: *1, 2, & 3*; Character: *Intensely Yin (with rising Yang)*; Crystals: *Yellow Jasper, Black Tourmaline*; Element: *Earth & Water*; Number: *5*

HISTORICAL USES: The distillation of vetiver is a painstaking, labor-intensive activity. The roots and rootlets of vetiver have been used in India as a perfume since antiquity.

OTHER POSSIBLE USES: Vetiver may help ACNE, ANOREXIA, ANXIETY, ARTHRITIS BREASTS (enlarge), CUTS, DEPRESSION (including postpartum), INSOMNIA, MUSCULAR RHEUMATISM, NERVOUSNESS (extreme), SKIN CARE (oily, aging, tired, irritated), SPRAINS, and STRESS.

BODY SYSTEM(S) AFFECTED: EMOTIONAL BALANCE, HORMONAL and NERVOUS SYSTEMS, SKIN.

AROMATIC INFLUENCE: Vetiver has a heavy, smokey, earthy fragrance reminiscent of patchouli with lemon-like undertones. Because of its PSYCHOLOGICALLY GROUNDING, CALMING, and STABILIZING properties, vetiver has also been valuable for relieving STRESS and helping people recover from EMOTIONAL

TRAUMAS and SHOCK. As a natural tranquilizer, it may help induce a RESTFUL SLEEP. It is known to affect the PARATHYROID GLAND. According to Susanne Fischer-Rizzi, "Sexual energies become more peaceful and grounded."

PPLICATION: Apply to VITA FLEX POINTS and/or directly on AREA of concern; diffuse. Also excellent in BATHS or in MASSAGE blends. A very small amount of vetiver oil is all that is needed in most applications. Mix with geranium and ylang ylang to help with breast enlargement.

RAL USE AS DIETARY SUPPLEMENT: Approved by the FDA for use as a Food Additive (FA) and Flavoring Agent (FL). *DILUTE one drop oil in 1 tsp. honey or 4 oz. of beverage (ie. soy/rice milk).* ***Not for children under 6 years old; use with CAUTION and in GREATER DILUTION for children 6 years old and over.***

AFETY DATA: Use with caution during PREGNANCY.

LENDS WITH: Clary sage, jasmine, lavender, patchouli, rose, sandalwood, ylang ylang.

DOR: Type: *Base Note (5-20% of the blend)*; Scent: *Heavy, earthy, balsamic, smoky, sweet undertones*; Intensity: *5*

Vitex

(*Vitex negundo*)

OTANICAL FAMILY: Labiatae (mint)

XTRACTION METHOD/ORIGIN: Steam distilled from the inner bark, small branches, and leaves of the Chaste tree (this essential oil is different from the extract of the chaste berry, which is used for PMS symptoms and hormone balance) — Turkey

HEMICAL CONSTITUENTS: Monoterpenes: limonene; Esters: α-terpinyl acetate; Oxides: 1,8 cineol, caryophyllene oxide.

ISTORICAL USES: Vitex has been historically used in Europe and Asia for its benefits relating to RHEUMATISM, HERNIAS, DEAFNESS, and MENTAL UNREST.

OSSIBLE USES: Currently, research is being conducted by Dr. Ulvie Zybeck, a professor of pharmacy from Ege University in Izmir, Turkey, on the use of vitex oil for reversing the symptoms of Parkinson's Disease.

RAL USE AS DIETARY SUPPLEMENT: None.

AFETY DATA: Use with caution during PREGNANCY.

Western Red Cedar

(***See Cedar, Western Red***)

White Fir

(*See Fir, White*)

White Lotus

(*Nymphaea lotus*)

BOTANICAL FAMILY: Nymphaeaceae

EXTRACTION METHOD/ORIGIN: Steam distilled from flower — Egypt

(NOTE: This oil is only available periodically in very small amounts.)

PROPERTIES: ANTI-CANCEROUS.

HISTORICAL USES: White lotus was traditionally used by the Egyptians for SPIRITUAL, EMOTIONAL, and PHYSICAL application; every recipe contained White lotus. Research in China found that White lotus contains ANTI-CANCEROUS and strong IMMUNE SUPPORTING properties.

OTHER POSSIBLE USES: EYES (inflamed), JAUNDICE, KIDNEYS, LIVER SPOTS, MENSTRUATION (promotes), PALPITATIONS, RHEUMATISM, SCIATICA, SPRAINS, SUNBURN, TOOTHACHES, TUBERCULOSIS, VOMITING.

BODY SYSTEM(S) AFFECTED: IMMUNE SYSTEM.

AROMATIC INFLUENCE: White lotus has a euphoric fragrance that LIFTS and STABILIZ the EMOTIONS, creating a powerful sense of EMOTIONAL, PHYSICAL, and SPIRITUAL WELL BEING.

ORAL USE AS DIETARY SUPPLEMENT: None.

BLENDS WITH: Most oils.

Wintergreen

(*Gaultheria procumbens*)

BOTANICAL FAMILY: Ericaceae (heather)

EXTRACTION METHOD/ORIGIN: Steam distillation from leaves — Canada

CHEMICAL CONSTITUENTS: Esters: methyl salicylate (>90%); Also: triacontane and various aldehydes, ketones, and alcohols.

PROPERTIES: ANALGESIC, ANTI-INFLAMMATORY, ANTI-RHEUMATIC, ANTISEPTIC, ANTISPASMODIC, DISINFECTANT, DIURETIC, STIMULANT (bone), and WARMING.

ESOTERIC USES/ACTIONS: Astrological: *Mercury & Moon*; Character: *Yin?*; Element: *Earth*; Color: *Yellow, reddish, colorless*; Odor: *strong characteristics*

HISTORICAL USES: Wintergreen oil has a strong, penetrating aroma. Wintergreen essential is almost identical in chemical constituents to birch essential oil (*Betula alleghaniensis*). The American Indians and early European settlers enjoyed a tea that was flavored with birch bark or wintergreen. According to Julia Lawless, "...this has been translated into a preference for 'root beer' flavourings [sic]." A synthetic methyl salicylate is now widely used as a flavoring agent, especially in 'root beer', chewing gum, toothpaste, etc. *In fact, the true essential oil is produced in such small quantities (compared to the very extensive uses of the synthetic methyl salicylate) that those desiring to use wintergreen essential oil for therapeutic uses should* ***verify the source*** *of their oil to make sure they have a true oil, not a synthetic one.*

ENCH MEDICINAL USES: RHEUMATISM, MUSCULAR PAIN, CRAMPS, ARTHRITIS, TENDONITIS, HYPERTENSION, INFLAMMATION.

THER POSSIBLE USES: This oil may be beneficial for ACNE, BLADDER INFECTION, CYSTITIS, DROPSY, ECZEMA, EDEMA, reducing FEVER, GALLSTONES, GOUT, INFECTION, reducing discomfort in JOINTS, KIDNEY STONES, draining and cleansing the LYMPHATIC SYSTEM, OBESITY, OSTEOPOROSIS, SKIN DISEASES, ULCERS, and URINARY TRACT DISORDERS. It is known for its ability to alleviate BONE PAIN. It has a cortisone-like action due to the high content of methyl salicylate. For nerve or tissue pain, use Relieve It.

DY SYSTEM(S) AFFECTED: MUSCLES and BONES.

ROMATIC INFLUENCE: It influences, elevates, opens, and increases AWARENESS in SENSORY SYSTEM (senses or sensations).

PLICATION: Apply to VITA FLEX POINTS and/or directly on AREA of concern; diffuse. Apply topically on location and use only small amounts (dilute with V-6 Mixing Oil for application on larger areas).

RAL USE AS DIETARY SUPPLEMENT: None.

FETY DATA: Avoid during PREGNANCY. Not for use by people with EPILEPSY. Some people are very allergic to methyl salicylate. TEST A SMALL AREA OF SKIN FIRST FOR ALLERGIES!

END CLASSIFICATION: Personifier and Enhancer

ENDS WITH: Basil, bergamot, chamomile, cypress, geranium, juniper, lavender, lemongrass, marjoram, peppermint, and rosewood.

Yarrow

(*Achillea millefolium*)

TANICAL FAMILY: Compositae (daisy)

XTRACTION METHOD/ORIGIN: Steam distilled from flowering top — Utah

HEMICAL CONSTITUENTS: Sesquiterpenes: chamazulene (up to 19%), germacrene-D (<8%), dihydroazulenes, trans-β-caryophyllene (<8%); Monoterpenes: α-pinene, β-pinene

(<7%), camphene, sabinene (<7%); Alcohols: borneol, terpineol; Oxides: 1,8-cineol (<6%); Ketones: isoartemisia ketone (up to 10%), camphor (up to 16%), thujones; Sesquiterpene lactones: achilline.

PROPERTIES: ANTI-INFLAMMATORY, ANTISEPTIC, ASTRINGENT, and STYPTIC.

FOLKLORE: The Greek Achilles, hero of the Trojan Wars, was said to have used yarrow to help cure the injury to his Achilles tendon. Yarrow was considered sacred by the Chine who recognized the harmony of the Yin and Yang energies within it. It has been said th the fragrance of yarrow makes possible the meeting of heaven and earth.

ESOTERIC USES/ACTIONS: Astrological: *Venus*; Character: *Yang (Yin when diluted), Ho 2nd Degree*; Crystals: *Amethyst*; Element: *Water*; Oriental: *Rising heat, internal wind*

HISTORICAL USES: Yarrow was used by Germanic tribes to treat battle wounds.

OTHER POSSIBLE USES: It is a powerful decongestant of the PROSTATE and helps to balance HORMONES. It may also help with ACNE, AMENORRHEA, APPETITE (la of), BLADDER or KIDNEY WEAKNESS, CELLULITE, COLDS, CATARRH, DIGESTION (poor), DYSMENORRHEA, ECZEMA, FEVERS, FLATULENCE, GALLBLADDER INFLAMMATION, GASTRITIS, GOUT, HAIR (promotes hair growth), HEADACHES, HEMORRHOIDS, HYPERTENSION, INJURIES, KIDNEY STONES, LIVER, MENOPAUSE PROBLEMS, NEURITIS, NEURALGIA, OPEN LEG SORES, PELVIC INFECTIONS, PROSTATITIS, RHEUMATISM, SCARRIN (reduces or prevents), SPRAINS, STOMACH FLU, SUNBURN, THROMBOSIS, ULCERS, URINARY INFECTIONS, VAGINITIS, VARICOSE VEINS, and WOUN (promotes healing).

BODY SYSTEM(S) AFFECTED: HORMONAL and IMMUNE SYSTEMS, SKIN.

AROMATIC INFLUENCE: Balancing highs and lows, both external and internal, yarrow ma allow us to have our heads in the clouds while our feet remain firm on the ground. Its BALANCING properties may also make it useful during MEDITATION. It is SUPPORTIVE to INTUITIVE ENERGIES and helps reduce CONFUSION and AMBIVALENCE. One source suggests that it may help open our awareness to COSM ENERGIES.

APPLICATION: Apply to VITA FLEX POINTS and/or directly on AREA of concern; diffus Also excellent for BATHS or MASSAGE blends.

ORAL USE AS DIETARY SUPPLEMENT: None.

SAFETY DATA: Repeated use can possibly result in CONTACT SENSITIZATION. Use with caution during PREGNANCY.

BLENDS WITH: Clary sage, hyssop, myrtle, pine, valerian, and vetiver.

ODOR: Type: *Middle Note (50-80% of the blend)*; Scent: *Sharp, woody, herbaceous, with a slight floral undertone*; Intensity: *4*

Ylang Ylang

(*Cananga odorata*)

OTANICAL FAMILY: Annonaceae (tropical trees and shrubs - custard-apple)

XTRACTION METHOD/ORIGIN: Steam distilled from flowers — Commores, Madagascar, Indonesia, Philippines *(Flowers are picked early in the morning to maximize oil yield. The highest quality oil is drawn from the first hour of distillation.)*

HEMICAL CONSTITUENTS: Mono- & Sesquiterpenes: α-farnesene (up to 12%), germacrene-D (up to 20%), pinenes, cadinene; Alcohols: linalol (up to 55%), farnesol, geraniol; Esters: benzyl acetate (<15%), geranyl acetate (>5%), benzyl benzoate (<6%), cinnamyl acetate (<5%), linalyl acetate; Phenols: methyl p-cresol (<9%), eugenol, isoeugenol (<5%).

ROPERTIES: ANTI-DEPRESSANT, ANTISEPTIC, ANTISPASMODIC, SEDATIVE, and TONIC.

SOTERIC USES/ACTIONS: Astrological: *Venus*; Body type: *Ectomorph*; Chakras: *2 & 3*; Character: *Strongly Yin*; Crystals: *Kunzite*; Element: *Earth & Water*; Number: *7*

ISTORICAL USES: Interestingly enough, the original wild flowers had no fragrance. Through selection and cloning, we have this unique fragrance today. Ylang ylang has been used to cover the beds of newlywed couples on their wedding night, for skin treatments, to soothe insect bites, and in hair preparations to promote thick, shiny, lustrous hair (it is also reported to help control split ends). It has also been used to treat colic, constipation, indigestion, stomachaches, and to regulate the heartbeat and respiration.

RENCH MEDICINAL USES: ANXIETY, ARTERIAL HYPERTENSION, DEPRESSION, DIABETES, FATIGUE (mental), FRIGIDITY, HAIR LOSS, HYPERPNEA (reduces), INSOMNIA, PALPITATIONS, TACHYCARDIA.

THER POSSIBLE USES: Ylang ylang may help balance MALE-FEMALE ENERGIES so one can move closer towards being in spiritual attunement and allow them to focus their thoughts together, filtering out the ever-present garbage. It may help lower BLOOD PRESSURE, rapid BREATHING, balance EQUILIBRIUM, FRUSTRATION, balance HEART FUNCTION, IMPOTENCE, INFECTION, INTESTINAL PROBLEMS, SEX DRIVE PROBLEMS, SHOCK, and SKIN PROBLEMS.

ODY SYSTEM(S) AFFECTED: EMOTIONAL BALANCE, CARDIOVASCULAR and HORMONAL SYSTEMS.

ROMATIC INFLUENCE: It influences SEXUAL ENERGY and enhances RELATIONSHIPS. It may help stimulate the adrenal glands. It is CALMING and RELAXING and may also help with ANGER and possibly RAGE and LOW SELF-ESTEEM. It brings back the feeling of SELF-LOVE, CONFIDENCE, JOY and PEACE.

PPLICATION: Apply to VITA FLEX POINTS and/or directly on AREA of concern; diffuse. It may be beneficial when applied over the THYMUS (to help stimulate the immune syste).

RAL USE AS DIETARY SUPPLEMENT: Generally regarded as safe (GRAS) for internal consumption by the FDA. *DILUTE one drop oil in 1 tsp. honey or 4 oz. of beverage (ie soy/rice milk).* ***Not for children under 6 years old; use with CAUTION and in GREATER DILUTION for children 6 years old and over.***

SAFETY DATA: Repeated use can possibly result in CONTACT SENSITIZATION.

BLEND CLASSIFICATION: Personifier and Modifier

BLENDS WITH: Anise, bergamot, cardamom, chamomile (Mixta), cumin, geranium, grapefrui lemon, marjoram, sandalwood, vetiver.

ODOR: Type: *Middle to Base Notes (20-80% of the blend)*; Scent: *Sweet, heavy, narcotic, cloying, tropical floral, with spicy-balsamic undertones*; Intensity: *5*

I am so grateful to have these oils!

My daughter, Haley, at age 18 was ill one Sunday, and later in the evening was feeling quite worse. When we checked, she had a fever of 105 degrees. I filled a gel capsule with 10 drops of Clove oil and had her take it with some water. In 1/2 an hour I checked her temperature again and it was down to 102. I gave her 5 more drops in another capsule and in another 1/2 hour, her fever was totally gone!!

-Submitted by Sally Donahue, Wilsonville, Oregon

Goodbye to Fibroid Lumps

I had suffered for 32 years with massive fibrocystic breast lumps. They were so painful that I could not even hug my children when they were young. I took vitamin E during those years which seemed to help. Then I heard about the research done on therapeutic grade essential oils and breast cancer. I stopped using deodorants with aluminum. I also mixed 40 drops of frankincense essential oil with 4oz of pure Apricot Oil and applied this mixture under my arms during the day as often as I would think about it. Every night before I went to bed, I applied 4-5 drops each of frankincense and lavender to both breasts. A little over 4 weeks later, all fibroid lumps, pain and tenderness were completely gone and have not returned.

-Submitted by Ann Gaither, Corpus Christi, Texas

Oil Blends

This section contains the authors' favorite commercial blends and detailed information ɔout each. Other commercial blends exist on the market but the authors (and many others) find ese blends to be superior in synergy and potency. An approximate frequency is indicated for any of the blends. However, please keep in mind that there are many variables involved in an l's frequency. Consequently, these numbers may be difficult to duplicate.

Abundance

This is a blend that was specifically designed to enhance MAGNETIC ENERGY and eate the law of attraction through the magnetic field around us, to enhance one's thoughts rough electrical stimulation of the somatides and the cells, and to put out a frequency charge of ROSPERITY and ABUNDANCE. It may ATTRACT RICHES to ONESELF. It also contains emendous ANTI-VIRAL and ANTI-FUNGAL properties, which may make it a very powerful UPPORT to the IMMUNE SYSTEM, possibly giving one an abundance of HEALTH as well.

INGLE OILS CONTAINED IN THIS BLEND:

Myrrh—is part of the formula the Lord gave Moses (Exodus 30:22-27). It is a TRUE GIFT. When we OPEN our HEARTS and MINDS to receive the gifts, they will be given.

Frankincense—contains sesquiterpenes, which may help OXYGENATE the PINEAL and PITUITARY GLANDS. It may help PROMOTE a POSITIVE ATTITUDE.

Patchouli—is SEDATING, CALMING, and RELAXING allowing it to reduce ANXIETY. It may have some particular influence on SEX, PHYSICAL ENERGY, and MONEY.

Orange—brings PEACE and HAPPINESS to the MIND and BODY and JOY to the HEART, which provide EMOTIONAL support.

Clove—may influence HEALING, improve MEMORY, and create a feeling of PROTECTION and COURAGE.

Ginger—is WARMING, UPLIFTING, and EMPOWERING. Emotionally, it may help influence PHYSICAL ENERGY, LOVE, and COURAGE. Because of its calming influence on the digestive system, it may help reduce feelings of NAUSEA, and MOTION SICKNESS.

Spruce—GROUNDS the BODY, creating the BALANCE and the OPENING necessary to RECEIVE and to GIVE. It may help DILATE the BRONCHIAL TRACT to IMPROVE the OXYGEN EXCHANGE. It also helps one release EMOTIONA BLOCKS.

BODY SYSTEM(S) AFFECTED: The oils in this blend may help it be effective for dealing wi various problems related to the IMMUNE and RESPIRATORY SYSTEMS, and to EMOTIONAL BALANCE.

AROMATIC INFLUENCE: When diffused, this oil creates harmonic energy around oneself.

APPLICATION: May be worn on the WRISTS, behind the EARS, on the NECK and FACE. Individuals with sensitive skin may want to blend with V-6 Mixing Oil, Genesis Hand an Body Lotion. May be worn as a PERFUME or COLOGNE or placed on the CHECKBOOK, CAR DASH, COMPUTER, PHONE, WALLET, or in your PURSE. Try COOKING with it. To create more business, one may want to add a ½ bottle of Abundance to 5 gallons of paint before painting the office.

SAFETY DATA:* *Repeated use can result in extreme CONTACT SENSITIZATION. Can be irritating to sensitive SKIN.

COMPANION OILS: Acceptance, Awaken, or Release may be used first to help release the emotions that stop us from receiving abundance. It may then be followed by Envision, In the Future, Joy, Magnify Your Purpose, Motivation, or Live with Passion.

FREQUENCY: Physical; approximately 78 MHz–same frequency as the brain.

BIBLE: "For as he thinketh in his heart, so [is] he . . ." (Proverbs 23:7). We can create the kind of abundance we want, even that of poverty by believing we can't receive.

Acceptance

This blend was formulated to help stimulate the mind to open up and ACCEPT NEW THINGS in LIFE, enabling us to reach toward our higher potential. It may also be beneficial in helping one OVERCOME DENIAL or PROCRASTINATION and to help create a feeling of SECURITY.

SINGLE OILS CONTAINED IN THIS BLEND:

Geranium—may help with HORMONAL BALANCE, LIVER and KIDNEY FUNCTIONS and the DISCHARGE of TOXINS from the LIVER that hold us back from having balance. Geranium OPENS the LIVER CHAKRA (Solar Plexus). Note: The liver is the place where fear and anger are stored.

Blue Tansy—may help CLEANSE the LIVER and CALM the LYMPHATIC SYSTEM to help rid one of ANGER and promote a feeling of SELF-CONTROL.

Frankincense—contains sesquiterpenes, which may help OXYGENATE the PINEAL an PITUITARY GLANDS. As one of the ingredients for the holy incense, it was used anciently to help ENHANCE one's COMMUNICATION WITH THE CREATOR. It may help PROMOTE a POSITIVE ATTITUDE.

Sandalwood—also, like frankincense, is high in sesquiterpenes, which were discovered to INCREASE the amount of OXYGEN around the PINEAL and PITUITARY GLANDS, thus helping to IMPROVE one's ATTITUDE. It ALLEVIATES DEPRESSION and assists in the removal of NEGATIVE PROGRAMMING from the cells of the body. It helps one ACCEPT OTHERS with an open heart while diminishing one's own egocentricity.

Neroli—has been regarded traditionally by the Egyptian people for its great attributes for HEALING the MIND, BODY and SPIRIT. It is CALMING and RELAXING to body and spirit. It may also help to STRENGTHEN and STABILIZE the emotions, and BRING RELIEF to seemingly hopeless situations. It encourages CONFIDENCE, COURAGE, JOY, PEACE, and SENSUALITY.

Rosewood—is SOOTHING to the SKIN, APPEASING to the MIND, RELAXING to the BODY, and creates a feeling of PEACE and GENTLENESS.

RRIER OIL CONTAINED IN BLEND: Almond Oil.

DY SYSTEM(S) AFFECTED: The oils in this blend may help it be effective for dealing with numerous problems related to the NERVOUS SYSTEM and EMOTIONAL BALANCE. Even when dealing with a physical problem, emotional "acceptance" of the present situation, rather than denial, helps one move forward in the healing process.

OMATIC INFLUENCE: When inhaled or diffused, this blend may help CALM a troubled mind and promote feelings of CONFIDENCE and COURAGE. By calming the raging storms of mental frustration, we are finally capable of viewing our true position in life. We can then accept where we are and move forward with confidence on our path to achieving loftier goals.

PLICATION: Best when rubbed over the LIVER (when the liver is toxic, the mind and emotions are lethargic), behind the EARS, on the CHEST, FACE, HEART, NECK, THYMUS, and WRISTS. It may also be applied over the SACRAL CHAKRA (base) and worn as a PERFUME or COLOGNE. It can be DIFFUSED for some great results.

EQUENCY: Physical and Emotional; approximately 102 MHz.

Aroma Life

This is a blend of oils which, through some extensive research, were found to help RENGTHEN and IMPROVE the CARDIOVASCULAR, LYMPHATIC, and RCULATORY SYSTEMS. This blend may also help to lower HIGH BLOOD PRESSURE, DUCE STRESS, and ALLEVIATE HEMORRHOIDS.

Oil Blends

SINGLE OILS CONTAINED IN THIS BLEND:

Cypress—is ANTI-INFECTIOUS, MUCOLYTIC, ANTISEPTIC, LYMPHATIC DECONGESTANT, REFRESHING, and RELAXING. It may help improve LUNG CIRCULATION and relieve other RESPIRATORY PROBLEMS.

Marjoram—is RELAXING, CALMING, and APPEASING to the MUSCLES that constrict and sometimes contribute to HEADACHES.

Helichrysum—may help CLEANSE the BLOOD and improve CIRCULATORY FUNCTIONS. It is ANTI-CATARRHAL in structure and nature. On a spirit level, it may help one LET GO OF ANGRY FEELINGS that prevent one from forgiving and moving forward in life.

Ylang Ylang—may help BALANCE the MALE-FEMALE ENERGIES so one can mo closer towards being in spiritual attunement and allow them to focus their thoug together, filtering out the ever-present garbage.

CARRIER OIL CONTAINED IN THIS BLEND: Sesame Seed Oil.

BODY SYSTEM(S) AFFECTED: The oils in this blend may help it be effective for dealing w various problems related to the CARDIOVASCULAR SYSTEM.

APPLICATION: Best when massaged over the HEART (left side of the chest). It can be dilut with V-6 Mixing Oil for a full body massage. It can also be applied to the VITA FLEX HEART points including, under the LEFT RING FINGER and the LEFT RING TOE, the left arm just ABOVE the ELBOW, and on the ARTERIES of the NECK. It may al help to apply this blend along the spine from the 1st to the 4th thoracic vertebrae, which correspond to the cardio-pulmonary nerves (*Refer to the Autonomic Nervous System ch in the Science and Application section of this book*).

COMPANION OILS: It may be beneficial to combine Joy with this blend when the heart is in stress or combine with Valor to give the heart courage. Adding some grapefruit oil to th blend may help improve circulation and dissolve fat more quickly. May also add helichrysum, rosemary, or ylang ylang.

FREQUENCY: Physical; approximately 84 MHz.

COMMENTS: This blend may work as a Natural Hemostat and Chelating agent. Red spots o the body may indicate a biotin deficiency. If so, using Super C may be beneficial.

Aroma Siez

The oils in this blend were selected specifically for their ability to RELAX, CALM and RELIEVE the TENSION of SPASTIC MUSCLES resulting from SPORTS INJURY, FATIGU or STRESS. This blend may also help to relieve HEADACHES.

NGLE OILS CONTAINED IN THIS BLEND:

Basil—has ANTI-INFLAMMATORY and ANTISPASMODIC properties. It is relaxing to SPASTIC MUSCLES, including those that contribute to HEADACHES and MIGRAINES.

Marjoram—is an ANTISPASMODIC and is RELAXING, CALMING, and APPEASING to the MUSCLES that constrict and sometimes contribute to HEADACHES. It has been useful for MUSCLE SPASMS, SPRAINS, BRUISES, MIGRAINES, and SORE MUSCLES.

Lavender—is an oil that has traditionally been known to BALANCE the BODY and to work wherever there is a need. It has ANTISPASMODIC and ANALGESIC properties. It may help with SPRAINS, SORE MUSCLES, HEADACHES, and general HEALING.

Peppermint—is an ANTI-INFLAMMATORY to the NERVES and helps REDUCE INFLAMMATION in DAMAGED TISSUE. It is SOOTHING, COOLING, and DILATING to the SYSTEM. It may help to REDUCE FEVERS, CANDIDA, NAUSEA, VOMITING, and strengthen the RESPIRATORY SYSTEM.

Cypress—is ANTI-INFECTIOUS, MUCOLYTIC, ANTISEPTIC, LYMPHATIC DECONGESTANT, REFRESHING, and RELAXING. It may help improve LUNG CIRCULATION as well as help relieve other RESPIRATORY PROBLEMS. It may also help relieve MUSCLE CRAMPS and improve overall CIRCULATION.

ODY SYSTEM(S) AFFECTED: The oils in this blend may help it be effective for dealing with various problems related to the RESPIRATORY SYSTEM and to MUSCLES and BONES.

PPLICATION: Best if applied on location for all MUSCLES and on back of NECK for STRESS HEADACHES. It may also be applied over the HEART or diluted with V-6 Mixing Oil for a full body MASSAGE. It is also beneficial when applied to the VITA FLEX points on FEET or placed in the BATH water.

OMPANION OILS: Basil, birch, elemi, helichrysum, Idaho tansy, marjoram, spruce, wintergreen. Ortho Ease Massage Oil or Ortho Sport Massage Oil may also be used to enhance the effects of this blend.

REQUENCY: Low (Physical); approximately 64 MHz.

Oil Blends

Australian Blue

With a base of Blue cypress oil, this blend has an exotic, tropical scent that is ROUNDING and STABILIZING, yet UPLIFTING and INSPIRING. Topically it may help lieve minor ACHES and PAINS. It may help calm ANGER and bring about SELF-CONTROL it balances and stabilizes the EMOTIONS.

SINGLE OILS CONTAINED IN THIS BLEND:

Blue Cypress (*Callitris intratropica*)—is an abundant source of sesquiterpenes. It is th only oil obtained from wood that contains guaiol and guaiazulene, which gives i deep blue color. It is grounding and stabilizing with a fragrance that uplifts and inspires.

Ylang Ylang—may help BALANCE the MALE-FEMALE ENERGIES so one can mov closer towards being in spiritual attunement and allow them to focus their thoug together, filtering out the ever-present garbage.

Cedarwood—was used traditionally by the North American Indians to enhance their potential for SPIRITUAL COMMUNICATION. It may help OPEN the PINEA GLAND.

Blue Tansy—may help CLEANSE the LIVER and CALM the LYMPHATIC SYSTEM to help rid one of ANGER and promote a feeling of SELF-CONTROL.

White Fir (*Abies grandis*)—creates a feeling of GROUNDING, ANCHORING, and EMPOWERMENT. It can STIMULATE the MIND while allowing the BODY to RELAX. Topically it helps relieve PAIN from INFLAMMATION.

BODY SYSTEM(S) AFFECTED: EMOTIONAL BALANCE.

AROMATIC INFLUENCE: When diffused, this special blend of oils can be CALMING and BALANCING to the emotions. It may help STRESS and ANGER, relieve ANXIETY and TENSION, and help RELAX the entire body. Mentally it can be STIMULATING and INSPIRING.

APPLICATION: Diffuse, wear as PERFUME or COLOGNE, or apply topically to areas of concern.

SAFETY DATA: Could possibly result in CONTACT SENSITIZATION or SKIN IRRITATION.

Awaken

This blend may help AWAKEN one to the possibility of their HIGHER POTENTIAL, that they may make the necessary transitions in their lives to achieve greater things. This blend may also be beneficial for SPIRITUAL and/or EMOTIONAL ENHANCEMENT.

OIL BLENDS CONTAINED IN THIS BLEND:

JOY—is a blend which may help to open the heart and promote feelings of SELF-LOVE and LOVE FOR OTHERS so one can experience ultimate joy.

FORGIVENESS—is a blend which was formulated to help move people into a mental state which may help them to forgive and forget. Inhaling this blend may stimulate one to FORGIVE THEMSELVES and OTHERS of TRANSGRESSION.

<u>DREAM CATCHER</u>—is an oil blend that was created to OPEN the MIND, to ENHANCE ones DREAMS, to help one VISUALIZE their dreams and HANG ONTO them until they become REALITY.

<u>PRESENT TIME</u>—is a blend of oils that was designed to bring one both mentally and emotionally into the PRESENT TIME. In order for us to AWAKEN to OUR HIGHER POTENTIAL, we must be living in the moment "NOW", not fretting about the past or daydreaming about the future.

<u>HARMONY</u>—Without HARMONY none of the other states of mind would come to be. We must be in HARMONY with ourselves, with our creator, and with the world and all those around us. When we have harmony in our lives, then many other things will come to balance and fruition.

ARRIER OIL CONTAINED IN THIS BLEND: Almond Oil.

ODY SYSTEM(S) AFFECTED: The oils in this blend may help it be effective for dealing with various problems related to EMOTIONAL BALANCE.

ROMATIC INFLUENCE: We enjoy diffusing this blend while sleeping at night because it helps us wake up INVIGORATED and REFRESHED.

PPLICATION: Best when applied on the CHEST, HEART, FOREHEAD, NECK, STERNUM (clearing allergies), TEMPLES, and WRISTS. It may be used as an AFTERSHAVE, a COLOGNE, or a PERFUME. It may also be diluted with V-6 Mixing Oil for a full BODY MASSAGE or added to the BATH water. <u>En-R-Gee</u> may be put on the feet and <u>Awaken</u> on the temples or cheeks for one to feel like they have had eight hours of sleep.

OMPANION OILS: <u>Dream Catcher</u>, <u>En-R-Gee</u>, <u>Envision</u>, <u>Harmony</u>, <u>Into the Future</u>, <u>Joy</u>, <u>Motivation</u>, <u>Live with Passion</u>, <u>Valor</u>, <u>White Angelica</u>

REQUENCY: Physical; approximately 89 MHz.

Believe

This blend has been specifically formulated to calm the spirit while stimulating the mind, llowing us to believe in our own limitless potential to create and improve. It is GROUNDING nd EMPOWERING, helping to promote positive action toward the accomplishment of goals and ılfillment of dreams.

INGLE OILS CONTAINED IN BLEND:

Idaho Balsam Fir—creates a feeling of GROUNDING, ANCHORING, and EMPOWERMENT. It can STIMULATE the MIND while allowing the BODY to RELAX. Topically it helps relieve OVERWORKED and TIRED MUSCLES and JOINTS.

Rosewood—may help improve SKIN ELASTICITY. It is SOOTHING to the SKIN, APPEASING to the MIND, RELAXING to the BODY, and creates a feeling of PEACE and GENTLENESS.

Frankincense—contains sesquiterpenes, which may help OXYGENATE the PINEAL ar PITUITARY GLANDS. As one of the ingredients for the holy incense, it was used anciently to help ENHANCE one's COMMUNICATION WITH THE CREATOR. It may help PROMOTE a POSITIVE ATTITUDE.

BODY SYSTEM(S) AFFECTED: The oils in this blend may help it be effective for dealing wi various problems related to the NERVOUS and IMMUNE SYSTEMS, MUSCLES and BONES, and to EMOTIONAL BALANCE.

AROMATIC INFLUENCE: This blend of oils has a CALMING, STABILIZING and MENTALLY ENERGIZING aroma. Diffusing this blend may help to RELEASE the unlimited POTENTIAL to CREATE and IMPROVE our surroundings. The mentally uplifting and energizing aroma may help PROMOTE BELIEF in ourselves and our capabilities.

APPLICATION: DIFFUSE or apply to the FOREHEAD, TEMPLES, and over the HEART. May also be worn as a PERFUME or COLOGNE.

COMPANION OILS: Humility, Gratitude, Grounding, Live with Passion, Motivation

Brain Power

This blend has been specifically formulated to include those oils that are high in sesquiterpene compounds. Research has shown that sesquiterpenes play a role in DISSOLVING PETROCHEMICALS along the receptor sites near the PITUITARY, PINEAL, and HYPOTHALAMUS. This helps to increase normal receptivity along those sites and increase the amount of oxygen in those areas. INCREASED OXYGEN around the pineal, pituitary, and hypothalamus can lead to INCREASED MENTAL CAPACITY, MENTAL CLARITY, and REDUCED SYMPTOMS of what has come to be known as "BRAIN FOG".

SINGLE OILS CONTAINED IN THIS BLEND:

Cedarwood—was used traditionally by the North American Indians to enhance their potential for SPIRITUAL COMMUNICATION. It may help OPEN the PINEA GLAND.

Sandalwood—also, like frankincense, is high in sesquiterpenes, which were discovered tc INCREASE the amount of OXYGEN around the PINEAL and PITUITARY GLANDS, thus helping to IMPROVE one's ATTITUDE. It ALLEVIATES DEPRESSION and assists in the removal of NEGATIVE PROGRAMMING from the cells of the body. It helps one ACCEPT OTHERS with an open heart while diminishing one's own egocentricity.

Frankincense—contains sesquiterpenes, which may help OXYGENATE the PINEAL and PITUITARY GLANDS. As one of the ingredients for the holy incense, it was used anciently to help ENHANCE one's COMMUNICATION WITH THE CREATOR. It may help PROMOTE a POSITIVE ATTITUDE.

Melissa—is an oil that is powerful as an ANTI-VIRAL agent, yet it is very gentle and very delicate because of the nature of the plant. It has the ability to work with and enhance the gentle aspects of the human body. It is CALMING and UPLIFTING and may also help to BALANCE the EMOTIONS. It may also help to remove EMOTIONAL BLOCKS and INSTILL a POSITIVE OUTLOOK on LIFE.

Blue Cypress (*Callitris intratropica*)—comes from Australia and has been shown to improve circulation and increase the flow of oxygen to the brain.

Lavender—is an oil that has traditionally been known to BALANCE the BODY and to work wherever there is a need. It has ANTISPASMODIC and ANALGESIC properties. It may help with SPRAINS, SORE MUSCLES, HEADACHES, and general HEALING.

Helichrysum—may help CLEANSE the BLOOD and improve CIRCULATORY FUNCTIONS. It is ANTI-CATARRHAL in structure and nature. On a spiritual level, it may help one LET GO OF ANGRY FEELINGS that prevent one from forgiving and moving forward in life.

)DY SYSTEM(S) AFFECTED: The oils in this blend may help it be effective for dealing with various problems related to the NERVOUS SYSTEM and to EMOTIONAL BALANCE.

ROMATIC INFLUENCE: This blend of oils has a POWERFULLY UPLIFTING and MENTALLY ENERGIZING aroma. Diffusing this blend may help to provide DEEP CONCENTRATION and FOCUS during strenuous MENTAL ACTIVITY.

PPLICATION: May be applied to the NECK, THROAT, under the NOSE, to the ROOF of the MOUTH using the thumb, or worn as a PERFUME or COLOGNE. May also be applied INSIDE the MOUTH with a finger, either UNDER the TONGUE or on the INSIDE of each CHEEK (*See SMELL in Personal Guide section of this book*).

)MPANION OILS: Clarity, Envision, RC, Raven

REQUENCY: Physical; approximately 78 MHz–same frequency as the brain.

Chivalry

This blend is a combination of four oil blends; Valor, Joy, Harmony, and Gratitude, each a lue that is embodied in the word "chivalry". This blend was created to be EMPOWERING and NNOBLING. It helps to open the ENERGY CENTERS and promote feelings of STRENGTH, :ACE, TRUSTWORTHINESS, and COURAGE.

Oil Blends

OIL BLENDS CONTAINED IN THIS BLEND:

VALOR—is emotionally uplifting and helps to empower the physical and spiritual bodie It helps to build COURAGE, CONFIDENCE, and SELF-ESTEEM while promoting CALMNESS, PEACE, and RELAXATION.

JOY—is a blend which may help to open the heart and promote feelings of SELF-LOVE and LOVE FOR OTHERS so one can experience ultimate joy.

HARMONY—Without HARMONY none of the other states of mind would come to be We must be in HARMONY with ourselves, with our creator, and with the world and all those around us. When we have harmony in our lives, then many other things will come to balance and fruition.

GRATITUDE—helps to ELEVATE, SOOTHE, and APPEASE the MIND while bringing RELIEF and RELAXATION to the body.

CARRIER OIL CONTAINED IN THIS BLEND: Almond Oil.

BODY SYSTEM(S) AFFECTED: EMOTIONAL BALANCE.

AROMATIC INFLUENCE: When diffused or worn as perfume, this special blend of oils help to BALANCE the emotions. It may help REVITALIZE and EMPOWER both body and mind promoting COURAGE, HONOR, and INTEGRITY.

APPLICATION: Rub over the HEART, and on FOREHEAD, and TEMPLES. DIFFUSE or wear as PERFUME or COLOGNE.

SAFETY DATA: Use with caution during PREGNANCY. Not for use by people with EPILEPSY. Use with caution if dealing with HIGH BLOOD PRESSURE. Avoid exposure to DIRECT SUNLIGHT for 3 to 6 hours after use.

COMPANION OILS: Magnify Your Purpose, Live with Passion

Christmas Spirit

This blend is effective for enhancing the FEELING and MEMORY of the beautiful time of CHRISTMAS and for enhancing the desire to be in that happy and joyful moment that Christmas brings. It may be very beneficial for PROTECTING against AIRBORNE VIRUSES and BACTERIA because it contains several very powerful ANTI-VIRAL and ANTISEPTIC oil It may also be quite SOOTHING and HEALING to the RESPIRATORY SYSTEM.

SINGLE OILS CONTAINED IN THIS BLEND:

Orange—spread a little sunshine on gloomy thoughts and depression. It may help encourage a positive outlook on life, bringing PEACE and HAPPINESS to the mind and body. Orange is ANTISEPTIC and ANTI-DEPRESSANT.

Cinnamon Bark—is part of the formula the Lord gave Moses (Exodus 30:22-27). It ha very specific purposes: (1) it is a POWERFUL PURIFIER, (2) it is a powerful OXYGENATOR, and (3) it ENHANCES the action and the activity of OTHER

OILS. It may have a STIMULATING and TONING effect on the whole body and particularly the circulatory system. It may also help bring about feelings of JOY. It is ANTISEPTIC, ANTI-BACTERIAL, and ANTI-VIRAL.

Spruce—GROUNDS the BODY, creating the balance and opening necessary to receive and to give. This oil is WARMING, HEALING, UPLIFTING, and SOOTHING. It may also help RELIEVE ANXIETY and act as an ANTISEPTIC.

ODY SYSTEM(S) AFFECTED: The oils in this blend may help it be effective for dealing with various problems related to the CARDIOVASCULAR and NERVOUS SYSTEMS and to EMOTIONAL BALANCE.

ROMATIC INFLUENCE: This blend of oils has a delightful FRAGRANCE and is wonderful for creating the FEELING of SECURITY that usually accompanies the HOLIDAY SEASON. It is also nice for AIR PURIFICATION.

PPLICATION: May be applied to the CROWN of the HEAD or worn as a PERFUME or COLOGNE. The beautiful fragrance of this blend can be further enhanced by placing it on pine boughs, pine cones, cedar chips, and on logs to burn in the fireplace. It makes an excellent addition to potpourri.

AFETY DATA: Repeated use on the skin can result in extreme CONTACT SENSITIVITY. Can cause extreme SKIN IRRITATION.

OMPANION OILS: Mandarin, clove, and nutmeg.

REQUENCY: Emotional and Spiritual; approximately 104 MHz.

Citrus Fresh

Citrus Fresh is a blend which may help to enhance the FEELING of WELL BEING in HILDREN. Because many of the oils contained in this blend are strong ANTISEPTICS, it may ork well for KILLING AIRBORNE BACTERIA. It may be useful for RELAXING, ALMING, and alleviating INSOMNIA. It may also help to BALANCE the SYSTEMS. It is a agrance that can be enjoyed by everyone. Flavoring ones water with this oil blend may help PEN the LYMPHATIC SYSTEM and STIMULATE the IMMUNE SYSTEM.

INGLE OILS CONTAINED IN THIS BLEND:

Orange—brings PEACE and HAPPINESS to the MIND and BODY and JOY to the HEART, which provide EMOTIONAL support to help one overcome depression.

Tangerine—contains esters and aldehydes which are SEDATING and CALMING to the NERVOUS SYSTEM. It is also a DIURETIC and a DECONGESTANT of the LYMPHATIC SYSTEM.

Mandarin—is APPEASING, GENTLE, and promotes HAPPINESS. It is also REFRESHING, UPLIFTING, and REVITALIZING. Because of its sedative and slightly hypnotic properties, it is very good for STRESS and IRRITABILITY.

Grapefruit—is an ANTI-DEPRESSANT, an ANTISEPTIC, and a DIURETIC. It is BALANCING and UPLIFTING to the mind, and may help to RELIEVE ANXIETY.

Lemon—promotes HEALTH, HEALING, PHYSICAL ENERGY, and PURIFICATION Its fragrance is INVIGORATING, ENHANCING, and WARMING.

Spearmint—is ANTI-FUNGAL and ANTISEPTIC. It also acts as an anti-depressant by relieving mental strain and fatigue, and by lifting one's spirits.

BODY SYSTEM(S) AFFECTED: The oils in this blend may help it be effective for dealing wi various problems related to the IMMUNE SYSTEM and to EMOTIONAL BALANCE.

AROMATIC INFLUENCE: This blend of oils may create an enjoyable aromatic fragrance in the HOME or WORK PLACE. Simple diffusion can be achieved by applying a few drop of this blend on a cotton ball and placing it on the desk at work or in an air vent.

APPLICATION: May be applied on the EARS, HEART, and WRISTS or worn as a PERFUME or COLOGNE. It may be diluted with V-6 Mixing Oil for a FULL BODY MASSAGE. It may also be added to water for a RELAXING BATH. This blend can also help PURIFY DRINKING WATER. Children may like to add this blend to water and freeze for POPSICLES. It is excellent for children, though dilution with V-6 Mixing Oil is highly recommended.

SAFETY DATA: Can cause extreme SKIN IRRITATION. Avoid exposure to direct SUNLIGHT for up to 12 hours after use.

FREQUENCY: Physical and Emotional; approximately 90 MHz.

COMMENTS: A university in Japan experimented with diffusing different oils in the office. When they diffused lemon there were 54% fewer errors, with jasmine there were 33% fewer errors, and with lavender there were 20% fewer errors. When oils are diffused whi studying and smelled during a test via a hanky or cotton ball, test scores may increase by as much as 50%. Different oils should be used for different tests, but the same oil should be used during the test as was used while studying for that particular test. The smell of th oil may help bring back the memory of what was studied.

Clarity

This blend may help with MEMORY RETENTION and MENTAL ALERTNESS; it ma even help OXYGENATE the BRAIN. One may want to STUDY with this blend, then smell it during a test to help recall what was studied earlier. It may also be a STIMULANT for LOW ENERGY and may help keep one from going into SHOCK.

SINGLE OILS CONTAINED IN THIS BLEND:

Basil—has been found beneficial for ALLEVIATING MENTAL FATIGUE. It may help SHARPEN the SENSES and ENCOURAGE CONCENTRATION. It may also STIMULATE the NERVES and the ADRENAL CORTEX.

Cardamom—is UPLIFTING, REFRESHING, and INVIGORATING. It may be beneficial for CLEARING CONFUSION.

Rosemary verbenon—may help BALANCE HEART FUNCTION, ENERGIZE the SOLAR PLEXUS, and REDUCE MENTAL FATIGUE. It also stimulates MEMORY and opens the CONSCIOUS MIND.

Peppermint—is an ANTI-INFLAMMATORY to the NERVES and helps REDUCE INFLAMMATION in DAMAGED TISSUE. It is SOOTHING, COOLING, and DILATING to the SYSTEM. Dr. Dembar, of the University of Cincinnati, discovered in a research study that inhaling peppermint oil INCREASED the MENTAL ACCURACY of the students tested by up to 28%.

Rosewood—may help improve SKIN ELASTICITY. It is SOOTHING to the SKIN, APPEASING to the MIND, RELAXING to the BODY, and creates a feeling of PEACE and GENTLENESS.

Geranium—may help with HORMONAL BALANCE, LIVER and KIDNEY FUNCTIONS and the DISCHARGE of TOXINS from the LIVER that hold us back from having balance. Geranium OPENS the LIVER CHAKRA.

Lemon—promotes HEALTH, HEALING, PHYSICAL ENERGY, and PURIFICATION. Its fragrance is INVIGORATING, ENHANCING, and WARMING.

Palmarosa—is valuable for all types of SKIN problems because it STIMULATES new CELL GROWTH, regulates oil production, MOISTURIZES and SPEEDS HEALING.

Ylang Ylang—may help BALANCE the MALE-FEMALE ENERGIES so one can move closer towards being in spiritual attunement and allow them to focus their thoughts together, filtering out the ever-present garbage and establishing a sense of relaxation. It brings back the feeling of SELF-LOVE, CONFIDENCE, JOY and PEACE.

Bergamot—is SOOTHING to the ENDOCRINE SYSTEM and the HORMONES of the body. It may UPLIFT and CALM the EMOTIONS to help relieve ANXIETY, STRESS, and TENSION.

Roman Chamomile—neutralizes ALLERGIES and helps to cleanse the BLOOD and EXPEL TOXINS from the LIVER.

Jasmine—is very UPLIFTING to the EMOTIONS; it may produce a feeling of CONFIDENCE, ENERGY, EUPHORIA, and OPTIMISM. As an ANTISPASMODIC, it has been used effectively for MENSTRUAL discomfort, MUSCLE SPASMS, and UTERINE disorders.

BODY SYSTEM(S) AFFECTED: The oils in this blend may help it be effective for dealing with various problems related to the NERVOUS SYSTEM and to EMOTIONAL BALANCE.

AROMATIC INFLUENCE: The oils in this blend are known for their ability to help increase MENTAL ALERTNESS. Simple diffusion can be achieved by applying a few drops of this blend on a cotton ball and placing it on the desk at work or in an air vent.

APPLICATION: Best when applied across the BROW, on the back of the NECK, on the TEMPLES, and on the WRISTS. This blend may be added to ones BATH water or worn as a PERFUME or COLOGNE.

SAFETY DATA: Can be irritating to sensitive SKIN. Use with caution during PREGNANCY. Avoid exposure to direct SUNLIGHT for up to 12 hours after use.

COMPANION OILS: This blend and En-R-Gee together may help one stay awake while driving late at night. Others include Brain Power, lemon, and peppermint.

FREQUENCY: Emotional; approximately 101 MHz.

COMMENTS: Since this blend contains cardamom and high levels of transphenol, it may cause headaches when inhaled if there is petrochemical or heavy metal accumulation in the brain

Di-Tone

This blend may be useful for IMPROVING the DIGESTIVE FUNCTION. The oils in this blend have been found to be beneficial in DIGESTING TOXIC MATERIAL and for ALLEVIATING INDIGESTION, STOMACH CRAMPS, UPSET STOMACH, BELCHING, BLOATING, and HEARTBURN. Placing a little of this blend behind the ears may help alleviate MORNING SICKNESS. It has been found to rid animals and people of PARASITES by applying it to their feet. It has also been reported that this blend helps to alleviate discomfort from parasites by massage and compress application across the stomach.

SINGLE OILS CONTAINED IN THIS BLEND:

Tarragon—may help to reduce ANOREXIA, DYSPEPSIA, FLATULENCE, INTESTINAL SPASMS, NERVOUS and SLUGGISH DIGESTION, and GENITAL URINARY TRACT INFECTION.

Ginger—is WARMING, UPLIFTING, and EMPOWERING. Emotionally, it may help influence PHYSICAL ENERGY, LOVE, and COURAGE. Because of its calming influence on the digestive system, it may help reduce feelings of NAUSEA, and MOTION SICKNESS.

Peppermint—is an ANTI-INFLAMMATORY to the PROSTATE and NERVES. It is SOOTHING, COOLING and DILATING to the SYSTEM. It may also be beneficial for FOOD POISONING, VOMITING, DIARRHEA, CONSTIPATION, FLATULENCE, HALITOSIS, COLIC, NAUSEA, and MOTION SICKNESS.

Juniper—has ANTISEPTIC, CLEANSING, and DETOXIFYING properties. It may help to IMPROVE CIRCULATION through the KIDNEYS.

Anise—may help CALM and STRENGTHEN the DIGESTIVE SYSTEM.

Fennel—may help SUPPORT the DIGESTIVE FUNCTION by SUPPORTING the LIVER. It may also help BALANCE the HORMONES.

Lemongrass—is a VASODILATOR, ANTISEPTIC, ANTI-BACTERIAL, ANTI-INFLAMMATORY, and SEDATIVE. It may help improve CIRCULATION, wake up the LYMPHATIC SYSTEM, and increase the flow of OXYGEN. It may also help to LIFT the SPIRIT.

Patchouli—is SEDATING, CALMING, and RELAXING allowing it to reduce ANXIETY. It is a digester of toxic material in the body.

)DY SYSTEM(S) AFFECTED: The oils in this blend may help it be effective for dealing with various problems related to the DIGESTIVE SYSTEM.

'PLICATION: May be applied to the VITA FLEX points on the FEET and ANKLES. It may also be applied topically over the STOMACH, as a COMPRESS on the ABDOMEN, on other VITA FLEX points on the BODY, and at the bottom of the THROAT (for gagging). As a DIETARY SUPPLEMENT, dilute one drop in 4 oz. of water or soy/rice milk and sip slowly. May also be used in a RETENTION ENEMA for ridding the COLON of PARASITES and for combating DIGESTIVE CANDIDA. Apply to ANIMAL PAWS for PARASITES.

.FETY DATA: Use with caution during PREGNANCY (only a drop massaged on the outer ear for morning sickness). Not for use by people with EPILEPSY.

)MPANION OILS: peppermint, and spearmint.

)MPANION SUPPLEMENTS: ComforTone, Essentialzyme, JuvaTone

:EQUENCY: Emotional; approximately 102 MHz.

Dragon Time

This is a blend of single oils that have historically been used to help ALLEVIATE PRE-ENSTRUAL and MENSTRUAL CRAMPS and discomfort. This blend may also help MEN th PROSTATE problems.

NGLE OILS CONTAINED IN THIS BLEND:

Clary Sage—is beneficial for REGULATING CELLS and BALANCING the HORMONES. It may help with MENSTRUAL CRAMPS, PMS, and PRE-MENOPAUSE symptoms. It may also help with CIRCULATORY PROBLEMS.

Fennel—may help SUPPORT the DIGESTIVE FUNCTION by SUPPORTING the LIVER. It may also help BALANCE the HORMONES.

Lavender—is an oil that has traditionally been known to BALANCE the BODY and to work wherever there is a need. It may help with PMS/MENOPAUSAL PROBLEMS, STRESS, STRETCH MARKS, TENSION, and WATER RETENTION.

Jasmine—is very UPLIFTING to the EMOTIONS; it may produce a feeling of CONFIDENCE, ENERGY, EUPHORIA, and OPTIMISM. As an

ANTISPASMODIC, it has been used effectively for MENSTRUAL discomfort MUSCLE SPASMS, and UTERINE disorders.

Yarrow—is a POWERFUL DECONGESTANT of the PROSTATE and a HORMONE BALANCER.

BODY SYSTEM(S) AFFECTED: The oils in this blend may help it be effective for dealing w various problems related to the HORMONAL SYSTEM and to EMOTIONAL BALANCE.

AROMATIC INFLUENCE: This blend of oils may be beneficial in times of HORMONAL STRESS. It may be diffused in the home, the office, or put a few drops on a cotton ball and place in the car vent.

APPLICATION: May be applied to the VITA FLEX points on the FEET and around the ANKLES, both inside and out. It may be diluted with V-6 Mixing Oil for application on the other VITA FLEX points on the BODY. It may also be applied as a hot COMPRES or rubbed over the ABDOMEN, across the LOWER BACK, or anywhere it HURTS.

SAFETY DATA: Use with caution during PREGNANCY.

COMPANION OILS: Combining this blend with Mister or EndoFlex may help ALLEVIATE HOT FLASHES (POWER SURGES) in women.

FREQUENCY: Physical; approximately 72 MHz.

Dream Catcher

This blend may help to open the MIND, to ENHANCE DREAMS, and to help one VISUALIZE their VISIONS and HANG ONTO them until they become REALITY. It may als serve to PROTECT one from the NEGATIVE DREAMS that tend to steal our VISION. Childr love the smell of this blend and it may even help them to sleep more soundly. Our little girl aske for this blend every night for a while, until she felt comfortable with sleeping in her own bed. Later, if she was having a bad dream, she would come ask for some to be put on her forehead an would go right back to bed and sleep soundly for the rest of the night.

SINGLE OILS CONTAINED IN THIS BLEND:

Sandalwood—also, like frankincense, is high in sesquiterpenes, which were discovered t INCREASE the amount of OXYGEN around the PINEAL and PITUITARY GLANDS, thus helping to IMPROVE one's ATTITUDE. It ALLEVIATES DEPRESSION and assists in the removal of NEGATIVE PROGRAMMING from the cells of the body.

Bergamot—is SOOTHING to the ENDOCRINE SYSTEM and the HORMONES of th body. It may UPLIFT and CALM the EMOTIONS to help relieve ANXIETY, STRESS, and TENSION.

Ylang Ylang—may help BALANCE the MALE-FEMALE ENERGIES so one can move closer towards being in spiritual attunement and allow them to focus their thoughts together, filtering out the ever-present garbage. It brings back the feeling of SELF-LOVE, CONFIDENCE, JOY and PEACE.

Juniper—evokes feelings of HEALTH, LOVE, and PEACE and may help to ELEVATE one's SPIRITUAL AWARENESS.

Blue Tansy—encourages an UPLIFTING FEELING, a POSITIVE ATTITUDE, and a general feeling of WELL BEING.

Tangerine—contains esters and aldehydes which are SEDATING and CALMING to the NERVOUS SYSTEM. It is also a DIURETIC and a DECONGESTANT of the LYMPHATIC SYSTEM.

Pepper, Black—may help STIMULATE the ENDOCRINE SYSTEM and INCREASE ENERGY. May help INCREASE CELLULAR OXYGENATION.

Anise—may help CALM and STRENGTHEN the DIGESTIVE SYSTEM.

ODY SYSTEM(S) AFFECTED: The oils in this blend may help it be effective for dealing with various problems related to EMOTIONAL BALANCE.

ROMATIC INFLUENCE: This blend may be diffused during the day, but seems to be most effective during sleep. This blend may also be useful during MEDITATION.

PPLICATION: Best when applied to the FOREHEAD (3rd EYE or BROW CHAKRA), EYE BROWS, TEMPLES, behind the EARS, and on the THROAT CHAKRA (base of neck). It may be worn as a PERFUME or COLOGNE. For a lasting aroma, place a drop under the NOSE or on the PILLOW. Add to BATH water.

AFETY DATA: Avoid exposure to direct SUNLIGHT for 3 to 6 hours after use.

OMPANION OILS: To enhance DREAM AWARENESS, put a couple drops of this blend on a PILLOW, Awaken on the TEMPLES, and Motivation on the CHEST. Other choices include Envision, Gathering, Into the Future, Live with Passion.

REQUENCY: Physical and Emotional; approximately 98 MHz.

OMMENTS: Indian dream catchers have been used to help keep bad dreams away. This blend may accomplish the same purpose. However, if bad dreams do come, continued use of this oil may be necessary as something in the subconscious may need to be processed. Hold onto your dreams and visualize them into reality by bringing them from the mind to the heart to make them come true.

En-R-Gee

En-R-Gee is a blend that may help IMPROVE ONE'S ENERGY in a natural way without erstimulating or creating problems that may be uncomfortable. It may also help with MENTAL LERTNESS.

SINGLE OILS CONTAINED IN THIS BLEND:

Rosemary cineol—may help BALANCE HEART FUNCTION, ENERGIZE the SOLA PLEXUS, and REDUCE MENTAL FATIGUE.

Juniper—has ANTISEPTIC, CLEANSING, and DETOXIFYING properties. It may help to IMPROVE CIRCULATION through the KIDNEYS.

Nutmeg—has adrenal cortex-like activity, which helps support the ADRENAL GLANI for INCREASED ENERGY.

Fir—may help create a feeling of GROUNDING, ANCHORING and EMPOWERMENT.

Pepper, Black—may help STIMULATE the ENDOCRINE SYSTEM and INCREASE ENERGY.

Lemongrass—is a VASODILATOR, ANTISEPTIC, ANTI-BACTERIAL, ANTI-INFLAMMATORY, and SEDATIVE. It may help improve CIRCULATION, wake up the LYMPHATIC SYSTEM, and increase the flow of OXYGEN. It may also help to LIFT the SPIRIT.

Clove—may influence HEALING, improve MEMORY, and create a feeling of PROTECTION and COURAGE. It may also help one overcome FATIGUE.

BODY SYSTEM(S) AFFECTED: The oils in this blend may help it be effective for dealing w various problems related to the NERVOUS SYSTEM and to EMOTIONAL BALANCI

AROMATIC INFLUENCE: This blend of oils may help boost one's ENERGY when diffused It is also PURIFYING. Simple diffusion can be achieved by applying a few drops of thi blend on a cotton ball and placing it in the air vent of a car or on the heat registers of the home or hotel room.

APPLICATION: Best when applied on the WRISTS and behind and on the EARS. It may als be massaged across the BASE of the NECK, TEMPLES, and rubbed on the FEET in th morning. Dilute with V-6 Mixing Oil for FULL BODY MASSAGE or wear as a PERFUME or COLOGNE.

***SAFETY DATA:* Can cause extreme SKIN IRRITATION. Use with caution if susceptible t EPILEPSY.**

COMPANION OILS: One may feel like they have had eight hours of sleep by rubbing this ble on the feet and Awaken on TEMPLES. This blend and Clarity together may help one st awake while driving late at night.

FREQUENCY: Emotional; approximately 106 MHz.

EndoFlex

This is a beautiful blend that may help provide overall BALANCE and SUPPORT to the ENDOCRINE SYSTEM and may work to IMPROVE the VITALITY of the body. It may SUPPORT the PINEAL and PITUITARY glands, PARATHYROID, THYMUS, and ADRENA glands. It may also help to ALLEVIATE HOT FLASHES and to STIMULATE WEIGHT LOSS by IMPROVING the METABOLIC FUNCTION. It may support the THYROID for METABOLIC and HORMONAL BALANCE.

SINGLE OILS CONTAINED IN THIS BLEND:

Spearmint—is an oil that may balance and increase METABOLISM; helping to BURN UP FATS and TOXINS in the body.

Sage—may help improve ESTROGEN and PROGESTERONE-TESTOSTERONE BALANCE. It is believed to contain elements that contribute to the SECRETION of PROGESTERONE-TESTOSTERONE.

Geranium—may help with HORMONAL BALANCE, LIVER and KIDNEY FUNCTIONS and the DISCHARGE of TOXINS from the LIVER that hold us back from having balance. Geranium OPENS the LIVER CHAKRA.

Myrtle—may help REGULATE THYROID FUNCTION. For HYPO-THYROID it may INCREASE ACTIVITY, and IMPROVE BALANCE.

Nutmeg—has adrenal cortex-like activity, which helps support the ADRENAL GLANDS for INCREASED ENERGY.

German Chamomile—has been found to help OPEN the LIVER, INCREASE LIVER FUNCTION and SECRETION, and SUPPORT the PANCREAS.

CARRIER OIL CONTAINED IN THIS BLEND: Sesame Seed Oil.

BODY SYSTEM(S) AFFECTED: The oils in this blend may help it be effective for dealing with various problems related to the HORMONAL (ENDOCRINE) SYSTEM.

APPLICATION: May be applied over the THYROID, KIDNEYS, LIVER (front right, 2" down from bra line), PANCREAS (front left), and all GLANDS. It may also work well when applied to the VITA FLEX points on the FEET including under the BIG TOE and on the THROAT or ENDOCRINE GLAND LOCATIONS.

SAFETY DATA: Can be irritating to sensitive SKIN. Use with caution if susceptible to EPILEPSY.

FREQUENCY: Emotional and Spiritual; approximately 138 MHz.

Envision

This blend is comprised of essential oils which provide powerful support and balance to the emotions. This type of emotional support is necessary for us to move forward with renewed faith in the future toward achieving our dreams and goals.

SINGLE OILS CONTAINED IN THIS BLEND:

Spruce—GROUNDS the BODY, creating the BALANCE and the OPENING necessary to RECEIVE and to GIVE. It may help DILATE the BRONCHIAL TRACT to

IMPROVE the OXYGEN EXCHANGE. It also helps one release EMOTIONAL BLOCKS.

Sage—may help improve ESTROGEN and PROGESTERONE-TESTOSTERONE BALANCE. It is believed to contain elements that contribute to the SECRETION of PROGESTERONE-TESTOSTERONE.

Rose—contains the highest frequency of the oils. It may help ENHANCE the FREQUENCY of every cell, which could help bring BALANCE and HARMONY to the body. It is thought by some to produce a magnetic energy that attracts LOVE and enhances the frequency of SELF-LOVE, bringing JOY to the heart.

Geranium—may help with HORMONAL BALANCE, LIVER and KIDNEY FUNCTIONS and the DISCHARGE of TOXINS from the LIVER that hold us back from having balance. Geranium OPENS the LIVER CHAKRA.

Orange—brings PEACE and HAPPINESS to the MIND and BODY and JOY to the HEART, which provide EMOTIONAL support to help one overcome depression.

Lavender—is an oil that has traditionally been known to BALANCE the BODY and to work wherever there is a need. It may help with PMS/MENOPAUSAL PROBLEMS, STRESS, STRETCH MARKS, TENSION, and WATER RETENTION.

BODY SYSTEM(S) AFFECTED: The oils in this blend may help it be effective for dealing wit various problems related to EMOTIONAL BALANCE.

AROMATIC INFLUENCE: This blend was structured specifically to EXPEL NEGATIVE EMOTIONS, ELEVATE the MIND, BALANCE, EMPOWER, and PROPEL one forward to achieve their desired goals.

APPLICATION: Apply to VITA FLEX points on FEET and/or directly on area of concern. This blend may also be DIFFUSED, applied to the WRISTS or TEMPLES, or added to warm BATH water (best when first combined with a bath gel base). For an uplifting massage, dilute first with a pure carrier oil.

SAFETY DATA: Because this blend contains sage, it should be used with caution by those individuals who are susceptible to HIGH BLOOD PRESSURE, EPILEPTIC SEIZURES, or who are PREGNANT.

COMPANION OILS: Acceptance, Clarity, Into the Future, Magnify Your Purpose, Motivation Valor.

FREQUENCY: Physical and Emotional; approximately 90 MHz.

Evergreen Essence

This blend is a combination of oils distilled from a variety of aromatic cedar, pine, and spruce trees. Now the PEACE, SERENITY, GROUNDING, and even SACRED FEELINGS of the evergreen forests can be brought into the home or workplace. All of these oils are grounding tc ne body, creating the BALANCE and OPENING necessary to receive and to give. This blend is IEALING, UPLIFTING, and SOOTHING. It may help RELIEVE ANXIETY and facilitate the ELEASE of EMOTIONAL BLOCKS, as well as promote feelings of PROTECTION, TRENGTH, and SECURITY. *More detailed information for many of these oils is not readily vailable. In those cases, only the common names and the latin names are listed.*

INGLE OILS CONTAINED IN THIS BLEND:

Colorado Blue Spruce (*Picea pungens*)

Ponderosa Pine (*Pinus ponderosa*)

Pine—may help DILATE and OPEN the RESPIRATORY SYSTEM, particularly the BRONCHIAL TRACT. It may also help IMPROVE CIRCULATION THROUGHOUT the LUNGS. It helps soothe MENTAL STRESS, relieve ANXIETY, and REVITALIZE the entire body.

Red Fir (*Abies magnifica*)

Cedar (*Cedrus canadensis*)

White Fir (*Abies grandis*)—creates a feeling of GROUNDING, ANCHORING, and EMPOWERMENT. It can STIMULATE the MIND while allowing the BODY to RELAX. Topically it helps relieve PAIN from INFLAMMATION.

Black Pine (*Pinus nigra*)

Piñon Pine (*Pinus edulis*)

Lodge Pole Pine (*Pinus contorta*)

May also contain Black spruce, fir, and cedarwood.

BODY SYSTEM(S) AFFECTED: The oils in this blend may help it be effective for dealing with various problems related to EMOTIONAL BALANCE.

AROMATIC INFLUENCE: When diffused, this blend of conifer oils, each with their own powerful antiseptic properties, helps to FRESHEN and DEODORIZE the air. It may help soothe MENTAL STRESS, relieve ANXIETY, and REVITALIZE the entire body. The individual oils in this blend have also been described as APPEASING, ELEVATING, and OPENING.

APPLICATION: Diffuse! Can also be sprinkled on logs in the fireplace or used to scent potpourri. Dilute well with V-6 Mixing Oil for any topical application.

SAFETY DATA: Could possibly result in CONTACT SENSITIZATION or SKIN IRRITATION.

Exodus II

This blend is comprised of many powerful and precious essential oils that are mentioned many times in the Bible (see Exodus, chapter 30). The intent behind this particular blend of oils was to enhance the ability of the body to EXPEL DISEASE and DEAD TISSUE. It was also specifically designed to work with the **Exodus** food supplement to help build ones defenses.

SINGLE OILS CONTAINED IN THIS BLEND:

Cinnamon Bark—is part of the formula the Lord gave Moses (Exodus 30:22-27). It has very specific purposes: (1) it is a POWERFUL PURIFIER, (2) it is a powerful OXYGENATOR, and (3) it ENHANCES the action and the activity of OTHER OILS. It may have a STIMULATING and TONING effect on the whole body and particularly the circulatory system. It is ANTISEPTIC, ANTI-BACTERIAL and ANTI-VIRAL.

Cassia—is part of the formula the Lord gave Moses (Exodus 30:22-27). It is ANTI-BACTERIAL, ANTI-COAGULANT, ANTI-INFECTIOUS and ANTIMICROBIAL.

Calamus—is part of the formula the Lord gave Moses (Exodus 30:22-27). It is ANTI-BACTERIAL, ANTISEPTIC, and ANTISPASMODIC. It was once highly regarded as an aromatic stimulant and a tonic for the digestive system.

Myrrh—is part of the formula the Lord gave Moses (Exodus 30:22-27). It is a TRUE GIFT. When we OPEN our HEARTS and MINDS to receive the gifts, they will be given.

Hyssop—was used by Moses during the Lord's Passover in Egypt (Exodus 12). It has ANTI-INFLAMMATORY and ANTI-VIRAL properties. It may also have the ability to OPEN up the RESPIRATORY SYSTEM and DISCHARGE TOXINS and MUCUS.

Frankincense—contains sesquiterpenes, which may help OXYGENATE the PINEAL an PITUITARY GLANDS. As one of the ingredients for the holy incense, it was used anciently to help ENHANCE one's COMMUNICATION WITH THE CREATOR. It was considered a prize possession and was given to Christ at his birth. It may help PROMOTE a POSITIVE ATTITUDE.

Spikenard—was highly prized in the Middle East during the time of Christ, and is referre to several times in the Bible. It is ANTIFUNGAL, ANTI-INFLAMMATORY, RELAXING, REGENERATIVE, and helpful for allergic skin reactions.

Galbanum—combined with frankincense was used biblically to make a holy incense that would ENHANCE ones COMMUNICATION with the CREATOR. It is recognized for its ANTI-VIRAL properties, its overall STRENGTHENING and SUPPORTING properties. It contains a low frequency in itself, but when combined with any other oils, such as frankincense or sandalwood, the frequency changes drastically.

CARRIER OIL CONTAINED IN THIS BLEND: Olive oil.

BODY SYSTEM(S) AFFECTED: The oils in this blend may help it be effective for dealing wit various problems related to the IMMUNE SYSTEM.

PPLICATION: Apply to VITA FLEX points on FEET and/or directly on area of concern. This blend may also be applied along the spine using the Raindrop Technique. **Dilution of this blend may be necessary due to the presence of cinnamon bark.**

AFETY DATA: Repeated use on the skin can result in extreme CONTACT SENSITIZATION. Can cause extreme SKIN IRRITATION. Avoid during PREGNANCY.

OMPANION SUPPLEMENTS: Exodus, ImmuneTune

REQUENCY: High (Spiritual); approximately 180 MHz.

IBLE: "Purge me with Hyssop and I shall be clean" (Psalms 51:7). Several of the oils in this blend come from Chapter 30 in the book of Exodus.

Forgiveness

The oils in this blend all have powerful emotional effects that may help people move past e barriers in life by bringing them into a HIGHER SPIRITUAL AWARENESS of their needs. his awareness leaves an angelic feeling in their soul that raises their frequency to the point where ey are almost compelled to FORGIVE, FORGET, LET GO, and go on with their lives.

INGLE OILS CONTAINED IN THIS BLEND:

Frankincense—contains sesquiterpenes, which may help OXYGENATE the PINEAL and PITUITARY GLANDS. As one of the ingredients for the holy incense, it was used anciently to help ENHANCE one's COMMUNICATION WITH THE CREATOR. It may help PROMOTE a POSITIVE ATTITUDE.

Sandalwood—also, like frankincense, is high in sesquiterpenes, which were discovered to INCREASE the amount of OXYGEN around the PINEAL and PITUITARY GLANDS, thus helping to IMPROVE one's ATTITUDE. It ALLEVIATES DEPRESSION and assists in the removal of NEGATIVE PROGRAMMING from the cells of the body. It helps one ACCEPT OTHERS with an open heart while diminishing one's own egocentricity.

Lavender—is an oil that has traditionally been known to BALANCE the BODY and to work wherever there is a need. It may help promote CONSCIOUSNESS, HEALTH, LOVE, PEACE, and a general sense of WELL BEING.

Melissa—is an oil that is powerful as an ANTI-VIRAL agent, yet it is very gentle and very delicate because of the nature of the plant. It has the ability to work with and enhance the gentle aspects of the human body. It is CALMING and UPLIFTING and may also help to BALANCE the EMOTIONS. It may also help to remove EMOTIONAL BLOCKS and INSTILL a POSITIVE OUTLOOK on LIFE.

Angelica—may help one RELEASE and LET GO of NEGATIVE FEELINGS.

Helichrysum—may help CLEANSE the BLOOD and improve CIRCULATORY FUNCTIONS. It is ANTI-CATARRHAL in structure and nature. On a spiritu level, it may help one LET GO OF ANGRY FEELINGS that prevent one from forgiving and moving forward in life.

Rose—contains the highest frequency of the oils. It may help ENHANCE the FREQUENCY of every cell, which could help bring BALANCE and HARMON to the body.

Rosewood—may help improve SKIN ELASTICITY. It is SOOTHING to the SKIN, APPEASING to the MIND, RELAXING to the BODY, and creates a feeling of PEACE and GENTLENESS.

Geranium—may help with HORMONAL BALANCE, LIVER and KIDNEY FUNCTIONS and the DISCHARGE of TOXINS from the LIVER that hold us back from having balance. Geranium OPENS the LIVER CHAKRA.

Lemon—promotes HEALTH, HEALING, PHYSICAL ENERGY, and PURIFICATIO Its fragrance is INVIGORATING, ENHANCING, and WARMING.

Palmarosa—is valuable for all types of SKIN problems because it STIMULATES new CELL GROWTH, regulates oil production, MOISTURIZES and SPEEDS HEALING.

Ylang Ylang—may help BALANCE the MALE-FEMALE ENERGIES so one can mov closer towards being in spiritual attunement and allow them to focus their thoug together, filtering out the ever-present garbage and establishing a sense of relaxation. It brings back the feeling of SELF-LOVE, CONFIDENCE, JOY an PEACE.

Bergamot—is SOOTHING to the ENDOCRINE SYSTEM and the HORMONES of th body. It may UPLIFT and CALM the EMOTIONS to help relieve ANXIETY, STRESS, and TENSION.

Roman Chamomile—neutralizes ALLERGIES and helps to cleanse the BLOOD and EXPEL TOXINS from the LIVER.

Jasmine—is very UPLIFTING to the EMOTIONS; it may produce a feeling of CONFIDENCE, ENERGY, EUPHORIA, and OPTIMISM. As an ANTISPASMODIC, it has been used effectively for MENSTRUAL discomfort, MUSCLE SPASMS, and UTERINE disorders.

CARRIER OIL CONTAINED IN THIS BLEND: Sesame Seed Oil.

BODY SYSTEM(S) AFFECTED: The oils in this blend may help it be effective for dealing wi various problems related to EMOTIONAL BALANCE.

AROMATIC INFLUENCE: When diffused, this blend of oils may stimulate one to feel the nee to FORGIVE themselves and others of transgression.

APPLICATION: Best when massaged clockwise over the NAVEL (key area, lasts longer) and the HEART, and also placed behind the EARS, and on the WRISTS. It may also be wor as a PERFUME or COLOGNE.

OMPANION OILS: Valor on the FEET, CHEEKS and FACE; Joy on the EARS and CHEST; Gathering on the FOREHEAD.

REQUENCY: High (Spiritual); approximately 192 MHz.

IBLE: Matthew 6:14-15

Gathering

The oils in this blend may help INCREASE the OXYGEN around the PITUITARY and INEAL GLANDS, bringing us more into a HARMONIC FREQUENCY to be a receptor of the ommunications that we desire to receive. As many of these single oils tend to move people in a rofound way, this blend may help BRING PEOPLE TOGETHER in SPIRITUAL ONENESS ith GOD. This blend may also HELP BRING not only the PHYSICAL but also the MOTIONAL and SPIRITUAL THOUGHTS and FEELINGS TOGETHER for GREATER OCUS and CLARITY. By helping to prevent the FRACTURING of THOUGHT ENERGY, this lend may help one find a greater PEACE and BALANCE in life. It may help to keep one OCUSED, GROUNDED, CONNECTED, and CLEAR, and may even help GATHER ones OTENTIAL for SELF-IMPROVEMENT. It may be a very powerful blend for SUPPORTING nd PROTECTING the BODY from OUTSIDE ATTACKS, especially when there has been a ACK of SLEEP. Because it tends to act as an AMPLIFIER, refer to the comments below egarding its use.

INGLE OILS CONTAINED IN THIS BLEND:

Galbanum—combined with frankincense was used biblically to make a holy incense that would ENHANCE ones COMMUNICATION with the CREATOR. It is recognized for its ANTI-VIRAL properties, its overall STRENGTHENING and SUPPORTING properties. It contains a low frequency in itself, but when combined with any other oils, such as frankincense or sandalwood, the frequency changes drastically.

Frankincense—contains sesquiterpenes, which may help OXYGENATE the PINEAL and PITUITARY GLANDS. As one of the ingredients for the holy incense, it was used anciently to help ENHANCE one's COMMUNICATION WITH THE CREATOR. It was considered a prize possession and was given to Christ at his birth. It may help PROMOTE a POSITIVE ATTITUDE.

Sandalwood—also, like frankincense, is high in sesquiterpenes, which were discovered to INCREASE the amount of OXYGEN around the PINEAL and PITUITARY GLANDS, thus helping to IMPROVE one's ATTITUDE. It ALLEVIATES DEPRESSION and assists in the removal of NEGATIVE PROGRAMMING from the cells of the body. It helps one ACCEPT OTHERS with an open heart while diminishing one's own egocentricity.

Lavender—is an oil that has traditionally been known to BALANCE the BODY and to work wherever there is a need. It may help promote CONSCIOUSNESS, HEALTH, LOVE, PEACE, and a general sense of WELL BEING.

Cinnamon Bark—is part of the formula the Lord gave Moses (Exodus 30:22-27). It ha very specific purposes: (1) it is a POWERFUL PURIFIER, (2) it is a powerful OXYGENATOR, and (3) it ENHANCES the action and the activity of OTHER OILS. It may have a STIMULATING and TONING effect on the whole body and particularly the circulatory system. It is ANTISEPTIC, ANTI-BACTERIA and ANTI-VIRAL.

Rose—contains the highest frequency of the oils. It may help ENHANCE the FREQUENCY of every cell, which could help bring BALANCE and HARMON to the body.

Spruce—GROUNDS the BODY, creating the BALANCE and the OPENING necessary to RECEIVE and to GIVE. It may help DILATE the BRONCHIAL TRACT to IMPROVE the OXYGEN EXCHANGE. It also helps one release EMOTIONA BLOCKS.

Geranium—may be HEALING, CALMING and BALANCING to the SKIN. It may help BALANCE the SEBUM which is the fatty secretion in the sebaceous glands of the skin that KEEP the SKIN SUPPLE. It helps OPEN and ELEVATE the MIND.

Ylang Ylang—may help BALANCE the MALE-FEMALE ENERGIES so one can move closer towards being in spiritual attunement and allow them to focus their though together, filtering out the ever-present garbage. It brings back the feeling of SELF-LOVE, CONFIDENCE, JOY and PEACE.

BODY SYSTEM(S) AFFECTED: The oils in this blend may help it be effective for dealing wi various problems related to EMOTIONAL BALANCE.

AROMATIC INFLUENCE: When diffused, this blend of oils may help one GATHER their THOUGHTS so they can become focused. It may also help the HEART and MIND to work harmoniously, allowing GOALS and DREAMS to be MANIFEST in PHYSICAL FORMS.

APPLICATION: Best when applied to the FOREHEAD, HEART, RIGHT TEMPLE across to the LEFT TEMPLE, bottom front of the NECK, THYMUS, FACE, CHEST, and on eac side of the upper chest NEAR the SHOULDERS. It can be applied anywhere on the bod or worn as a PERFUME or COLOGNE.

COMPANION OILS: Forgiveness on the NAVEL, Sacred Mountain on the CROWN (to bring person with a negative attitude to a clear space). This blend also works well with Valor (crown or feet), 3 Wise Men (crown), Clarity (temples), and Dream Catcher.

FREQUENCY: Physical and Emotional; approximately 99 MHz.

BIBLE: Galbanum and frankincense are talked about in Exodus and were used by Moses as the holy incense. Cinnamon is part of the formula that the Lord gave Moses to help him "become single unto God".

)MMENTS: Gathering has a specific purpose for each individual use. One must use this blend with the right intent as it may amplify negative as well as positive attitudes. Wear with caution when feeling negative because it may amplify the negative feelings. It may be necessary to use Sacred Mountain first in order to bring oneself to a clear space before using Gathering.

Gentle Baby

This is a wonderful blend, designed specifically for EXPECTANT MOTHERS and EWBORN BABIES. It is COMFORTING, SOOTHING, and RELAXING. It may help ELIEVE STRESS during PREGNANCY and may even be BENEFICIAL during the RTHING PROCESS. It helps to ENHANCE the YOUTHFUL APPEARANCE of the SKIN d may be beneficial for men to use on CHAPPED SKIN and as an AFTERSHAVE. It may also lp with SKIN ELASTICITY and STRETCH MARKS. Every oil in **Gentle Baby** is for SKIN EGENERATION and may help to PREVENT and RETARD WRINKLES. This blend is so ntle and soothing to the skin that it could possibly be used for DIAPER RASHES (dilute at least ½).

INGLE OILS CONTAINED IN THIS BLEND:

Rose Geranium (*Pelargonium x asperum*)—may be HEALING, CALMING and BALANCING to the SKIN. It may help BALANCE the SEBUM which is the fatty secretion in the sebaceous glands of the skin that KEEP the SKIN SUPPLE.

Rosewood—may help improve SKIN ELASTICITY. It is SOOTHING to the SKIN, APPEASING to the MIND, RELAXING to the BODY, and creates a feeling of PEACE and GENTLENESS.

Palmarosa—is valuable for all types of SKIN problems because it STIMULATES new CELL GROWTH, regulates oil production, MOISTURIZES and SPEEDS HEALING.

Lavender—is an oil that has traditionally been known to BALANCE the BODY and to work wherever there is a need. It may help prevent SCARRING and STRETCH MARKS and promote a general sense of WELL BEING.

Roman Chamomile—neutralizes ALLERGIES and helps in SKIN REGENERATION. It may also help reduce IRRITABILITY and minimize NERVOUSNESS in children, especially HYPERACTIVE CHILDREN.

Ylang Ylang—may help BALANCE the MALE-FEMALE ENERGIES so one can move closer towards being in spiritual attunement and allow them to focus their thoughts together, filtering out the ever-present garbage. It brings back the feeling of SELF-LOVE, CONFIDENCE, JOY and PEACE.

Rose—has a BEAUTIFUL FRAGRANCE and contains the highest frequency of the oil It may help ENHANCE the FREQUENCY of every cell, which could help brin BALANCE and HARMONY to the body.

Lemon—promotes HEALTH, HEALING, PHYSICAL ENERGY, and PURIFICATIO Its fragrance is INVIGORATING, ENHANCING, and WARMING.

Bergamot—is SOOTHING to the ENDOCRINE SYSTEM and the HORMONES of th body. It may UPLIFT and CALM the EMOTIONS to help relieve ANXIETY, STRESS, and TENSION.

Jasmine—is very UPLIFTING to the EMOTIONS; it may produce a feeling of CONFIDENCE, ENERGY, EUPHORIA, and OPTIMISM.

BODY SYSTEM(S) AFFECTED: The oils in this blend may help it be effective for dealing w various problems related to EMOTIONAL BALANCE and to the SKIN.

AROMATIC INFLUENCE: The aroma of this blend of oils is very RELAXING and CALMING. It may also help one CREATE a SPACE for BEING in ones CHILDHOO again.

APPLICATION: Best when applied to the VITA FLEX points on the INNER ANKLES, acros the LOWER BACK and ABDOMEN (to reduce cramping and stretch marks), and on th FEET, FACE and NECK areas. Dilute with V-6 Mixing Oil for FULL BODY MASSAGE or wear as a PERFUME or COLOGNE. It may also be added to BATH water.

BABY—When using on a baby dilute at least by ½. Dilute with V-6 Mixing Oil for FULL BODY MASSAGE. It may also be applied to the FEET, ABDOMEN, LOWER BACK, FACE, and NECK areas.

DELIVERY—Massage it on the PERINEUM to help it STRETCH and possibly help AVOID an EPISIOTOMY.

FREQUENCY: High (Spiritual); approximately 152 MHz.

Gratitude

This blend was specifically formulated to ELEVATE, SOOTHE, and APPEASE the MIND while BRINGING RELIEF and RELAXATION to the body. While the body is relaxing, the heart and mind can be opened to receive the gifts that are given each day.

SINGLE OILS CONTAINED IN THIS BLEND:

Idaho Balsam Fir—creates a feeling of GROUNDING, ANCHORING, and EMPOWERMENT. It can STIMULATE the MIND while allowing the BODY to RELAX. Topically it helps relieve OVERWORKED and TIRED MUSCLES and JOINTS.

Frankincense—contains sesquiterpenes, which may help OXYGENATE the PINEAL and PITUITARY GLANDS. As one of the ingredients for the holy incense, it was used anciently to help ENHANCE one's COMMUNICATION WITH THE CREATOR. It was considered a prize possession and was given to Christ at his birth. It may help PROMOTE a POSITIVE ATTITUDE.

Rosewood—is SOOTHING to the SKIN, APPEASING to the MIND, RELAXING to the BODY, and creates a feeling of PEACE and GENTLENESS.

Myrrh—is part of the formula the Lord gave Moses (Exodus 30:22-27). It promotes SPIRITUAL AWARENESS and is a TRUE GIFT. When we OPEN our HEARTS and MINDS to receive the gifts, they will be given.

Galbanum—combined with frankincense was used biblically to make a holy incense that would ENHANCE ones COMMUNICATION with the CREATOR. It is recognized for its ANTI-VIRAL properties, its overall STRENGTHENING and SUPPORTING properties. It contains a low frequency in itself, but when combined with any other oils, such as frankincense or sandalwood, the frequency changes drastically.

Ylang Ylang—may help BALANCE the MALE-FEMALE ENERGIES so one can move closer towards being in spiritual attunement and allow them to focus their thoughts together, filtering out the ever-present garbage. It brings back the feeling of SELF-LOVE, CONFIDENCE, JOY and PEACE.

ODY SYSTEM(S) AFFECTED: The oils in this blend may help it be effective for dealing with various problems related to the NERVOUS and IMMUNE SYSTEMS, MUSCLES and BONES, and to EMOTIONAL BALANCE.

ROMATIC INFLUENCE: This blend of oils may help SOOTHE and APPEASE the MIND. It is RELAXING and ELEVATING, promoting a sense of gratitude for blessings received.

PPLICATION: Rub over the HEART, and on FOREHEAD, and TEMPLES. DIFFUSE or wear as PERFUME or COLOGNE.

OMPANION OILS: Acceptance, Believe, Forgiveness, Inner Child, Inspiration, Peace & Calming

Grounding

This blend may help to STABILIZE and GROUND us in order TO DEAL WITH EALITY in a logical, peaceful manner. It can be easy for us to disconnect from reality. We are ther excited about new ideas or want to escape into our own fantasy world. However, doing this lows us to make choices that can lead to some very unfortunate circumstances. This blend may ELP US DEAL with REALITY.

SINGLE OILS CONTAINED IN THIS BLEND:

Juniper—evokes feelings of HEALTH, LOVE, and PEACE and may help to ELEVAT one's SPIRITUAL AWARENESS.

Angelica—may help one RELEASE and LET GO of NEGATIVE FEELINGS.

Ylang Ylang—may help BALANCE the MALE-FEMALE ENERGIES so one can mo closer towards being in spiritual attunement and allow them to focus their thoug together, filtering out the ever-present garbage. It brings back the feeling of SELF-LOVE, CONFIDENCE, JOY and PEACE.

Cedarwood—was used traditionally by the North American Indians to enhance their potential for SPIRITUAL COMMUNICATION. It may help OPEN the PINE GLAND.

Pine—may help DILATE and OPEN the RESPIRATORY SYSTEM, particularly the BRONCHIAL TRACT. It may also help IMPROVE CIRCULATION THROUGHOUT the LUNGS. It helps soothe MENTAL STRESS, relieve ANXIETY, and REVITALIZE the entire body.

Spruce—GROUNDS the BODY, creating the BALANCE and the OPENING necessar to RECEIVE and to GIVE. It may help DILATE the BRONCHIAL TRACT t IMPROVE the OXYGEN EXCHANGE. It also helps one release EMOTION BLOCKS.

Fir—may help create a feeling of GROUNDING, ANCHORING and EMPOWERMENT.

BODY SYSTEM(S) AFFECTED: The oils in this blend may help it be effective for dealing w various problems related to EMOTIONAL BALANCE.

AROMATIC INFLUENCE: The aroma of this blend of oils may help GROUND and BALANCE the EMOTIONS.

APPLICATION: Best when worn on the back of the NECK and on the TEMPLES.

SAFETY DATA: Could possibly result in SKIN IRRITATION.

FREQUENCY: Emotional and Spiritual; approximately 140 MHz.

Harmony

This blend may help to establish SPIRITUAL and EMOTIONAL HARMONY within u We must be in HARMONY with ourselves, our creator, others, and the world around us before can truly feel and OVERCOME our NEGATIVE EMOTIONS. When we have HARMONY in our lives, many other things will come to balance and fruition. It may promote PHYSICAL and EMOTIONAL HEALING by bringing about a HARMONIC BALANCE to the CHAKRAS (ENERGY CENTERS) of the BODY, allowing us to RELAX and feel SAFE and SECURE. Balancing and unblocking the CHAKRAS may allow the energy to flow more efficiently through the body, helping to REDUCE STRESS and create a general overall FEELING of WELL BEIN

INGLE OILS CONTAINED IN THIS BLEND:

Hyssop—was used by Moses during the Lord's Passover in Egypt (Exodus 12). It may help stimulate MEDITATION and promote CENTERING.

Spruce—GROUNDS the BODY, creating the BALANCE and the OPENING necessary to RECEIVE and to GIVE. It also helps one release EMOTIONAL BLOCKS.

Lavender—is an oil that has traditionally been known to BALANCE the BODY and to work wherever there is a need. It may help promote CONSCIOUSNESS, HEALTH, LOVE, PEACE, and a general sense of WELL BEING.

Frankincense—contains sesquiterpenes, which may help OXYGENATE the PINEAL and PITUITARY GLANDS. As one of the ingredients for the holy incense, it was used anciently to help ENHANCE one's COMMUNICATION WITH THE CREATOR. It was considered a prize possession and was given to Christ at his birth. It may help PROMOTE a POSITIVE ATTITUDE.

Geranium—may help with HORMONAL BALANCE, LIVER and KIDNEY FUNCTIONS and the DISCHARGE of TOXINS from the LIVER that hold us back from having balance. Geranium OPENS the LIVER CHAKRA (Solar Plexus). Note: The liver is the place where fear and anger are stored.

Ylang Ylang—may help BALANCE the MALE-FEMALE ENERGIES so one can move closer towards being in spiritual attunement and allow them to focus their thoughts together, filtering out the ever-present garbage. It brings back the feeling of SELF-LOVE, CONFIDENCE, JOY and PEACE.

Orange—brings PEACE and HAPPINESS to the MIND and BODY and JOY to the HEART, which provide EMOTIONAL support to help one overcome depression.

Sandalwood—also, like frankincense, is high in sesquiterpenes, which were discovered to INCREASE the amount of OXYGEN around the PINEAL and PITUITARY GLANDS, thus helping to IMPROVE one's ATTITUDE. It ALLEVIATES DEPRESSION and assists in the removal of NEGATIVE PROGRAMMING from the cells of the body. It helps one ACCEPT OTHERS with an open heart while diminishing one's own egocentricity.

Angelica—may help one RELEASE and LET GO of NEGATIVE FEELINGS.

Sage Lavender—has been shown to increase both estradiol and testosterone levels. It may also help HARMONIZE and BALANCE the EMOTIONS and reduce STRESS-RELATED conditions .

Rose—has BEAUTIFUL FRAGRANCE and contains the highest frequency of the oils. It may help ENHANCE the FREQUENCY of every cell, which could help bring BALANCE and HARMONY to the body.

Rosewood—may help improve SKIN ELASTICITY. It is SOOTHING to the SKIN, APPEASING to the MIND, RELAXING to the BODY, and creates a feeling of PEACE and GENTLENESS.

Lemon—promotes HEALTH, HEALING, PHYSICAL ENERGY, and PURIFICATION. Its fragrance is INVIGORATING, ENHANCING, and WARMING.

Palmarosa—is valuable for all types of SKIN problems because it STIMULATES new CELL GROWTH, regulates oil production, MOISTURIZES and SPEEDS HEALING.

Bergamot—is SOOTHING to the ENDOCRINE SYSTEM and the HORMONES of the body. It may UPLIFT and CALM the EMOTIONS to help relieve ANXIETY, STRESS, and TENSION.

Roman Chamomile—neutralizes ALLERGIES and helps in SKIN REGENERATION. may also help reduce IRRITABILITY and minimize NERVOUSNESS in children, especially HYPERACTIVE CHILDREN.

Jasmine—is very UPLIFTING to the EMOTIONS; it may produce a feeling of CONFIDENCE, ENERGY, EUPHORIA, and OPTIMISM.

BODY SYSTEM(S) AFFECTED: The oils in this blend may help it be effective for dealing wit various problems related to EMOTIONAL BALANCE.

AROMATIC INFLUENCE: The fragrance of this blend of oils may help one establish and maintain a POSITIVE ATTITUDE, which is essential for PHYSICAL and EMOTIONA HEALING.

APPLICATION: Best when applied on EACH CHAKRA (or rub this blend between the hands i a circular, clockwise motion and place over the chakras), on the EARS, FEET, over the HEART, and over areas of poor CIRCULATION. One may want to start at the FEET and go up the ENERGY CENTERS and then over the CROWN. Application of this blen to each chakra or "energy center" will help open them and balance the electrical fields surrounding the body. Wear it as PERFUME or COLOGNE. If there is an ALLERGY or irritation to the smell of an oil, do the following:

1. Rub this blend between both hands in a circular, clockwise motion.
2. Put one hand over the NAVEL and the other hand over the THYMUS (above the heart). Hold for 20 SECONDS. CHANGE HANDS and REPEAT.

SAFETY DATA:* *Use with caution during PREGNANCY. Not for use by people with EPILEPSY. Use with caution if dealing with HIGH BLOOD PRESSURE. Avoid exposure to DIRECT SUNLIGHT for 3 to 6 hours after use.

FREQUENCY: Emotional; approximately 101 MHz.

Highest Potential

This blend contains the biblical oils of frankincense, galbanum, cedarwood, and sandalwood to help you tap into the divine power within yourself, EMPOWERING and ENABLING you to achieve your full potential. In addition, ylang ylang and lavender help to balance physical and emotional energies to help focus on the higher goal, while the emotionally uplifting scent of jasmine helps to promote confidence and energy to reach that goal. This unique blend of oils is UPLIFTING and INSPIRING while promoting feelings of STABILITY and PEACE.

BLENDS AND SINGLE OILS CONTAINED IN THIS BLEND:

AUSTRALIAN BLUE—is emotionally uplifting and helps to empower the physical and spiritual bodies. It helps to build COURAGE, CONFIDENCE, and SELF-ESTEEM while promoting CALMNESS, PEACE, and RELAXATION.

GATHERING—helps to keep one FOCUSED, GROUNDED, CONNECTED, and CLEAR, and may even help GATHER ones POTENTIAL for SELF-IMPROVEMENT.

Ylang Ylang—may help BALANCE the MALE-FEMALE ENERGIES so one can move closer towards being in spiritual attunement and allow them to focus their thoughts together, filtering out the ever-present garbage. It brings back the feeling of SELF-LOVE, CONFIDENCE, JOY and PEACE.

Jasmine—is very UPLIFTING to the EMOTIONS; it penetrates the deepest layers of the soul, opening doors to our emotions. It produces feelings of CONFIDENCE, ENERGY, and OPTIMISM.

BODY SYSTEM(S) AFFECTED: EMOTIONAL BALANCE.

AROMATIC INFLUENCE: When diffused or worn as perfume, this special blend of oils helps to BALANCE the emotions. It may help relieve ANXIETY, REVITALIZE the entire body, and EMPOWER both mind and soul.

APPLICATION: Rub over the HEART, and on FOREHEAD, and TEMPLES. DIFFUSE or wear as PERFUME or COLOGNE.

COMPANION OILS: Magnify Your Purpose, Live with Passion, Chivalry

Hope

The single oils in this blend have the ability to help SUPPORT THE BODY PHYSICALLY AND MENTALLY to give us HOPE. These oils when inhaled together may give us the feeling of GOING FORWARD with HOPE and ACHIEVEMENT. It reconnects us with a feeling of STRENGTH and GROUNDING. It may also help RELIEVE DEPRESSION and SUICIDAL THOUGHTS.

SINGLE OILS CONTAINED IN THIS BLEND:

Melissa—is an oil that is powerful as an ANTI-VIRAL agent, yet it is very gentle and very delicate because of the nature of the plant. It has the ability to work with and enhance the gentle aspects of the human body. It is CALMING and UPLIFTING and may help to BALANCE the EMOTIONS. It may also help to remove EMOTIONAL BLOCKS and INSTILL a POSITIVE OUTLOOK on LIFE.

Myrrh—is part of the formula the Lord gave Moses (Exodus 30:22-27). It is a TRUE GIFT. When we OPEN our HEARTS and MINDS to receive the gifts, they will be given.

Juniper—evokes feelings of HEALTH, LOVE, and PEACE and may help to ELEVATE one's SPIRITUAL AWARENESS.

Spruce—GROUNDS the BODY, creating the BALANCE and the OPENING necessary to RECEIVE and to GIVE. It may help DILATE the BRONCHIAL TRACT to IMPROVE the OXYGEN EXCHANGE. It also helps one release EMOTIONAL BLOCKS.

CARRIER OIL CONTAINED IN THIS BLEND: Almond Oil.

BODY SYSTEM(S) AFFECTED: The oils in this blend may help it be effective for dealing wit various problems related to EMOTIONAL BALANCE.

AROMATIC INFLUENCE: This blend of oils may be instrumental in giving one the feelings o PEACE, SECURITY, HOPE and ACHIEVEMENT.

APPLICATION: Apply on EARS (outer edge). It may also be placed on the CHEST, HEART, TEMPLES, SOLAR PLEXUS, across the NAPE of the NECK (in back), FEET, WRISTS, or ANY PLACE on the BODY. For SUICIDE THOUGHTS, use on EARS and WRISTS. Wear as PERFUME or COLOGNE.

FREQUENCY: Physical and Emotional; approximately 98 MHz.

COMMENTS: The first time this blend was used was for a lady in Arkansas for whom they could not find a diagnosis. She was dying from a mysterious disease. She was given Hop and her life was spared. At different times in our lives we may experience the feeling of hopelessness which can cause us to lose the vision of our goals and desires. Hope helps u reconnect with a feeling of strength and grounding, which may restore hope for tomorrow and help us go forward in life.

Humility

Having humility and forgiveness HELPS US HEAL OURSELVES AND OUR EARTH. It is an integral ingredient in having forgiveness and seeking a closer relationship with God. Through its frequency and fragrance, you may find that special place where your own healing may begin.

SINGLE OILS CONTAINED IN THIS BLEND:

Geranium—may help with HORMONAL BALANCE, LIVER and KIDNEY FUNCTIONS and the DISCHARGE of TOXINS from the LIVER that hold us back from having balance. Geranium OPENS the LIVER CHAKRA (Solar Plexus). It may help EASE NERVOUS TENSION and STRESS, BALANCE th EMOTIONS, LIFT the SPIRIT, and foster PEACE, WELL BEING, and HOPE.

Ylang Ylang—may help BALANCE the MALE-FEMALE ENERGIES so one can move closer towards being in spiritual attunement and allow them to focus their thought together, filtering out the ever-present garbage. It brings back the feeling of SELF-LOVE, CONFIDENCE, JOY and PEACE.

Frankincense—contains sesquiterpenes, which may help OXYGENATE the PINEAL and PITUITARY GLANDS. As one of the ingredients for the holy incense, it was used anciently to help ENHANCE one's COMMUNICATION WITH THE CREATOR. It was considered a prize possession and was given to Christ at his birth. It may help PROMOTE a POSITIVE ATTITUDE.

Spikenard—was highly prized in the Middle East during the time of Christ, and is referred to several times in the Bible. It is ANTIFUNGAL, ANTI-INFLAMMATORY, RELAXING, REGENERATIVE, and helpful for allergic skin reactions.

Myrrh—is part of the formula the Lord gave Moses (Exodus 30:22-27). It promotes SPIRITUAL AWARENESS and is a TRUE GIFT. When we OPEN our HEARTS and MINDS to receive the gifts, they will be given.

Rose—contains the highest frequency of the oils. It may help ENHANCE the FREQUENCY of every cell, which could help bring BALANCE and HARMONY to the body.

Rosewood—is SOOTHING to the SKIN, APPEASING to the MIND, RELAXING to the BODY, and creates a feeling of PEACE and GENTLENESS.

Melissa—is an oil that is powerful as an ANTI-VIRAL agent, yet it is very gentle and very delicate because of the nature of the plant. It has the ability to work with and enhance the gentle aspects of the human body. It is CALMING and UPLIFTING and may help to BALANCE the EMOTIONS. It may also help to remove EMOTIONAL BLOCKS and INSTILL a POSITIVE OUTLOOK on LIFE.

Neroli—has been regarded traditionally by the Egyptian people for its great attributes for HEALING the MIND, BODY and SPIRIT. It is CALMING and RELAXING to body and spirit. It may also help to STRENGTHEN and STABILIZE the emotions, and BRING RELIEF to seemingly hopeless situations. It encourages CONFIDENCE, COURAGE, JOY, PEACE, and SENSUALITY. It brings everything into the FOCUS of one and at the moment.

ARRIER OIL CONTAINED IN THIS BLEND: Sesame Seed Oil.

ODY SYSTEM(S) AFFECTED: The oils in this blend may help it be effective for dealing with various problems related to EMOTIONAL BALANCE.

ROMATIC INFLUENCE: This blend of oils may help one find that special, peaceful place where healing can begin.

PPLICATION: Rub over the HEART, on NECK, TEMPLES, etc.

OMPANION OILS: Acceptance, Envision, Forgiveness, Inner Child, Inspiration, Peace & Calming

REQUENCY: Physical and Emotional; approximately 88 MHz.

Oil Blends

Immupower

This is a powerful oil blend for BUILDING, STRENGTHENING and PROTECTING BODY and supporting its defense mechanism. This blend raises the frequency of the IMMUNE SYSTEM which helps one overcome the FLU, COLDS, RESPIRATORY PROBLEMS, INFECTIONS, etc. It should be worn and diffused in the home daily, especially during the seasons of cold and flu. It should be used to PROTECT the HOME ENVIRONMENT.

SINGLE OILS CONTAINED IN THIS BLEND:

Cistus—has ANTI-BACTERIAL, ANTI-INFECTIOUS, and ANTI-VIRAL properties. Because it is high in oxygenating molecules, it may assist the AUTO-IMMUNE SYSTEM; it may help strengthen the IMMUNE SYSTEM

Frankincense—contains sesquiterpenes, which may help OXYGENATE the PINEAL a PITUITARY GLANDS. As one of the ingredients for the holy incense, it was used anciently to help ENHANCE one's COMMUNICATION WITH THE CREATOR. It may help PROMOTE a POSITIVE ATTITUDE and has ANTI INFECTIOUS and ANTISEPTIC properties.

Hyssop—was used by Moses during the Lord's Passover in Egypt (Exodus 12). It has ANTI-INFLAMMATORY and ANTI-VIRAL properties. It may also have the ability to OPEN up the RESPIRATORY SYSTEM and DISCHARGE TOXIN and MUCUS.

Ravensara—is a powerful ANTI-VIRAL, ANTI-BACTERIAL, ANTI-FUNGAL, and ANTI-INFECTIOUS oil. It may help DILATE, OPEN, and STRENGTHEN t RESPIRATORY SYSTEM. As a cross between clove and nutmeg, it may also help support the ADRENAL GLANDS.

Mountain Savory—has IMMUNE-STIMULANT, ANTI-VIRAL, ANTI-FUNGAL, ANTI-INFECTIOUS, ANTIMICROBIAL, AND ANTI-PARASITIC propertie

Oregano—has ANTI-BACTERIAL, ANTI-FUNGAL, ANTISEPTIC, ANTI-VIRAL, and IMMUNE-STIMULANT properties. It strengthens one's feeling of SECURITY.

Clove—is ANTI-PARASITIC, ANTI-TUMORAL, ANTI-VIRAL and IMMUNE-STIMULANT.

Cumin—is an ANTISEPTIC and an IMMUNE-STIMULANT.

Idaho Tansy—is ANTI-VIRAL and may help support the IMMUNE SYSTEM.

BODY SYSTEM(S) AFFECTED: The oils in this blend may help it be effective for dealing w various problems related to the IMMUNE SYSTEM.

AROMATIC INFLUENCE: This blend of oils should be worn and diffused every other day (alternate with Thieves), especially during COLD and FLU season.

APPLICATION: To protect oneself from our chemical environment and during the cold and fl season, diffuse ImmuPower in the morning and again in the evening and apply Thieves t the feet. The next day, alternate with Thieves. Diffuse Thieves and apply ImmuPower to the THROAT, CHEST, SPINE, and FEET (best to DILUTE for topical application - see Safety Data below). Apply two to three drops on THYMUS in a clockwise motion. Stimulate by tapping the Thymus with energy fingers (pointer and middle). Also apply oil on JUGULAR VEINS in NECK and on ARM PITS. Use ImmuPower by Raindrop Technique up the spine for a FEVER, VIRUS, or to strengthen the IMMUNE SYSTEM.

***AFETY DATA:** Can be irritating to sensitive SKIN, best to DILUTE with V-6 Mixing Oil or Massage Oil Base for topical application. Use with caution during PREGNANCY. Use with caution if susceptible to EPILEPSY.*

OMPANION OILS: Thieves or Exodus II (good to alternate with ImmuPower). Single oils that may be added for extra strength include the following: Cistus, clove, frankincense, melissa, Mountain savory, oregano, rosewood.

OMPANION SUPPLEMENTS: ComforTone, Essentialzyme, Exodus, ImmuGel, ImmuneTune, Super C / Super C Chewable.

REQUENCY: Physical and Emotional; approximately 89 MHz.

Oil Blends

Inner Child

This blend has a fragrance that may STIMULATE MEMORY RESPONSE and help one ECONNECT WITH their inner-self or OWN IDENTITY, which is one of the first steps to ıding EMOTIONAL BALANCE. When children have been abused and misused, they become sconnected from their inner child, or identity, which causes confusion. This can contribute to ultiple personalties. These problems may not manifest themselves until early- to mid-adult years, ten labeled as mid-life crisis.

NGLE OILS CONTAINED IN THIS BLEND:

Orange—is UPLIFTING and CALMING. It brings PEACE and HAPPINESS to the MIND and BODY and JOY to the HEART, which provide EMOTIONAL support to help one overcome depression.

Tangerine—contains esters and aldehydes which are SEDATING and CALMING to the NERVOUS SYSTEM. It is also a DIURETIC and a DECONGESTANT of the LYMPHATIC SYSTEM.

Jasmine—is very UPLIFTING to the EMOTIONS; it may produce a feeling of CONFIDENCE, ENERGY, EUPHORIA, and OPTIMISM.

Ylang Ylang—may help BALANCE the MALE-FEMALE ENERGIES so one can move closer towards being in spiritual attunement and allow them to focus their thoughts together, filtering out the ever-present garbage. It brings back the feeling of SELF-LOVE, CONFIDENCE, JOY and PEACE.

Spruce—GROUNDS the BODY, creating the BALANCE and the OPENING necessary to RECEIVE and to GIVE. It also helps one release EMOTIONAL BLOCKS.

Sandalwood—also, like frankincense, is high in sesquiterpenes, which were discovered t INCREASE the amount of OXYGEN around the PINEAL and PITUITARY GLANDS, thus helping to IMPROVE one's ATTITUDE. It ALLEVIATES DEPRESSION and assists in the removal of NEGATIVE PROGRAMMING from the cells of the body. It helps one ACCEPT OTHERS with an open heart while diminishing one's own egocentricity.

Lemongrass—is a VASODILATOR, ANTISEPTIC, ANTI-BACTERIAL, ANTI-INFLAMMATORY, and SEDATIVE. It may help improve CIRCULATION, wake up the LYMPHATIC SYSTEM, and increase the flow of OXYGEN. It may also help to LIFT the SPIRIT.

Neroli—has been regarded traditionally by the Egyptian people for its great attributes fo HEALING the MIND, BODY and SPIRIT. It is CALMING and RELAXING body and spirit. It may also help to STRENGTHEN and STABILIZE the emotions, and BRING RELIEF to seemingly hopeless situations. It encourages CONFIDENCE, COURAGE, JOY, PEACE, and SENSUALITY. It brings everything into FOCUS and into the moment.

BODY SYSTEM(S) AFFECTED: The oils in this blend may help it be effective for dealing w various problems related to EMOTIONAL BALANCE.

AROMATIC INFLUENCE: The oils in this blend are very CALMING to the NERVES and EMOTIONS when diffused.

APPLICATION: Apply around NAVEL, on CHEST, TEMPLES, and NOSE.

SAFETY DATA: Avoid exposure to direct SUNLIGHT for up to 12 hours after use. Could possibly result in SKIN IRRITATION.

COMPANION OILS: Acceptance, Awaken, Citrus Fresh, Envision, Forgiveness, Gentle Baby, Surrender

FREQUENCY: Physical and Emotional; approximately 98 MHz.

Inspiration

This blend includes oils that have been combined to help ENHANCE those desirous in COMMUNICATING WITH and getting closer to the CREATOR and enjoying the spiritual aspects of life. It RELIEVES NEGATIVE THOUGHTS and ENHANCES SPIRITUAL AWARENESS. It creates a space for PRAYER and INNER AWARENESS during meditation and prayer.

SINGLE OILS CONTAINED IN THIS BLEND:

Cedarwood—was used traditionally by the North American Indians to enhance their potential for SPIRITUAL COMMUNICATION. It may help OPEN the PINEA GLAND.

Spruce—GROUNDS the BODY, creating the BALANCE and the OPENING necessary to RECEIVE and to GIVE. It also helps one release EMOTIONAL BLOCKS. It was used by the Lakota Indians to enhance their communication with the Great Spirit. It may also OPEN the PINEAL GLAND.

Rosewood—is SOOTHING to the SKIN, APPEASING to the MIND, RELAXING to the BODY, and creates a feeling of PEACE and GENTLENESS.

Sandalwood—also, like frankincense, is high in sesquiterpenes, which were discovered to INCREASE the amount of OXYGEN around the PINEAL and PITUITARY GLANDS, thus helping to IMPROVE one's ATTITUDE. It ALLEVIATES DEPRESSION and assists in the removal of NEGATIVE PROGRAMMING from the cells of the body. It helps one ACCEPT OTHERS with an open heart while diminishing one's own egocentricity.

Frankincense—contains sesquiterpenes, which may help OXYGENATE the PINEAL and PITUITARY GLANDS. As one of the ingredients for the holy incense, it was used anciently to help ENHANCE one's COMMUNICATION WITH THE CREATOR.

Myrtle—is a DECONGESTANT of the RESPIRATORY SYSTEM. It is EUPHORIC, ELEVATING, and may help to soother ANGER.

Mugwort (*Artemisia vulgaris*)—was seen as a protective charm against danger and evil and anciently believed to increase psychic powers.

ODY SYSTEM(S) AFFECTED: The oils in this blend may help it be effective for dealing with various problems related to EMOTIONAL BALANCE.

ROMATIC INFLUENCE: When diffused, this blend of oils is wonderful for creating a spiritual environment in the home during times of PRAYER, MEDITATION, or when seeking INSPIRATION and direction. Put on cotton ball near vent in the car.

PPLICATION: Apply to HORNS (right and left sides of FOREHEAD), CROWN, SHOULDERS, along SPINE, and on back of NECK.

OMPANION OILS: Acceptance, Forgiveness, Humility, Surrender, 3 Wise Men

REQUENCY: High (Spiritual); approximately 141 MHz.

Into the Future

This blend may help one leave the past behind in order to go forward with vision and xcitement. The single oils contained in this blend are all invigorating and uplifting. So many imes we find ourselves settling for mediocrity and sacrificing one's own potential and success ecause of the fear of the unknown and what the future may or may not hold. This blend was ormulated to SUPPORT the EMOTIONS IN helping us create the feeling of MOVING ORWARD and not being afraid to let determination and that pioneering spirit come through. iving on the edge with tenacity and integrity brings the excitement of the challenge and the joy of uccess.

Oil Blends

SINGLE OILS CONTAINED IN THIS BLEND:

Frankincense—contains sesquiterpenes, which may help OXYGENATE the PINEAL ar PITUITARY GLANDS. As one of the ingredients for the holy incense, it was used anciently to ENHANCE COMMUNICATION with the CREATOR.

Jasmine—is very UPLIFTING to the EMOTIONS; it may produce a feeling of CONFIDENCE, ENERGY, EUPHORIA, and OPTIMISM.

Clary Sage—may be beneficial for REGULATING CELLS and BALANCING the HORMONES. It may calm and enhance the DREAM STATE, helping to bring about a feeling of EUPHORIA.

Juniper—may help to IMPROVE CIRCULATION through the KIDNEYS. It has ANTISEPTIC, ANTISPASMODIC, ASTRINGENT, CLEANSING, DETOXIFYING, DIURETIC, STIMULANT, and TONIC properties.

Idaho Tansy—is ANTI-VIRAL and may help support the IMMUNE SYSTEM.

Fir—may help create a feeling of GROUNDING, ANCHORING and EMPOWERMENT.

Ylang Ylang—may help BALANCE the MALE-FEMALE ENERGIES so one can move closer towards being in spiritual attunement and allow them to focus their though together, filtering out the ever-present garbage. It brings back the feeling of SELF-LOVE, CONFIDENCE, JOY and PEACE.

May also contain orange, cedarwood, and White lotus.

CARRIER OIL CONTAINED IN THIS BLEND: Almond Oil.

BODY SYSTEM(S) AFFECTED: The oils in this blend may help it be effective for dealing wi various problems related to EMOTIONAL BALANCE.

AROMATIC INFLUENCE: Diffusing this blend of oils may helps LIFT the SPIRIT and STABILIZE the EMOTIONS making it easier for one to recognize their own potential.

APPLICATION: DIFFUSE, put in BATH water, over the HEART, on WRISTS, NECK, as a COMPRESS, and dilute with V-6 Mixing Oil for full BODY MASSAGE.

COMPANION OILS: Awaken, Clarity, Dream Catcher, Envision, Inspiration, Magnify Your Purpose, Live with Passion

FREQUENCY: Physical and Emotional; approximately 88 MHz.

Joy

This blend is a beautiful complimentary blend of oils. When inhaled, it brings back MEMORIES of BEING LOVED, BEING HELD, SHARING LOVING TIMES, feeling and opening those blocks in our lives where perhaps we have shut down to love or receiving love or love of self. When there is grief, the adenoids and the adrenal glands shut down; JOY opens these glands.

NGLE OILS CONTAINED IN THIS BLEND:

Lemon—promotes HEALTH, HEALING, PHYSICAL ENERGY, and PURIFICATION. Its fragrance is INVIGORATING, ENHANCING, and WARMING.

Mandarin—is APPEASING, GENTLE, and promotes HAPPINESS. It is also REFRESHING, UPLIFTING, and REVITALIZING. Because of its sedative and slightly hypnotic properties, it is very good for STRESS and IRRITABILITY.

Bergamot—is SOOTHING to the ENDOCRINE SYSTEM and the HORMONES of the body. It may UPLIFT and CALM the EMOTIONS to help relieve ANXIETY, STRESS, and TENSION.

Ylang Ylang—may help BALANCE the MALE-FEMALE ENERGIES so one can move closer towards being in spiritual attunement and allow them to focus their thoughts together, filtering out the ever-present garbage. It brings back the feeling of SELF-LOVE, CONFIDENCE, JOY and PEACE.

Rose—contains the highest frequency of the oils. It may help ENHANCE the FREQUENCY of every cell, which could help bring BALANCE and HARMONY to the body. It is thought by some to produce a magnetic energy that attracts LOVE and enhances the frequency of SELF-LOVE, bringing JOY to the heart.

Rosewood—may help improve SKIN ELASTICITY. It is SOOTHING to the SKIN, APPEASING to the MIND, RELAXING to the BODY, and creates a feeling of PEACE and GENTLENESS.

Geranium—may help with HORMONAL BALANCE, LIVER and KIDNEY FUNCTIONS and the DISCHARGE of TOXINS from the LIVER that hold us back from having balance. Geranium OPENS the LIVER CHAKRA (Solar Plexus). It may help EASE NERVOUS TENSION and STRESS, BALANCE the EMOTIONS, LIFT the SPIRIT, and foster PEACE, WELL BEING, and HOPE.

Palmarosa—is valuable for all types of SKIN problems because it STIMULATES new CELL GROWTH, regulates oil production, MOISTURIZES and SPEEDS HEALING.

Roman Chamomile—neutralizes ALLERGIES and helps in SKIN REGENERATION. It may also help reduce IRRITABILITY and minimize NERVOUSNESS in children, especially HYPERACTIVE CHILDREN.

Jasmine—is very UPLIFTING to the EMOTIONS; it may produce a feeling of CONFIDENCE, ENERGY, EUPHORIA, and OPTIMISM.

ODY SYSTEM(S) AFFECTED: The oils in this blend may help it be effective for dealing with various problems related to EMOTIONAL BALANCE.

ROMATIC INFLUENCE: The fragrance of this blend of oils promotes the feelings of LOVE, SELF-LOVE, and CONFIDENCE. Emotional blockages to love may produce a dislike to the fragrance of this blend (see *HARMONY; APPLICATION* for method of correcting fragrance dislikes). Remember, the ENERGY of LOVE is the true source of all healing!

PPLICATION: Rub over HEART, EARS, NECK, THYMUS, HEART CHAKRAS, TEMPLES, ACROSS BROW, and WRISTS. Apply on HEART VITA FLEX POINT.

Oil Blends

Put four drops in KidScents Lotion for an aftershave. Put in BATH water. Use as COMPRESS; dilute with V-6 Mixing Oil for a full BODY MASSAGE. Place on AREA of POOR CIRCULATION. Wear as PERFUME or COLOGNE especially over the hea Put two drops on a wet cloth and put in the dryer for GREAT SMELLING CLOTHES.

SAFETY DATA: Avoid exposure to direct SUNLIGHT for up to 12 hours after use.

COMPANION OILS: Hope, Magnify Your Purpose, Motivation, Live with Passion, Valor

FREQUENCY: High (Spiritual); approximately 188 MHz.

Juva Cleanse

In today's chemically polluted environment, there is a desperate need for natural, effecti products that CLEANSE and DETOXIFY the LIVER. This blend was created with three of the most powerful and effective liver cleansing oils.

SINGLE OILS CONTAINED IN THIS BLEND:

Helichrysum—may help CLEANSE the BLOOD and improve CIRCULATORY FUNCTIONS. It is ANTI-CATARRHAL in structure and nature. In the last f years, research has documented its ANTIOXIDANT and LIVER PROTECTIV properties.

Celery Seed—is ANTI-OXIDATIVE and ANTISEPTIC to the URINARY TRACT. It helps DECONGEST the LIVER by stimulating drainage. It has also been show to aid LYMPHATIC DRAINAGE and may help BALANCE the ENDOCRINE SYSTEM.

Ledum—has a long history of use as a tea by the natives of North America where it was used to fight CANCER, SCURVY, and URINARY PROBLEMS. It may be a wonderful support to the URINARY TRACT and a powerful LIVER support a detoxifier.

BODY SYSTEM(S) AFFECTED: DIGESTIVE SYSTEM.

APPLICATION: Apply to VITA FLEX points on FEET and especially over the LIVER.

SAFETY DATA: Can be irritating to sensitive SKIN (test first for sensitivity).

JuvaFlex

This blend contains oils that have been recognized medically and traditionally for aiding the body in CLEANSING the LIVER and BUILDING a STRONGER SYSTEM. It may help DETOXIFY the LYMPHATIC SYSTEM and provide DIGESTIVE SUPPORT. Anger and hat are stored in the liver, which creates extreme toxicity. Liver cancer is caused by solidified hate.

ıvaFlex supports GETTING OFF ADDICTIONS. The helichrysum contained in JuvaFlex is for ıelating and may possess the ability to cut through ANGER BARRIERS.

INGLE OILS CONTAINED IN THIS BLEND:

Fennel—may help SUPPORT the DIGESTIVE FUNCTION by SUPPORTING the LIVER. It is an ANTISEPTIC and a TONIC for the LIVER. It may break up FLUIDS and TOXINS and help CLEANSE the TISSUES in the body. It may also help BALANCE the HORMONES.

Geranium—may help with HORMONAL BALANCE, LIVER and KIDNEY FUNCTIONS and the DISCHARGE of TOXINS from the LIVER that hold us back from having balance. Geranium OPENS the LIVER CHAKRA (Solar Plexus). It may help DILATE the BILIARY DUCTS for LIVER DETOXIFICATION.

Rosemary cineol—may help BALANCE HEART FUNCTION, ENERGIZE the SOLAR PLEXUS, and REDUCE MENTAL FATIGUE. It is an ANTISEPTIC and may help decongest the LIVER.

Roman Chamomile—NEUTRALIZES ALLERGIES and increases the ability of the SKIN to REGENERATE. It may help the LIVER to REJECT and DISCHARGE POISONS. This oil is SOOTHING, RELAXING, CALMING, and may help REMOVE FEARS.

Blue Tansy—may help CLEANSE the LIVER and CALM the LYMPHATIC SYSTEM.

Helichrysum—may help CLEANSE the BLOOD and improve CIRCULATORY FUNCTIONS. It is ANTI-CATARRHAL in structure and nature. On a spiritual level, it may help one LET GO OF ANGRY FEELINGS that prevent one from forgiving and moving forward in life.

ARRIER OIL CONTAINED IN THIS BLEND: Sesame Seed Oil.

ODY SYSTEM(S) AFFECTED: The oils in this blend may help it be effective for dealing with various problems related to the DIGESTIVE SYSTEM and to EMOTIONAL BALANCE.

PPLICATION: Apply to VITA FLEX points on FEET, SPINE (using the Raindrop Technique), and especially over the LIVER. Also over the ENTIRE BODY (dilute with V-6 Mixing Oil).

AFETY DATA: Can be irritating to sensitive SKIN.

OMPANION OILS: Enhance results by using this blend with Di-Tone.

OMPANION SUPPLEMENTS: Use JuvaTone and ComforTone together with this blend for maximum results. Best taken an hour apart. Also Essentialzyme to help digest expelled toxins.

REQUENCY: Physical; approximately 82 MHz.

Lady Sclareol

This blend was formulated to have a SEDUCTIVE and ALLURING scent with oils that are beneficial for the SKIN as well.

SINGLE OILS CONTAINED IN THIS BLEND:

Rosewood—is SOOTHING to the SKIN, APPEASING to the MIND, RELAXING to t BODY, and creates a feeling of PEACE and GENTLENESS.

Vetiver—is ANTISPASMODIC and locally WARMING. Vetiver has also been valuab for relieving STRESS and helping people recover from EMOTIONAL TRAUMAS and SHOCK. According to Susanne Fischer-Rizzi, "Sexual energie become more peaceful and grounded."

Geranium—may help with HORMONAL BALANCE, LIVER and KIDNEY FUNCTIONS and the DISCHARGE of TOXINS from the LIVER.

Orange—is rich in compounds noted for their STRESS-REDUCING effects. It brings PEACE and HAPPINESS to the MIND and BODY and JOY to the HEART.

Clary Sage—is beneficial for REGULATING CELLS and BALANCING the HORMONES. It may help with MENSTRUAL CRAMPS, PMS, and PRE-MENOPAUSE symptoms. It may also help with CIRCULATORY PROBLEM

Ylang Ylang—may help BALANCE the MALE-FEMALE ENERGIES so one can mov closer towards being in spiritual attunement and allow them to focus their though together, filtering out the ever-present garbage. It brings back the feeling of SELF-LOVE, CONFIDENCE, JOY and PEACE.

Sandalwood—helps to ALLEVIATE DEPRESSION and assists in the removal of NEGATIVE PROGRAMMING from the cells of the body. It helps one ACCEP OTHERS with an open heart while diminishing one's own egocentricity.

Sage Lavender—has been shown to increase both estradiol and testosterone levels. It may also help HARMONIZE and BALANCE the EMOTIONS and reduce STRESS-RELATED conditions .

Jasmine—is very UPLIFTING to the EMOTIONS; it penetrates the deepest layers of the soul, opening doors to our emotions. It produces feelings of CONFIDENCE, ENERGY, and OPTIMISM.

Idaho Tansy—is ANTI-VIRAL and may help support the IMMUNE SYSTEM. Its aroma is UPLIFTING and promotes a general sense of WELL-BEING.

BODY SYSTEM(S) AFFECTED: EMOTIONAL BALANCE, SKIN.

AROMATIC INFLUENCE: Because the aroma of this blend of oils is so SEDUCTIVE and AROUSING, it promotes feelings of EXCITEMENT and ROMANCE.

APPLICATION: Apply on LOCATION (most effective when applied by the male partner), use for MASSAGE, and add to your Bath and Shower Gel Base. May also be used with a COMPRESS over the abdomen. DIFFUSE or wear as a PERFUME.

Legacy
(The Master Blend)

This is an incredible, comprehensive blend of 90 essential oils. Its exquisite aroma fine-tunes and energies the entire body.

SINGLE OILS CONTAINED IN THIS BLEND: (*Botanical names are found under each individual oil in the Single Oils section*)

Angelica
Balsam Fir
Basil
Bergamot
Black Pepper
Blue Tansy
Buplevere *(Bupleurum fruticosum)*
Cajeput
Cardamom
Carrot Seed
Canadian Red Cedar
Cedar Leaf
Cedarwood
Cinnamon Bark
Cistus
Citronella
Clary Sage
Clove
Coriander
Cumin
Cypress
Dill
Douglas Fir
Elemi
Eucalyptus citriodora
Eucalyptus dives
Eucalyptus globulus
Eucalyptus polybractea
Eucalyptus radiata
Fennel
Fleabane
Frankincense
Galbanum
Geranium
German Chamomile
Ginger
Goldenrod
Grapefruit
Helichrysum
Hyssop
Idaho Balsam Fir
Idaho Tansy
Jasmine
Juniper
Laurel
Lavender
Ledum
Lemon
Lemongrass
Lime
Mandarin
Marjoram
Melaleuca alternifolia
Melaleuca ericifolia
Melissa
Mountain Savory
Myrrh
Myrtle
Neroli
Nutmeg
Orange
Oregano
Palmarosa
Patchouli
Peppermint
Petitgrain
Pine
Ravensara
Red Fir (*Abies magnifica*)
Roman Chamomile
Rose
Rosehip (*Rosa canina*)
Rosemary cineol
Rosewood
Sage
Sandalwood
Spearmint
Spikenard
Spruce
Tangerine
Tarragon
Thyme linalol
Tsuga
Valerian
Vetiver
White Fir
Wintergreen
Yarrow
Yellow Pine (*Pinus ponderosa*)
Ylang Ylang

BODY SYSTEM(S) AFFECTED: The oils in this blend may help it be effective for dealing with various problems related to EMOTIONAL BALANCE.

AROMATIC INFLUENCE: Because of all the oils contained in this blend, it is EMPOWERING and ENERGIZING, not just for the emotions, but for the entire body.

APPLICATION: Apply to VITA FLEX points on FEET and/or directly on area of concern. This blend may also be DIFFUSED.

SAFETY DATA:* *Because of the diversity of the oils that exist in this blend, it should be used with caution by those individuals who are susceptible to EPILEPTIC SEIZURES or who are PREGNANT. Repeated use could possibly result in CONTACT SENSITIZATION or SKIN IRRITATION. For TOPICAL use only.

COMPANION OILS: Every single oil.

Live with Passion

The oils in this blend are all EMOTIONALLY BALANCING and UPLIFTING, helping to enhance our PASSION for life. By STRENGTHENING and STABILIZING the emotions, not only may this blend help BRING RELIEF to seemingly hopeless situations, but it may also help to instill a POSITIVE ATTITUDE that can bring back the passion in our lives to help PROPEL us toward ACCOMPLISHING OUR GOALS.

SINGLE OILS CONTAINED IN THIS BLEND:

Melissa—is an oil that is powerful as an ANTI-VIRAL agent, yet it is very gentle and very delicate because of the nature of the plant. It has the ability to work with and enhance the gentle aspects of the human body. It is CALMING and UPLIFTING and may help to BALANCE the EMOTIONS. It may also help to remove EMOTIONAL BLOCKS and INSTILL a POSITIVE OUTLOOK on LIFE.

Helichrysum—may help CLEANSE the BLOOD and improve CIRCULATORY FUNCTIONS. It is ANTI-CATARRHAL in structure and nature. As a powerful ANTI-INFLAMMATORY, it may even help reduce inflammation in the meninges of the brain. On a spiritual level, it may help one LET GO OF ANGRY FEELINGS that prevent one from forgiving and moving forward.

Clary Sage—is beneficial for REGULATING CELLS and BALANCING the HORMONES. It may help with MENSTRUAL CRAMPS, PMS, and PRE-MENOPAUSE symptoms. It may also help with CIRCULATORY PROBLEMS.

Cedarwood—was used traditionally by the North American Indians to enhance their potential for SPIRITUAL COMMUNICATION. It may help OPEN the PINEAL GLAND.

Angelica—is referred to by the German people as the "oil of angels". It may help one RELEASE and LET GO of NEGATIVE FEELINGS.

Ginger—is WARMING, UPLIFTING, and EMPOWERING. Emotionally, it may help influence PHYSICAL ENERGY, LOVE, and COURAGE. Because of its calming influence on the digestive system, it may help reduce feelings of NAUSEA, and MOTION SICKNESS.

Neroli—has been regarded traditionally by the Egyptian people for its great attributes for HEALING the MIND, BODY and SPIRIT. It is CALMING and RELAXING to body and spirit. It may also help to STRENGTHEN and STABILIZE the emotions, and BRING RELIEF to seemingly hopeless situations. It encourages CONFIDENCE, COURAGE, JOY, PEACE, and SENSUALITY. It brings everything into the FOCUS of one and at the moment.

Sandalwood—also, like frankincense, is high in sesquiterpenes, which were discovered to INCREASE the amount of OXYGEN around the PINEAL and PITUITARY GLANDS, thus helping to IMPROVE one's ATTITUDE. It ALLEVIATES DEPRESSION and assists in the removal of NEGATIVE PROGRAMMING from the cells of the body.

Patchouli—is SEDATING, CALMING, and RELAXING allowing it to reduce ANXIETY.

Jasmine—is very UPLIFTING to the EMOTIONS; it may produce a feeling of CONFIDENCE, ENERGY, EUPHORIA, and OPTIMISM.

)DY SYSTEM(S) AFFECTED: The oils in this blend may help it be effective for dealing with various problems related to the NERVOUS SYSTEM and to EMOTIONAL BALANCE.

ROMATIC INFLUENCE: This blend is UPLIFTING, EMPOWERING, and STABILIZING to the emotions. It may help to improve one's ATTITUDE by encouraging CONFIDENCE and COURAGE.

PPLICATION: Apply on the WRISTS, TEMPLES, CHEST AREA, and FOREHEAD. Add two to four drops in BATH water. May also be worn as PERFUME or COLOGNE.

OMPANION OILS: Acceptance, Clarity, Gathering, Harmony, Inspiration, Magnify Your Purpose, Motivation, 3 Wise Men

REQUENCY: Physical and Emotional; approximately 89 MHz.

Longevity

This blend contains oils that have powerful antioxidant properties. As measured on the RAC (oxygen radical absorbent capacity) scale, this blend has scored near 150,000! When taken a dietary supplement, it may help to promote longevity and prevent premature aging. For easier pplement use, refer to Longevity Capsules in the Supplements section of this book.

NGLE OILS CONTAINED IN THIS BLEND:

Thyme CT Thymol—has been shown in studies to DRAMATICALLY BOOST GLUTATHIONE LEVELS in the heart, liver, and brain. Because it can also help to PREVENT the OXIDATION of FATS in the body, it may help to slow the aging process. It is also ANTI-FUNGAL and ANTI-VIRAL.

Orange—is rich in compounds noted for their STRESS-REDUCING effects; lipid-solub traits; ANTIOXIDANT properties which ENHANCE VITAMIN ABSORPTIO

Clove—has one of the highest ORAC (oxygen radical absorbent capacity) scores. It is ANTI-BACTERIAL, ANTI-FUNGAL, ANTI-INFECTIOUS, ANTI-PARASITIC, a strong ANTISEPTIC, ANTI-VIRAL, and an IMMUNE STIMULANT; helps preserve integrity of fatty acids. Clove may also influence HEALING and help improve MEMORY.

Frankincense—has powerful ANTI-TUMORAL and ANTI-INFLAMMATORY properties. It has been used in several clinical applications for fighting cancer. Frankincense also contains sesquiterpenes, which may help OXYGENATE the PINEAL and PITUITARY GLANDS.

BODY SYSTEM(S) AFFECTED: The oils in this blend may help it be effective for dealing w various problems related to the CARDIOVASCULAR SYSTEM.

APPLICATION: Can be taken as a dietary supplement by diluting one drop in 4 oz. of liquid (i soy/rice milk); Diffuse. This blend of oils has been put into gel capsules for easier consumption as a dietary supplement (refer to Longevity Capsules in the Supplements section of this book).

SAFETY DATA: Repeated use can possibly result in CONTACT SENSITIZATION. Can b irritating to sensitive SKIN. Avoid eye contact. Avoid exposure to direct SUNLIGH for 3 to 6 hours after use.

M-Grain

This blend contains single oils that have traditionally been proven to help RELIEVE MIGRAINE and STRESS HEADACHES. This blend may also help with NAUSEA and DEPRESSION.

SINGLE OILS CONTAINED IN THIS BLEND:

Basil—has ANTIDEPRESSANT, ANTI-INFLAMMATORY, and ANTISPASMODIC properties. It is relaxing to SPASTIC MUSCLES, including those that contribu to HEADACHES and MIGRAINES.

Marjoram—is RELAXING, CALMING, and APPEASING to the MUSCLES that constrict and sometimes contribute to HEADACHES.

Lavender—is an oil that has traditionally been known to BALANCE the BODY and to work wherever there is a need. It has ANTISPASMODIC and ANALGESIC properties. It may help with SPRAINS, SORE MUSCLES, HEADACHES, an general HEALING.

Peppermint—is ANTI-INFLAMMATORY to the NERVES. It has a SOOTHING and COOLING EFFECT on HEADACHES. It is PURIFYING and STIMULATING to the CONSCIOUS MIND.

Roman Chamomile—is ANTI-INFLAMMATORY and ANTISPASMODIC. It is CALMING and RELAXING and helps to relieve MUSCLE TENSION and STRESS that can lead to migraine headaches.

Helichrysum—may help CLEANSE the BLOOD and improve CIRCULATORY FUNCTIONS. It is ANTI-CATARRHAL in structure and nature. As a powerful ANTI-INFLAMMATORY, it may even help reduce inflammation in the meninges of the brain. On a spiritual level, it may help one LET GO OF ANGRY FEELINGS that prevent one from forgiving and moving forward.

ODY SYSTEM(S) AFFECTED: The oils in this blend may help it be effective for dealing with various problems related to the NERVOUS SYSTEM and to MUSCLES and BONES.

ROMATIC INFLUENCE: It is very effective for clearing HEADACHES when inhaled.

PPLICATION: It is most effective when INHALED; for MIGRAINES, place two drops in PALMS of HANDS then cup over nose and INHALE. MASSAGE along the BRAIN STEM or through the THUMBS. Have someone cross their hands and rub your thumbs using their middle finger to push toward your hand. Also put on FOREHEAD, CROWN, SHOULDERS, BACK of NECK, TEMPLES, and VITA FLEX points on the FEET.

OMPANION OILS: Aroma Siez, Clarity, PanAway.

REQUENCY: Physical; approximately 72 MHz.

Oil Blends

Magnify Your Purpose

The emotionally uplifting properties of the single oils in this blend make it excellent for elping us to OVERCOME NEGATIVE EMOTIONS and such self-defeating behaviors as rocrastination and self-pity. By helping us to deal with belittling feelings like abandonment, ejection, and betrayal, we are able to more fully understand and MAGNIFY our life's purpose.

INGLE OILS CONTAINED IN THIS BLEND:

Sandalwood—also, like frankincense, is high in sesquiterpenes, which were discovered to INCREASE the amount of OXYGEN around the PINEAL and PITUITARY GLANDS, thus helping to IMPROVE one's ATTITUDE. It ALLEVIATES DEPRESSION and assists in the removal of NEGATIVE PROGRAMMING from the cells of the body. It helps one ACCEPT OTHERS with an open heart while diminishing one's own egocentricity.

Nutmeg—has adrenal cortex-like activity, which helps support the ADRENAL GLANDS for INCREASED ENERGY.

Rosewood—is SOOTHING to the SKIN, APPEASING to the MIND, RELAXING to t BODY, and creates a feeling of PEACE and GENTLENESS.

Cinnamon Bark—is part of the formula the Lord gave Moses (Exodus 30:22-27). It ha very specific purposes: (1) it is a POWERFUL PURIFIER, (2) it is a powerful OXYGENATOR, and (3) it ENHANCES the action and the activity of OTHER OILS. It may have a STIMULATING and TONING effect on the whole body and particularly the circulatory system. It is ANTISEPTIC, ANTI-BACTERIA and ANTI-VIRAL.

Ginger—is WARMING, UPLIFTING, and EMPOWERING. Emotionally, it may help influence PHYSICAL ENERGY, LOVE, and COURAGE. Because of its calming influence on the digestive system, it may help reduce feelings of NAUSEA, and MOTION SICKNESS.

Sage—may help improve ESTROGEN and PROGESTERONE-TESTOSTERONE BALANCE. It is believed to contain elements that contribute to the SECRETIO of PROGESTERONE-TESTOSTERONE.

BODY SYSTEM(S) AFFECTED: The oils in this blend may help it be effective for dealing wi various problems related to the NERVOUS SYSTEM and to EMOTIONAL BALANCE

AROMATIC INFLUENCE: Because of the oils contained in this blend, it is EMPOWERING and UPLIFTING, helping us to rise above our negative emotions.

APPLICATION: Apply to VITA FLEX points on FEET and/or directly on area of concern. This blend may also be DIFFUSED, applied to the WRISTS or TEMPLES, or added to warm BATH water (best when first combined with a bath gel base). For an uplifting massage, dilute first with a pure carrier oil.

SAFETY DATA:* *Because of the existing contra-indications for nutmeg, cinnamon bark, and sage, this blend should be used with caution by those individuals who are susceptible to EPILEPTIC SEIZURES or who are PREGNANT. Repeated use could possibly result in CONTACT SENSITIZATION or SKIN IRRITATION.

COMPANION OILS: Clarity, Harmony, Gathering, Into the Future, Live with Passion, Sensation

FREQUENCY: Physical and Emotional; approximately 99 MHz.

Melrose

The strong antiseptic properties of the single oils in this blend make it excellent for cleansing and healing CUTS, BRUISES, SCRAPES, INSECT BITES; but primarily, for helping with TISSUE REGENERATION from damage or injury. It also helps with SKIN ABRASIONS BURNS, RASHES, EARACHES, GUMS, COLD SORES, CANKER SORES, and CANDIDA. It fights INFECTION and kills ANAEROBIC BACTERIA and FUNGUS. It has been used to help horses (and other animals) with skin cuts. ***Avoid use on cats.***

SINGLE OILS CONTAINED IN THIS BLEND:

Melaleuca—has ANTI-BACTERIAL, ANTI-FUNGAL, ANTI-INFECTIOUS, ANTI-VIRAL, STRONG ANTISEPTIC, and TISSUE REGENERATING properties.

Melaleuca quinquenervia—is a very strong, very powerful ANTI-FUNGAL, ANTI-VIRAL and ANTI-BACTERIAL oil. It may help PROTECT against RADIATION and is a STRONG TISSUE REGENERATOR.

Rosemary cineol—may help BALANCE HEART FUNCTION, ENERGIZE the SOLAR PLEXUS, and REDUCE MENTAL FATIGUE. It has ANALGESIC, ANTISEPTIC, and ANTI-INFECTIOUS properties.

Clove—is ANTI-BACTERIAL, ANTI-INFECTIOUS, ANTI-INFLAMMATORY, a STRONG ANTISEPTIC, DISINFECTANT, IMMUNE-STIMULANT, and TOPICAL ANESTHETIC.

Oil Blends

BODY SYSTEM(S) AFFECTED: The oils in this blend may help it be effective for dealing with various problems related to the RESPIRATORY SYSTEM and to the SKIN.

AROMATIC INFLUENCE: Dispels ODORS.

APPLICATION: Rub across BROW, THUMB VITA FLEX points, and LIVER. Apply topically on CUTS, SCRAPES, BURNS, RASHES, or ANY INFECTION. Put one to two drops on a piece of cotton and place in the EAR for earaches.

SAFETY DATA: Repeated use can possibly result in CONTACT SENSITIZATION. Can be irritating to sensitive SKIN.

COMPANION OILS: *Melaleuca ericifolia.*

COMPANION PRODUCTS: Rose Ointment (delays evaporation of oil and promotes healing)

FREQUENCY: Very Low (Physical); approximately 48 MHz.

Mister

This blend was initially formulated to help BALANCE MALE ENERGY and help REGULATE PROSTATE FUNCTION. However, it has also been used successfully in eliminating HOT FLASHES FOR WOMEN. Generally, **MISTER** is good for WOMEN AGE 30-45, while ENDOFLEX is for WOMEN AGE 45+ and DRAGON TIME is for WOMEN up to AGE 30.

SINGLE OILS CONTAINED IN THIS BLEND:

Sage—may help improve ESTROGEN and PROGESTERONE-TESTOSTERONE BALANCE. It is believed to contain elements that contribute to the SECRETION of PROGESTERONE-TESTOSTERONE.

Fennel—may help SUPPORT the DIGESTIVE FUNCTION by SUPPORTING the LIVER. It may also help BALANCE the HORMONES.

Lavender—is an oil that has traditionally been known to BALANCE the BODY and to work wherever there is a need. It is ANTI-INFLAMMATORY and may help reduce inflammation of the PROSTATE.

Myrtle—is a DECONGESTANT of the PROSTATE and RESPIRATORY SYSTEM.

Yarrow—is a POWERFUL DECONGESTANT of the PROSTATE and a HORMONE BALANCER.

Peppermint—is ANTI-INFLAMMATORY to the PROSTATE.

CARRIER OIL CONTAINED IN THIS BLEND: Sesame Seed Oil.

BODY SYSTEM(S) AFFECTED: The oils in this blend may help it be effective for dealing with various problems related to the HORMONAL SYSTEM.

APPLICATION: Apply to VITA FLEX points on ANKLES, LOWER PELVIS as a COMPRESS and VITA FLEX points on BODY. Use directly on area of concern. Use on PROSTATE (may want to dilute).

SAFETY DATA: Avoid during PREGNANCY. Use with caution if susceptible to EPILEPSY

COMPANION OILS: Dragon Time is a good companion with Mister for ladies. Single oils may include sage and Clary sage.

COMPANION SUPPLEMENTS: FemiGen (capsules), Estro (tincture)

FREQUENCY: High (Spiritual); approximately 147 MHz.

Motivation

The single oils in this blend were combined to help people overcome FEAR and PROCRASTINATION and take action in their lives. The authors of this book have used this blend several times to help push us through the difficult tasks of reformatting and editing.

SINGLE OILS CONTAINED IN THIS BLEND:

Roman Chamomile—was used by the ancient Romans traditionally to EMPOWER them to go into battle. It was also to give them a CLEAR MIND. This oil is SOOTHING, RELAXING, CALMING, and may help REMOVE FEARS.

Ylang Ylang—may help BALANCE the MALE-FEMALE ENERGIES so one can move closer towards being in spiritual attunement and allow them to focus their thoughts together, filtering out the ever-present garbage. It brings back the feeling of SELF-LOVE, CONFIDENCE, JOY and PEACE.

Spruce—GROUNDS the BODY, creating the BALANCE and the OPENING necessary to RECEIVE and to GIVE. This is EMPOWERING, ANCHORING and ENCOURAGING.

Lavender—is an oil that has traditionally been known to BALANCE the BODY and to work wherever there is a need. It may help promote CONSCIOUSNESS, HEALTH, LOVE, PEACE, and a general sense of WELL BEING.

ODY SYSTEM(S) AFFECTED: The oils in this blend may help it be effective for dealing with various problems related to the NERVOUS SYSTEM and to EMOTIONAL BALANCE.

ROMATIC INFLUENCE: This blend of oils is wonderful for helping to OVERCOME the FEAR of ACHIEVING GOALS and DREAMS and for MOTIVATING the BODY and MIND into action.

PPLICATION: Wear on the CHEST or the NAPE of the NECK to stimulate the mind to want to take action. Place on SOLAR PLEXUS, STERNUM (key area), FEET (especially the BIG TOE), NAVEL area, EARS (on and behind), WRIST, PALMS of HANDS, and UNDER NOSE (sniff). Wear as PERFUME or COLOGNE.

REQUENCY: Emotional; approximately 103 MHz.

PanAway

Due to the aspirin-like properties of wintergreen and the powerful anti-inflammatory roperties of the other oils, this blend helps to REDUCE PAIN. It also STIMULATES UICKER HEALING by the INDUCTION of OXYGEN into the TISSUE SITE. It has been sed to RELIEVE PAIN DURING SURGERY with no anesthetic (helichrysum and clove were lso used). It alleviates the symptoms of SCIATICA, relieves BONE PAIN, ARTHRITIS, HEUMATISM, and promotes HEALTHY CIRCULATION. It also helps with SPORTS NJURIES, SPRAINS, MUSCLE SPASMS, BUMPS, and BRUISES.

INGLE OILS CONTAINED IN BLEND:

Wintergreen—contains 99% methyl salicylate which gives it cortisone-like properties. It may be beneficial for ARTHRITIS, RHEUMATISM, TENDINITIS, and any other discomfort that is related to the inflammation of BONES, MUSCLES, and JOINTS.

Helichrysum—may help CLEANSE the BLOOD and improve CIRCULATORY FUNCTIONS. It is ANTI-CATARRHAL in structure and nature. As a powerful ANTI-INFLAMMATORY, it may even help reduce inflammation in the meninges of the brain. On a spiritual level, it may help one LET GO OF ANGRY FEELINGS that prevent one from forgiving and moving forward.

Clove—is ANTI-INFECTIOUS, ANTI-INFLAMMATORY, a STRONG ANTISEPTIC, DISINFECTANT, IMMUNE-STIMULANT, and TOPICAL ANESTHETIC. It is also good for ARTHRITIS, INFECTION, and RHEUMATISM.

Peppermint—is ANTI-INFLAMMATORY to the PROSTATE and to DAMAGED TISSUES. It has a SOOTHING and COOLING effect which may help ARTHRITIS and RHEUMATISM.

BODY SYSTEM(S) AFFECTED: The oils in this blend may help it be effective for dealing with various problems related to the NERVOUS SYSTEM and to MUSCLES and BONES.

APPLICATION: Apply as a COMPRESS on SPINE and to VITA FLEX points on FEET. Apply on location for MUSCLES, CRAMPS, BRUISES, or any place that hurts.

COMPANION OILS: Add helichrysum (to enhance), birch/wintergreen (for bone pain), or use with Ortho Ease or Ortho Sport Massage Oil. For deep tissue pain use Relieve It.

FREQUENCY: Emotional; approximately 112 MHz.

Peace & Calming

The oils in this blend have historically been used to help reduce DEPRESSION, ANXIETY, STRESS and TENSION. This blend may help HYPERACTIVE CHILDREN get of RITALIN. It may also help children with HYPERTENSION. It may be useful at the end of a stressful day to promote RELAXATION and PEACE or to relieve INSOMNIA.

SINGLE OILS CONTAINED IN THIS BLEND:

Tangerine—contains esters and aldehydes which are SEDATING and CALMING to the NERVOUS SYSTEM. It is also a DIURETIC and a DECONGESTANT of the LYMPHATIC SYSTEM.

Orange—brings PEACE and HAPPINESS to the MIND and BODY and JOY to the HEART, which provide EMOTIONAL support to help overcome depression.

Ylang Ylang—may help BALANCE the MALE-FEMALE ENERGIES so one can move closer towards being in spiritual attunement and allow them to focus their though together, filtering out the ever-present garbage. It brings back the feeling of SELF-LOVE, CONFIDENCE, JOY and PEACE.

Patchouli—is SEDATING, CALMING, and RELAXING allowing it to reduce ANXIETY.

Blue Tansy—may help CLEANSE the LIVER and CALM the LYMPHATIC SYSTEM

BODY SYSTEM(S) AFFECTED: The oils in this blend may help it be effective for dealing wi various problems related to the NERVOUS SYSTEM and to EMOTIONAL BALANCE.

AROMATIC INFLUENCE: This blend of oils is perfect for CALMING the NERVES or EMOTIONS at the end of a long day or in times of stress. It may help one RELAX befor going to bed. By helping the body relax, more blood is able to circulate to the brain, allowing GOALS and DREAMS to be visualized more vividly and accurately.

APPLICATION: Apply UNDER NOSE, back of NECK, BACK (dilute with V-6 Mixing Oil), and FEET. Put in BATH water. Apply to NAVEL, FEET, or BACK of NECK for INSOMNIA. Wear as PERFUME or COLOGNE.

SAFETY DATA: Avoid exposure to direct SUNLIGHT for 3 to 6 hours after use.

COMPANION OILS: Lavender (add for INSOMNIA), chamomile (for calming)

FREQUENCY: Emotional; approximately 105 MHz.

Present Time

This blend was specifically created to helped BRING PEOPLE into the MOMENT. We ıst live in the moment in order to heal. We cannot live yesterday; we cannot live tomorrow; we ve to live TODAY.

NGLE OILS CONTAINED IN THIS BLEND:

Neroli—has been regarded traditionally by the Egyptian people for its great attributes for HEALING the MIND, BODY and SPIRIT. It is CALMING and RELAXING to body and spirit. It may also help to STRENGTHEN and STABILIZE the emotions, and BRING RELIEF to seemingly hopeless situations. It encourages CONFIDENCE, COURAGE, JOY, PEACE, and SENSUALITY. It brings everything into the FOCUS of one and at the moment.

Spruce—GROUNDS the BODY, creating the BALANCE and the OPENING necessary to RECEIVE and to GIVE. It also helps one release EMOTIONAL BLOCKS. It was used by the Lakota Indians to enhance their communication with the Great Spirit.

Ylang Ylang—may help BALANCE the MALE-FEMALE ENERGIES so one can move closer towards being in spiritual attunement and allow them to focus their thoughts together, filtering out the ever-present garbage. It brings back the feeling of SELF-LOVE, CONFIDENCE, JOY and PEACE.

ARRIER OIL CONTAINED IN THIS BLEND: Almond Oil.

ODY SYSTEM(S) AFFECTED: The oils in this blend may help it be effective for dealing with various problems related to EMOTIONAL BALANCE.

PPLICATION: It is most effective when rubbed clockwise over the THYMUS (down the sternum—middle front of ribs) in a circular motion, close eyes and tap three times with energy fingers (pointer and middle). Also apply to NECK and FOREHEAD.

OMPANION OILS: Harmony, Hope.

REQUENCY: Physical and Emotional; approximately 98 MHz.

Purification

The individual oils in this blend have some powerful antiseptic, anti-bacterial, anti-fungal, ıd sanitizing properties. This blend is therefore useful for KILLING ODORS and their ACTERIA, MOLDS and FUNGUS. It KILLS ANAEROBIC BACTERIA. It PURIFIES and LEANSES BACTERIA in the AIR, neutralizes MILDEW, CIGARETTE SMOKE, and other oxious ODORS. It REPELS BUGS, INSECTS, and MICE that like to live in homes, offices, ıd other confined areas. It has also been beneficial in NEUTRALIZING POISON FROM

INSECT BITES; such as SPIDERS, BEES, HORNET, and WASPS. It is good for first-aid in sterilizing WOUNDS and CUTS.

SINGLE OILS CONTAINED IN THIS BLEND:

Citronella—has ANTISEPTIC, ANTI-BACTERIAL, ANTISPASMODIC, ANTI-INFLAMMATORY, DEODORIZING, INSECTICIDAL, PURIFYING, and SANITIZING properties.

Lemongrass—is a VASODILATOR, ANTISEPTIC, ANTI-BACTERIAL, ANTI-INFLAMMATORY, and SEDATIVE. It may help improve CIRCULATION, wake up the LYMPHATIC SYSTEM, and increase the flow of OXYGEN. It may also help to LIFT the SPIRIT.

Rosemary cineol—may help BALANCE HEART FUNCTION, ENERGIZE the SOLA PLEXUS, and REDUCE MENTAL FATIGUE. It may IMPROVE CIRCULATION and help STIMULATE the NERVES. It is ANTISEPTIC an ANTI-INFECTIOUS.

Melaleuca—may help BALANCE HEART FUNCTION and act as a CLEANSER and DETOXIFIER of the BLOOD. It has ANTI-BACTERIAL, ANTI-FUNGAL, ANTI-INFECTIOUS, ANTISEPTIC, ANTI-VIRAL, and IMMUNE-STIMULANT properties.

Lavandin—is an ANTI-FUNGAL, an ANTI-BACTERIAL, a STRONG ANTISEPTIC and a TISSUE REGENERATOR.

Myrtle—is a DECONGESTANT of the RESPIRATORY SYSTEM. It may help IMPROVE OXYGENATION and work as an EXPECTORANT in DISCHARGING MUCUS. It is ANTISEPTIC and ANTI-BACTERIAL, and i EUPHORIC and ELEVATING.

BODY SYSTEM(S) AFFECTED: The oils in this blend may help it be effective for dealing w various problems related to the DIGESTIVE SYSTEM, to EMOTIONAL BALANCE, and to the SKIN.

AROMATIC INFLUENCE: This blend is great for AIR PURIFICATION when diffused. When illness is in the HOME, diffuse for one hour then wait for two. Repeat this pattern as desired. Diffuse in the OFFICE, BARN, GARBAGE AREAS, or put on cotton ball and place in an air vent to freshen the CAR.

APPLICATION: APPLY to VITA FLEX points of the BODY, EARS, FEET, and TEMPLES Apply topically for infections and cleansing. Put on cotton balls and place in air vents fo an INSECT REPELLANT at home or at work. Can also be added to PAINT to help REDUCE FUMES.

SAFETY DATA:* *Repeated use can possibly result in CONTACT SENSITIZATION. Can be irritating to sensitive SKIN.

COMPANION OILS: Citrus Fresh, Melrose, Thieves

FREQUENCY: Very Low (Physical); approximately 46 MHz.

Raven

The properties of the individual oils in this blend make it well suited to help alleviate the ymptoms of TUBERCULOSIS and PNEUMONIA. It goes beyond RC for UPPER ESPIRATORY PROBLEMS and is especially useful for VIRAL infections. It has been very eneficial for alleviating the symptoms of ASTHMA.

INGLE OILS CONTAINED IN THIS BLEND:

Ravensara—is a powerful ANTI-VIRAL, ANTI-BACTERIAL, ANTI-FUNGAL, and ANTI-INFECTIOUS oil. It may help DILATE, OPEN, and STRENGTHEN the RESPIRATORY SYSTEM. As a cross between clove and nutmeg, it may also help support the ADRENAL GLANDS.

Eucalyptus radiata—may have a profound ANTI-VIRAL effect upon the RESPIRATORY SYSTEM. It may also help reduce INFLAMMATION of the NASAL MUCOUS MEMBRANE.

Peppermint—is ANTISEPTIC, ANTISPASMODIC, and ANTI-INFLAMMATORY. It is SOOTHING, COOLING, and DILATING to the SYSTEM.

Wintergreen—contains 99% methyl salicylate which gives it cortisone-like properties. It may be beneficial for ARTHRITIS, RHEUMATISM, TENDINITIS, and any other discomfort that is related to the inflammation of BONES, MUSCLES, and JOINTS. It is also a LYMPHATIC CLEANSER.

Lemon—promotes HEALTH, HEALING, PHYSICAL ENERGY, and PURIFICATION. Its fragrance is INVIGORATING, ENHANCING, and WARMING. It is an ANTISEPTIC and is great for the RESPIRATORY SYSTEM.

ODY SYSTEM(S) AFFECTED: The oils in this blend may help it be effective for dealing with various problems related to the RESPIRATORY SYSTEM and to the SKIN.

ROMATIC INFLUENCE: This blend of oils is excellent for opening the RESPIRATORY SYSTEM when diffused or inhaled.

PPLICATION: Apply to VITA FLEX points of the BODY. Apply topically to LUNGS and THROAT. Put on pillow at night. It was traditionally used in SUPPOSITORY or ENEMA application with V-6 Mixing Oil and retained throughout the night. This method of application can directly benefit the LUNGS within seconds.

AFETY DATA: Can be irritating to sensitive SKIN.

OMPANION OILS: Melrose, RC, Thieves.

REQUENCY: Physical; approximately 70 MHz.

RC

Although not as powerful against viral infections as RAVEN, the properties of the oils in this blend make it extremely effective against ALLERGIES, COLDS, BRONCHITIS, RESPIRATORY CONGESTION, FLU, COLD SORES, PNEUMONIA, SINUSITIS, SORE THROAT, MUCUS, and BONE SPURS.

SINGLE OILS CONTAINED IN THIS BLEND:

Eucalyptus (four types including *E. globulus*, *E. radiata*, *E. australiana*, and *E. citriodora*)—may have a profound ANTI-VIRAL effect upon the RESPIRATORY SYSTEM. They also have STRONG ANTI-BACTERIAL, ANTI-CATARRHAL, and ANTISEPTIC properties.

Myrtle—is a DECONGESTANT of the RESPIRATORY SYSTEM. It may help IMPROVE OXYGENATION and work as an EXPECTORANT in DISCHARGING MUCUS. It is ANTISEPTIC and ANTI-BACTERIAL, and is EUPHORIC and ELEVATING.

Marjoram—is RELAXING, CALMING, and APPEASING to the MUSCLES that constrict and sometimes contribute to HEADACHES. As an ANTISPASMODIC, it may help relieve spasms in the RESPIRATORY SYSTEM.

Pine—may help DILATE and OPEN the RESPIRATORY SYSTEM, particularly the BRONCHIAL TRACT. It may also help IMPROVE CIRCULATION THROUGHOUT the LUNGS.

Cypress—is ANTI-INFECTIOUS, MUCOLYTIC, ANTISEPTIC, LYMPHATIC DECONGESTANT, REFRESHING, and RELAXING. It may help improve LUNG CIRCULATION as well as help relieve other RESPIRATORY PROBLEMS.

Lavender—is an oil that has traditionally been known to BALANCE the BODY and to work wherever there is a need. It may help promote CONSCIOUSNESS, HEALTH, LOVE, PEACE, and a general sense of WELL BEING.

Spruce—GROUNDS the BODY, creating the BALANCE and the OPENING necessary to RECEIVE and to GIVE. It may help DILATE the BRONCHIAL TRACT to IMPROVE the OXYGEN EXCHANGE. It also helps one release EMOTIONAL BLOCKS.

Peppermint—is ANTISEPTIC, ANTISPASMODIC, and ANTI-INFLAMMATORY. It is SOOTHING, COOLING, and DILATING to the SYSTEM.

BODY SYSTEM(S) AFFECTED: The oils in this blend may help it be effective for dealing with various problems related to the RESPIRATORY SYSTEM.

ROMATIC INFLUENCE: RC is very beneficial in the diffuser to DECONGEST and RELIEVE ALLERGY-TYPE symptoms such as COUGHS, SORE THROAT, and LUNG CONGESTION.

PPLICATION: Diffuse. Dilute with V-6 Mixing Oil and MASSAGE on the CHEST, BACK, and FEET. It can be used as a COMPRESS over the CHEST and BACK. Put on SINUSES and NASAL PASSAGES (put oil on a Q-tip and rub on inside of NASAL PASSAGES). Rub around EARS, FEET, NECK, and THROAT. Apply to VITA FLEX points on BODY. It can be exchanged and alternated effectively with Raven.

OMPANION OILS: Raven on feet, RC on throat and chest, alternate morning and night. Run hot steaming water in sink, put Raven, RC and birch/wintergreen in water, put towel over head and INHALE to open sinuses for FLU, COLDS or PNEUMONIA. Another companion oil is Thieves.

REQUENCY: Physical; approximately 75 MHz.

Release

This is a powerful blend for enhancing the RELEASE of MEMORY TRAUMA from the lls of the liver, where anger and hate emotions are stored. The frequency of the oils in Release ay aid in the LETTING GO of NEGATIVE EMOTIONS so one can progress in a more effective d efficient way. It helps to RELEASE FRUSTRATION.

NGLE OILS CONTAINED IN THIS BLEND:

Ylang Ylang—may help BALANCE the MALE-FEMALE ENERGIES so one can move closer towards being in spiritual attunement and allow them to focus their thoughts together, filtering out the ever-present garbage. It brings back the feeling of SELF-LOVE, CONFIDENCE, JOY and PEACE.

Lavandin—is an ANTI-FUNGAL, an ANTI-BACTERIAL, a STRONG ANTISEPTIC, and a TISSUE REGENERATOR.

Geranium—may help with HORMONAL BALANCE, LIVER and KIDNEY FUNCTIONS and the DISCHARGE of TOXINS from the LIVER that hold us back from having balance. Geranium OPENS the LIVER CHAKRA (Solar Plexus). It may help DILATE the BILIARY DUCTS for LIVER DETOXIFICATION. It may also help foster PEACE, WELL BEING, and HOPE.

Sandalwood—also, like frankincense, is high in sesquiterpenes, which were discovered to INCREASE the amount of OXYGEN around the PINEAL and PITUITARY GLANDS, thus helping to IMPROVE one's ATTITUDE. It ALLEVIATES DEPRESSION and assists in the removal of NEGATIVE PROGRAMMING from the cells of the body. It helps one ACCEPT OTHERS with an open heart while diminishing one's own egocentricity.

Blue Tansy—may help CLEANSE the LIVER thereby helping to release ANGER and NEGATIVE EMOTIONS.

CARRIER OIL CONTAINED IN THIS BLEND: Olive Oil.

BODY SYSTEM(S) AFFECTED: The oils in this blend may help it be effective for dealing w various problems related to EMOTIONAL BALANCE.

APPLICATION: Apply over LIVER or as a COMPRESS. Put on EARS, bottom of FEET, especially VITA FLEX points of FEET. Wear as PERFUME OR COLOGNE.

COMPANION OILS: Put Valor on FEET first, then put Harmony (for balance) on FEET, JuvaFlex on FEET, Release on LIVER, rotate the oil used each day.

FREQUENCY: Emotional; approximately 102 MHz.

Relieve It

The pepper oil along with the other deep penetrating oils in this blend, make it effective f the relief of DEEP TISSUE PAIN. This extraordinary blend, with its high ANTI-INFLAMMATORY action, seems to go beyond **PanAway** in some pain applications, especially when alternated with PanAway and/or helichrysum. It may also help with SCIATICA and ARTHRITIC PAIN (Try birch or wintergreen too!) **PanAway** is more for BONE PAIN.

SINGLE OILS CONTAINED IN THIS BLEND:

Spruce—GROUNDS the BODY, creating the BALANCE and the OPENING necessary to RECEIVE and to GIVE. It may help DILATE the BRONCHIAL TRACT to IMPROVE the OXYGEN EXCHANGE. It also helps one release EMOTIONA BLOCKS.

Pepper, Black—may help STIMULATE the ENDOCRINE SYSTEM and INCREASE ENERGY. It is an ANTI-INFLAMMATORY and was traditionally used for RHEUMATOID ARTHRITIS. It may also help INCREASE CELLULAR OXYGENATION.

Hyssop—was used by Moses during the Lord's Passover in Egypt (Exodus 12). It has ANTI-INFLAMMATORY and ANTISPASMODIC properties. It may also hav the ability to OPEN up the RESPIRATORY SYSTEM and DISCHARGE TOXINS and MUCUS.

Peppermint—is ANTISEPTIC, ANTISPASMODIC, and ANTI-INFLAMMATORY. I is SOOTHING, COOLING, and DILATING to the SYSTEM.

BODY SYSTEM(S) AFFECTED: The oils in this blend may help it be effective for dealing wi various problems related to MUSCLES and BONES.

APPLICATION: Apply on location, anywhere there is DEEP TISSUE PAIN.

FETY DATA: Can be irritating to sensitive SKIN. Use with caution during PREGNANCY. Use with caution if susceptible to EPILEPSY or HIGH BLOOD PRESSURE.

MPANION OILS: PanAway is a great companion to Relieve It, especially when there is BONE PAIN. Other companion oils may include Aroma Siez, Melrose, cypress, and helichrysum.

EQUENCY: Very Low (Physical); approximately 56 MHz.

Sacred Mountain

The predominance of conifer oils in this blend creates a feeling of PROTECTION, IPOWERMENT, and GROUNDING. This blend may help one find SECURITY and CREDNESS within ONESELF. In addition, it is ANTI-BACTERIAL and very SOOTHING he RESPIRATORY SYSTEM.

NGLE OILS CONTAINED IN THIS BLEND:

Spruce—GROUNDS the BODY, creating the BALANCE and the OPENING necessary to RECEIVE and to GIVE. It also helps one release EMOTIONAL BLOCKS. It was used by the Lakota Indians to enhance their communication with the Great Spirit.

Ylang Ylang—may help BALANCE the MALE-FEMALE ENERGIES so one can move closer towards being in spiritual attunement and allow them to focus their thoughts together, filtering out the ever-present garbage. It brings back the feeling of SELF-LOVE, CONFIDENCE, JOY and PEACE.

Idaho Balsam Fir—may help create a feeling of GROUNDING, ANCHORING and EMPOWERMENT.

Cedarwood—was used traditionally by the North American Indians to enhance their potential for SPIRITUAL COMMUNICATION. It may help OPEN the PINEAL GLAND.

DDY SYSTEM(S) AFFECTED: The oils in this blend may help it be effective for dealing with various problems related to EMOTIONAL BALANCE.

ROMATIC INFLUENCE: The aroma of this blend of oils creates a feeling of STRENGTH, EMPOWERMENT, GROUNDING, and PROTECTION.

PLICATION: DIFFUSE. Apply to SOLAR PLEXUS, BRAIN STEM, CROWN of HEAD, back of NECK, behind EARS, THYMUS, and WRISTS. Wear as PERFUME or COLOGNE.

FETY DATA: Can be irritating to sensitive SKIN.

REQUENCY: High (Spiritual); approximately 176 MHz.

COMMENTS: The three conifer oils have been traditionally used by the North American Indi symbolically to represent the umbrella they create in protecting the earth and bringing energy in from the universe. At night the animals in the wild lie under a tree for the protection, recharging and rejuvenation the trees bring to them.

SARA

The oils in this blend produce such a beautiful fragrance as may allow one to relax into mental state whereby they may be able to RELEASE and let go of the NEGATIVE EMOTION and MEMORY of TRAUMATIC EXPERIENCES. Although created specifically to provide re from the MEMORY TRAUMA of SEXUAL and/or RITUAL ABUSE, it may also work well f other traumatic experiences.

SINGLE OILS CONTAINED IN THIS BLEND:

Blue Tansy—may help CLEANSE the LIVER and CALM the LYMPHATIC SYSTE

Rose—has a BEAUTIFUL FRAGRANCE and contains the highest frequency of the oi It may help ENHANCE the FREQUENCY of every cell, which could help brin BALANCE and HARMONY to the body. It is thought by some to produce a magnetic energy that attracts LOVE and enhances the frequency of SELF-LOV bringing JOY to the heart.

Lavender—is an oil that has traditionally been known to BALANCE the BODY and to work wherever there is a need. It may help promote CONSCIOUSNESS, HEALTH, LOVE, PEACE, and a general sense of WELL BEING.

Geranium—may help with HORMONAL BALANCE, LIVER and KIDNEY FUNCTIONS and the DISCHARGE of TOXINS from the LIVER that hold us back from having balance. Geranium OPENS the LIVER CHAKRA (Solar Plexus). It may help DILATE the BILIARY DUCTS for LIVER DETOXIFICATION. It may also help foster PEACE, WELL BEING, and HOPE by promoting the release of NEGATIVE MEMORIES.

Orange—brings PEACE and HAPPINESS to the MIND and BODY and JOY to the HEART, which provide EMOTIONAL support to help overcome depression.

Cedarwood—was used traditionally by the North American Indians to enhance their potential for SPIRITUAL COMMUNICATION. It may help OPEN the PINEA GLAND.

Ylang Ylang—may help BALANCE the MALE-FEMALE ENERGIES so one can mo closer towards being in spiritual attunement and allow them to focus their thoug together, filtering out the ever-present garbage. It brings back the feeling of SELF-LOVE, CONFIDENCE, JOY and PEACE.

White Lotus—was traditionally used by the Egyptians for spiritual, emotional, and physical applications. It has a euphoric fragrance that LIFTS and STABILIZES the EMOTIONS, creating a powerful sense of EMOTIONAL, PHYSICAL, and SPIRITUAL WELL BEING.

ODY SYSTEM(S) AFFECTED: The oils in this blend may help it be effective for dealing with various problems related to EMOTIONAL BALANCE.

ROMATIC INFLUENCE: The aroma of this blend of oils creates a feeling of PEACE and FREEDOM to move forward in life with JOY.

PPLICATION: Apply over ENERGY CENTERS, on VITA FLEX points, TEMPLES, NOSE, and AREAS of ABUSE.

OMPANION OILS: Forgiveness, Hope, Inner Child, Inspiration, Joy, Magnify Your Purpose, 3 Wise Men, Trauma Life, Valor, White Angelica

REQUENCY: Emotional; approximately 102 MHz.

OMMENTS: One individual muscle tested positive for this oil for the purpose of overcoming the emotions related to having a twin brother die early in gestation, but remain in the womb until full-term delivery.

SclarEssence

This blend was formulated to support the HORMONES and increase estradiol and stosterone levels. When taken as a dietary supplement, it may also help improve DIGESTION, duce BLOATING, and help balance the body's pH.

INGLE OILS CONTAINED IN THIS BLEND:

Clary Sage—is beneficial for REGULATING CELLS and BALANCING the HORMONES. It may help with MENSTRUAL CRAMPS, PMS, and PRE-MENOPAUSE symptoms. It may also help with CIRCULATORY PROBLEMS.

Peppermint—is an ANTI-INFLAMMATORY to the PROSTATE and NERVES. It is SOOTHING to the STOMACH, COOLING, and DILATING to the SYSTEM.

Sage Lavender—has been shown to increase both estradiol and testosterone levels. It may help HARMONIZE and BALANCE the EMOTIONS and reduce STRESS-RELATED conditions. It may also help decongest the LIVER.

Fennel—may help SUPPORT the DIGESTIVE FUNCTION by SUPPORTING the LIVER. It may also help BALANCE the HORMONES.

ODY SYSTEM(S) AFFECTED: HORMONAL and DIGESTIVE SYSTEMS.

RAL USE AS DIETARY SUPPLEMENT: *Put 1-20 drops in a capsule. Ingest 1 capsule daily as needed.* ***Not recommended for children.***

Sensation

Because of the incredibly beautiful aromas of ylang ylang, rosewood, and jasmine, this blend is extremely UPLIFTING, REFRESHING, and AROUSING. It is very beneficial for SKI PROBLEMS of any kind as it is very nourishing and hydrating for the skin.

SINGLE OILS CONTAINED IN THIS BLEND:

Rosewood—is SOOTHING to the SKIN, APPEASING to the MIND, RELAXING to t BODY, and creates a feeling of PEACE and GENTLENESS.

Ylang Ylang—may help BALANCE the MALE-FEMALE ENERGIES so one can mov closer towards being in spiritual attunement and allow them to focus their thougl together, filtering out the ever-present garbage. It brings back the feeling of SELF-LOVE, CONFIDENCE, JOY and PEACE.

Jasmine—is very UPLIFTING to the EMOTIONS; it may produce a feeling of CONFIDENCE, ENERGY, EUPHORIA, and OPTIMISM.

BODY SYSTEM(S) AFFECTED: The oils in this blend may help it be effective for dealing wi various problems related to the HORMONAL SYSTEM and to EMOTIONAL BALANCE.

AROMATIC INFLUENCE: Because the aroma of this blend of oils is so UPLIFTING and AROUSING, it creates a feeling EXCITEMENT and ROMANCE which may help move one to new heights of SELF-EXPRESSION and AWARENESS.

APPLICATION: Apply on LOCATION, use for MASSAGE, and add to your Sensation Bath and Shower Gel. May also be used with a COMPRESS over the abdomen, or just worn a COLOGNE or PERFUME.

COMPANION OILS: Awaken, Dream Catcher, Into the Future, Joy, Live with Passion

FREQUENCY: Physical and Emotional; approximately 88 MHz.

Surrender

Most of the single oils in this blend are CALMING, RELAXING, and BALANCING to the emotions, making it effective for those with DOMINANT PERSONALITIES who at times may become UNFOCUSED or OVERBEARING. By BALANCING the EMOTIONS, CLEARING the MIND, and reducing feelings of ANXIETY and STRESS, this blend may help such individuals recover EQUILIBRIUM, and calm INNER STRENGTH.

SINGLE OILS CONTAINED IN THIS BLEND:

Lavender—is an oil that has traditionally been known to BALANCE the BODY and to work wherever there is a need. It may help promote CONSCIOUSNESS, HEALTH, LOVE, PEACE, and a general sense of WELL BEING.

Roman Chamomile—eliminates some of the emotional charge of ANXIETY, IRRITABILITY, and NERVOUSNESS. Because it is CALMING and RELAXING, it can combat STRESS.

German Chamomile—can dispel ANGER, stabilize the EMOTIONS, and help release emotions liked to the past. It may also help to SOOTHE and CLEAR the MIND creating an atmosphere of PEACE and PATIENCE.

Angelica—is referred to by the German people as the "oil of angels". It may help one RELEASE and LET GO of NEGATIVE FEELINGS.

Mountain Savory—has IMMUNE-STIMULANT, ANTIMICROBIAL, and ANTI-PARASITIC properties. It is also a powerful ENERGIZER and MOTIVATOR.

Lemon—promotes HEALTH, HEALING, PHYSICAL ENERGY, and PURIFICATION. Its fragrance is INVIGORATING, ENHANCING, and WARMING.

Spruce—GROUNDS the BODY, creating the BALANCE and the OPENING necessary to RECEIVE and to GIVE. It may help DILATE the BRONCHIAL TRACT to IMPROVE the OXYGEN EXCHANGE. It also helps one release EMOTIONAL BLOCKS.

ODY SYSTEM(S) AFFECTED: The oils in this blend may help it be effective for dealing with various problems related to the NERVOUS SYSTEM and to EMOTIONAL BALANCE.

ROMATIC INFLUENCE: May help to reduce ANXIETY and calm NERVOUSNESS and IRRITABILITY. It may also help to BALANCE the EMOTIONS and CLEAR the MIND.

PPLICATION: Apply on the FOREHEAD, along the RIM of the EARS, at the NAPE of the NECK, on the CHEST, and on the SOLAR PLEXUS. May also be added to BATH water.

AFETY DATA: Because of some of the oils contained within this blend, it should be used with caution by individuals who are PREGNANT. Repeated use could possibly result in SKIN IRRITATION.

OMPANION OILS: Clarity, Forgiveness, Grounding, Peace & Calming, Sacred Mountain

REQUENCY: Physical and Emotional; approximately 98 MHz.

Thieves

The highly anti-viral, antiseptic properties of the single oils contained in this blend help rotect the body from the onset of FLU, CANDIDA, COLDS, etc. It may also help with INUSITIS, BRONCHITIS, PNEUMONIA, COUGHS, STREP, SORE THROATS, ERIODONTAL (GUM) DISEASE, TEETHING, COLD SORES, CANKER SORES, RUISES, CUTS, INFECTION, SLIVERS and SPLINTERS (pulls to surface). It is considered NTI-PLAGUE as it was used by thieves in England to protect them from the plague when ealing from the sick and dying.

SINGLE OILS CONTAINED IN THIS BLEND:

Clove—is ANTI-BACTERIAL, ANTI-FUNGAL, ANTI-INFECTIOUS, ANTI-PARASITIC, a STRONG ANTISEPTIC, ANTI-VIRAL, and an IMMUNE STIMULANT. It may influence HEALING and help create a feeling of PROTECTION and COURAGE.

Lemon—promotes HEALTH, HEALING, PHYSICAL ENERGY, and PURIFICATIO Its fragrance is INVIGORATING, ENHANCING, and WARMING. It is an ANTISEPTIC and is great for the RESPIRATORY SYSTEM.

Cinnamon Bark—is part of the formula the Lord gave Moses (Exodus 30:22-27). It ha very specific purposes: (1) it is a POWERFUL PURIFIER, (2) it is a powerful OXYGENATOR, and (3) it ENHANCES the action and the activity of OTHER OILS. It may have a STIMULATING and TONING effect on the whole body and particularly the circulatory system. It is ANTI-BACTERIAL, ANTI-FUNGAL, ANTI-INFECTIOUS, ANTI-INFLAMMATORY, ANTIMICROBIAL, ANTI-PARASITIC, ANTISEPTIC, ANTISPASMODIC, ANTI-VIRAL, ASTRINGENT, IMMUNE-STIMULANT, SEXUAL STIMULANT, and WARMING.

Eucalyptus radiata—may have a profound ANTI-VIRAL effect upon the RESPIRATORY SYSTEM. It also has STRONG ANTI-BACTERIAL, ANTI-CATARRHAL, and ANTISEPTIC properties.

Rosemary cineol—may help BALANCE HEART FUNCTION, ENERGIZE the SOLA PLEXUS, and REDUCE MENTAL FATIGUE. It may IMPROVE CIRCULATION and help STIMULATE the NERVES. It is ANTISEPTIC and ANTI-INFECTIOUS.

BODY SYSTEM(S) AFFECTED: The oils in this blend may help it be effective for dealing wi various problems related to the IMMUNE SYSTEM.

AROMATIC INFLUENCE: Diffuse this blend of oils periodically for 20-25 minutes at a time to help protect the body against the onset of FLU, COLDS, and VIRUSES.

APPLICATION: Massage bottom of FEET, THROAT, STOMACH, and INTESTINES. Dilute one drop of Thieves in 15 drops of V-6 Mixing Oil and massage the THYMUS to stimulate the IMMUNE SYSTEM and massage UNDER the ARMS to stimulate the LYMPHATIC SYSTEM. It is best applied to the bottom of the feet as it may be caustic to the skin. **Always dilute with V-6 Mixing Oil**.

SAFETY DATA: Repeated use can result in extreme CONTACT SENSITIZATION. Can cause extreme SKIN IRRITATION. Use with caution during PREGNANCY.

COMPANION OILS: Put ImmuPower on the THROAT and Thieves on the FEET, then alternate by putting Thieves on the THROAT and ImmuPower on the FEET. Can also alternate ImmuPower with Exodus II.

FREQUENCY: Emotional and Spiritual; approximately 150 MHz.

COMMENTS: Studies conducted by Weber State University (Ogden, UT) during 1997 showed the antibacterial effectiveness of this blend (Thieves) against airborne microorganisms.

One study showed a 90% reduction in the number of gram positive *Micrococcus luteus* organisms after diffusing Thieves for 12 minutes. After diffusing Thieves for a total of 20 minutes, there was a 99.3% reduction. Another study against the gram negative *Pseudomonas aeruginosa* showed a kill rate of 99.96% after just 12 minutes of diffusion.

3 Wise Men

The highly spiritual nature of the oils in this blend allow it to OPEN the CROWN IAKRA and facilitate the release of negative emotions. This blend brings a sense of .OUNDING and UPLIFTING through MEMORY RECALL. It also keeps negative energy and gative emotions from reattaching to the body.

NGLE OILS CONTAINED IN THIS BLEND:

Sandalwood—also, like frankincense, is high in sesquiterpenes, which were discovered to INCREASE the amount of OXYGEN around the PINEAL and PITUITARY GLANDS, thus helping to IMPROVE one's ATTITUDE. It ALLEVIATES DEPRESSION and assists in the removal of NEGATIVE PROGRAMMING from the cells of the body. It helps one ACCEPT OTHERS with an open heart while diminishing one's own egocentricity.

Juniper—evokes feelings of HEALTH, LOVE, and PEACE and may help to ELEVATE one's SPIRITUAL AWARENESS.

Frankincense—contains sesquiterpenes, which may help OXYGENATE the PINEAL and PITUITARY GLANDS. As one of the ingredients for the holy incense, it was used anciently to help ENHANCE one's COMMUNICATION WITH THE CREATOR. It was considered a prize possession and was given to Christ at his birth by the three wise men. It may help PROMOTE a POSITIVE ATTITUDE.

Spruce—GROUNDS the BODY, creating the BALANCE and the OPENING necessary to RECEIVE and to GIVE. It also helps one release EMOTIONAL BLOCKS. It was used by the Lakota Indians to enhance their communication with the Great Spirit.

Myrrh—is part of the formula the Lord gave Moses (Exodus 30:22-27). It promotes SPIRITUAL AWARENESS and is a TRUE GIFT (one of the gifts that was brought for the Christ child). When we OPEN our HEARTS and MINDS to receive the gifts, they will be given.

ARRIER OIL CONTAINED IN THIS BLEND: Almond Oil.

)DY SYSTEM(S) AFFECTED: The oils in this blend may help it be effective for dealing with various problems related to EMOTIONAL BALANCE.

ROMATIC INFLUENCE: Diffusing this blend of oils may help to create a feeling of REVERENCE and heightened SPIRITUAL CONSCIOUSNESS.

APPLICATION: Apply to the CROWN of the HEAD in a clockwise motion to create an ener of opening and releasing, followed by receiving the energy of the oils to FILL the NEW VOID. Put on NECK, EYE BROW, SOLAR PLEXUS, and THYMUS (clockwise). Wear as PERFUME or COLOGNE.

COMPANION OILS: Frankincense, myrrh, sandalwood, juniper, and spruce.

FREQUENCY: Physical; approximately 72 MHz.

COMMENTS: When all or any of the companion oils are combined with 3 Wise Men, a sense GROUNDING and UPLIFTMENT come through the release of memory recall. In addition, when the oil is placed on the crown, it elevates ones spiritual consciousness.

Transformation

Many of the oils in this blend are powerfully ENERGIZING and STIMULATING to th CONSCIOUS MIND allowing for the SUPPORT necessary when making changes, especially MENTAL and EMOTIONAL CHANGES.

SINGLE OILS CONTAINED IN THIS BLEND:

Lemon—promotes HEALTH, HEALING, PHYSICAL ENERGY, and PURIFICATIC Its fragrance is INVIGORATING, ENHANCING, and WARMING.

Peppermint—is ANTI-INFLAMMATORY to the NERVES. It has a SOOTHING an COOLING EFFECT on HEADACHES. It is PURIFYING and STIMULATI to the CONSCIOUS MIND.

Sandalwood—also, like frankincense, is high in sesquiterpenes, which were discovered INCREASE the amount of OXYGEN around the PINEAL and PITUITARY GLANDS, thus helping to IMPROVE one's ATTITUDE.

Frankincense—contains sesquiterpenes, which may help OXYGENATE the PINEAL PITUITARY GLANDS. As one of the ingredients for the holy incense, it was used anciently to help ENHANCE one's COMMUNICATION WITH THE CREATOR. It may help PROMOTE a POSITIVE ATTITUDE.

Clary Sage—may calm and enhance the DREAM STATE, helping to bring about a feeling of EUPHORIA.

Balsam Fir—creates a feeling of GROUNDING, ANCHORING, and EMPOWERMENT. It can STIMULATE the MIND while allowing the BODY to RELAX.

Rosemary cineol—may help BALANCE HEART FUNCTION, ENERGIZE the SOL PLEXUS, and REDUCE MENTAL FATIGUE. It may IMPROVE CIRCULATION and help STIMULATE the NERVES.

Cardamom—is UPLIFTING, REFRESHING, and INVIGORATING. It may be beneficial for CLEARING CONFUSION.

)DY SYSTEM(S) AFFECTED: The oils in this blend may help it be effective for dealing with various problems related to EMOTIONAL BALANCE.

ROMATIC INFLUENCE: When diffused or worn as perfume, this blend of oils may help STIMULATE one's mind and STRENGTHEN one's resolve when dealing with difficult decisions, especially when related to a change in ATTITUDE or a change in one's BELIEF SYSTEM.

PPLICATION: DIFFUSE or apply to the FOREHEAD ("third eye" chakra) and over the HEART, helping to unite heart and mind.

)MPANION OILS: Hope, Humility, Into the Future.

REQUENCY: Physical and Emotional; approximately 92 MHz.

Trauma Life

Many of the oils in this blend are powerfully CALMING and GROUNDING, helping JRGE the STRESS and UPROOT the TRAUMAS that are often at the heart of our physical tigue and over-burdened immune system. Others are SPIRITUALLY UPLIFTING, bringing us oser to our CREATOR and helping us to see our TRIALS from the PROPER PERSPECTIVE. ometimes, physical and mental difficulties are a result of unreleased trauma. For example, our e year old daughter would continuously babble until she fell down a flight of stairs. Although e was not physically hurt from the fall, we soon noticed that the babbling had stopped. One plication of this blend brought back the constant babbling.

NGLE OILS CONTAINED IN THIS BLEND:

Citrus hystrix **(Leech-lime)**—is very high in aldehydes and esters, making it very SEDATING and CALMING.

Davana—is ANTI-INFECTIOUS and may stimulate the ENDOCRINE SYSTEM and improve HORMONAL BALANCE.

Geranium—may help with HORMONAL BALANCE, LIVER and KIDNEY FUNCTIONS and the DISCHARGE of TOXINS from the LIVER that hold us back from having balance. Geranium OPENS the LIVER CHAKRA (Solar Plexus). It may help DILATE the BILIARY DUCTS for LIVER DETOXIFICATION, which may help one let go of ANGER and NEGATIVE EMOTIONS.

Spruce—GROUNDS the BODY, creating the BALANCE and the OPENING necessary to RECEIVE and to GIVE. It may help DILATE the BRONCHIAL TRACT to IMPROVE the OXYGEN EXCHANGE. It also helps one release EMOTIONAL BLOCKS.

Helichrysum—may help CLEANSE the BLOOD and improve CIRCULATORY FUNCTIONS. It is ANTI-CATARRHAL in structure and nature. As a powerful ANTI-INFLAMMATORY, it may even help reduce inflammation in the meninges of the brain. On a spiritual level, it may help one LET GO OF ANGRY FEELINGS that prevent one from forgiving and moving forward.

Rose—contains the highest frequency of the oils. It may help ENHANCE the FREQUENCY of every cell, which could help bring BALANCE and HARMON to the body. It is thought by some to produce a magnetic energy that attracts LOVE and enhances the frequency of SELF-LOVE, bringing JOY to the heart.

Sandalwood—also, like frankincense, is high in sesquiterpenes, which were discovered INCREASE the amount of OXYGEN around the PINEAL and PITUITARY GLANDS, thus helping to IMPROVE one's ATTITUDE.

Frankincense—contains sesquiterpenes, which may help OXYGENATE the PINEAL a PITUITARY GLANDS. As one of the ingredients for the holy incense, it was used anciently to help ENHANCE one's COMMUNICATION WITH THE CREATOR. It may help PROMOTE a POSITIVE ATTITUDE.

Lavender—is an oil that has traditionally been known to BALANCE the BODY and to work wherever there is a need. It may help promote CONSCIOUSNESS, HEALTH, LOVE, PEACE, and a general sense of WELL BEING.

Valerian—has a powerful sedative effect. It is also ANTISPASMODIC, DEPRESSAN to the central nervous system, and somewhat HYPNOTIC. It may help minimiz the shock, the feeling of anxiety, and the stress that accompanies traumatic situations.

BODY SYSTEM(S) AFFECTED: The oils in this blend may help it be effective for dealing w various problems related to EMOTIONAL BALANCE.

AROMATIC INFLUENCE: When diffused, this blend of oils may help promote the CALMIN and BALANCING effect that is necessary in overcoming TRAUMA.

APPLICATION: Best when applied to the SPINE using the Raindrop Technique. It is also beneficial when placed on the bottom of the FEET, on the CHEST, behind the EARS, or the nap of the NECK, or in the center of the FOREHEAD ("third eye" chakra).

COMPANION OILS: Peace & Calming, Joy, Hope, Into the Future.

FREQUENCY: Physical and Emotional; approximately 92 MHz.

Valor

This blend has been used to help EMPOWER the PHYSICAL and SPIRITUAL BODIE It helps us OVERCOME FEAR and OPPOSITION so we can stand tall during adversity. It ma help build COURAGE, CONFIDENCE, and SELF-ESTEEM. It brings a feeling of CALMNESS, PEACE and RELAXATION. It may be used in place of PEACE and CALMING for HYPERACTIVITY and ATTENTION DEFICIT DISORDER in CHILDREN. It has been found beneficial in helping to ALIGN the PHYSICAL STRUCTURE of the BODY, RELIEVIN PAIN along SPINE. It also BALANCES and ALIGNS ELECTRICAL ENERGIES within the BODY. It is best applied with six drops on each foot or massaged in along the spine using the aindrop Technique. Valor has been touted as a CHIROPRACTOR in a bottle. It has improved COLIOSIS in as little as 30 minutes, though this should not be considered normal. Some dividuals require several months of application before any improvement is seen. *Valor has also een shown to change anaerobic mutated cells back to their aerobic natural state.*

INGLE OILS CONTAINED IN THIS BLEND:

Spruce—GROUNDS the BODY, creating the BALANCE and the OPENING necessary to RECEIVE and to GIVE. It may help DILATE the BRONCHIAL TRACT to IMPROVE the OXYGEN EXCHANGE. It also helps one release EMOTIONAL BLOCKS.

Rosewood—is SOOTHING to the SKIN, APPEASING to the MIND, RELAXING to the BODY, and creates a feeling of PEACE and GENTLENESS.

Blue Tansy—may help CLEANSE the LIVER and CALM the LYMPHATIC SYSTEM to help rid one of ANGER and promote a feeling of SELF-CONTROL.

Frankincense—contains sesquiterpenes, which may help OXYGENATE the PINEAL and PITUITARY GLANDS. As one of the ingredients for the holy incense, it was used anciently to help ENHANCE one's COMMUNICATION WITH THE CREATOR. It may help PROMOTE a POSITIVE ATTITUDE.

:ARRIER OIL CONTAINED IN THIS BLEND: Almond Oil.

ODY SYSTEM(S) AFFECTED: The oils in this blend may help it be effective for dealing with various problems related to MUSCLES and BONES, SKIN, the NERVOUS SYSTEM, and EMOTIONAL BALANCE.

ROMATIC INFLUENCE: This blend of oils may help BALANCE the ELECTRICAL ENERGIES in the body. Diffuse wherever and whenever possible.

PPLICATION: It WORKS BEST on BOTTOM of FEET. Put six drops of Valor on BOTTOM of FEET. Put Valor on HEART, THROAT CHAKRA, WRISTS, SOLAR PLEXUS from NECK to THYMUS. To BALANCE LEFT and RIGHT BRAIN, put Valor on LEFT FINGERS and rub on RIGHT TEMPLE or put Valor on RIGHT FINGERS and rub on LEFT TEMPLE OR CROSS ARMS and rub VITA FLEX points on bottom of FEET. To RELIEVE PAIN along the SPINE, apply Valor to VITA FLEX points on FEET and on SPINE using the RAINDROP TECHNIQUE. Wear as PERFUME or COLOGNE.

:OMPANION OILS: BALANCE with Valor and PROTECT with White Angelica.

'REQUENCY: VERY LOW to balance and align the physical body; aligns the skeletal system; approximately 47 MHz.

:OMMENTS: This blend is the most important oil in any application. It helps balance electrical energies within the body, giving courage, confidence, and self-esteem. Most importantly, it builds the bridge between the body and the oils allowing higher frequency oils to raise the frequency of the body thus promoting physical, emotional, and spiritual well being. (*Refer to the Vita Flex Therapy part of the Science and Application section of this book for the importance of using this blend and how to use it to balance the body's energy*).

White Angelica

This unique blend of 10 different oils helps create a frequency field to WARD OFF the BOMBARDMENT of NEGATIVE ENERGY. It is important for use in EMOTIONAL CLEANSING. It may help INCREASE the AURA around the body, bringing a delicate sense of STRENGTH and PROTECTION and a greater AWARENESS of ONE'S POTENTIAL. It may also help with ANGER, DEPRESSION, HEADACHES (especially when flying), HEMORRHOIDS, CIRCULATION, and LOWERING HIGH BLOOD PRESSURE.

SINGLE OILS CONTAINED IN THIS BLEND:

Geranium—may help with HORMONAL BALANCE, LIVER and KIDNEY FUNCTIONS and the DISCHARGE of TOXINS from the LIVER that hold us back from having balance. Geranium OPENS the LIVER CHAKRA (Solar Plexus). It may help DILATE the BILIARY DUCTS for LIVER DETOXIFICATION, which may help one let go of ANGER and NEGATIVE EMOTIONS.

Spruce—GROUNDS the BODY, creating the BALANCE and the OPENING necessary to RECEIVE and to GIVE. It also helps one release EMOTIONAL BLOCKS.

Myrrh—is part of the formula the Lord gave Moses (Exodus 30:22-27). It promotes SPIRITUAL AWARENESS and is a TRUE GIFT (one of the gifts that was brought for the Christ child). When we OPEN our HEARTS and MINDS to receive the gifts, they will be given.

Ylang Ylang—may help BALANCE the MALE-FEMALE ENERGIES so one can move closer towards being in spiritual attunement and allow them to focus their thought together, filtering out the ever-present garbage. It brings back the feeling of SELF-LOVE, CONFIDENCE, JOY and PEACE.

Hyssop—was used by Moses during the Lord's Passover in Egypt (Exodus 12). It has ANTI-INFLAMMATORY and ANTI-VIRAL properties. It may have the ability to OPEN up the RESPIRATORY SYSTEM and DISCHARGE TOXINS and MUCUS. It may also stimulate MEDITATION and promote CENTERING.

Bergamot—is SOOTHING to the ENDOCRINE SYSTEM and the HORMONES of the body. It may UPLIFT and CALM the EMOTIONS to help relieve ANXIETY, STRESS, and TENSION.

Melissa—is an oil that is powerful as an ANTI-VIRAL agent, yet it is very gentle and very delicate because of the nature of the plant. It has the ability to work with and enhance the gentle aspects of the human body. It is CALMING and UPLIFTING and may help to BALANCE the EMOTIONS. It may also help to remove EMOTIONAL BLOCKS and INSTILL a POSITIVE OUTLOOK on LIFE.

Sandalwood—also, like frankincense, is high in sesquiterpenes, which were discovered to INCREASE the amount of OXYGEN around the PINEAL and PITUITARY GLANDS, thus helping to IMPROVE one's ATTITUDE. It ALLEVIATES

DEPRESSION and assists in the removal of NEGATIVE PROGRAMMING from the cells of the body.

Rose—contains the highest frequency of the oils. It may help ENHANCE the FREQUENCY of every cell, which could help bring BALANCE and HARMONY to the body. It is thought by some to produce a magnetic energy that attracts LOVE and enhances the frequency of SELF-LOVE, bringing JOY to the heart.

Rosewood—may help bring a synergism to all the oils. It is SOOTHING to the SKIN, APPEASING to the MIND, RELAXING to the BODY, and creates a feeling of PEACE and GENTLENESS.

ARRIER OIL CONTAINED IN THIS BLEND: Almond Oil.

ODY SYSTEM(S) AFFECTED: The oils in this blend may help it be effective for dealing with various problems related to EMOTIONAL BALANCE.

ROMATIC INFLUENCE: The aroma of this blend of oils may be a tremendous aid in times of MEDITATION.

PPLICATION: Apply on SHOULDERS, CROWN, CHEST, behind the EARS, NECK, FOREHEAD, and WRISTS. Add to BATH water. Wear as PERFUME or COLOGNE.

AFETY DATA: Avoid exposure to direct SUNLIGHT for 3 to 6 hours after use.

OMPANION OILS: BALANCE with Valor and PROTECT with White Angelica. Use with Inspiration, Awaken, and Sacred Mountain to create a feeling of wholeness in the realm of one's own spirituality and oneness with the CREATOR. When the heart is stressed, use Joy and Aroma Life with White Angelica.

REQUENCY: Physical and Emotional; approximately 89 MHz.

Oil Blends

A Great Help for Alzheimer's Disease

When my mother who has Alzheimer's came to live with us, she didn't sleep at night but was up cleaning out drawers, slamming doors and being generally noisy all night. We were introduced to Young Living Oils and started putting Peace & Calming in a cool mist vaporizer 3-4 times during the day in the living area where she spent her time. In two weeks, she began sleeping ALL NIGHT!!! We've continued using a variety of oils (Lavender, Brain Power, Lemon, Clarity) and she is now in better health than she's been in 20 years. She still has Alzheimer's but her mood is mostly stabilized.

-Submitted by E. Pinar (July 2004)

Animal Scents™ Pet Shampoo

Stop bathing your pet in chemical-laden products. This product gives you natural ingredients, mixed with essential oils, to pamper your pet. Not only will it keep your pet clean, it will also assist in cleansing and healing their cuts and scratches.

Ingredients: Demineralized water; saponified oils of coconut and olive, essential oils (as shown below), vegetable gum, aloe vera, and rosemary extract.

Essential Oils:

Citronella—deodorant; insect repellant; also good for oily skin.

Lavandin—is an anti-fungal, an anti-bacterial, a strong antiseptic, and a tissue regenerator.

Lemon—helps promote leukocyte formation; antiseptic.

Geranium—improves blood flow, regenerates tissue and nerves, cleans oily skin, and ma even liven up pale skin.

Spikenard—anti-bacterial and anti-fungal; helps with staph infections.

Suggested Use: Pour a small amount of Animal Scents' Shampoo into palm and rub gently between hands. Massage thoroughly into pet's wet coat. Lather. Rinse thoroughly. Repeat if necessary.

Body System(s) Affected: SKIN

Precautions: Animal Scents' Shampoo is highly concentrated. If necessary, dilute with water.

Animal Scents™ Pet Ointment

Instead of the harmful chemicals and antibiotics, give your pet the same natural ingredier and powerful germ fighting essential oils that you've come to rely on. This products is wonderfu blend of wholesome herbs and essential oils designed for helping your pet heal from minor skin irritations, cuts, and scrapes. It sure seems to work great on humans as well.

ngredients: Mink oil, lecithin, beeswax, lanolin, sesame seed oil, wheat germ oil, and essential oils as shown below.

> **Not Just for Animals**
> I am a nursing mother and have used geranium and helichrysum applied neat to my nipples followed by Animal Scents Ointment to combat thrush, and have used Animal Scents Ointment to help treat sore nipples, heal diaper rash and prevent stretch marks during pregnancy.
> **-Submitted by A. Cornn, Machesney Park, Illinois (July 2004)**

ssential Oils:

Rosewood—antiseptic and antibacterial; tissue regenerative; soothing to the skin and increases elasticity.

Palmarosa—stimulates new cell growth, regulates oil production, moisturizes and speeds healing.

Patchouli—helps digest toxic material; tones / tightens skin; helps prevent wrinkles.

Myrrh—is soothing to the skin; used for chapped and cracked skin and wrinkles.

Carrot seed—a natural phytonutrient that is rich in beta carotene; helps to reduce wrinkles and dryness.

Melaleuca alternifolia—tissue regenerative; helps promote the healing of wounds.

Rosehip seed—helps reduce scarring and prevent premature aging of the skin.

Geranium—improves blood flow, regenerates tissue and nerves, cleans oily skin, and may even liven up pale skin.

Idaho Balsam Fir—is a rich source of the antioxidant limonene which has been shown to help relieve overworked and tired muscles and joints.

uggested Use: Clean the affected area. Apply as needed. If using additional essential oils, apply oils prior to application of Animal Scents Pet Ointment.

ody System(s) Affected: SKIN

AromaGuard Deodorants

This is one of the most unique deodorant products on the market today. Made with natural ngredients (no toxic aluminum salts or propylene glycol) and bacteria fighting essential oils, these leodorants will help keep your skin clean and fresh while not interfering with the body's natural cooling system. The formulation is also clean and evaporative, with no sticky residue.

ngredients: Coconut oil, white beeswax, pure vegetable esters (34 and 40 from palm kernel and coconut oils), zinc oxide, natural mixed tocopherols (vitamin E), and essential oils as follows:

Mountain Mint Essential Oils:

Lemon—helps promote leukocyte formation; antiseptic.

Rosemary cineol—highly anti-infectious; antifungal and anti-bacterial; good for various skin conditions.

Clove—is anti-bacterial, anti-fungal, anti-infectious, anti-parasitic, a strong antiseptic, anti-viral, and an immune stimulant. It may influence healing and help create a feeling of protection and courage.

Cedarwood—rejuvenating and refreshing; antiseptic and beneficial to the skin.

Blue Cypress (*Callitris intratropica*)—is an abundant source of sesquiterpenes. It is grounding and stabilizing with a fragrance that uplifts and inspires.

May also contain peppermint, eucalyptus, and/or white fir.

Meadow Mist Essential Oils:

Lemon—helps promote leukocyte formation; antiseptic.

Geranium—can be used on almost any kind of skin; cleansing, refreshing, astringent, and a mild skin tonic; used to balance hyposecretion of androgens or estrogens which frequently occurs during menopause.

Rosewood—antiseptic and antibacterial; tissue regenerative; soothing to the skin and increases elasticity.

Rosemary cineol—highly anti-infectious; antifungal and anti-bacterial; good for various skin conditions.

Lavender—balancing and calming; works wherever there is a need; useful for any type of skin condition.

Melaleuca alternifolia—tissue regenerative; helps promote the healing of wounds.

Melaleuca quinquenervia—is powerfully anti-fungal, anti-viral, anti-bacterial; may help protect against radiation and is a strong tissue regenerator.

Clove—is anti-bacterial, anti-fungal, anti-infectious, anti-parasitic, a strong antiseptic, anti-viral, and an immune stimulant. It may influence healing and help create a feeling of protection and courage.

May also contain peppermint, eucalyptus, and/or white fir.

Suggested Use: After bath or shower, apply 3-4 light strokes of AromaGuard to underarms.

Body System(s) Affected: SKIN

Precautions: Skin test first for sensitivity. Note: The authors of this book use these deodorants, and when first beginning to use them, the Mountain Mint deodorant would produce an itchy rash under the arms. The Meadow Mist would not produce the rash. After a few weeks of using the Meadow Mist product, the application of Mountain Mint would not produce the rash and has not since. It seems, therefore, that when switching from chemical-laden commercial products to these deodorants, a cleansing process is required and the Meadow Mist product is recommended for the first while.

Boswellia Wrinkle Creme

Ingredients: Deionized water, calendula extract, chamomile extract, rosebud extract, orange blossom extract, St. John's wort extract, aloe vera gel, kelp extract, *Ginkgo biloba* extract, grapeseed extract, ASC 111, goat's cream, glyceryl stearate, caprylic/capric triglyceride, shea butter, essential oils (as shown below), wolfberry seed oil, stearic acid, stearyl alcohol, sodium PCA, sodium hyaluronate, allantoin, panthenol, retinyl palmitate (vitamin A), and tocopheryl acetate (vitamin E).

Essential Oils:

Frankincense—is high in sesquiterpenes; helps deliver oxygen to the pineal and pituitary glands; improves hGH production; increases leukocyte production,

Sandalwood—helps strengthen the lymphatic systems; revitalizes the skin.

Myrrh—is soothing to the skin; used for chapped and cracked skin and wrinkles.

Geranium—improves blood flow, regenerates tissue and nerves, cleans oily skin, and may even liven up pale skin.

Ylang Ylang—balances secretion of sebum (a waxy oil produced by the skin); energizing and uplifting.

Instructions: Apply directly to skin. Boswellia Wrinkle Creme is a collagen builder. Used daily, it will help minimize and prevent wrinkles. Put small amount in hand, emulsify, and apply to face and neck using upward strokes.

Body System(s) Affected: SKIN.

Cinnamint Lip Balm

Ingredients: Sweet almond oil, beeswax, MSM, wolfberry (*Lycium barbarum*) seed oil, essential oils (as shown below), hemp seed oil, orange wax, orange oil, tocopheryl palmitate (vitamin E), ascorbyl palmitate (vitamin A), ascorbic acid (vitamin C), and citric acid.

Essential Oils:

Peppermint—enhances the effect of the other oils; cooling and soothing sensations; invigorates the skin and helps with nerve regeneration. It also enhances digestion and increases endurance.

Spearmint—brings soothing relief to dry skin.

Cinnamon Bark—is a powerful purifier and a powerful oxygenator; it enhances the actic and the activity of the other oils while its warming action balances the cooling effect of the mint oils to bring comfortable relief to dry, chapped lips.

Instructions: To soften and moisturize lips, apply Cinnamint Lip Balm as often as needed.

Body System(s) Affected: SKIN.

ClaraDerm

This product, packaged in a spray bottle, is a blend of essential oils that are most soothin and nourishing to the skin. Designed to be used topically on skin that is stressed before and after childbirth, these oils help to relieve skin irritation and itching, and may also improve skin elasticit

Essential Oils:

Myrrh—is soothing to the skin; used for chapped and cracked skin and wrinkles.

Melaleuca alternifolia—tissue regenerative; helps promote the healing of wounds.

Lavender—balancing and calming; works wherever there is a need; useful for any type o skin condition.

Frankincense—is high in sesquiterpenes; helps deliver oxygen to the pineal and pituitary glands; improves hGH production; increases leukocyte production,

Roman Chamomile—helps increase the regenerative ability of the skin; blood cleanser.

Helichrysum—may help cleanse the blood and improve circulatory functions. It is anti-catarrhal in structure and nature.

Ingredients: Essential oils come in a base of fractionated coconut oil.

Suggested Use: Spray topically on location.

Body System(s) Affected: SKIN

Dentarome/Dentarome Plus Toothpaste

A revolutionary antimicrobial essential-oil-fortified toothpaste. It is an all-natural toothpaste that includes a highly antimicrobial blend of pure plant-derived essential oils. It contains no sugar, saccharine, sodium lauryl sulfate, or synthetic chemicals, colors, or eservatives of any kind. This formula was tested at Weber State University and found to have tent antimicrobial properties against a wide range of oral microbes including *streptococcus alis, streptococcus pneumoniae, bramunella catarrhalis, and candida albicans.* Other studies nfirm the plaque-fighting and antimicrobial attributes of the essential oils included in Dentarome d Dentarome Plus, including one study published in the International Journal of Food icrobiology that found the essential oils of thyme, clove, and cinnamon to exhibit antimicrobial fects. Another study listed peppermint as one of the most potent essential oils against plaque-using elements. **The added thymol and eugenol in Dentarome Plus are derived from pure yme (*Thymus vulgaris*) and clove (*Eugenia caryophyllata*) oils and enhance its antimicrobial tency**.

gredients:

Baking Soda—a mild abrasive and fast-acting cleansing agent.

Deionized Water—added for consistency.

Vegetable Glycerin—used as a moistener.

Xanthum Gum—a natural thickener.

Ionic Minerals—added as a nutritional supplement and together with the essential oil of wintergreen, help to strengthen teeth.

Thymol & Eugenol—added to Dentarome Plus for more powerful antiseptic and antimicrobial effects. Thymol is derived from thyme oil (*thymus vulgaris*) and eugenol is derived from clove oil (*eugenia caryophyllata*).

Stevioside—a natural, intensely sweet extract from a tropical plant native to South America.

ssential Oils:

Wintergreen—used here to help strengthen teeth. Also antimicrobial in nature.

Peppermint—used as a natural flavoring, breath-freshening agent.

Thieves—a proprietary blend of clove, lemon, cinnamon bark, *Eucalyptus radiata*, rosemary, and other essential oils which has been documented to be highly antibacterial and antimicrobial in nature.

Dentarome Ultra Toothpaste

This product contains a revolutionary formula of all-natural, edible ingredients. Created to gentle on teeth enamel, the calcium carbonate and zinc oxide in this toothpaste are substantially aller in particle size than other popular commercial toothpastes. Add to that the germ and cavity ghting power of the essential oils and other ingredients, and this toothpaste is ultimate in dental re.

Personal Care Products

Ingredients: Calcium carbonate, essential oil concentrate containing peppermint essential oil, Thieves essential oil blend, zinc oxide, deionized water with papain, xylitol, vegetable glycerine, essential oil base (thymol from *Thymus vulgaris*, *Eucalyptus globulus*, and methyl salycilate from wintergreen), xanthum gum, zinc citrate, and stevioside.

Essential Oils:

Peppermint—used as a natural flavoring, breath-freshening agent.

Thieves—a proprietary blend of clove, lemon, cinnamon bark, *Eucalyptus radiata*, rosemary, and other essential oils which has been documented to be highly antibacterial and antimicrobial in nature.

Thyme—contains 46% thymol–one of the most potently antimicrobial natural substance known. It has been studied in Europe for its effects against bronchitis, laryngitis and tonsillitis.

Eucalyptus—contains eucalyptol, also known as 1,8-cineol.

Wintergreen—used here to help strengthen teeth. Also antimicrobial in nature.

Essential Waters (Hydrosols)

Essential waters (hydrosols) are the by-product of the steam distillation process for essential oils. They have similar properties to those of the essential oils, but in lower concentrations. This makes them gentle enough to be used by all age groups, even babies and children. Essential waters are rehydrating, nurturing, and protective to the skin. They are also uniquely uplifting, calming, soothing, relaxing, and restorative.

Caution: DO NOT SPRAY DIRECTLY INTO EARS OR EYES.

How to Use:

1. Diffuse using the Essential Mist Diffuser.
2. Mist into the air to freshen the home or office.
3. Mist into the dryer to lightly scent clothing and linen.
3. Mist in an airplane or other enclosed environment to dispel and sanitize stale air.
4. Mist on the face to energize, and overcome fatigue and drowsiness.
5. Drink undiluted or diluted to taste with water or juice.
6. Mist on animals to deter pests.
7. Mist on plants to deter pests.

Lavender Essential Water—is soothing to the skin and is gently calming and relaxing. Spray o skin or mist in air to promote sleep. Can also be used in hair or makeup routines.

elissa Essential Water—is exquisitely relaxing and uplifting. It can be used to help with herpes sores. In lab tests, it has been shown to be antimicrobial against *Streptococcus haemolytica*, which can colonize in the throat and esophagus.

ountain Essence Essential Water—is a hydrosol of White fir (*Abies grandis*). It is antibacterial, energizing, and helps to enhance the respiratory action. It is wonderful for refreshing and sanitizing stale hotel rooms.

eppermint Essential Water—is uplifting, energizing, cooling, refreshing, and soothing to digestion. It also increases endurance.

ed Cedar Essential Water—is a hydrosol of Western Red cedar leaf and is antiseptic and calming. It can also have powerful effects on the unconscious and subconscious mind.

asil Essential Water—has antidepressant, anti-inflammatory, and antispasmodic properties; relaxing to spastic muscles, including those that contribute to headaches and migraines.

lary Sage Essential Water—may be beneficial for regulating cells and balancing the hormones. It may calm and enhance the dream state, helping to bring about a feeling of euphoria.

daho Tansy Essential Water—is anti-viral and may help support the immune system. Its aroma is uplifting and promotes a general sense of well-being.

pearmint Essential Water—acts as an anti-depressant by relieving mental strain and fatigue, and by lifting one's spirits.

Fresh Essence Mouthwash

The ultimate oral rinse, formulated with antimicrobial therapeutic-grade essential oils that aturally contain compounds which have been clinically proven to kill microbes that can cause bad reath, plaque, and periodontal diseases like gingivitis. It is formulated with a patented liposome chnology (using soy-derived lecithin), which binds the essential oils to the mucus membrane side the mouth to provide long-lasting germ-killing and breath-freshening protection. As an all-atural mouth and gum care product, Fresh Essence Antiseptic Mouthwash contains absolutely **no yes, no alcohol, no saccharin, and no synthetic flavors or preservatives**.

Unlike some commercially available products which contain just the active constituents of ıymol, eucalyptol, methyl salicylate, and menthol, Fresh Essence Antiseptic Mouthwash uses the ntire essential oil. The complete oil exhibits far stronger antimicrobial power than its active onstituents alone. From his research on the essential oil of eucalyptus, Jean Valnet, M.D. made e following statement. "The antiseptic properties of the essences of eucalyptus were much more owerful than those of its principle constituent, eucalyptol." The whole oil is also safer because it ontains a natural balance of elements that make it relatively harmless to human tissue.

Essential Oils:

Thyme—contains 46% thymol–one of the most potently antimicrobial natural substance known. It has been studied in Europe for its effects against bronchitis, laryngitis and tonsillitis.

Eucalyptus—contains eucalyptol, also known as 1,8 cineol.

Wintergreen—contains methyl salicylate.

Peppermint—contains natural menthol.

Thieves—is a proprietary blend of clove, lemon, cinnamon bark, *Eucalyptus radiata*, rosemary, and other essential oils which has been documented to be highly antibacterial and antimicrobial in nature.

Ingredients: Other ingredients include deionized water, lecithin, steviocide (a naturally sweet plant extract), and 1/3 of 1% poloxamer 407 (a food-grade dispersing agent).

Instructions: Gargle with each morning and before bed.

Fresh Essence Plus Mouthwash

The ultimate oral rinse with an extra boost. Formulated the same as Fresh Essence Mouthwash, but with the liposome concentrate containing larger amounts of the following:

Essential Oils:

Peppermint—contains natural menthol; helps reduce pain; helps calm the stomach. It also enhances digestion and increases endurance.

Thieves—is a proprietary blend of clove, lemon, cinnamon bark, *Eucalyptus radiata*, rosemary, and other essential oils which has been documented to be highly antibacterial and antimicrobial in nature.

Spearmint—used as a natural flavoring, breath-freshening agent.

Vetiver—is high in sesquiterpenes; fixative; helps stabilize essential oils.

Ingredients: Other ingredients include deionized water, peppermint floral water, melissa floral water, and colloidal silver.

Genesis Hand & Body Lotion

The essential oils in this product are beneficial for feeding, nurturing, and hydrating the skin. Excellent for rough, dry skin, wrinkles, and premature aging.

Ingredients: Deionized water, MSM, glyceryl stearate, stearic acid, glycerin, grapeseed extract, sodium hyaluronate, sorbitol, rosehip seed oil, shea butter, mango butter, wheat germ oil, kukui nut oil, lecithin, safflower oil, apricot oil, almond oil, tocopheryl acetate (vitamin E), retinyl palmitate (vitamin A), jojoba oil, sesame oil, calendula extract, orage blossom extract, St. John's wort extract, algae extract, aloe vera gel, ascorbic acid (vitamin C), ginkgo biloba extract, essential oils (as shown below), and honeysuckle and gardenia fragrance oils.

Essential Oils:

Bergamot—helps to relieve anxiety, stress, and tension; helps to balance the hormones.

Geranium—can be used on almost any kind of skin; cleansing, refreshing, astringent, and a mild skin tonic; used to balance hyposecretion of androgens or estrogens which frequently occurs during menopause.

Jasmine—deeply penetrating effect on the skin; produces a feeling of confidence, energy, euphoria, and optimism.

Lemon—helps promote leukocyte formation; antiseptic.

Palmarosa—stimulates new cell growth, regulates oil production, moisturizes and speeds healing.

Roman Chamomile—helps increase the regenerative ability of the skin; blood cleanser.

Rosewood—antiseptic and antibacterial; tissue regenerative; soothing to the skin and increases elasticity.

Ylang Ylang—stimulating; helps to balance male-female energies.

May also contain patchouli.

Instructions: Dispense in hand and apply directly to skin.

Body System(s) Affected: SKIN.

Warning: Avoid eye contact. If contact occurs, rinse thoroughly with water.

KidScents Lotion

An extraordinarily gentle and safe lotion with the ideal pH for moisturizing, softening, and protecting young skin. It contains all natural ingredients and therapeutic-grade essential oils with no mineral oils, synthetic perfumes, artificial colorings, or toxic ingredients.

Ingredients: Deionized water, methylsulfonylmethane (MSM), glyceryl stearate, stearic acid, glycerin, grape (*Vitis vinifera*) seed extract, sodium hyaluronate, sorbitol, rose (*Rosa rugosa*) hip seed oil, shea butter, mango (*Mangifera indica*) butter, wheat germ oil, kukui

(*Aleurites moluccana*) nut oil, lecithin, safflower (*Carthamus tinctorius*) oil, apricot (*Prunus armeniaca*) kernal oil, almond (*Prunus amygdalus dulcis*) oil, tocopheryl acetate (vitamin E), retinyl palmitate (vitamin A), jojoba (*Buxus chinensis*) oil, seasame (*Sesamum indicum*) oil, *Calendula officinalis* extract, chamomile (*Anthemis nobilis*) extract, orange (*Citrus aurantium dulcis*) blossom extract, St. John's Wort (*Hypericum perforatum*) extract, algae (*Gellidiela acerosa*) extract, aloe vera (*Aloe barbadensis*) gel ascorbic acid (vitamin C), *Ginkgo biloba* extract, and pure therapeutic-grade essential oil (as listed below).

Essential Oils:

Cedarwood—rejuvenating and refreshing; antiseptic and beneficial to the skin.

Western Red Cedar—anti-bacterial; antiseptic; calming.

Rosewood—antiseptic and antibacterial; tissue regenerative; soothing to the skin and increases elasticity.

Geranium—improves blood flow, regenerates tissue and nerves, cleans oily skin, and ma even liven up pale skin.

Instructions: Apply KidScents Lotion liberally to the skin.

Common Sense Caution: While KidScents products contain no harmful ingredients, store out of reach of children to prevent messy spills. Children do not like lotion in their mouth or eyes. Use with gentle care.

KidScents Tender Tush

This product is a mild, soothing, and gentle ointment designed to protect and nourish young skin and promote healing. It contains all natural ingredients and therapeutic-grade essential oils with no mineral oils, synthetic perfumes, artificial colorings, or toxic ingredients. It is particularly useful for diaper rash and other skin irritations.

Ingredients: Coconut (*Cocos nucifera*) oil, cocoa (*Theobroma cacao*) butter, bees wax, wheat germ oil, olive (*Olea europaea*) oil, almond (*Prunus amygdalus dulcis*) oil, and pure therapeutic-grade essential oils (as listed below).

Essential Oils:

Sandalwood—helps strengthen the lymphatic systems; revitalizes the skin.

Rosewood—antiseptic and antibacterial; tissue regenerative; soothing to the skin and increases elasticity.

Roman Chamomile—helps increase the regenerative ability of the skin; blood cleanser.

Lavender—balancing and calming; works wherever there is a need; useful for any type of skin condition.

Cistus—has anti-bacterial, anti-infectious, and anti-viral properties. Because it is high in oxygenating molecules, it may assist the auto-immune system and may help strengthen the immune system.

Blue Tansy—may help cleanse the liver and calm the lymphatic system to help rid one of anger and promote a feeling of self-control.

Frankincense—is anti-inflammatory; high in sesquiterpenes; helps deliver oxygen to the pineal and pituitary glands; improves hGH production; increases leukocyte production.

Instructions: Apply liberally to the skin on the bottom or wherever it is needed.

Common Sense Caution: While KidScents products contain no harmful ingredients, store out of reach of children to prevent messy spills. Children do not like ointments in their mouth or eyes. Use with gentle care.

Body System(s) Affected: SKIN.

KidScents Toothpaste

This product is a completely safe and natural alternative to other commercial toothpastes. It is fluoride free and contains all natural ingredients and therapeutic-grade essential oils with no synthetic dyes or flavorings. It is safe to swallow with a great Bubble Gum flavor.

Ingredients: Calcium carbonate (tooth health agent), deionized water (consistency), colloidal silver (tooth health agent), strawberry flavor (natural flavor), vegetable glycerin (moistener), zinc oxide (tooth health agent), xanthum gum (natural thickener), ionic minerals (tooth and gum support), xylitol (tooth and gum support), stevioside (natural flavor), and pure therapeutic-grade essential oils (as listed below).

Essential Oils:

Peppermint—used as a natural flavoring, breath-freshening agent.

Spearmint—used as a natural flavoring, breath-freshening agent.

Orange—used as a natural flavor, it also contains over 91% d-limonene (which helps to promote normal cell life cycles); rich in stress-reducing compounds.

Lemon—used as a natural flavor, it also contains over 65% d-limonene (which helps to promote normal cell life cycles); helps promote leukocyte formation; helps to dissolve cholesterol and fats.

Thieves—is a proprietary blend of clove, lemon, cinnamon bark, *Eucalyptus radiata*, rosemary, and other essential oils which has been documented to be highly antibacterial and antimicrobial in nature.

Instructions: Brush teeth and gums thoroughly morning and night.

Common Sense Caution: While KidScents products contain no harmful ingredients, store out of reach of children to prevent messy spills. Use with gentle care.

LavaDerm Cooling Mist

This Cooling Mist provides wonderful relief to any type of burn, from the lightest sunburn to the most serious 3rd degree burn. It quickly cools and hydrates the skin and speeds healing and tissue regeneration.

Ingredients: Re-structured water, lavender floral water, aloe vera gel, and lavender essential oil.

Instructions: Mist directly on area of concern as often as needed to keep the skin cool and promote regeneration.

Body System(s) Affected: EMOTIONAL BALANCE, SKIN.

Lavender Volume Conditioner

This is a fabulous nourishing, volumizing rinse that utilizes vitamins, amino acids, MSM, and essential oils to support and feed fine hair.

Ingredients: Natural vegetable fatty acid base (saponified coconut oil), MSM, milk protein, phospholipids, amino acids cysteine (and) cysteine 8 methionine, glyco protein (glycogen and mucopolysaccharides), quinoa extract, rosemary extract, sage extract, horsetail extract, coltsfoot extract, hydrolyzed wheat protein, hydrolyzed soy protein, retinyl palmitate (vitamin A), ascorbic acid (vitamin C), tocopheryl acetate (vitamin E), panthenol (vitamin B5), grapeseed extract, and essential oils (as shown below).

Essential Oils:

Lavender—balancing and calming; works wherever there is a need; useful for any type of skin condition.

Clary Sage—astringent; good for cell regulation, cholesterol, and dry skin.

Lemon—helps promote leukocyte formation; antiseptic.

Jasmine—deeply penetrating effect on the skin; produces a feeling of confidence, energy, euphoria, and optimism.

structions: Apply Lavender Volume Conditioner through the hair. Leave on hair for a few seconds for light conditioning or for several minutes for deep conditioning. Rinse well. *For maximum benefit, leave on 2 to 5 minutes.*

Lavender Volume Shampoo

As this shampoo is formulated for the gentle cleansing of fine hair, it makes an excellent ampoo for babies and children.

gredients: Coconut oil, decyl polyglucose, MSM, vegetable protein (wheat, oat, and soya), deionized water, nettle extract, mushroom extract, billberry extract, sugar cane extract, lemon extract, sugar maple extract, orange extract, essential oils (as shown below), aloe vera gel, retinyl palmitate (vitamin A), ascorbic acid (vitamin C), tocopheryl acetate (vitamin E), panthenol (vitamin B5), grapeseed extract, inositol, and niacin.

ssential Oils:

Lavender—balancing and calming; works wherever there is a need; useful for any type of skin condition.

Clary Sage—astringent; good for cell regulation, cholesterol, and dry skin.

Lemon—helps promote leukocyte formation; antiseptic.

Jasmine—deeply penetrating effect on the skin; produces a feeling of confidence, energy, euphoria, and optimism.

structions: Wet hair thoroughly. Apply small amount of Lavender Volume Shampoo. Massage thoroughly into hair and scalp. Rinse well. Repeat if desired. *For maximum benefit, leave on 2 to 5 minutes.*

Lemon Sage Clarifying Conditioner

This is a fabulous clarifying rinse that utilizes vitamins, amino acids, MSM, and essential ils to support and feed hair of all types without buildup.

ngredients: Natural vegetable fatty acid base (saponified coconut oil), MSM, milk protein, phospholipids, Chenopodium quinoa extract, rosemary extract, sage extract, horsetail extract, coltsfoot extract, hydrolyzed wheat protein, hydrolyzed soy protein, retinyl palmitate (vitamin A), ascorbic acid (vitamin C), essential oils (as shown below), amino acids cysteine (and) cysteine 8 methionine, glyco protein (glycogen and mucopolysaccharides), grapeseed extract, tocopheryl acetate (vitamin E), and panthenol (vitamin B5).

Essential Oils:

Lemon—helps promote leukocyte formation; antiseptic.

Pine—was used by the American Indians to repel lice and flees; antimicrobial and antiviral; may also be good against skin parasites.

Lime—helps remove dead skin cells; tightens skin and connective tissue.

Geranium—improves blood flow, regenerates tissue and nerves, cleans oily skin, and m even liven up pale skin.

Roman Chamomile—helps increase the regenerative ability of the skin; blood cleanser.

Ylang Ylang—has been used historically in hair preparations to promote thick, shiny, lustrous hair and to help control split ends.

Sage—helps balance hormone levels; may also help with dandruff and hair loss.

Instructions: Apply Lemon Sage Clarifying Conditioner through the hair. Leave on hair for a few seconds for light conditioning or for several minutes for deep conditioning. Rinse well. *For maximum benefit, leave on 2 to 5 minutes.*

Lemon Sage Clarifying Shampoo

This shampoo is formulated with herbal extracts, vitamins, and essential oils to naturally remove buildup of styling products and return hair to its natural healthy shine.

Ingredients: Coconut oil, olive oil, decylpolyglucose, MSM, vegetable protein (wheat, oat, soya deionized water, nettle extract, mushroom extract, billberry extract, sugar cane extract, lemon extract, sugar maple extract, orange extract, essential oils (as shown below), aloe vera gel, retinyl palmitate (vitamin A), ascorbic acid (vitamin C), tocopheryl acetate (vitamin E), panthenol (vitamin B5), grapeseed extract, inositol, and niacin.

Essential Oils:

Lemon—helps promote leukocyte formation; antiseptic.

Lime—helps remove dead skin cells; tightens skin and connective tissue.

Pine—was used by the American Indians to repel lice and flees; antimicrobial and antiviral; may also be good against skin parasites.

Geranium—improves blood flow, regenerates tissue and nerves, cleans oily skin, and ma even liven up pale skin.

Roman Chamomile—helps increase the regenerative ability of the skin; blood cleanser.
Ylang Ylang—has been used historically in hair preparations to promote thick, shiny, lustrous hair and to help control split ends.
Sage—helps balance hormone levels; may also help with dandruff and hair loss.

nstructions: Wet hair thoroughly. Apply small amount of Lemon Sage Clarifying Shampoo. Massage thoroughly into hair and scalp. Rinse well. Repeat if desired. *For maximum benefit, leave on 2 to 5 minutes.*

NeuroGen

Moisturizing Lotion

An excellent moisturizing lotion for deeper layers of the skin that can be damaged by xcessive sun and wind exposure. By providing the proper nutrients to tissue layers beneath the urface of the skin, moisture and natural health is restored. Additionally, many of the ingredients nd essential oils in this lotion contain properties that may help support and even regenerate amaged nerves.

ngredients: Deionized water, pregnenolone, lecithin, MSM, essential oils (as shown below), caprylic/capric triglyceride, sorbitol, wolfberry seed oil, shea butter, glyceryl stearate, linseed oil, aloe barbadensis gel, sodium PCA, stearic acid, *Calendulla officinalis* extract, German chamomile extract, rosebud extract, orange flower extract, wild yam extract, algae extract, tocopheryl acetate (vitamin E), hydrolyzed wheat protein, locust bean gum, allantoin, natural progesterone (from soybean extract), kelp, retinyl palmitate (vitamin A), tocopheryl linoleate (vitamin E), and ascorbic acid (vitamin C).

ssential Oils:

Lemongrass—helps repair connective tissue; it helps stimulate the agents in the tissue to rejuvenate and reconnect; helps regulate the parasympathetic nervous system and strengthen vascular walls.
Peppermint—invigorating to the skin; soothing and relaxing to tired muscles; may also help with nerve regeneration. It also enhances digestion and increases endurance.
Douglas Fir—calming to tired and overworked joints; very soothing to sore muscles.
Juniper—antispasmodic; helps reduce muscle aches/pains; may also help nerve function and regeneration.
May also contain helichrysum, frankincense, and spearmint essential oils.

ody System(s) Affected: HORMONAL and NERVOUS SYSTEMS, MUSCLES and BONES.

Personal Care Products

Orange Blossom Facial Wash

Ingredients: Deionized water, calendula extract, chamomile extract, rosebud extract, orange blossom extract, St. John's wort extract, algae, aloe vera gel, kelp extract, *Ginkgo bilobc* extract, grapeseed extract, decyl polyglucose, MSM, wolfberry seed oil, essential oils (as shown below), multifruit acid complex, hydrolyzed wheat protein, citric acid, dimethyl lauramine oleate.

Essential Oils:

Lavender—balancing and calming; works wherever there is a need; useful for any type c skin condition.

Lemon—helps promote leukocyte formation; helps brighten a pale, dull complexion by removing the dead skin cells.

Rosemary verbenon—is milder than rosemary cineol and better suited for skin care.

Patchouli—helps digest toxic material; tones / tightens skin; helps prevent wrinkles.

Instructions: Apply warm water to the face to moisten skin. Apply wash directly to the face anc gently massage in a gentle circular motion creating a lather. Rinse thoroughly and gently pat dry. For best results, use Orange Blossom Facial Wash twice daily. Follow up with Sandalwood Toner and Sandalwood Moisture Creme to promote younger and healthier looking skin.

Body System(s) Affected: SKIN.

Prenolone / Prenolone+

Moisturizing Cream

This cream utilizes natural pregnenolone (called the "Master Hormone" because it is a precursor to all the other hormones produced within the body including progesterone, estrogen, an testosterone) and a small amount of natural progesterone (derived from soy) to replenish and softe dry or irritated skin. With the help of the essential oils that are included in this formulation, the pregnenolone is quickly and efficiently transferred to the cellular level where it can be converted into the appropriate hormone that the body needs at that particular time. Unlike many natural progesterone creams, there is not the need to regulate the use of this cream as the body can eliminate what is not needed without any side effects. Also, unlike other natural hormone creams, this one can also be used by men. Similar natural hormone creams have been found to help with the following: wrinkles, libido (restores), blood sugar levels (normalizes), cell oxygen levels (restores), bone density (improves), weight control (helps use fat for energy), zinc and copper levels (normalizes), blood clotting (normalizes), thyroid action, breast cancer and fibroids (protect ainst), headaches, asthma, backaches, infertility, hair loss, depression, hypoglycemia, lammation, exhaustion, insomnia, arthritis, and more. **The regular Prenolone contains all the ne ingredients as Prenolone+ without the addition of DHEA.**

gredients: Deionized water, MSM, caprylic/capric triglyceride, sorbitol, pregnenolone, lecithin, wolfberry seed oil, shea butter, glyceryl stearate, aloe vera gel, sodium PCA, stearic acid, calendula extract, chamomile extract, rosebud extract, orange blossom extract, St. John's wort extract, *Ginkgo biloba* extract, grapeseed extract, algae extract, tocopheryl acetate (vitamin E), hydrolyzed wheat protein, locust bean gum, ionic trace minerals, flax seed oil, vitamin E (from wheat germ oil), ylang ylang essential oil (see below), allantoin, wild yam, ginseng, Clary sage essential oil (see below), blue cohosh, black cohosh, kelp, retinyl palmitate (vitamin A), tocopheryl linoleate, essential oils of bergamot, fennel, geranium, sage, and yarrow (see below), DHEA (only in Prenolone+), progesterone, and ascorbic acid (vitamin C).

sential Oils:

Geranium—can be used on almost any kind of skin; cleansing, refreshing, astringent, and a mild skin tonic; used to balance hyposecretion of androgens or estrogens which frequently occurs during menopause.

> "...Geranium is an adrenal cortex stimulant. The hormones secreted by the adrenal cortex are primarily regulators, governing the balance of hormones secreted by other organs, including male and female sex hormones; so it is of great assistance in menopausal problems and all conditions where fluctuating hormone balance is indicated. In particular, geranium may be used to relieve pre-menstrual tension, and here its diuretic properties also enter into play, helping to relieve the excessive fluid retention which many women experience premenstrually."
> –Patricia Davis

Ylang Ylang—stimulating and helps to balance male-female energies.

Clary Sage—helps balance the hormones; tonic to the reproductive system.

Bergamot—helps to relieve anxiety, stress, and tension; helps to balance the hormones.

Fennel—helps balance the hormones.

Sage—contains estriol and has estrogen-like properties; believed to contain elements that contribute to the secretion of progesterone.

Yarrow—anti-inflammatory; antiseptic; excellent for menstrual problems.

May also contain fleabane essential oil.

structions: Apply ¼ to ½ tsp. one to two times daily for 21 continuous days. Discontinue use for 7 days and repeat. Massage cream thoroughly into soft tissue areas of the body (inside thigh, stomach, breasts, etc.) until absorbed. Individual needs may vary.

Body System(s) Affected: EMOTIONAL BALANCE, HORMONAL and NERVOUS SYSTEMS, MUSCLES and BONES, SKIN.

Warnings: Application is intended for external use. If pregnant or under a doctor's care, consu your physician. Keep in a cool, dry place. Do not expose to excessive heat. Keep out o the reach of children.

Companion Products: FemiGen (an herbal complex for supporting the female reproductive system), Dragon Time oil blend, Thyromin (for thyroid support).

Progessence Cream

This cream contains natural progesterone (derived from soy), MSM, and wolfberry oil t moisturize and nourish dry skin. With the help of the essential oils that are included in this formulation, the progesterone is quickly and efficiently transferred to the cellular level where it c be utilized by the body. Natural hormone creams like this one have been found to help with the following: wrinkles, libido (restores), blood sugar levels (normalizes), cell oxygen levels (restore bone density (improves), weight control (helps use fat for energy), zinc and copper levels (normalizes), blood clotting (normalizes), thyroid action, breast cancer and fibroids (protects against), headaches, asthma, backaches, infertility, hair loss, depression, hypoglycemia, inflammation, exhaustion, insomnia, arthritis, and more.

Ingredients: Deionized water, MSM, caprylic/capric triglyceride, sorbitol, wolfberry oil, shea butter, glyceryl stearate, aloe vera gel, sodium PCA, stearic acid, calendula extract, chamomile extract, rosebud extract, orange blossom, St. John's wort extract, *Ginkgo biloba* extract, grapeseed extract, algae extract, tocopheryl acetate (vitamin E), hydrolyz wheat protein, locus bean gum, allantoin, lecithin, kelp, retinyl palmitate (vitamin A), tocopheryl linoleate, ascorbic acid (vitamin C), progesterone (from soybean extract), eleuthero (*Eleuthero coccus senticosus*), trace minerals complex, ylang ylang essential c (see below), Clary sage essential oil (see below), Canadian fleabane essential oil (see below), flax seed oil, wheat germ oil, wild yam extract, black cohosh, blue cohosh, and t essential oils of geranium, fennel, yarrow, and sage (see below).

Essential Oils:

Ylang Ylang—stimulating and helps to balance male-female energies.

Clary Sage—helps balance the hormones; tonic to the reproductive system.

Canadian Fleabane—is a rare essential oil studied for its ability to stimulate the pancre and liver and counteract retarded puberty. It is a mood enhancer and promoter c hGH.

Geranium—can be used on almost any kind of skin; cleansing, refreshing, astringent, and a mild skin tonic; used to balance hyposecretion of androgens or estrogens which frequently occurs during menopause.

Fennel—helps balance the hormones.

Yarrow—anti-inflammatory; antiseptic; excellent for menstrual problems.

Sage—contains estriol and has estrogen-like properties; believed to contain elements that contribute to the secretion of progesterone.

structions: Apply ¼ to ½ tsp. one to two times daily for 21 continuous days. Discontinue use for 7 days and repeat. Massage cream thoroughly into soft tissue areas of the body (inside thigh, stomach, etc.) until absorbed. Individual needs may vary.

ody System(s) Affected: EMOTIONAL BALANCE, HORMONAL and NERVOUS SYSTEMS, MUSCLES and BONES, SKIN.

arnings: Application is intended for external use. If pregnant or under a doctor's care, consult your physician. Keep in a cool, dry place. Do not expose to excessive heat. Keep out of the reach of children.

ompanion Products: FemiGen (an herbal complex for supporting the female reproductive system), Dragon Time oil blend, Thyromin (for thyroid support).

Protec

Designed for topical use only, it should never be taken orally. This formula was esigned to accompany the nightlong retention enema. It helps buffer the prostate from flammation, enlargement, and tumor activity. Also suitable for women as a nightlong retention ouche.

gredients:

Olive Oil—moisturizing agent.

Grape Seed Oil—antioxidant; rich in bioflavonoids; helps maintain pH balance.

Sweet Almond Oil—nourishes the skin will reducing friction for smoother application.

Wheat Germ Oil—high in natural vitamins E and B and lecithin; natural antioxidant; useful for reducing scar tissue and stretch marks; acts as a preservative for the other base oils.

Vitamin E Oil—natural antioxidant; protects and promotes regeneration of the skin.

Essential Oils:

Frankincense—anti-tumoral and anti-inflammatory; good for prostate problems.

Myrrh—anti-inflammatory and antiseptic; helps to decongest the prostate gland.

Sage—contains estriol and has estrogen-like properties; may help improve estrogen and progesterone-testosterone balance.

Cumin—anti-bacterial; antispasmodic; some anti-tumoral properties.

Instructions: For the retention enema or douche, use ½ to 1 oz. and hold all night long for 21 consecutive nights. If irritation occurs, discontinue use for three days before restarting.

Body System(s) Affected: HORMONAL SYSTEM.

Regenolone

Moisturizing Cream

This cream utilizes natural pregnenolone (called the "Master Hormone" because it is a precursor to all the other hormones produced within the body including progesterone, estrogen, a testosterone) and a small amount of natural progesterone (derived from soy) to replenish and soft dry or irritated skin. With the essential oils that are included, this product may be effective in promoting the regeneration of damaged nerves and tissues.

Ingredients: Deionized water, MSM, caprylic/capric triglyceride, sorbitol, wolfberry oil, shea butter, glyceryl stearate, aloe vera gel, sodium PCA, stearic acid, calendula extract, chamomile extract, rosebud extract, orange blossom extract, St. John's wort extract, *Gingko biloba* extract, grapeseed extract, algae extract, tocopheryl acetate (vitamin E), hydrolyzed wheat protein, locust bean gum, allantoin, lecithin, kelp, retinyl palmitate, tocopheryl linoleate, ascorbic acid (vitamin C), progesterone, pregnenolone, wild yam, ginseng, flax seed, trace minerals, vitamin E (from wheat germ), blue cohosh, and essent oils (as shown below).

Essential Oils:

Wintergreen—has a cortisone-like action that helps to reduce inflammation in the tissue contains methyl salicylate.

Douglas Fir—calming to tired and overworked joints; very soothing to sore muscles.

Peppermint—invigorating to the skin; soothing and relaxing to tired muscles; may also help with nerve regeneration.

Oregano—powerful antimicrobial; anti-inflammatory; locally warming.

May also contain spearmint essential oil.

ıstructions: Apply ⅛ to ¼ tsp. on location as needed. Individual needs may vary. May be best not to use more than 5 times a day.

ody System(s) Affected: HORMONAL and NERVOUS SYSTEMS, MUSCLES and BONES, SKIN.

Varnings: Application is intended for external use. If pregnant or under a doctor's care, consult your physician. Keep in a cool, dry place. Do not expose to excessive heat. Keep out of the reach of children.

:ompanion Oils: Oregano, thyme, Dragon Time, Mister.

:ompanion Products: Prenolone/Prenolone+, ThermaMist Oral Spray, Thyromin (for thyroid support).

Rose Ointment

Dramatically improves the effectiveness of other essential oils that are applied for skin onditions. When applied on top of oils such as PanAway, lavender, helichrysum, and Melrose, ıis product seals in the volatile constituents of the essential oil, increasing their effectiveness by rolonging their contact with the skin. It also helps maintain the natural pH balance of the skin, onserve its acid mantle, and balance the slight drying effect that some essential oils may have on ıe skin.

ngredients: Lecithin (natural dispersing agent; used in place of sodium lauryl sulfate), lanolin (taken from sheep wool; excellent for skin care), beeswax (used as the thickening and stabilizing agent), mink oil (nurture and regenerate the skin), sesame seed oil (high in linoleic acid; maintains pH balance of the skin), vitamin E oil (antioxidant; excellent for the skin and the cells of the skin), rosehip seed oil (helps reduce scarring and premature aging), and essential oils (as shown below).

:ssential Oils:

Carrot seed—a natural phytonutrient that is rich in beta carotene; helps to reduce wrinkles and dryness.

Melaleuca—tissue regenerative; helps promote the healing of wounds.

Myrrh—helps to heal chapped or cracked skin and reduce inflammation.

Palmarosa—stimulates new cell growth, regulates oil production, moisturizes and speeds healing.

Patchouli—for protection against UV radiation and for tissue regeneration; helps tighten loose skin and prevent wrinkles.
Rosewood—tissue regenerative; soothing to the skin and increases elasticity.
Rose otto—brings balance and harmony by enhancing the frequency of every cell.

Instructions: Apply directly to skin.

Body System(s) Affected: SKIN.

Rosewood Moisturizing Conditioner

This is a fabulous nourishing, moisturizing rinse that utilizes vitamins, amino acids, MSM and essential oils to support and feed dry hair.

Ingredients: Natural vegetable fatty acid base, MSM, milk protein, phospholipids, amino acids cysteine (and) cysteine 8 methionine, glyco protein (glycogen and mucopolysaccharides), quinoa extract, rosemary extract, sage extract, horsetail extract, coltsfoot extract, hydrolyzed wheat protein, hydrolyzed soy protein, retinyl palmitate (vitamin A), ascorbic acid (vitamin C), tocopheryl acetate (vitamin E), panthenol (vitamin B5), grapeseed extract, and essential oils (as shown below).

Essential Oils:
Bergamot—may help with oily complexion, eczema, and psoriasis. It calms the emotion to helps relieve anxiety, stress, and tension.
Wintergreen—has a cortisone-like action that helps to reduce inflammation in the tissues
Geranium—improves blood flow, regenerates tissue and nerves, cleans oily skin, and ma even liven up pale skin.
Sandalwood—helps strengthen the lymphatic systems; revitalizes the skin.
Clary Sage—astringent; good for cell regulation, cholesterol, and dry skin.
Rosewood—skin cell regenerative; soothing to the skin and promotes elasticity; appeasin to the mind and relaxing to the body.

Instructions: Apply Rosewood Moisturizing Conditioner through the hair. Leave on hair for a few seconds for light conditioning or for several minutes for deep conditioning. Rinse well. *For maximum benefit, leave on 2 to 5 minutes.*

Rosewood Moisturizing Shampoo

This shampoo is formulated for the gentle cleansing of dry hair while nourishing and oisturizing it with herbal extracts, vitamins, and essential oils.

ıgredients: Coconut oil, olive oil, decyl polyglucose, MSM, vegetable protein (wheat, soya, and/or oat), deionized water, nettle extract, mushroom extract (*Grandoderma lucidum* and *Trametes veriscolor*), billberry extract, sugar cane extract, lemon extract, sugar maple extract, orange extract, essential oils (as shown below), aloe vera gel, retinyl palmitate (vitamin A), ascorbic acid (vitamin C), grapeseed extract, inositol, and niacin.

ssential Oils:

Bergamot—may help with oily complexion, eczema, and psoriasis. It calms the emotions to helps relieve anxiety, stress, and tension.

Wintergreen—has a cortisone-like action that helps to reduce inflammation in the tissues.

Geranium—improves blood flow, regenerates tissue and nerves, cleans oily skin, and may even liven up pale skin.

Sandalwood—helps strengthen the lymphatic systems; revitalizes the skin.

Clary Sage—astringent; good for cell regulation, cholesterol, and dry skin.

Rosewood—skin cell regenerative; soothing to the skin and promotes elasticity; appeasing to the mind and relaxing to the body.

ıstructions: Wet hair thoroughly. Apply small amount of Rosewood Moisturizing Shampoo. Massage thoroughly into hair and scalp. Rinse well. Repeat if desired. *For maximum benefit, leave on 2 to 5 minutes.*

Sandalwood Moisture Creme

ıgredients: Deionized water, calendula extract, chamomile extract, rosebud extract, orange blossom extract, St. John's wort extract, aloe vera gel, kelp, *Ginkgo biloba* extract, grapeseed extract, caprylic/capric triglyceride, sorbitol, shea butter, goat's cream, glyceryl stearate, essential oils (as shown below), wolfberry seed oil, rosehip seed oil, sodium PCA, algae extract, stearic acid, allantoin, lecithin, retinyl palmitate (vitamin A), tocopheryl acetate (vitamin E), ascorbic acid (vitamin C), locust bean gum, hydrolyzed wheat protein, sodium hyaluronate, and tocopheryl linoleate.

ssential Oils:

Myrrh—is soothing to the skin; used for chapped and cracked skin and wrinkles.

Sandalwood—helps strengthen the lymphatic systems; revitalizes the skin.

Rosewood—skin cell regenerative; soothing to the skin and promotes elasticity; appeasin to the mind and relaxing to the body.

Lavender—balancing and calming; works wherever there is a need; useful for any type o skin condition.

Rosemary verbenon—is milder than rosemary cineol and better suited for skin care.

Instructions: For best results, use Sandalwood Moisture Creme after cleansing and toning the face and neck to promote younger, healthier skin. Put small amount in hand, emulsify, ar apply to face and neck using upward strokes.

Body System(s) Affected: SKIN.

Sandalwood Toner

Ingredients: Deionized water, MSM, glycerin, sorbitol, sodium PCA, allantoin, aloe vera gel, cucumber extract, chamomile extract, rosemary extract, echinacea extract, gotu kola extract, sodium hyaluronate, arnica extract, witch hazel extract, horse chestnut extract, wolfberry seed oil, and essential oils (as shown below).

Essential Oils:

Sandalwood—helps strengthen the lymphatic systems; revitalizes the skin.

Roman Chamomile—helps increase the regenerative ability of the skin; blood cleanser.

Rosewood—skin cell regenerative; soothing to the skin and promotes elasticity; appeasin to the mind and relaxing to the body.

Myrrh—is soothing to the skin; used for chapped and cracked skin and wrinkles.

Instructions: After cleansing face thoroughly, pour a small amount in palm, rub between hands, and pat on face. Or, apply to a cotton facial puff and pat on face. For best results, follov up with Sandalwood Moisture Creme.

Body System(s) Affected: SKIN.

Satin Hand & Body Lotion

Ingredients: Deionized water, MSM, glyceryl stearate (vegetable based), stearic acid, glycerin, goat's cream, sorbitol, wolfberry seed oil, essential oils (as shown below), safflower oil, apricot oil, almond oil, jojoba oil, sesame oil, calendula extract, chamomile extract, orang blossom extract, St. John's wort extract, algae extract, aloe vera gel, *Ginkgo biloba* extract, grapeseed extract, tocopheryl acetate (vitamin E), retinyl palmitate (vitamin A), ascorbic acid (vitamin C), and sodium hyaluronate.

sential Oils:

Geranium—improves blood flow, regenerates tissue and nerves, cleans oily skin, and may even liven up pale skin.

Rosewood—skin cell regenerative; soothing to the skin and promotes elasticity; appeasing to the mind and relaxing to the body.

Ylang Ylang—balances secretion of sebum (a waxy oil produced by the skin); energizing and uplifting.

Jasmine—deeply penetrating effect on the skin; produces a feeling of confidence, energy, euphoria, and optimism.

Sandalwood—helps strengthen the lymphatic systems; revitalizes the skin.

Peppermint—enhances the effect of the other oils; cooling and soothing sensations; invigorates the skin and helps with nerve regeneration.

Roman Chamomile—helps increase the regenerative ability of the skin; blood cleanser.

Melaleuca alternifolia—tissue regenerative; helps promote the healing of wounds.

structions: To moisturize the skin, promote healing, and leave the skin feeling soft, silky and smooth, apply Satin Hand & Body Lotion to hands, body, and feet. Also good for scars, burns, rashes, itching, and sunburns.

›dy System(s) Affected: SKIN.

Satin Facial Scrub (Mint)

As a gentle exfoliating scrub designed for **normal skin**, Mint Satin Facial Scrub gently minates layers of dead skin cells with a revolutionary formula of jojoba beads and other natural gredients. It can be used as a drying face mask to draw impurities from the skin. Peppermint sential oil is added to soothe and refresh the skin.

gredients: Deionized water, glycerin, caprylic/capric triglyceride, jojoba (*Buxus chinensis*) wax beads, methylsulfonylmethane (MSM), sorbitol, glyceryl stearate, peppermint (*Mentha piperita*) oil, aloe vera (*Aloe barbadensis*) gel, stearic acid, algae (*Gellidiela acerosa*) extract, rosemary (*Rosmarinus officinalis*) extract, chamomile (*Anthemis nobilis*) extract, tocopheryl acetate (vitamin E), retinyl palmitate (vitamin A), sodium PCA, shea butter, grape (*Vitis vinifera*) seed extract, titanium dioxide, mango (*Mangifera indica*) butter, ascorbic acid (vitamin C), sodium hyaluronate, tocopheryl linoleate, allantoin, hydrolyzed wheat protein, and hydrolyzed soy protein.

Essential Oils:

Peppermint—is invigorating to the skin; may also help with nerve regeneration.

Instructions: Apply warm water to the face to moisten the skin. Apply scrub directly to the face and gently massage in a gentle circular motion, creating a lather. Rinse thoroughly and gently pat dry. May also be mixed with Orange Blossom Facial Wash for a milder scrub Mix ½ tsp. of both in palm of hand before applying. Use four or five times weekly, depending on need.

Body System(s) Affected: SKIN.

Sensation Hand & Body Lotion

Ingredients: Deionized water, cocoa butter, glyceryl stearate, cetyl alcohol, lanolin oil, floral water, vitamin E, and essential oils (as shown below).

Essential Oils:

Rosewood—antiseptic and antibacterial; tissue regenerative; soothing to the skin and increases elasticity.

Ylang Ylang—stimulating and helps to balance male-female energies.

Jasmine—deeply penetrating effect on the skin; produces a feeling of confidence, energy euphoria, and optimism.

Instructions: Dispense in hand and apply directly to skin.

Warning: Avoid eye contact. If contact occurs, rinse thoroughly with water. For external use only. Keep out of reach of children.

Sunsation Suntan Oil

Natural sunscreen and insect repellent. This product helps filter out ultraviolet rays without blocking the absorption of vitamin D, which is important to skin and bone development. SPF 6.

Ingredients: Coconut oil, cocoa butter, mink oil, wheat germ oil, vitamin E, essential oils (as shown below), and coconut fragrance oil.

sential Oils:

Lavender—balancing and calming; works wherever there is a need; useful for any type of skin condition.

Melaleuca—strong antiseptic; tissue regenerator

Lemongrass—helps repair connective tissue; it helps stimulate the agents in the tissue to rejuvenate and reconnect; also good as an insect repellant.

Citronella—deodorant; insect repellant; also good for oily skin.

ution: This is not a sunblock! For fair skin, this will generally prevent sunburn for approximately 1½ hours.

Thieves Cleaning Products

These new antiseptic products utilize the documented bacteria killing power of the Thieves blend. Throw away those chemical-laden cleaning products and fight those germs with these werful, natural products.

gredients:

Thieves Household Cleaner: Proprietary suspension base of safe surfactants (wetting agents) and Thieves essential oil blend.

Thieves Spray: Pure grain alcohol, deionized water, Thieves essential oil blend, coconut oil, and soy lecithin.

Thieves Wipes: Pure grain alcohol, deionized water, Thieves essential oil blend, coconut oil and soy lecithin.

ggested Use: Follow label directions.

dy System(s) Affected: IMMUNE SYSTEM.

ecautions: Keep out of reach of children. Not recommended for use on infants or sensitive areas of the body.

Thieves Lozenges

Freshen your breath and soothe the sore throat, while fighting bacteria with these natural zenges. This all natural lozenge is made from natural ingredients including the sweeteners of rbitol (derived from fruit and shown not to contribute to tooth decay) and xylitol (shown to inhibit plaque growth). The essential oils of lemon, orange and peppermint provide natural flavoring and germ fighting ability, especially when combined with the essential oil blend of Thieves.

Ingredients: Xylitol, sorbitol, orange essential oil (*Citrus aurantium*), the essential oil blend of Thieves (a blend of clove, lemon, cinnamon, *Eucalyptus radiata*, and rosemary), peppermint essential oil (*Mentha piperita*), cellulose, silicon dioxide, magnesium silicate and vegetable-grade lubricant (sugar cane and palm oil).

Suggested Use: Dissolve 1 lozenge in mouth as needed.

Body System(s) Affected: IMMUNE SYSTEM and oral hygiene.

Precautions: Keep out of reach of children. Swallowing lozenges whole may cause choking.

Wolfberry Eye Creme

Ingredients: Deionized water, aloe vera gel, caprylic/capric triglyceride, MSM, sorbitol, glycer glyceryl stearate, goat's cream, avocado oil, shea butter, kukui nut oil, rosehip seed oil, essential oils (as shown below), wolfberry seed oil, hydrocotyl extract, coneflower extra sodium PCA, lecithin, dipalmitoyl hydroxyproline, phenoxyethanol, beta-sitosterol, linol acid, tocopheryl, sodium ascorbate, mannitol, almond oil, jojoba oil, mango butter, sodi hyaluronate, cucumber extract, green tea extract, tocopherol acetate, tocopherol palmitat (vitamin E), ascorbyl palmitate (vitamin A), ascorbic acid (vitamin C), citric acid, soy protein, wheat protein, allantoin, witch hazel extract, and horse chestnut extract.

Essential Oils:

Lavender—balancing and calming; works wherever there is a need; useful for any type skin condition.

Rosewood—skin cell regenerative; soothing to the skin and promotes elasticity; appeasi to the mind and relaxing to the body.

Roman Chamomile—helps increase the regenerative ability of the skin; blood cleanser.

Frankincense—is high in sesquiterpenes; helps deliver oxygen to the pineal and pituitar glands; improves hGH production; increases leukocyte production.

Geranium—improves blood flow, regenerates tissue and nerves, cleans oily skin, and m even liven up pale skin.

Instructions: Apply a tiny amount of Wolfberry Eye Creme under eye area and on the eyelid before bed. Repeat in morning if desired.

Bath and Shower Gels

All of the following bath and shower products (gels and bar soaps) have a base that is om a unique, proprietary soap-making process. This base contains saponified oils of palm, ɔconut, and/or olive. Saponification is a process by which sodium hydroxide is combined with the ıtty acids from the palm, coconut, and olive oils to create a soap. By altering the amounts of the ifferent oils, different textures of this soap base are produced. It is the same process which yields ıe soap bases for both the bath & shower gels and the bar soaps that follow, with only slight ıodifications in the formulation of the soap base. The wonderful thing about this process is that ıe resulting soap is vegetable-based with more than 50 percent moisturizers. Add to that liquid loe vera extract for added moisturizing effect and rosemary extract for its antioxidant properties ıd you have a soap that doesn't just clean but nourishes the skin.

Aqua Essence

Aqua Essence bath packets utilize hydro-diffusion technology to slowly and efficiently iffuse essential oils into shower or bath water.

łow to Use: Just place any number of packets into your bath while filling it with warm water. After a short time, the oils begin to diffuse into the bath water. The packets can also be placed on the soap tray in the shower where the warm moist air will pick up the aroma of the oils being diffused to create the soothing and rejuvenating experience desired.

oy—brings back memories of being loved, being held, and sharing loving times. It is uplifting and inspiring as it brings joy to the heart. The single oils contained in this blend include lemon, mandarin, bergamot, ylang ylang, rose, rosewood, geranium, palmarosa, Roman chamomile, and jasmine.

'eace & Calming—is exquisitely relaxing to the senses. It is extremely useful at the end of a stressful day to promote relaxation and peace and to help relieve insomnia. The single oils contained in this blend include tangerine, orange, ylang ylang, patchouli, and Blue tansy.

acred Mountain—helps to create a feeling of protection, empowerment, and grounding. It is soothing to the respiratory system and may help one find security and sacredness within oneself. The single oils contained in this blend include spruce, ylang ylang, Idaho Balsam fir, and cedarwood.

Valor—is emotionally uplifting and helps to empower the physical and spiritual bodies. It helps build courage, confidence, and self-esteem while promoting calmness, peace, and relaxation. The single oils contained in this blend include spruce, rosewood, Blue tansy, and frankincense.

Bath Gel Base

Add your favorite oils to create your own fragrance or therapeutic action.

Ingredients: Saponified oils of coconut and olive, guar gum, aloe vera, rosemary extract, and glycerin.

Dragon Time

For the relief of those monthly aches and pains.

Ingredients: Saponified oils of coconut and olive, guar gum, aloe vera, rosemary extract, and glycerin.

Essential Oils:

Bergamot—sedative; helps to relieve anxiety, stress, and tension.

Clary Sage—helps balance the hormones; tonic to the reproductive system.

Geranium—helps balance the hormones; tissue and nerve regenerative.

Jasmine—deeply penetrating effect on the skin; produces a feeling of confidence, energy, euphoria, and optimism.

Lemon—helps promote leukocyte formation; helps brighten a pale, dull complexion by removing the dead skin cells.

Palmarosa—stimulates new cell growth, regulates oil production, moisturizes and speeds healing.

Roman Chamomile—helps increase the regenerative ability of the skin; blood cleanser.

Rosewood—antiseptic and antibacterial; tissue regenerative; soothing to the skin and increases elasticity.

Lavender—helps balance body systems.

Blue Tansy—calms the lymphatic system; promotes a feeling of self-control.

Mandarin—good for skin problems, stretch marks, nervous tension, and restlessness.

Sage—contains estriol and has estrogen-like properties; believed to contain elements that contribute to the secretion of progesterone.

Fennel—helps balance the hormones.

Ylang Ylang—stimulating and helps to balance male-female energies.

dy System(s) Affected: EMOTIONAL BALANCE, HORMONAL SYSTEM, SKIN.

Evening Peace

Perfect for that evening bath or shower, to help you relax after a very stressful day.

gredients: Saponified oils of coconut and olive, guar gum, aloe vera, rosemary extract, and glycerin.

sential Oils:

Bergamot—sedative; helps to relieve anxiety, stress, and tension.

Roman Chamomile—calming and relaxing; helps increase the regenerative ability of the skin; blood cleanser.

Clary Sage—helps balance the hormones; tonic to the reproductive system.

Geranium—helps balance the hormones; tissue and nerve regenerative.

Jasmine—deeply penetrating effect on the skin; produces a feeling of confidence, energy, euphoria, and optimism.

Lemon—helps promote leukocyte formation; helps brighten a pale, dull complexion by removing the dead skin cells.

Palmarosa—stimulates new cell growth, regulates oil production, moisturizes and speeds healing.

Rosewood—antiseptic and antibacterial; tissue regenerative; soothing to the skin and increases elasticity.

Blue Tansy—calms the lymphatic system; promotes a feeling of self-control.

Sandalwood—helps strengthen the lymphatic systems; revitalizes the skin.

Ylang Ylang—stimulating and helps to balance male-female energies.

dy System(s) Affected: EMOTIONAL BALANCE, SKIN.

KidScents Bath Gel

A shower gel with a neutral pH, perfect for young skin. It is gentle, mild, and safe. It ntains all natural ingredients and therapeutic-grade essential oils with no mineral oils, synthetic rfumes, artificial colorings, or toxic ingredients.

gredients: Deionized water, decylpolyglugose, glycerin, sorbitol, methylsulfonylmethane (MSM), aloe vera (*Aloe barbadensis*) gel, pure therapeutic-grade essential oils (as listed below), panthenol, tocopheryl acetate (vitamin E), chamomile (*Anthemis nobilis*) extract PG-hydroxethylcellulose cocodimonium chloride, purple coneflower (*Echinacea purpure* extract, kukui (*Aleurites moluccana*) nut oil, jojoba (*Buxus chinensis*) oil, citrus seed extract, babassu oil, grape seed (*Vitis vinifera*) extract, dimethicone copolyol meadowfoamate, soap bark extract, soapwort extract, hyaluronic acid, wheat germ oil, keratin, linoleic acid, and linolenic acid.

Essential Oils:

Cedarwood—rejuvenating and refreshing; antiseptic and beneficial to the skin; astringe diuretic; helps reduce oily secretions.

Geranium—can be used on almost any kind of skin; cleansing, refreshing, astringent, ar a mild skin tonic.

Instructions: Apply a small amount of KidScents Bath Gel to a washcloth or directly to the skin Rub gently, then rinse.

Common Sense Caution: While KidScents products contain no harmful ingredients, store out o reach of children to prevent messy spills. Children do not like soap in their mouth or eye Use with gentle care.

KidScents Shampoo

This shampoo contains the finest natural ingredients for gently cleansing young, delicate hair. It is perfectly pH-balanced and contains all natural ingredients and therapeutic-grade essential oils with no mineral oils, synthetic perfumes, artificial colorings, or toxic ingredients.

Ingredients: Deionized water, decylpolyglucose, methylsulfonylmethane (MSM), aloe vera (*Alo barbadensis*) gel, pure therapeutic-grade essential oils (as listed below), panthenol, tocopheryl acetate (vitamin E), chamomile (*Anthemis nobilis*) extract, purple coneflowe (*Echinacea purpurea*) extract, kukui (*Aleurites moluccana*) nut oil, jojoba (*Buxus chinensis*) oil, citrus seed extract, babassu (*Orbignya oleifera*) oil, grape (*Vitis vinifera*) seed extract, dimethicone copolyol medowfoamate, hyaluronic acid, wheat germ oil, keratin, linoleic acid, and linolenic acid.

Essential Oils:

Tangerine—calming to the nervous system; also a decongestant of the lymphatic system

Lemon—promotes leukocyte formation; helps remove the dead skin cells.

Blue Tansy—helps cleanse the liver and promote a feeling of self-control.

Instructions: Apply a small amount of KidScents Shampoo to the hair. Lather, then rinse.

Common Sense Caution: While KidScents products contain no harmful ingredients, store out of reach of children to prevent messy spills. Children do not like shampoo in their mouth or eyes. Use with gentle care.

Morning Start

For an invigorating bath or shower, to physically and emotionally prepare you for another hectic day. Due to the deep penetrating, cleansing action of the oils in this product, Morning Start may actually help dissolve and wash away oil and grease from the skin.

Ingredients: Saponified oils of coconut and olive, guar gum, aloe vera, rosemary extract, and glycerin.

Essential Oils:

Lemongrass—helps stimulate the agents in the tissue to rejuvenate and reconnect.
Rosemary cineol—highly anti-infectious; good for various skin conditions.
Juniper— evokes feelings of health and peace and elevates one's spiritual awareness.
Peppermint—is invigorating to the skin; may also help with nerve regeneration.

Body System(s) Affected: EMOTIONAL BALANCE, SKIN.

Sensation

The exquisite, sensual fragrance of this bath gel is a wonderful addition to those romantic evenings.

Ingredients: Saponified oils of coconut and olive, guar gum, aloe vera, rosemary extract, and glycerin.

Essential Oils:

Rosewood—antiseptic and antibacterial; tissue regenerative; soothing to the skin and increases elasticity.
Ylang Ylang—stimulating and helps to balance male-female energies.
Jasmine—deeply penetrating effect on the skin; produces a feeling of confidence, energy, euphoria, and optimism.

Body System(s) Affected: EMOTIONAL BALANCE, HORMONAL SYSTEM, SKIN.

Bar Soaps

Lavender Rosewood

Moisturizing Soap

Contains oils that nourish the skin while their fragrance is calming and relaxing.

Ingredients: Saponified oils of palm, coconut, wolfberry seed, and olive, therapeutic-grade essential oils (as listed below), liquid aloe vera extract (moisturizing agent), rosemary extract (antioxidant), and organic oatmeal (mild abrasive to stimulate pores).

Essential Oils:

Lavender—helps balance body systems.

Rosewood—antiseptic and antibacterial; tissue regenerative; soothing to the skin and increases elasticity.

Lemon Sandalwood

Cleansing Soap

Contains oils that deep clean and revitalize the skin with an invigorating fragrance.

Ingredients: Saponified oils of palm, coconut, wolfberry seed, and olive, therapeutic-grade essential oils (as listed below), liquid aloe vera extract (moisturizing agent), rosemary extract (antioxidant), and organic oatmeal (mild abrasive to stimulate pores).

Essential Oils:

Lemon—helps promote leukocyte formation; helps brighten a pale, dull complexion by removing the dead skin cells.

Sandalwood—helps strengthen the lymphatic systems; revitalizes the skin.

Melaleuca Geranium
Moisturizing Soap

Contains oils that are antiseptic and revitalizing to the skin with a calming fragrance.

Ingredients: Saponified oils of palm, coconut, wolfberry seed, and olive, therapeutic-grade essential oils (as listed below), liquid aloe vera extract (moisturizing agent), rosemary extract (antioxidant), and organic oatmeal (mild abrasive to stimulate pores).

Essential Oils:

Melaleuca—is anti-fungal, antiseptic, anti-bacterial; tissue regenerative.

Geranium—can be used on almost any kind of skin; cleansing, refreshing, astringent, and a mild skin tonic.

Melaleuca ericifolia—is very gentle and non-irritating to the skin; well suited for youth and others who may be more sensitive to the oils.

Vetiver—antispasmodic and locally warming; good for arthritis, muscular rheumatism, and sprains.

Morning Start
Moisturizing Soap

Patterned after the popular Bath and Shower Gel, this soap is uplifting and energizing.

Ingredients: Saponified oils of palm, coconut, wolfberry seed, and olive, therapeutic-grade essential oils (as listed below), liquid aloe vera extract (moisturizing agent), rosemary extract (antioxidant), and organic oatmeal (mild abrasive to stimulate pores).

Essential Oils:

Lemongrass—helps repair connective tissue; it helps stimulate the agents in the tissue to rejuvenate and reconnect; also good as an insect repellant.

Rosemary cineol—highly anti-infectious; antifungal and anti-bacterial; good for various skin conditions.

Peppermint—invigorating to the skin; may also help with nerve regeneration.

Juniper—evokes feelings of health, love, and peace and may help to elevate one's spiritual awareness.

Peppermint Cedarwood
Moisturizing Soap

Contains oils that purify and invigorate the skin with a calming fragrance.

Ingredients: Saponified oils of palm, coconut, wolfberry seed, and olive, therapeutic-grade essential oils (as listed below), liquid aloe vera extract (moisturizing agent), rosemary extract (antioxidant), and organic oatmeal (mild abrasive to stimulate pores).

Essential Oils:

Peppermint—invigorates skin and enhances effects of cedarwood.

Cedarwood—rejuvenating and refreshing; antiseptic and beneficial to the skin.

Sacred Mountain
Moisturizing Soap for Oily Skin

Contains extra abrasives to remove dead skin cells and oils that are antiseptic, purifying, and calming.

Ingredients: Saponified oils of palm, coconut, wolfberry seed, and olive, therapeutic-grade essential oils (as listed below), liquid aloe vera extract (moisturizing agent), rosemary extract (antioxidant), and organic oatmeal (mild abrasive to stimulate pores).

Essential Oils:

Spruce—helps to open and release emotional blocks.

Ylang Ylang—stimulating and helps to balance male-female energies.

Idaho Balsam Fir—antiseptic; helps create a feeling of grounding, anchoring, and empowerment.

Cedarwood—rejuvenating and refreshing; antiseptic and beneficial to the skin.

Thieves
Cleansing Soap

Contains oils that are high in antiseptic properties.

Ingredients: Saponified oils of palm, coconut, wolfberry seed, and olive, therapeutic-grade essential oils (as listed below), liquid aloe vera extract (moisturizing agent), rosemary extract (antioxidant), and organic oatmeal (mild abrasive to stimulate pores).

ssential Oils:

Clove—is anti-bacterial, anti-fungal, anti-infectious, anti-parasitic, a strong antiseptic, anti-viral, and an immune stimulant. It may influence healing and help create a feeling of protection and courage.

Lemon—helps promote leukocyte formation; helps brighten a pale, dull complexion by removing the dead skin cells.

Cinnamon Bark—is anti-bacterial, anti-fungal, anti-infectious, anti-inflammatory, antimicrobial, anti-parasitic, antiseptic, antispasmodic, anti-viral, astringent, immune-stimulant, sexual stimulant, and warming.

Eucalyptus radiata—has strong anti-bacterial, anti-catarrhal, and antiseptic properties.

Rosemary cineol—may improve circulation and help stimulate the nerves. It is antiseptic and anti-infectious.

Valor

Moisturizing Soap

Contains the oil blend of Valor which is soothing and nourishing for the skin with a alancing and calming fragrance.

gredients: Saponified oils of palm, coconut, wolfberry seed, and olive, therapeutic-grade essential oils (as listed below), liquid aloe vera extract (moisturizing agent), rosemary extract (antioxidant), and organic oatmeal (mild abrasive to stimulate pores).

ssential Oils:

Spruce—grounds the body, creating the balance and the opening necessary to receive and to give; may help dilate the bronchial tract to improve the oxygen exchange; helps one release emotional blocks.

Rosewood—is soothing to the skin, appeasing to the mind, relaxing to the body, and creates a feeling of peace and gentleness.

Blue Tansy—may help cleanse the liver and calm the lymphatic system to help rid one of anger and promote a feeling of self-control.

Frankincense—contains sesquiterpenes, which may help oxygenate the pineal and pituitary glands; may help promote a positive attitude.

Tinctures

Chelex

An herbal tincture synergistically formulated to help rid the body of heavy metals and other immune-damaging free radicals. Heavy metals absorbed from the air, water, food, skin car products, etc., lodge and store in the fatty layers of the body and give off toxic gases in the syster which may create allergic symptoms. Ridding our bodies of heavy metals is extremely important order to have healthy immune function, especially if we have mercury fillings. This formula contains the essential oil of helichrysum, which may help the body in the elimination of heavy metals because of its natural chelating action.

Ingredients: Essential oils (as shown below), with extracts of astragalus, garlic, wild sarsaparil Siberian ginseng, red clover, and royal jelly. Extracted in a 1:4 ratio of grain alcohol anc water.

Essential Oils:

Eucalyptus—is highly antiseptic (eucalyptol) and antimicrobial.

Helichrysum—may help cleanse the blood and improve circulatory functions. It is anti-catarrhal in structure and nature.

Roman Chamomile—helps increase the regenerative ability of the skin; blood cleanser.

Rosemary cineol—helps balance heart function, stimulates nerves, and decongests the liver.

Suggested Use: One to three droppers (25-75 drops) three times daily in distilled water or as desired.

Body System(s) Affected: IMMUNE SYSTEM.

Estro

Designed with plant-derived phytoestrogens to safely help harmonize the female hormone levels. Works well with Prenolone or Prenolone+.

gredients: Extracts of black cohosh, blue cohosh, royal jelly, and essential oils (as shown below). Extracted in a 1:4 ratio of grain alcohol and water.

ssential Oils:

Fennel—helps balance the hormones.
Lavender—helps balance body systems.
Clary Sage—helps balance the hormones; tonic to the reproductive system.

uggested Use: Start with one dropper two to three times daily. Increase as needed to as much as three droppers daily. Estro may take as long as four weeks to reach maximum effectiveness.

ody System(s) Affected: HORMONAL SYSTEM.

HRT

This formula was created out of specially selected herbs and oils to give nutritional ıpport to help overcome deficiencies and irregularities of the heart.

ngredients: Water, hawthorn berry juice, vegetable glycerin, blackberry brandy, lobelia extract, garlic extract, cayenne extract, and essential oils (as shown below). Extracted in a 1:4 ratio of grain alcohol and water.

ssential Oils:

Lemon—helps promote leukocyte formation; helps to dissolve cholesterol and fats.
Rosewood—antiseptic and antibacterial; tissue regenerative; helps increase elasticity.
Ylang Ylang—is a nutrient that has been found to help support heart function.
Cypress—astringent, lymphatic decongestant; strengthens connective tissue.

uggested Use: One to three droppers (25-75 drops) three times daily in distilled water or as desired.

ody System(s) Affected: CARDIOVASCULAR SYSTEM.

K & B

The herbs contained in this supplement, combined with oils, have been traditionally used to ɜlp the kidneys and bladder in cases of irregularity, infection and bed wetting.

Ingredients: Extracts of juniper berries, parsley, uva ursi, dandelion root, German chamomile, royal jelly, and essential oils (as shown below). Extracted in a 1:4 ratio of grain alcohol and water.

Essential Oils:

Clove—anti-infectious, antiviral, anti-fungal, and anti-parasitic.

Juniper—cleanser, detoxifier, diuretic; helps the body release fluids.

Sage—diuretic; contains estriol and has estrogen-like properties; believed to contain elements that contribute to the secretion of progesterone.

Fennel—diuretic; may break up fluids and toxins, and cleanse the tissues.

Geranium—cleansing, refreshing, astringent, diuretic; helps support the kidney and bladder functions and helps with stone removal.

Roman Chamomile—blood cleanser; helps liver discharge toxins.

Suggested Use: Take one to three droppers (25-75 drops) three times daily in distilled water or a desired.

Body System(s) Affected: DIGESTIVE SYSTEM.

Rehemogen

This formula contains herbs that were used by Chief Sundance to clean the blood, fight free radicals and give support to the blood cells and immune system.

Ingredients: Essential oils (as shown below), extracts of red clover blossom, licorice root, poke root, peach bark, Oregon grape root, stillingia, sarsparilla, cascara sagrada, prickly ash bark, burdock root, buckthorn bark, and royal jelly. Extracted in a 1:4 ratio of grain alcohol and water.

Essential Oils:

Roman Chamomile—blood cleanser; helps liver discharge toxins.

Rosemary cineol—helps balance heart function, stimulates nerves, and decongests the liver.

Thyme—anti-inflammatory; anti-fungal; antiseptic; anti-viral.

Melaleuca—anti-fungal, antiseptic, anti-bacterial; tissue regenerative.

Suggested Use: One to three droppers (25-75 drops) three times daily in distilled water or as desired.

Body System(s) Affected: CARDIOVASCULAR and DIGESTIVE SYSTEMS.

Cel-Lite Magic

Shake well before using.

Ingredients:

Fractionated Coconut Oil—is distilled from pure coconut oil to create an odorless, colorless vegetable oil. Because the oil's completely saturated fatty acid triglycerides are smaller, with no double bonds, the oil never goes rancid and is more readily absorbed by the skin. It easily washes out of clothes and sheets with no staining.

Grape Seed Oil—antioxidant; rich in bioflavonoids; helps maintain pH balance.

Wheat Germ Oil—high in natural vitamins E and B and lecithin; natural antioxidant; useful for reducing scar tissue and stretch marks; acts as a preservative for the other base oils.

Sweet Almond Oil—nourishes the skin will reducing friction for smoother application.

Olive Oil—moisturizing agent.

Vitamin E Oil—natural antioxidant; protects and promotes regeneration of the skin.

Essential Oils:

Grapefruit—excellent for fluid retention and cellulite; diuretic, detoxifier, and stimulant of the lymphatic system; important as an antidepressant.

Cypress—mucolytic, astringent, diuretic, lymphatic decongestant; reduces cellulite and strengthens connective tissue.

Cedarwood—astringent; diuretic; helps reduce oily secretions.

Juniper—cleanser, detoxifier, diuretic; helps the body release fluids.

Clary Sage—astringent; good for cell regulation, cholesterol, and dry skin.

Suggested Use: Massage on location.

Warning: Avoid eye contact. If contact occurs, rinse thoroughly with water. For external use only. Keep out of reach of children.

Body System(s) Affected: SKIN.

Chivalry

Shake well before using.

Ingredients:

Fractionated Coconut Oil—is distilled from pure coconut oil to create an odorless, colorless vegetable oil. Because the oil's completely saturated fatty acid triglycerides are smaller, with no double bonds, the oil never goes rancid and is more readily absorbed by the skin. It easily washes out of clothes and sheets with no staining.

Grape Seed Oil—antioxidant; rich in bioflavonoids; helps maintain pH balance.

Wheat Germ Oil—high in natural vitamins E and B and lecithin; natural antioxidant; useful for reducing scar tissue and stretch marks; acts as a preservative for the other base oils.

Olive Oil—moisturizing agent.

Sweet Almond Oil—nourishes the skin will reducing friction for smoother application.

Essential Oil Blends:

Valor—is emotionally uplifting and helps to empower the physical and spiritual bodies. I helps to build courage, confidence, and self-esteem while promoting calmness, peace, and relaxation.

Joy—is a blend which may help to open the heart and promote feelings of self-love and love for others so one can experience ultimate joy.

Harmony—Without harmony none of the other states of mind would come to be. We must be in harmony with ourselves, with our creator, and with the world and all those around us. When we have harmony in our lives, then many other things wil come to balance and fruition.

Gratitude—helps to elevate, soothe, and appease the mind while bringing relief and relaxation to the body.

Suggested Use: Massage on location.

Warning: Avoid eye contact. If contact occurs, rinse thoroughly with water. For external use only. Keep out of reach of children.

Body System(s) Affected: EMOTIONAL BALANCE.

Dragon Time

Shake well before using.

Ingredients:

Fractionated Coconut Oil—is distilled from pure coconut oil to create an odorless, colorless vegetable oil. Because the oil's completely saturated fatty acid triglycerides are smaller, with no double bonds, the oil never goes rancid and is more readily absorbed by the skin. It easily washes out of clothes and sheets with no staining.

Grape Seed Oil—antioxidant; rich in bioflavonoids; helps maintain pH balance.

Sweet Almond Oil—nourishes the skin will reducing friction for smoother application.

Olive Oil—moisturizing agent.

Wheat Germ Oil—high in natural vitamins E and B and lecithin; natural antioxidant; useful for reducing scar tissue and stretch marks; acts as a preservative.

Vitamin E Oil—natural antioxidant; protects and promotes regeneration of the skin.

Essential Oils:

Clary Sage—helps balance the hormones; tonic to the reproductive system.

Fennel—helps balance the hormones.

Lavender—helps balance body systems.

Jasmine—helps relieve menstrual pains; good for uterine disorders.

Sage—contains estriol and has estrogen-like properties; believed to contain elements that contribute to the secretion of progesterone.

Ylang Ylang—stimulates adrenal glands; helps balance male/female energies.

Yarrow—anti-inflammatory; antiseptic; excellent for menstrual problems.

Warning: Avoid eye contact. If contact occurs, rinse thoroughly with water. For external use only. Keep out of reach of children.

Body System(s) Affected: EMOTIONAL BALANCE, HORMONAL SYSTEM, SKIN.

Massage Oil Base

Ingredients:

Wheat Germ Oil—high in natural vitamins E and B and lecithin; natural antioxidant; useful for reducing scar tissue and stretch marks; acts as a preservative.

Grape Seed Oil—antioxidant; rich in bioflavonoids; helps maintain pH balance.

Sweet Almond Oil—nourishes the skin will reducing friction for smoother application.
Olive Oil—moisturizing agent.
Vitamin E Oil—natural antioxidant; protects and promotes regeneration of the skin.

Ortho Ease

Ingredients:

Fractionated Coconut Oil—is distilled from pure coconut oil to create an odorless, colorless vegetable oil. Because the oil's completely saturated fatty acid triglycerides are smaller, with no double bonds, the oil never goes rancid and is more readily absorbed by the skin. It easily washes out of clothes and sheets with no staining.

Grape Seed Oil—antioxidant; rich in bioflavonoids; helps maintain pH balance.

Wheat Germ Oil—high in natural vitamins E and B and lecithin; natural antioxidant; useful for reducing scar tissue and stretch marks; acts as a preservative.

Sweet Almond Oil—nourishes the skin will reducing friction for smoother application.

Olive Oil—moisturizing agent.

Essential Oils:

Wintergreen—locally warming; contains methyl salicylate; has a cortisone-like action that helps to reduce inflammation in the joints and tissue.

Juniper—antispasmodic; helps reduce muscle aches/pains.

Peppermint—enhances the effect of the other oils; high in natural menthol, for a wonderful mentholatum-type of sensation.

Eucalyptus australiana—wonderful as an anti-inflammatory.

Lemongrass—helps repair connective tissue; when combined with marjoram, it helps stimulate the agents in the tissue to rejuvenate and reconnect.

Marjoram—powerful muscle relaxant and anti-inflammatory; relaxing and soothing to cartilage tissue.

Thyme—anti-inflammatory; anti-fungal; antiseptic; anti-viral.

Vetiver—antispasmodic and locally warming; good for arthritis, muscular rheumatism, and sprains.

Warning: Avoid eye contact. If contact occurs, rinse thoroughly with water. For external use only. Keep out of reach of children.

Body System(s) Affected: MUSCLES and BONES, SKIN.

Ortho Sport

This massage oil is an enhanced version of Ortho Ease, super-charged for the more manding athlete or sportsman.

gredients:

Fractionated Coconut Oil—is distilled from pure coconut oil to create an odorless, colorless vegetable oil. Because the oil's completely saturated fatty acid triglycerides are smaller, with no double bonds, the oil never goes rancid and is more readily absorbed by the skin. It easily washes out of clothes and sheets with no staining.

Grape Seed Oil—antioxidant; rich in bioflavonoids; helps maintain pH balance.

Sweet Almond Oil—nourishes the skin will reducing friction for smoother application.

Olive Oil—moisturizing agent.

ssential Oils:

Wintergreen—locally warming; contains methyl salicylate; has a cortisone-like action that helps to reduce inflammation in the joints and tissue.

Peppermint—enhances the effect of the other oils; high in natural menthol, for a wonderful mentholatum-type of sensation.

Oregano—powerful antimicrobial; anti-inflammatory; locally warming.

Eucalyptus globulus—wonderful as an anti-inflammatory.

Elemi—very powerful anti-inflammatory; similar to helichrysum as a topical anesthetic.

Vetiver—antispasmodic and locally warming; good for arthritis, muscular rheumatism, and sprains.

Lemongrass—helps repair connective tissue; when combined with marjoram, it helps stimulate the agents in the tissue to rejuvenate and reconnect.

Thyme—anti-inflammatory; anti-fungal; antiseptic; anti-viral.

'arning: Avoid eye contact. If contact occurs, rinse thoroughly with water. For external use only. Keep out of reach of children.

ody System(s) Affected: MUSCLES and BONES.

Relaxation

Shake well before using.

Ingredients:

Fractionated Coconut Oil—is distilled from pure coconut oil to create an odorless, colorless vegetable oil. Because the oil's completely saturated fatty acid triglycerides are smaller, with no double bonds, the oil never goes rancid and is more readily absorbed by the skin. It easily washes out of clothes and sheets wi no staining.

Grape Seed Oil—antioxidant; rich in bioflavonoids; helps maintain pH balance.

Wheat Germ Oil—high in natural vitamins E and B and lecithin; natural antioxidant; useful for reducing scar tissue and stretch marks; acts as a preservative for the other base oils.

Sweet Almond Oil—nourishes the skin will reducing friction for smoother application.

Olive Oil—moisturizing agent.

Essential Oils:

Tangerine—sedating and calming to the nervous system; also a diuretic and a decongestant of the lymphatic system.

Lavender—sedative; balances body systems and promotes a general sense of well being

Peppermint—purifying and stimulating to the conscious mind; anti-inflammatory; helps with nerve regeneration.

Spearmint—acts as an anti-depressant by relieving mental strain and fatigue, and by lifting one's spirits.

Rosewood—appeasing to the mind and relaxing to the body.

Ylang Ylang—anti-depressant; calming and relaxing; balances male/female energies.

Warning: Avoid eye contact. If contact occurs, rinse thoroughly with water. For external use only. Keep out of reach of children.

Body System(s) Affected: EMOTIONAL BALANCE, SKIN.

Sensation

Shake well before using.

Ingredients:

Fractionated Coconut Oil—is distilled from pure coconut oil to create an odorless, colorless vegetable oil. Because the oil's completely saturated fatty acid triglycerides are smaller, with no double bonds, the oil never goes rancid and is more readily absorbed by the skin. It easily washes out of clothes and sheets with no staining.

Grape Seed Oil—antioxidant; rich in bioflavonoids; helps maintain pH balance.

Wheat Germ Oil—high in natural vitamins E and B and lecithin; natural antioxidant; useful for reducing scar tissue and stretch marks; acts as a preservative for the other base oils.

Sweet Almond Oil—nourishes the skin will reducing friction for smoother application.

Olive Oil—moisturizing agent.

Essential Oils:

Rosewood—skin cell regenerative; soothing to the skin and promotes elasticity; appeasing to the mind and relaxing to the body.

Ylang Ylang—balances secretion of sebum (a waxy oil produced by the skin); energizing and uplifting.

Jasmine—deeply penetrating effect on the skin; produces a feeling of confidence, energy, euphoria, and optimism.

Warning: Avoid eye contact. If contact occurs, rinse thoroughly with water. For external use only. Keep out of reach of children.

Body System(s) Affected: EMOTIONAL BALANCE, HORMONAL SYSTEM.

V-6
Advanced Vegetable Oil Complex

This new formulation of mixing oil contains the same nourishing oils but with an increase shelf life and virtually no color or odor. Food Grade.

Ingredients:

Fractionated Coconut Oil—is distilled from pure coconut oil to create an odorless, colorless vegetable oil. Because the oil's completely saturated fatty acid triglycerides are smaller, with no double bonds, the oil never goes rancid and is more readily absorbed by the skin. It easily washes out of clothes and sheets with no staining.

Sesame Seed Oil (certified organic)—is high in linoleic acid; contains vitamins, minerals, amino acids, lecithin, and natural vegetable proteins; moisturizing; easily absorbs into the skin.

Grapeseed Oil (kosher)—nourishes the skin; antioxidant; rich in bioflavonoids; helps maintain pH balance.

Almond Oil (certified organic)—contains natural vitamin D; well suited for massage.

Wheatgerm Oil (non GMO)—high in lecithin and natural E and B vitamins; natural antioxidant; useful for reducing scar tissue and stretch marks; acts as a preservative for the other base oils.

Sunflower Seed Oil (certified organic)—contains natural vitamin E; antioxidant; suitable for a variety of skin types.

Olive Oil (Extra Virgin & certified organic)—is a moisturizing agent.

Directions: Suggested blending is 15-30 drops of essential oil to 1 oz. mixing oil. V-6 Mixing O is good for mixing massage oils, creating your own blends and formulas, for cooking and making salad dressings, etc.

Supplements and Vitamins

This section contains product information about the authors' favorite food supplements. ost of this information was obtained from the product labels. We chose to review these pplements because they are the only products, known to the authors, that contain both herbs and sential oils. The essential oils in these products act as catalysts to deliver oxygen and nutrients ough the cell walls while assisting the body in the removal of toxic waste.

When taking supplements, it is important to give the body a rest one or two days a week. king supplements only five or six days out of the week gives the body time to regain its own lance and allow its own healing powers to operate rather than rely solely on the supplements ing taken. These supplements are usually dissolved and assimilated by the body within a couple urs so the effectiveness of the supplements can be increased by taking them throughout the day stead of all at once.

An approximate frequency is indicated for some of the supplements. However, please ep in mind that there are many variables involved in determining frequency. Consequently, these mbers may be difficult to duplicate.

Using Essential Oil Food Supplements
to
Cleanse, Build, and Support the Body
Summary of an article written by Rita Anderson, Wellness Consultan

1. Start with the **Cleansing Trio** of Essentialzyme, ComforTone, and ICP.
   - A. Begin immediately to take **Essentialzyme** before each meal. It may also be take between meals to help lessen allergy symptoms.
   - B. Take enough **ComforTone** each morning and before bedtime to allow your body to have several smooth bowel movements each day.

     Comments: If I began using **ComforTone** and actually felt clogged the first da or two, I would increase my **ComforTone** intake until I had very good movements two to three times a day. I would also increase my water intake to help my cells wash away the toxins.
   - C. Once you are having several smooth bowel movements each day, begin taking **IC** fiber beverage in juice or water. Warm water seems to help it "slide" down. Do not use citrus juices as they are too acidic.
2. Two weeks after the **Cleansing Trio** is working smoothly, start on the **Body Balancing Trio** (Bodygize, Vita Green, and Master Formula His (or Master Formula Hers)) to re-nutrient and fortify the body.
3. Two weeks after starting on the **Body Balancing Trio**, start using **Mineral Essence** and **ImmuneTune** to support the immune system.

Comments: Anyone who has not worked with a cleansing program in the past two years may want to continue on the **Cleansing Trio** for at least 90 days in a very consistent manner t rid the body of all stages of parasites. **Di-Tone** may also be used on the digestive Vita Flex points of the feet or as a hot compress over the abdominal area to help relax intestin spasms and expel parasites. Apply full strength; if your skin is sensitive, it may be necessary to dilute with V-6 Mixing Oil. If you have a degenerative disease you will wa to stay on the **Cleansing Trio** for at least a year.

NOTE: *Learn to feed the body by taking supplements throughout the day.*

AD&E

This product contains Vitamins A, D, and E. These vitamins are known as powerful :ioxidants. They contain the essential nutrients for supporting immune function. They may also ·p nourish the eyes, hair, nails, skin, and be instrumental in bone development. These vitamins : extremely important to the metabolism and elasticity of cells for increased longevity.

gredients: Vitamins A, D, and E, beta carotene, grapeseed oil, mixed tocopherals.

ggested Use: Take five droppers once a day in distilled water or as desired.

dy System(s) Affected: IMMUNE and NERVOUS SYSTEMS, SKIN.

Agave

This product is an organically grown, kosher certified sweetener that is 50% sweeter than ›le sugar with fewer calories. Because it is scientifically proven to have a low glycemic index ırrently at 39), it becomes the sweetener of choice for diabetics and hypoglycemics who need to ntrol their blood sugar levels. It also helps to support normal intestinal function.

gredients: This Agave product is a blend of nectars from two plant varieties: *Agave salmiana*, and *Agave angustifolia*. When possible, may include nectar from *Agave tequiliana*.

ggested Use: Can be used in beverages and food recipes as a sugar replacement. Because Agave is sweeter than table sugar, use only 3/4 the amount of Agave as table sugar. It also makes a delicious replacement for honey in sandwiches and on toast. Can also be used like honey on cereals and in beverages.

ompanion Products: Essential Manna, and Power Meal.

ody System(s) Affected: HORMONAL SYSTEM, MUSCLES and BONES.

AlkaLime

A precisely-balanced acid-neutralizing mineral formulation designed to combat yeast and ngus overgrowth and preserve the body's proper pH balance - the cornerstone of health. This ecially designed alkalizing mineral powder contains an array of high-alkaline salts and other yeast/fungus-fighting elements such as citric acid and essential oils. By boosting blood alkalinit yeast and fungus are deprived of the acidic terrain they require to flourish. The effectiveness of other Essential Oils is enhanced when the body's blood and tissues are alkaline.

Ingredients: Sodium bicarbonate, calcium carbonate, magnesium citrate, citric acid, potassiun bicarbonate, sea salts, and essential oils (as shown below).

Essential Oils:

Lemon—helps promote leukocyte formation; helps to dissolve cholesterol and fats.

Lime—helps remove dead skin cells; tightens skin and connective tissue. Lemon and lin both become alkaline when absorbed by the body.

Suggested Use: Take one rounded teaspoon in 6 to 8 oz. of distilled or purified water. **Mix onl with water.** Drink immediately. For best results, drink one hour before or after eating. To balance pH, take one to three times per day one hour before meals or before retiring. As an antacid, AlkaLime may be taken as needed. Otherwise, an ideal time to take AlkaLime would be prior to bedtime.

Body System(s) Affected: CARDIOVASCULAR and DIGESTIVE SYSTEMS, MUSCLES a BONES.

Companion Products: Essentialzyme, Mineral Essence, Royaldophilus, VitaGreen.

Companion Oils: Valor, 3 Wise Men, Harmony, Forgiveness, Joy, Present Time, Release, Inne Child, Grounding, Hope, SARA, White Angelica, Di-Tone, Purification, Thieves, peppermint, and spearmint.

ALKALIME may help reduce the following signs of acid-based yeast and fungus dominance: Fatigue/low energy, unexplained aches and pains, overweight conditions, low resistance to illness, allergies, unbalanced blood sugar, headaches, irritability/mood swings, indigestion, colitis/ulcers, diarrhea/constipation, urinary tract infections, rectal/vaginal itch.

Allerzyme

A vegetable enzyme complex designed to provide some relief from occasional symptoms such as fullness, pressure, bloating, gas, pain, and/or minor cramping that occur after eating. It may also help combat allergies, fermentation, fatigue, and irritable bowel syndrome. Allerzyme contains a powerful combination of sugar-splitting and starch-splitting enzymes, as well as a sma nount of fat-digesting and protein-digesting enzymes, which help to promote proper digestion for ›ople with sensitive stomachs.

ıgredients: Amylase, bromelain, peptidase, protease, invertase, phytase, lipase, lactase, cellulase, alpha-galactosidase, maltase, plantain (sulfite-free), pure therapeutic-grade essential oils (as listed below), sucrase, vegetable cellulose, rice bran, deionized water, barley sprout powder, and silica.

ssential Oils:

Tarragon—may help reduce anorexia, dyspepsia, flatulence, intestinal spasms, nervous and sluggish digestion, and genital urinary tract infection.

Ginger—is warming, uplifting, and empowering; helps reduce feelings of nausea, and motion sickness.

Peppermint—purifying and stimulating to the conscious mind; anti-inflammatory; helps with nerve regeneration. It also enhances digestion and increases endurance.

Juniper—antispasmodic; helps reduce muscle aches/pains.

Fennel—anti-parasitic; promotes the removal of toxic wastes; may break up fluids and toxins, and cleanse the tissues.

Lemongrass—helps repair connective tissue; it helps stimulate the agents in the tissue to rejuvenate and reconnect; helps regulate the parasympathetic nervous system and strengthen vascular walls.

Patchouli—protects against UV radiation and promotes tissue regeneration; helps tighten loose skin and prevent wrinkles.

Anise—may help calm and strengthen the digestive system.

uggested Use: Take 1-2 capsules three times daily just prior to all meals. Can also be sprinkled on food or in beverages.

ody System(s) Affected: DIGESTIVE and RESPIRATORY SYSTEMS.

ompanion Products: ComforTone, JuvaTone, Sulfurzyme, Royaldophilus, and Power Meal.

ompanion Oils: Di-Tone and JuvaFlex.

Varning: Do not give this product to children under 12 years of age except under the supervision of a doctor. If symptoms persist, discontinue use of this product and consult your physician. Keep in a cool, dry place. Do no expose to excessive heat or direct sunlight. If pregnant or under a doctor's care, consult your physician.

AminoTech

This energizing formula provides all the amino acids necessary for strength and energy. The amino acids of L-glutamine, L-arginine, L-alanine, and L-taurine stimulate the production of hGH (human growth hormone) which has been shown in studies to increase lean body mass while reducing fat deposits. The reduction of fat is also aided by the Chinese wolfberry while the increase in muscle tissue is aided by creatine. Together these and other synergistic ingredients all combine to lengthen physical workouts, enhance endurance, increase strength, and build muscle.

Ingredients: Creatine monohydrate, L-glutamine, L-arginine, L-alanine, L-taurine, MSM, calcium alpha-ketoglutarate, potassium bicarbonate, magnesium phosphate, alpha-lipoic acid, RNA, zinc citrate, chromium polynicotinate, L-selenometionine, fructooligosaccharides (FOS), Chinese wolfberry, and essential oils (as listed below).

Essential Oils:

Lemon—helps promote leukocyte formation; helps to dissolve cholesterol and fats.

Lime—helps remove dead skin cells; tightens skin and connective tissue. Lemon and lim both become alkaline when absorbed by the body.

Suggested Use: Take one to two heaping scoop(s) daily mixed with water. For additional flavor mix with rice or almond milk. *Maximum benefits are achieved when AminoTech is used in combination with exercise.*

Body System(s) Affected: MUSCLES and BONES.

Companion Products: Be-Fit, ThermaBurn, Ultra Young, WheyFit.

ArthroTune

This whole food herbal formula may help arthritis and rheumatoid conditions. Active OPC's 85+ Proanthocyanidins (Pycnogenol). **Natural antioxidant.**

Ingredients: Butcher's broom, alfalfa powder, alfalfa sprouts, *Uncaria tomentosa* root, alpha-keto-glutaric acid, yucca root, magnesium citrate, capsicum (cayenne), active grape seed extract, cellulose, calcium citrate, gelatin, and essential oils (shown below).

Essential Oils:

Wintergreen—locally warming; contains methyl salicylate; has a cortisone-like action that helps to reduce inflammation in the joints and tissue.

Basil—has antidepressant, anti-inflammatory, and antispasmodic properties; relaxing to spastic muscles, including those that contribute to headaches and migraines.

Marjoram—powerful muscle relaxant and anti-inflammatory; relaxing and soothing to cartilage tissue.

Juniper—antispasmodic; helps reduce muscle aches/pains.

Spruce—anti-inflammatory, antispasmodic, cortisone-like; helps with joint pain.

Fir—antiseptic; helps create a feeling of grounding, anchoring, and empowerment.

Helichrysum—may help cleanse the blood and improve circulatory functions. It is anti-catarrhal in structure and nature.

Black Pepper—increases cellular oxygenation; stimulates the endocrine and circulatory systems.

Cypress—mucolytic, astringent, diuretic, lymphatic decongestant; reduces cellulite and strengthens connective tissue.

uggested Use: Take one capsule before meals. With sensitive digestion, take with meals.

ody System(s) Affected: MUSCLES and BONES.

ompanion Products: Essentialzyme, Ortho Ease and Ortho Sport Massage Oils, Royaldophilus, Sulfurzyme, and VitaGreen.

ompanion Oils: Relieve It, PanAway.

Be-Fit

A high-powered formula for enhancing strength and endurance and promoting muscle ›rmation. Several ingredients are utilized in this product to help build muscle tissue.

ngredients: Wolfberry powder *(Refer to the Wolfberry Bar at the end of this section for more information on the benefits of the Chinese Wolfberry)*, HMB (beta-hydroxy beta-methylbutyrate), Eleuthero (*Eleuthero-ciccus senticoccus*), ginkgo biloba extract, L-arginine, L-lysine, creatine monohydrate, cayenne, essential oils (as shown below), and gelatin.

ssential Oils:

Nutmeg—supports adrenal glands; anti-inflammatory; stimulates immune function.

Lemongrass—helps repair connective tissue; when combined with marjoram, it helps stimulate the agents in the tissue to rejuvenate and reconnect.

Rosemary cineol—helps balance heart function, stimulates nerves, and decongests the liver.

Wintergreen—locally warming; contains methyl salicylate; has a cortisone-like action that helps to reduce inflammation in the joints and tissue.

Suggested Use: Two capsules morning and evening.

Body System(s) Affected: MUSCLES and BONES.

Companion Products: Master Formula His/Hers, Power Meal, Ultra Young, Wolfberry Bars.

Companion Oils: Brain Power, En-R-Gee, EndoFlex, Envision, Live with Passion, Valor.

Berrygize Nutrition Bars

A delicious nutrition bar, made with the Chinese Wolfberry and other nutrient packed, natural ingredients. The **Wolfberry** is high in the branched-chain amino acid L-leucine. When metabolized, L-leucine produces a muscle-building compound in the body called HMB (beta-hydroxy beta-methylbutyrate). **Amaranth** is a high-protein grain (over 16% protein by weight) containing large amounts of another essential amino acid called L-lysine. Both L-leucine (found i the Wolfberry) and L-lysine (from the amaranth) work together synergistically to build muscle. With over 15 grams of protein per serving, this bar makes an ideal meal replacement or even an energizing supplement while exercising.

Ingredients: Soy/whey protein, almond butter, agave nectar (*Agave salmiana/angustifolia*), Ningxia wolfberry, FOS (fructooligosaccharides), xylitol, orange/lemon powders (freeze-dried - rich in vitamin C), creatine monohydrate, L-arginine, phenylalanine, alpha lipoic acid (powerful antioxidant), amaranth, chromium.

Suggested Use: Take 1 bar a day or as a meal alternative or a high-energy snack.

Body System(s) Affected: DIGESTIVE and IMMUNE SYSTEMS, MUSCLES and BONES.

Companion Products: Be-Fit, Berry Young Juice, ComforTone, Essential Manna, Essentialzym ICP, JuvaPower, JuvaSpice, Master Formula His/Hers, KidScents Mighty Mist/Vites, Thyromin, VitaGreen.

Companion Oils: Abundance, Citrus Fresh, EndoFlex, Envision, Juva Cleanse, Live with Passion, Magnify Your Purpose.

Berry Young Juice

A powerful blend of the highest known antioxidant fruit juices with the strongest anti-ing effects. With an ORAC (Oxygen Radical Absorbence Capacity) score of over 5,500, it has ore powerful antioxidant properties than even Tahitian Noni Juice. The Chinese wolfberry also ntains the highest levels of immune-stimulating polysaccharides.

gredients: Ningxia wolfberry (*Lycium barbarum*) juice, blueberry juice, pomegranate juice, agave (as a sweetener), apricot juice, raspberry juice, natural blueberry flavor, ascorbic acid, potassium sorbate, sodium benzoate, and pure therapeutic-grade essential oils (as listed below).

sential Oils:

Lemon—contains over 65% d-limonene (which helps to promote normal cell life cycles); helps promote leukocyte formation; helps to dissolve cholesterol and fats.

Orange—contains over 91% d-limonene (which helps to promote normal cell life cycles); rich in compounds noted for their stress-reducing effects.

ggested Use: Take 1 teaspoon mixed in one cup of juice or water, twice daily or as needed between meals.

dy System(s) Affected: IMMUNE SYSTEM.

mpanion Products: Berry Young Cookies, Ultra Young, Essential Manna, and Power Meal.

mpanion Oils: En-R-Gee, EndoFlex, Envision, JuvaFlex, Magnify Your Purpose, Longevity, and Valor.

BLM

Protect your mobility by providing your bones and joints with the proper nutritional pport. This product synergistically combines some of the most potent ingredients known. vailable in both powder and capsule form.

gredients: **Manganese citrate** (catalyst to synergize ingredients), potassium chloride, and a proprietary blend of glucosamine sulfate (helps formation of cartilage), **type II collagen** (joint-supporting proteoglycans, also contains cartilage matrix glycoprotein (CMGP), which can help reduce oxidative damage to joints), **MSM** (sulfur - restores flexibility tc cell membranes, slows breakdown of cartilage), and essential oils as shown below.

Essential Oils:

Idaho Balsam Fir—is a rich source of the antioxidant limonene which has been shown help relieve OVERWORKED and TIRED MUSCLES and JOINTS.

Wintergreen—contains 99% methyl salicylate which gives it cortisone-like properties. may be beneficial for ARTHRITIS, RHEUMATISM, TENDINITIS, and any other discomfort that is related to the inflammation of BONES, MUSCLES, anc JOINTS.

Clove—as an antioxidant it has one of the highest ORAC (oxygen radical absorbent capacity) scores. It helps preserve the integrity of fatty acids and has been used a numbing agent in dentistry.

Suggested Use:

Capsules: If you weigh **less than 120 lbs**, take 1 capsule three times a day. If you wei **between 120 and 200 lbs**, take 1 capsule four times a day. If you weigh **more than 200 lbs**, take 1 capsule five times a day.

Powder: If you weigh **less than 120 lbs**, take 1/4 teaspoon three times a day. If you weigh **between 120 and 200 lbs**, take 1/4 teaspoon four times a day. If you we **more than 200 lbs**, take 1/4 teaspoon five times a day.

Body System(s) Affected: MUSCLES and BONES.

Bodygize

Bodygize is a nutritional drink mix with a complete profile of essential amino acids, vitamins, and minerals for improved balance and lymphatic decongestion. The purpose of Bodygize is to help balance the body at its ideal weight. Advanced technology has made low heat glass-pack pasteurization of nonfat dry milk possible, leaving the enzymes intact. Fructose (sug derived from fruit) is a perfect sweetener and contains a proper digestive balance. The essential oils provide its unique flavor and act as a **natural antioxidant**. European research has found tha the oils in Bodygize may help dissolve hard fatty deposits and decongest the lymphatic system. The high level of protein in this product may help your body maintain a good food supply for muscle tissue.

Ingredients: Non-fat dry milk, ultrafiltered whey protein, fructose, potassium citrate, vanilla, lecithin, silicon dioxide, guar gum, sodium chloride, potassium chloride, magnesium citrate, ascorbic acid (vitamin C), zinc citrate, mixed tocopherols (vitamin E), niacinami (vitamin B3), essential oil of grapefruit (as shown below), vitamin B5 (as calcium pantothenate), copper (as amino acid chelate), vitamin A (palmitate), folic acid, vitamin B6 (as pyrodoxine HCl), riboflavin (vitamin B2), thiamin (vitamin B1), lutein, lycopene, vitamin B12, biotin, potassium iodine, essential oils of lemon, tangerine, orange, mandarin, and lime (as shown below), vitamin D3 (as cholecalciferol), selenium (as selenomethionine), and essential oil of cypress (as shown below).

sential Oils:

Grapefruit—excellent for fluid retention and cellulite; diuretic, detoxifier, and stimulant of the lymphatic system; important as an antidepressant.

Lemon—helps promote leukocyte formation; helps to dissolve cholesterol and fats.

Tangerine—sedating and calming to the nervous system; also a diuretic and a decongestant of the lymphatic system..

Orange—is rich in compounds noted for their stress-reducing effects.

Mandarin—helps to strengthen the digestive function and the liver.

Lime—turns alkaline during digestion; helps to dissolve cholesterol and fats.

Cypress—mucolytic, astringent, diuretic, lymphatic decongestant; reduces cellulite and strengthens connective tissue.

ggested Use: One measuring scoop to 8-10 oz. of purified water, juice or low fat milk. Blend in blender for 30 seconds. Ice cubes may be added to thicken like a shake. Bodygize works with all juices. It is a pre-digested protein and can be taken at any time. For optimum results, take with Master Formula His or Hers, and Thyromin supplements.

1. ***For Fast Weight Loss:*** Enjoy Bodygize as a replacement for breakfast and dinner. Eat a sensible, low-fat, well-balanced lunch which includes vegetables, fruits, and whole grains. As with any weight loss program, fats, sugars, and high-calorie foods should be omitted from your diet. Raw vegetables are excellent snacks.
2. ***For Weight Gain:*** Enjoy Bodygize mixed with rice/almond milk or apple juice. Add a banana or a pear and drink after each meal.
3. ***For Good Health and Weight Maintenance:*** After you have achieved your ideal weight, enjoy a Bodygize shake as a meal replacement daily, possibly for breakfast. Bodygize can also be used as a filling and nutritious snack for the entire family.

fety Data: Anyone who is pregnant or nursing, has health problems, or wants to lose more than 50 pounds or more than 20% of their body weight should consult their physician before starting this or any other weight loss program.

dy System(s) Affected: DIGESTIVE and IMMUNE SYSTEMS, MUSCLES and BONES.

Frequency: Approximately 87 MHz.

Companion Products: Be-Fit, Cel-Lite Magic Massage Oil, ComforTone, Master Formula His/Hers, Mineral Essence, Super B, Super Cal, Thyromin.

Companion Oils: Citrus Fresh, EndoFlex, Envision, Live with Passion, Magnify Your Purpose

Comments: The authors of this book enjoy mixing Bodygize with a glass of Rice Dream (a bro rice beverage). May also be mixed with soy or almond beverages.

Carbozyme

A carbohydrate-digestive blend of active ingredients that aids digestion and enhances the absorption of nutrients. Carbozyme may provide relief of occasional symptoms such as fullness, pressure, bloating, gas, pain, and/or minor cramping that may occur after eating.

Ingredients: Amylase, bee pollen, pure therapeutic-grade essential oils (as listed below), trace minerals, rice bran, vegetable cellulose, and deionized water.

Essential Oils: Thieves Blend, containing the following oils:

Clove—is anti-bacterial, anti-fungal, anti-infectious, anti-parasitic, a strong antiseptic, anti-viral, and an immune stimulant; helps preserve integrity of fatty acids.

Lemon—helps to dissolve cholesterol and fats.

Cinnamon Bark—anti-fungal, anti-bacterial, and antiviral.

Eucalyptus radiata—has strong anti-bacterial, anti-catarrhal, and antiseptic properties.

Rosemary cineol—helps balance heart function, stimulates nerves, and decongests the liver.

Suggested Use: Take 1-2 capsules three times daily just before meals containing carbohydrates or as needed.

Body System(s) Affected: DIGESTIVE SYSTEM.

Companion Products: ComforTone, JuvaTone, Sulfurzyme, Royaldophilus, and Power Meal.

Companion Oils: Di-Tone and JuvaFlex.

Warning: Do not give this product to children under 12 years of age except under the supervision of a doctor. If symptoms persist, discontinue use of this product and consult your physician. Keep in a cool, dry place. Do not expose to excessive heat or direct sunlight. If pregnant or under a doctor's care, consult your physician.

CardiaCare

Strengthens and supports the heart and cardiovascular system.

Ingredients: Chinese wolfberry powder *(Refer to the Wolfberry Bar at the end of this section for more information on the benefits of the Chinese Wolfberry)*, hawthorn berry (may help increase blood circulation in the heart), magnesium citrate, vitamin E (d alpha succinate, naturally derived), coenzyme Q10 (CoQ10), rhododendron caucasicum extract (contains phenylpropanoids which have been shown in clinical studies to increase the efficiency of the cardiovascular system—*refer to comment below on rhododendron caucasicum*), essential oils (as shown below), and gelatin.

Essential Oils:

Helichrysum—is a natural blood thickness regulator, allowing for better passage of the blood between vessels and tissues.

Lemon—helps to dissolve cholesterol and fats.

Marjoram—provides support for the smooth muscles of the heart.

Ylang Ylang—is a nutrient that has been found to help support heart function.

Suggested Use: Three capsules, twice daily.

Body System(s) Affected: CARDIOVASCULAR SYSTEM.

Companion Products: AD&E tincture, HRT tincture, and Mineral Essence.

Companion Oils: Aroma Life, Forgiveness, Harmony, Joy, Live with Passion.

Comments: *Rhododendron caucasicum* contains some powerful and highly beneficial antioxidant flavonoids and polyphenols similar to those found in pine bark extract. One study showed that Rhododendron possessed the same antioxidant activity as the powerful antioxidant, Pycnogenol. Some of the clinically researched benefits of rhododendron include significant effects on physical endurance and the cardiovascular system by increasing the blood supply to the muscles and the brain, diminished heart and chest pains, normalized blood pressure, improved heart circulation, lowered blood serum cholesterol levels, improved systolic blood pressure levels, inhibition of the enzyme hyaluronidase (which may play a role in the cause of arthritis and colon cancer), increased uric acid elimination (which may help provide relief from gout).

ComforTone

Herbal formula with Bentonite, Apple Pectin, and herbal extracts which may relieve constipation, enhance colon function, and dispel parasites and toxins. The addition of essential oils may enhance the flavor as well as the activity of the herbs contained in this formula. This product was designed as a cleanser for any type of bowel irregularity.

Ingredients: German chamomile flowers, cascara sagrada, bentonite, diatomacious earth, psyllium seed, fennel, burdock root, garlic, barberry, *Echinacea purpurea* root, ginger root, apple pectin, licorice root, cayenne pepper, essential oils (as shown below), and gelatin.

Essential Oils:

Rosemary cineol—helps balance heart function, stimulates nerves, and decongests the liver.

Tarragon—may help reduce anorexia, dyspepsia, flatulence, intestinal spasms, nervous and sluggish digestion, and genital urinary tract infection.

Peppermint—purifying and stimulating to the conscious mind; anti-inflammatory; helps with nerve regeneration. It also enhances digestion and increases endurance.

Ginger—is warming, uplifting, and empowering; helps reduce feelings of nausea, and motion sickness.

Anise—may help calm and strengthen the digestive system.

Mugwort (*Artemisia vulgaris*)—has been used to help calm nerves.

Tangerine—sedating and calming to the nervous system; also a diuretic and a decongestant of the lymphatic system..

German Chamomile—has been found to help open the liver, increase liver function and secretion, and support the pancreas.

Suggested Use: Start with two to five capsules first thing in the morning (½ hour before breakfast) and two to five capsules just before bed. Drink eight to ten 8 oz. glasses of purified or distilled water per day for best results. If you get cramps, skip the next morning or day, and start up again with two capsules in the morning and two in the evening. After starting ComforTone, you may cut back, but don't stop completely becaus all the toxins that have been pulled out of the system will go back into the system. Take at least one in the morning and one in the evening, but don't stop once you start.

ComforTone can be taken every day without becoming addictive. For maximum results, use with JuvaTone and Essentialzyme. *CAUTION: Do not take ComforTone at the same time as JuvaTone! When taken together, possible reactions include bloating, gas, diaphragm and chest pains (heartburn or acid reflux). If a reaction occurs, Di-Tone or JuvaFlex applied around the navel or center of the spine has helped. It is best to take ComforTone and JuvaTone at least one hour apart from each other.*

ıfety Data: ComforTone can be taken during pregnancy as long as you don't get diarrhea. Diarrhea can cause cramping which could bring on labor.

›dy System(s) Affected: DIGESTIVE and IMMUNE SYSTEMS.

omments: ComforTone may be used to get rid of parasites. It breaks up the encrustation along the colon wall and relaxes spasms that may occur. Use Di-Tone when there is nausea. If constipation is increased with five ComforTone, increase the water intake (or a spasm in the colon may cause more constipation) and decrease or stop taking ICP. If a person has a history of chronic constipation, don't start ICP and ComforTone at the same time. Start ComforTone until the system is open, then start ICP with ten glasses of water per day. One woman was paralyzed by surgery and had to have a colonic two times a day. When she started taking ComforTone, she was able to have natural bowel movements.

·equency: Approximately 43 MHz.

ompanion Supplements: Essentialzyme and ICP, JuvaTone, Chelex, ParaFree.

ompanion Oils: Di-Tone (use with hot compress on abdomen or rub on feet), JuvaFlex, Purification, Release, Thieves.

Coral Sea

This product is a potent calcium supplement that contains 58 trace minerals necessary for aintaining optimal bone and joint health. Studies have shown this type of calcium to be better ›sorbed and more efficient in cell preservation than regular calcium carbonate. It is especially eal for mixed diets, high fiber/high grain diets, or diets that are high in carbonated beverages. *ːfer to the chart shown under MegaCal in this same section for a comparison of Coral Sea to egaCal and SuperCal.*

ıgredients: The organic coral calcium in this product comes from ancient coral that is mined from the island of Okinawa off the coast of Japan. The living coral is not used.

Suggested Use: Take one teaspoon mixed in one cup of juice or water, twice daily or as needed *between* meals.

Body System(s) Affected: MUSCLES and BONES.

Companion Products: Essential Manna, Power Meal, Prenolone/Prenolone+, PD 80/20.

CortiStop
(Men's)

This product is formulated specifically for men and is designed to modulate the productic of cortisol (the "Death" hormone) in the body, thereby helping to maintain the natural balance an harmony of other important substances like testosterone. The negative effects of high amounts of cortisol are also diminished by providing nutrients that influence glandular balance.

Ingredients: Zinc citrate (important for prostate health), 4 androstene-3,17diol (testosterone precursor), tribulus (*T. terrestris*) fruit (activates the anterior pituitary which increases production of testosterone), l-a-lysophosphatidyl choline (Epikuron 100E) (blocks cortisc production), l-a-phosphatidyl choline (LECI-PC 35P) (blocks cortisol production), yohimbe (*Pausinystalia yohimbe*) bark extract (helps decrease the production of fat and removes fat from storage to be used as fuel), DHEA (dioscorea villosa) (testosterone precursor - shown to enhance memory and increase muscle strength and lean body mass) therapeutic-grade essential oils as listed below, rice flour and gelatin.

Essential Oils:

Fleabane (*Conyza canadensis*)—is a rare essential oil studied by Daniel Pénoël, M.D. fc its ability to stimulate the pancreas and liver and counteract retarded puberty. It a mood enhancer and promoter of hGH.

Peppermint—purifying and stimulating to the conscious mind; anti-inflammatory; helps with nerve regeneration. It also enhances digestion and increases endurance.

Frankincense—anti-tumoral and anti-inflammatory; increases activity of leukocytes. It also enhances the function of the pituitary and hypothalamus.

Suggested Use: Take one capsule before retiring. If desired, for extra benefits, take another capsule in the morning before breakfast. Use daily for 8 weeks. Discontinue use for 2-4 weeks before resuming.

Precautions: Keep in a cool, dry place. Keep out of reach of children. If pregnant or under a doctor's care, consult your physician.

Comments: The natural pro-hormone activity of this formulation has led to restriction of use by some athletic organizations.

Body System(s) Affected: HORMONAL SYSTEM.

Companion Products: Essential Manna, PD 80/20, Power Meal, Prenolone/Prenolone+, Super C, Wolfberry Bars.

CortiStop
(Women's)

This product is formulated specifically for women and is designed to modulate the production of cortisol (the "Death" hormone) in the body, thereby helping to maintain the natural balance and harmony of other important substances like estrogen and progesterone. The negative effects of high amounts of cortisol are also diminished by providing nutrients that influence glandular balance.

Ingredients: Pregnenolone (promotes glandular balance, improves energy, and reduces stress), l-a-lysophosphatidyl choline (Epikuron 100E) (blocks cortisol production), l-a-phosphatidyl choline (LECI-PC 35P) (blocks cortisol production), Black cohosh (has estrogen-like functions; helps with hot flashes and other menopausal problems), DHEA (dioscorea villosa) (estrogen precursor - shown to enhance memory and increase muscle strength and lean body mass), therapeutic-grade essential oils as listed below, rice flour and gelatin.

Essential Oils:

Fleabane (*Conyza canadensis*)—is a rare essential oil studied by Daniel Pénoël, M.D. for its ability to stimulate the pancreas and liver and counteract retarded puberty. It is a mood enhancer and promoter of hGH

Peppermint—purifying and stimulating to the conscious mind; anti-inflammatory; helps with nerve regeneration. It also enhances digestion and increases endurance.

Clary Sage—helps balance the hormones; tonic to the reproductive system.

Fennel—helps balance the hormones.

Frankincense—anti-tumoral and anti-inflammatory; increases activity of leukocytes. It also enhances the function of the pituitary and hypothalamus.

Suggested Use: Take one capsule before retiring. If desired, for extra benefits, take another capsule in the morning before breakfast. Use daily for 8 weeks. Discontinue use for 2-4 weeks before resuming.

Precautions: Keep in a cool, dry place. Keep out of reach of children. If pregnant or under a doctor's care, consult your physician.

Comments: The natural pro-hormone activity of this formulation has led to restriction of use by some athletic organizations.

Body System(s) Affected: HORMONAL SYSTEM.

Companion Products: Essential Manna, PD 80/20, Power Meal, Prenolone/Prenolone+, Super C Wolfberry Bars.

Detoxzyme

A vegetable enzyme complex designed to promote detoxification of the body and to support and maintain a healthy intestinal environment. Because it combines essential oils with enzymes that are meant to digest starches, sugars, proteins, and fats, it may also provide relief of occasional symptoms such as fullness, pressure, bloating, gas, pain, and/or minor cramping that occur after eating. By facilitating the optimal absorption of nutrients from foods and supplements the aging process is delayed and energy levels enhanced.

Ingredients: Amylase, glucoamylase, alpha-galactosidase, invertase, lactase, cellulase, protease, bromelain, lipase, phytase, pure therapeutic-grade essential oils (as listed below), rice bran, vegetable cellulose, deionized water, cumin seed extract, and silica.

Essential Oils:

Cumin—anti-bacterial; antispasmodic; some anti-tumoral properties.

Anise—may help calm and strengthen the digestive system.

Fennel—anti-parasitic; promotes the removal of toxic wastes; may break up fluids and toxins, and cleanse the tissues.

Suggested Use: Take 2-3 capsules three times daily between meals. This product may be used in conjunction with a cleansing/detoxifying program. Can also be sprinkled on food or in beverages.

Body System(s) Affected: DIGESTIVE and IMMUNE SYSTEMS.

Companion Products: ComforTone, JuvaTone, Sulfurzyme, Royaldophilus, and Power Meal.

Companion Oils: Di-Tone and JuvaFlex.

Warning: Do not give this product to children under 12 years of age except under the supervision of a doctor. If symptoms persist, discontinue use of this product and consult your physician. Keep in a cool, dry place. Do not expose to excessive heat or direct sunlight. If pregnant or under a doctor's care, consult your physician.

Comments: This formula contains trace minerals that can help to detoxify the body and assist in the reduction of cholesterol and triglycerides. It also helps to open the gallbladder duct, cleanse the liver, and regulate pH levels, thereby reducing acidification which helps to prevent candida and yeast overgrowth as well as parasite colonization and infestation. It may also help provide relief from diarrhea, constipation, heartburn, and food allergies.

Essential Manna

This super food has been adapted from the diet of the Hunza people, who are one of the few groups of people that live past 100 years of age with excellent health. All of the following ingredients are in their raw form.

Ingredients: Apricots, barley, Chinese wolfberries, pineapple, buckwheat, almonds, brown rice, papaya, pumpkin seeds, apricot concentrate, walnuts, amaranth, unsweetened coconut, millet, filberts, sesame seeds, rolled oats, pecans, Brazil nuts, potassium sorbate, fructooligosaccharides (FOS), sodium ascorbate, citric acid, L-lysine, and frankincense powder. May also contain cashews and stevia.

Flavors: As of July 2002, available in Apricot, Carob (additional carob chips), Carob Mint (additional carob chips and peppermint essential oil), and Spice (additional cinnamon powder).

Suggested Use: Snack on Essential Manna throughout the day whenever you feel hungry.

Body System(s) Affected: DIGESTIVE and IMMUNE SYSTEMS, MUSCLES and BONES.

Companion Products: Essentialzyme, JuvaTone, Mineral Essence, Power Meal, Sulfurzyme.

Companion Oils: Exodus II, En-R-Gee, EndoFlex, Envision, JuvaFlex, Magnify Your Purpose, Valor.

Essential Omegas

This unique blend of organic fatty acids and essential oils as shown below is much needed in most diets today. Organic flaxseed oil is not only rich in lignans (supports normal cardiovascular and colon function), but also provides one of the richest food sources for the omega 3 essential fatty acid. Black currant oil is not only rich in essential fatty acids but also provides an excellent source of gamma linoleic acid (supports function of the heart, brain, and circulatory system).

Ingredients: Black currant oil, organic flaxseed oil, agave (dark; low-glycemic sweetner; rich in magnesium, potassium, and calcium), FOS (NutriFlora), and essential oils (as shown below).

Essential Oils:

Orange—is rich in compounds noted for their stress-reducing effects; lipid-soluble traits; antioxidant properties which enhance vitamin absorption.

Clove—is anti-bacterial, anti-fungal, anti-infectious, anti-parasitic, a strong antiseptic, anti-viral, and an immune stimulant; helps preserve integrity of fatty acids.

Body System(s) Affected: CARDIOVASCULAR and NERVOUS SYSTEMS, SKIN.

Essentialzyme

A high-quality enzyme complex which may improve and aid digestion and the elimination of toxic waste from the body. Essentialzyme was formulated to help supply the enzymes to people who have difficulty digesting or assimilating food. Helps promote and re-establish proper enzyme balance in the digestive system and throughout the body. Also helps to retard the aging process. Flavor enhanced with Essential Oils. **Natural antioxidant**.

Ingredients: Betaine HCI, pancrelipase, pancreatin 4x (porcine pancreas glands originating in the United States), bromelain, trypsin, thyme (*Thymus vulgaris*) leaf, carrot (*Daucus carota*) root powder, alfalfa (*Medicago sativa*) sprouts and leaf, papain, cumin (*Cuminum cyminum*) seeds, essential oils (as shown below), dicalcium phosphate, stearic acid, croscarmellose sodium, and magnesium stearate.

Essential Oils:

Anise—may help calm and strengthen the digestive system.

Fennel—diuretic; may break up fluids and toxins, and cleanse the tissues.

Peppermint—is antispasmodic, and anti-inflammatory; soothing, cooling, and dilating to the system. It also enhances digestion and increases endurance.
Tarragon—may help reduce anorexia, dyspepsia, flatulence, intestinal spasms, nervous and sluggish digestion, and genital urinary tract infection.
Clove—anti-infectious, antiviral, anti-fungal, and anti-parasitic.

ggested Use: Take three tablets, three times daily prior to or with meals (more may be taken for larger meals), or as needed. Take Essentialzyme with meals, especially protein meals after 3 p.m. as it will help lessen the burden on the digestive system. Also helps with digestive functions in the liver.

dy System(s) Affected: DIGESTIVE SYSTEM.

equency: Approximately 83 MHz.

mpanion Products: ComforTone, JuvaTone, Mineral Essence, Royaldophilus, Power Meal.

mpanion Oils: Di-Tone, Harmony, JuvaFlex.

Exodus

Exodus is the ultimate supercharged antioxidant containing a Biblical Blend of Essential ls and other valuable herbs that provide important support for the body's defenses.

gredients: *Uncaria tomentosa* root (or Cat's Claw), OPC grapeseed extract (highly-praised antioxidant), *Echinacea purpurea* root (boosts activity of T-cells), yucca root (good for osteoarthritis and rheumatoid arthritis), pantothenic acid, vitamin A (as mixed carotenoids), amino acid complex (includes alanine, cystine, argenine, glycine, lycine, threonine, and thorine), ionic minerals, and essential oils (as shown below).

sential Oils:
Frankincense—anti-tumoral and anti-inflammatory; increases activity of leukocytes. It also enhances the function of the pituitary and hypothalamus.
Hyssop—helps with viral infections and expelling parasites.
Laurel (*Laurus nobilis)*—anti-fungal and antiseptic.
Spikenard—anti-bacterial and anti-fungal; helps with staph infections.

Comments: Some of the company literature states that myrrh (anti-infectious and antiseptic) ma also be included.

Suggested Use: Take three capsules two to three times daily.

Body System(s) Affected: IMMUNE SYSTEM.

Companion Products: ComforTone, Essential Manna, ImmuneTune, Power Meal, Super C, VitaGreen.

Companion Oils: Exodus II, ImmuPower, Purification, Thieves.

FemiGen

An herbal formula, with glandular substances and amino acids, which helps build and balance the reproductive system and maintain better hormonal balance for developmental years all the way through menopause. When one has experienced mood swings, PMS, and symptoms related to menopause, it is an indication that the body is nutritionally out of balance. FemiGen acts as a natural estrogen and helps balance the hormones.

Ingredients: Vitamin A, vitamin C, calcium, magnesium, damiana (blood purifier), epimedium aerial parts (detoxifies kidneys), wild yam root, dong quai root, muira-puama root (potency wood), American ginseng root, licorice root, black cohosh, L-carnitine, dimethyglycine, L-phenylalanine, cramp bark, squaw vine aerial parts, L-cystine, L-cysteine HCl, essential oils (as shown below), and gelatin.

Essential Oils:

Fennel—helps balance the hormones.

Clary Sage—helps balance the hormones; tonic to the reproductive system.

Sage—contains estriol and has estrogen-like properties; believed to contain elements tha contribute to the secretion of progesterone.

Ylang Ylang—stimulates adrenal glands; helps balance male/female energies.

Suggested Use: Take two capsules with breakfast and two capsules with lunch. A maintenance dose of two capsules may be taken three times a day for ten days before a period.

Body System(s) Affected: HORMONAL SYSTEM.

ompanion Products: Dragon Time Massage Oil.

ompanion Oils: Dragon Time, Mister, PanAway, Peace & Calming, Relieve It.

Fiberzyme

A fiber-digestive blend of active ingredients that aids digestion and enhances the sorption of nutrients. Fiberzyme may provide relief of occasional symptoms such as fullness, essure, bloating, gas, pain, and/or minor cramping that may occur after eating.

gredients: Cellulase, bee pollen, trace mineral powder, pure therapeutic-grade essential oils (as listed below), rice bran, vegetable cellulose, and deionized water.

ssential Oils:

Tarragon—may help reduce anorexia, dyspepsia, flatulence, intestinal spasms, nervous and sluggish digestion, and genital urinary tract infection.

Ginger—is warming, uplifting, and empowering; helps reduce feelings of nausea, and motion sickness.

Peppermint—purifying and stimulating to the conscious mind; anti-inflammatory; helps with nerve regeneration. It also enhances digestion and increases endurance.

Juniper—antispasmodic; helps reduce muscle aches/pains.

Fennel—anti-parasitic; promotes the removal of toxic wastes; may break up fluids and toxins, and cleanse the tissues.

Lemongrass—helps repair connective tissue; it helps stimulate the agents in the tissue to rejuvenate and reconnect; helps regulate the parasympathetic nervous system and strengthen vascular walls.

Anise—may help calm and strengthen the digestive system.

Patchouli—protects against UV radiation and promotes tissue regeneration; helps tighten loose skin and prevent wrinkles.

iggested Use: Take 1-2 capsules three times daily just prior to meals containing fruits and/or vegetables or as needed.

ody System(s) Affected: DIGESTIVE SYSTEM.

ompanion Products: ComforTone, JuvaTone, Sulfurzyme, Royaldophilus, and Power Meal.

ompanion Oils: Di-Tone and JuvaFlex.

Warning: Do not give this product to children under 12 years of age except under the supervisic of a doctor. If symptoms persist, discontinue use of this product and consult your physician. Keep in a cool, dry place. Do not expose to excessive heat or direct sunlight If pregnant or under a doctor's care, consult your physician.

H_2Oils

H_2Oils packets utilize hydro-diffusion technology to slowly and efficiently diffuse essent oils into drinking water. This provides a great-tasting, natural way to add the zing of essential oi to your drinking water. Children simply love the taste.

How to Use: Just place one or more packets into the Young Living Hydro Diffusion Dispenser other container) and fill with water. Within a few minutes, the oils will begin to diffuse into the water. The packets are re-usable until all of the oils have diffused out of the packet.

Peppermint—is refreshing and invigorating, especially on hot days. It enhances digestion and increases endurance.

Lemon—is refreshing and purifying. It helps to promote a sense of well being while alkalizing a cleansing the digestive and lymphatic systems.

Lemon-Grapefruit—is stimulating and invigorating. It helps to detoxify the system and promot the removal of excess fat.

Lemon-Orange—is uplifting and refreshing. It helps to calm the nerves while lowering cholesterol and reducing water retention.

ICP

Fiber Beverage - a unique source of fiber and bulk for the diet, which helps speed the transit time of waste matter through the intestinal tract. The psyllium, oat bran, flax, and rice br are specifically balanced to eliminate allergy symptoms that many people experience when taking psyllium alone. Essential oils enhance the flavor and may help to dispel gas and discomfort. Designed as both a cleanser and a builder, this formula is unsurpassed as an aid in enhancing normal bowel function.

Ingredients: Psyllium seed powder, oat bran (binds up fat), flax seed (roto-rooter; strong antioxidant), fennel seed (anti-parasitic), rice bran (roto-rooter), guar gum (opens colon), yucca root (anti-cancerous), plant cellulose, vegetarian protease enzyme formula (aids digestion), aloe vera extract (natural laxative), and essential oils (as shown below).

Essential Oils:

Fennel, Tarragon, Ginger, Lemongrass, and **Rosemary cineol**—all anti-parasitic by nature and promote the removal of toxic wastes.

Anise—as an anti-spasmodic and relaxant, it helps relax the muscles of the colon wall.

Suggested Use: Take five times a week for maintenance (½ cup water, ½ cup apple juice, and one heaping teaspoon (tsp.) of ICP). Take more often for cleansing (start with one heaping teaspoon (tsp.) two to three times a day with carrot juice or other vegetable juices. When things are going well, increase to three teaspoons (tsp.) three times a day). ICP dilutes better in warm water. Drink immediately as this product tends to thicken quickly when added to liquid. Sprinkle on yogurt, cereal, or other foods. Drink 8 to 16 oz. of fluid per teaspoon. ICP may be added to Bodygize or Power Meal.

Comments: For best results, take ComforTone first then ICP morning and night. If added to Citrus Juices, it creates more acid. Best to use other juices. ICP absorbs toxins so that it can build and improve the wave-like movement of the intestinal walls.

Frequency: Approximately 56 MHz.

Body System(s) Affected: CARDIOVASCULAR and DIGESTIVE SYSTEMS.

Companion Products: Bodygize, ComforTone, Essentialzyme, JuvaTone, ParaFree, Power Meal.

Companion Oils: Di-Tone, JuvaFlex, Purification, Thieves.

ImmuGel

ImmuGel is a unique blend of naturally occurring liquid amino acids, ionic-charged trace minerals, and herbal extracts with essential oils. This blend creates one of nature's most powerful antioxidant and antimicrobial formulas. It may aid in destroying fungi and bacteria, thereby boosting the immune defenses. Amino acids have a unique ability to neutralize and help eliminate free radicals in the system. This formula is used for general maintenance and one should increase their use during times of fatigue, depression, or when a cold is beginning. It is also used as a support in eliminating candida. It is a great companion to ImmuPower, Thieves, Super C, and ImmuneTune.

Ingredients: Deionized water (cleanses and purifies tissues), methylcellulose, hydrolyzed vegetable protein (contains amino acids of alanine, arginine, aspartic acid, glutamic acid, glycine, histidine, hydroxyproline, leucine and isoleucine, lycine, methionine, and phenylalanine), German chamomile extract, trace minerals (restore electrolyte balance), and essential oils (as shown below).

Essential Oils:

Cinnamon Bark—anti-fungal, anti-bacterial, and antiviral.

Clove—anti-infectious, antiviral, anti-fungal, and anti-parasitic.

Rosemary cineol—helps balance heart function, stimulates nerves, and decongests the liver.

Lemon—helps promote leukocyte formation

Thyme—anti-inflammatory; anti-fungal; antiseptic; anti-viral.

Oregano—powerful antimicrobial; anti-inflammatory; locally warming.

Suggested Use: Take ¼ to ½ tsp. three times daily. May be taken with water if desired. Refrigerate after opening.

Body System(s) Affected: IMMUNE and RESPIRATORY SYSTEMS.

Comments: One individual used ½ tsp. of ImmuGel per day and was able to clear up candida on the brain in one week.

Companion Products: ImmuneTune, Super C, Exodus, and JuvaTone.

Companion Oils: ImmuPower, Thieves, Exodus II, JuvaFlex, Purification, Release, Valor.

ImmuneTune

A super antioxidant and dietary supplement to support the body's immune defense system and fight against free radicals that are the primary cause of disease. The curcuminoid blend in this product has been found to be 60 percent stronger in antioxidant activity than pine bark or grape pi extract. However, synergism is the key to obtaining maximum effect. Through the combining of curcuminoids and grape pit extract, the antioxidant frequency is almost doubled. The minerals are added to maintain cell electrolyte and pH balance. Chromium supports the metabolism and selenium supports the nervous system while its antioxidant ability adds to the synergism of the formula. Yucca and echineaca lend their support to the immune system and their antioxidant and anti-infectious attributes increase the nutrient support. The essential oil of orange increases the avonoid activity; pine and fir oils increase the anti-inflammatory action; and cistus, ravensara, nd lemon oils add immune system support. **Natural antioxidant.**

ngredients: Turmeric extract, magnesium citrate, yucca root, potassium citrate, Echinacea root, calcium citrate, wild yam, pantothenic acid, grapeseed extract, selenium, chromium, alpha lipoic acid, ginger extract, essential oils (as shown below), and gelatin.

ssential Oils:

Orange—is rich in compounds noted for their stress-reducing effects.

Pine—was used by the American Indians to repel lice and flees; antimicrobial, antiviral, and anti-inflammatory; may also be good against skin parasites.

Ravensara—is a powerful anti-viral, anti-bacterial, anti-fungal, and anti-infectious oil. It may help dilate, open, and strengthen the respiratory system. As a cross between clove and nutmeg, it may also help support the adrenal glands.

Lemon—helps promote leukocyte formation; helps to dissolve cholesterol and fats.

Fir—antiseptic and anti-inflammatory; helps create a feeling of grounding, anchoring, and empowerment.

Cistus—has anti-bacterial, anti-infectious, and anti-viral properties. Because it is high in oxygenating molecules, it may assist the auto-immune system and may help strengthen the immune system.

uggested Use: For slow metabolism, take two to three capsules daily. For fast metabolism, take three to six capsules daily. Best taken on an empty stomach. For stomach sensitivity, take with meals.

ody System(s) Affected: IMMUNE SYSTEM.

requency: Approximately 108 MHz.

ompanion Products: Exodus, ImmuGel, ParaFree, Super C.

ompanion Oils: ImmuPower (on throat and chest), Thieves (on feet), Envision, Exodus II, Release.

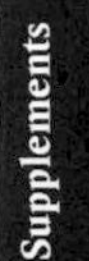

ImmuPro

ImmuPro is a unique blend of five powerful polysaccharides—natural immune system nhancers that aid in normal immune function and support the body's ability to fight illness. This egan formula comes in a chewable tablet with a great strawberry taste.

Ingredients: Zinc (as zinc citrate), selenium (as selenomethionine), copper (as copper chelate), Ningxia wolfberry (*Lycium barbarum*) polysaccharide), Reishi (*Ganoderma lucidum*) mycelia, Maitake (*Grifola frondosa*) mycelia, *Agaricus blazei* mycelia, arabinogalactin (larch tree extract), limonene (from orange essential oil), melatonin, organic strawberry powder, fructose, raspberry juice, pure lemon powder, and silicon dioxide.

Suggested Use: Chew one tablet before retiring. If under stress, chew 2-4 tablets before retiring or one tablet as needed.

Precautions: May cause drowsiness. Keep out of reach of children. If pregnant, lactating or under a doctor's care, consult your physician. Keep in a cool, dry place.

Body System(s) Affected: IMMUNE SYSTEM

Companion Products: ImmuneTune, Super C, Exodus, and JuvaTone.

Companion Oils: ImmuPower, Thieves, Exodus II, JuvaFlex, Purification, Release, Valor.

JuvaPower

This new food supplement is packed with ingredients that have a dual purpose, to cleanse both the liver and the intestines simultaneously. Many of the ingredients in this supplement are some of the most powerful acid-binding foods, packed into this formulation to help support and cleanse the liver by helping to remove acids from the body. Not only does it fortify with optimum nutrition, but it also tastes great. Sprinkle some on a baked potato or some scrambled eggs and you'll be providing your body with some much needed support for proper digestion.

Ingredients: Rice seed bran, spinach leaf, tomato fruit, beet root, flax seed, oat seed bran, brocco floret, cucumber fruit, dill seed, sprouted barley seed, ginger root and rhizome, slippery elm bark, L-taurine, psyllium seed husk, essential oils (as shown below), aloe vera inner leaf extract, and peppermint leaf.

Essential Oils:

Anise—may help calm and strengthen the digestive system.

Fennel—anti-parasitic; promotes the removal of toxic wastes; may break up fluids and toxins, and cleanse the tissues.

ggested Use: Sprinkle 1 tablespoon on food (i.e., baked potato, salad, rice, eggs, etc.) or add to 4-8 oz. Purified water or rice/almond milk and drink. Use three times daily for maximum benefits.

dy System(s) Affected: DIGESTIVE SYSTEM (especially the LIVER).

ompanion Products: ComforTone, JuvaTone, Mineral Essence, Royaldophilus, Power Meal.

ompanion Oils: Di-Tone, Harmony, Juva Cleanse, JuvaFlex.

JuvaSpice

Contains all the same ingredients as JuvaPower, spiced up with some potassium, ealSalt™, and cayenne pepper. Great for adding both nutritional support and flavor to your vorite dishes. Sprinkle some on a baked potato or some scrambled eggs and you'll be providing ur body with some much needed support for proper digestion.

gredients: Rice seed bran, spinach leaf, tomato fruit, beet root, flax seed, oat seed bran, broccoli floret, cucumber fruit, potassium chloride, Redmond RealSalt™, dill leaf, sprouted barley seed, cayenne pepper fruit (*Capsicum annum*), ginger root and rhizome, slippery elm bark, L-taurine, psyllium seed husk, essential oils (as shown below), aloe vera inner leaf extract, and peppermint leaf.

ssential Oils:

Anise—may help calm and strengthen the digestive system.

Fennel—anti-parasitic; promotes the removal of toxic wastes; may break up fluids and toxins, and cleanse the tissues.

uggested Use: Sprinkle ⅓ - ½ teaspoon on food (i.e., baked potato, salad, rice, eggs, etc.) or add to 4-8 oz. Purified water or rice/almond milk and drink.

ody System(s) Affected: DIGESTIVE SYSTEM (especially the LIVER).

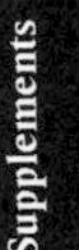

ompanion Products: ComforTone, JuvaTone, Mineral Essence, Royaldophilus, Power Meal.

ompanion Oils: Di-Tone, Harmony, Juva Cleanse, JuvaFlex.

JuvaTone

Amino acid herbal complex with trace minerals and essential oils for enhanced liver function, diminished addictions and skin improvement in a synergistic suspension isolation proce This product was designed specifically as a cleanser of the liver. The same essential oils that are included in this product are also included in the JuvaFlex oil blend making it the perfect topically applied companion to JuvaTone.

Ingredients: Calcium, copper citrate, sodium, choline bitartrate, dl-methionine, beet root, inosit raw dandelion root, L-cysteine HCl, alfalfa sprouts, Oregon grape root, parsley leaves, b propolis 5x, sodium copper chlorophyllin, echinacea root, essentials oils (as shown belov cellulose, stearic acid, croscarmellose sodium, silicon dioxide, magnesium stearate, and cellulose film coat.

Essential Oils:

Lemon—helps promote leukocyte formation; helps to dissolve cholesterol and fats.

German Chamomile—has been found to help open the liver, increase liver function and secretion, and support the pancreas.

Geranium—cleansing, refreshing, astringent, diuretic; helps support the kidney and bladder functions and helps with stone removal.

Rosemary cineol—helps balance heart function, stimulates nerves, and decongests the liver.

Myrtle—is a decongestant of the respiratory system. It may help improve oxygenation and work as an expectorant in discharging mucus.

Blue Tansy—calms the lymphatic system; promotes a feeling of self-control.

Suggested Use: Take three capsules mid-morning and three capsules mid-afternoon. For maximum results, use with ComforTone. *CAUTION: Do not take ComforTone* ***at the same time*** *as JuvaTone! When taken together, possible reactions include bloating, gas diaphragm and chest pains (heartburn or acid reflux). If a reaction occurs, Di-Tone or JuvaFlex applied around the navel or center of the spine has helped.* ***It is best to take ComforTone and JuvaTone at least one hour apart from each other***. Also apply JuvaFlex over the liver, on the spine, or on the feet.

Body System(s) Affected: DIGESTIVE and IMMUNE SYSTEMS.

Frequency: Approximately 140 MHz.

Companion Products: ComforTone, Essentialzyme, ICP, ParaFree, Power Meal.

Companion Oils: JuvaFlex, Di-Tone, Forgiveness, Release, Surrender, Thieves.

omments: JuvaTone goes through five stages of isolation when made so it won't upset an empty stomach. The liver plays a major role in helping the body to detoxify. The final products of digestion are transported through the portal vein from the colon to the liver to be cleansed. People have reported that while using JuvaTone, addictions to coffee, tea, tobacco, sugar, or alcohol are diminished.

KidScents Mighty Mist

A multi-vitamin antioxidant complex with wolfberry polysaccharides.

ngredients: Vitamin A (solubilized), vitamin C (ascorbic acid), vitamin D (cholecalciferol), vitamin E (d-tocopheryl acetate), vitamin K (menadione), thiamin (vitamin B1), riboflavin (vitamin B2), niacin, vitamin B6 (pyridoxine HCl), folic acid, vitamin B12 (cyanocobalamin), biotin, pantothenic acid (Ca pantothenate), magnesium, zinc (zinc gluconate), selenium (selenomethionine), manganese, *Echinacea purpurea* extract, wolfberry polysaccharide, aloe vera, distilled water, vegetable glycerin, trace mineral complex, amino acid complex, phosphatidycholine, ginkgo biloba, PABA (para-amino benzoic acid), inositol, stevia extract, and natural fruit flavoring.

uggested Use: Spray 3 mists inside cheeks, three times daily or as needed. Shake well before using.

ody System(s) Affected: EMOTIONAL BALANCE, CARDIOVASCULAR, IMMUNE, and NERVOUS SYSTEMS.

KidScents Mighty Vites

A great-tasting, chewable multi-vitamin for kids. The essential oils of lime, mandarin, and range, along with the Chinese wolfberry and the stevia extract, give this vitamin supplement a aste that makes children ask for more.

Supplements

ngredients: Vitamin A (retinyl palmitate), vitamin C (sodium ascorbate and ascorbic acid), vitamin D3 (cholecalciferol), vitamin E (d-alpha tocopheryl acid succinate), thiamin (vitamin B1), riboflavin (vitamin B2), niacin (niacin and niacinamide), vitamin B6 (pyroxidoxine HCl), folic acid, vitamin B12 (cyanocobalamin), biotin, pantothenic acid (d-calcium pantothenate), calcium, iodine (potassium iodine), magnesium, zinc, selenium, copper, manganese, chromium, potassium (potassium citrate), fructose, sorbitol, Chinese wolfberry (*Lycium barbarum*), bee pollen, inositol, pure therapeutic-grade essential oils (as listed below), wolfberry polysaccharides, and stevia extract.

Note: The calcium, iron, magnesium, zinc, selenium, copper, manganese, and chromium were derived from hydrolyzed protein complex.

Essential Oils:

Lime—helps remove dead skin cells; tightens skin and connective tissue.
Mandarin—good for skin problems, stretch marks, nervous tension, and restlessness.
Orange—is rich in compounds noted for their stress-reducing effects.

Suggested Use: Chew 3 tablets with breakfast daily.

Body System(s) Affected: EMOTIONAL BALANCE, CARDIOVASCULAR, IMMUNE, and NERVOUS SYSTEMS.

KidScents MightyZyme

With a special micro-encapsulation process to give the enzyme capsule a subtle peppermint flavor and sweetened with pure apple syrup, this vegetarian formula is sure to appeal to every child. It will also provide them with the natural enzymes to unlock and metabolize the vitamins, minerals and amino acids they desperately need for their growing bodies. It's **chewable** as well.

Ingredients: Calcium, folic acid, protease (3.0, 4.5, & 5.0), amylase, bromelain, cellulase, peptidase, lipase, phytase, alfalfa leaf, carrot root, peppermint (*Mentha piperita*) leaf, fructose, apple syrup, coconut oil, and silicon dioxide.

Suggested Use: Take 1 tablet, three times daily prior to or with meals.

Body System(s) Affected: DIGESTIVE SYSTEM.

Lipozyme

A fat-digestive blend of active ingredients that aids digestion and enhances the absorption of nutrients. Lipozyme may provide relief of occasional symptoms such as fullness, pressure, bloating, gas, pain, and/or minor cramping that may occur after eating.

gredients: Lipase, bee pollen, pancreatin 10x, pure therapeutic-grade essential oils (as listed below), trace minerals, vegetable cellulose, and deionized water.

sential Oils:

Tarragon—may help reduce anorexia, dyspepsia, flatulence, intestinal spasms, nervous and sluggish digestion, and genital urinary tract infection.

Ginger—is warming, uplifting, and empowering; helps reduce feelings of nausea, and motion sickness.

Peppermint—purifying and stimulating to the conscious mind; anti-inflammatory; helps with nerve regeneration. It also enhances digestion and increases endurance.

Juniper—antispasmodic; helps reduce muscle aches/pains.

Fennel—anti-parasitic; promotes the removal of toxic wastes; may break up fluids and toxins, and cleanse the tissues.

Lemongrass—helps repair connective tissue; it helps stimulate the agents in the tissue to rejuvenate and reconnect; helps regulate the parasympathetic nervous system and strengthen vascular walls.

Anise—may help calm and strengthen the digestive system.

Patchouli—protects against UV radiation and promotes tissue regeneration; helps tighten loose skin and prevent wrinkles.

ıggested Use: Take 1-2 capsules three daily just prior to meals containing fat or as needed.

ɔdy System(s) Affected: DIGESTIVE SYSTEM.

ompanion Products: ComforTone, JuvaTone, Sulfurzyme, Royaldophilus, and Power Meal.

ompanion Oils: Di-Tone and JuvaFlex.

ʼarning: Do not give this product to children under 12 years of age except under the supervision of a doctor. If symptoms persist, discontinue use of this product and consult your physician. Keep in a cool, dry place. Do not expose to excessive heat or direct sunlight. If pregnant or under a doctor's care, consult your physician.

Supplements

Longevity Capsules

(Longevity oil blend in gel capsules)

This blend of therapeutic-grade essential oils, as measured on the ORAC (oxygen radical ɔsorbent capacity) scale, has scored near 150,000! 100 mg of this blend of oils has been placed in gelatin capsules for easier consumption as a dietary supplement. It may help to promote longevity and prevent premature aging. For the regular oil blend, refer to Longevity in the Blend section of this book.

Ingredients: Pure therapeutic-grade essential oils (as listed below), lecithin (from soy), gelatin, and glycerin.

Essential Oils:

Thyme CT Thymol—has been shown in studies to DRAMATICALLY BOOST GLUTATHIONE LEVELS in the heart, liver, and brain. Because it can also he to PREVENT the OXIDATION of FATS in the body, it may help to slow the aging process. It is also ANTI-FUNGAL and ANTI-VIRAL.

Orange—is rich in compounds noted for their STRESS-REDUCING effects; lipid-solu traits; ANTIOXIDANT properties which ENHANCE VITAMIN ABSORPTIC

Clove—has one of the highest ORAC (oxygen radical absorbent capacity) scores. It is ANTI-BACTERIAL, ANTI-FUNGAL, ANTI-INFECTIOUS, ANTI-PARASITIC, a strong ANTISEPTIC, ANTI-VIRAL, and an IMMUNE STIMULANT; helps preserve integrity of fatty acids. Clove may also influence HEALING and help improve MEMORY.

Suggested Use: Take one capsule once daily or as needed.

Body System(s) Affected: CARDIOVASCULAR SYSTEM.

Companion Products: Essential Manna, Power Meal, Wolfberry Bars.

Companion Oils: Longevity

Precautions: Keep in a cool, dry place. Do not expose to excessive heat or direct sunlight. If pregnant or under a doctor's care, consult your physician.

Master Formula Hers and His

In addition to the following list of ingredients, each of these formulations has their own additional ingredients to customize them to the needs of either females or males.

Ingredients: Vitamin A (retinyl palmitate), vitamin C (sodium ascorbate and ascorbic acid), vitamin D3 (cholecalciferol), vitamin E (d-alpha tocopheryl acid succinate), thiamin (vitamin B1), riboflavin (vitamin B2), niacin (vitamin B3), vitamin B6, folic acid, vitami

B12, biotin, pantothenic acid, calcium, iron, iodine, magnesium, zinc, selenium, copper, manganese, chromium, potassium, choline bitartrate, PABA, betaine HCl, cellulose, maltodextrin, croscarmellose sodium, stearic acid, magnesium stearate, cellulose film coat in a Synergistic Suspension Isolation, L-cystine, L-cysteine, L-lysine, L-aspartic acid, L-glutamic acid, L-methionine, L-leucine, L-isoleucine, L-arganine, L-alanine, L-threonine, L-glutamine, L-tyrosine, L-valine, L-histadine, L-phenylalanine, L-serine, L-proline, L-hydroxyproline, L-citruline, and molybdenum.

ggested Use: For slow metabolism, three to six tablets daily. For fast metabolism, six to eight tablets daily. Take half of the daily amount with breakfast and half with dinner. Best taken before meals.

dy System(s) Affected: EMOTIONAL BALANCE, CARDIOVASCULAR, IMMUNE, and NERVOUS SYSTEMS.

te: Free of allergens. Contains no artificial flavors, preservatives, sugar, cornstarch, corn, wheat, yeast, or soy products.

Master Formula Hers

This high-potency, time released multi-vitamin and mineral supplement (with all the amins and minerals as listed previously) was formulated specifically for women with more gnesium, calcium, and B vitamins. It also contains silica (from hydrolyzed soy protein chelate), rus flavonoid complex, and glycine. It has been found to reduce the symptoms of PMS as well increase energy levels in general. This product was designed to help build and feed the productive system and because of the specific ingredients, it may also help women who have had hysterectomy. **Natural antioxidant.**

fety Data: If pregnant or under a doctor's care, please contact your physician.

equency: Approximately 88 MHz.

mpanion Products: Be-Fit, Estro, FemiGen, VitaGreen.

mpanion Oils: Dragon Time (contains more Clary sage and fennel), Mister (more estrogen-like oils—may be better for women who have had an hysterectomy), Abundance, Harmony, Joy, Magnify Your Purpose.

Master Formula His

This high-potency, time released multi-vitamin and mineral supplement, designed specifically for men, includes all the vitamins and minerals listed previously with more zinc. It a contains citrus bioflavonoids, montmorillonite, maltodextrin, silicon dioxide, alfalfa sprouts, rut inositol, and L-glycine. This product was designed to build and feed the male reproductive orga **Natural antioxidant**.

Suggested Use: Three tablets with breakfast and three with lunch (take before meals).

Frequency: Approximately 86 MHz.

Companion Products: Be-Fit, Essential Manna, Mineral Essence, ProGen, Power Meal, Sulfurzyme, VitaGreen, Wolfberry Bars.

Companion Oils: Mister, Envision, Magnify Your Purpose, Sacred Mountain.

MegaCal

Calcium is important for proper health. 98% of the calcium in the body is found in the bones and 1% in the teeth. The other 1% supports these crucial metabolic functions: Steady heartbeat, muscle contraction, transmission of nerve impulses, and blood clotting. If this last 1% not available from ones diet, it is pulled from the bones, creating osteoporosis. Current statistics indicate that 25 million American women and 5 million American men are affected by osteoporosis, showing just how difficult it has become to obtain enough calcium and other miner through diet alone.

MegaCal differs from the other two calcium supplements in this book (SuperCal and Co Sea) as follows:

	MegaCal	SuperCal	Coral Sea
Calcium per serving	618 mg	242 mg	1300 mg
Type of calcium	lactate pentahydrate, carbonate, glycerophosphate, ascorbate	citrate	carbonate
Calcium to magnesium ratio	1:1	3:1	30:1

	MegaCal	SuperCal	Coral Sea
Additional minerals/nutrients	Magnesium (carbonate, citrate, and sulfate), potassium, zinc gluconate, copper gluconate, manganese sulfate, xylitol, vitamin C	Potassium, zinc, boron	Magnesium, potassium, zinc, selenium, 60 other micronutrient minerals

This particular product is formulated into a time-released mineral complex and is ideal for ıose who already have adequate calcium levels due to high consumption of dairy products. It may elp alleviate osteoporosis and muscle cramps and support normal thyroid function.

ngredients: Xylitol, calcium, magnesium, zinc, manganese, copper, fractionated coconut oil, and lemon (*Citrus limon*) therapeutic-grade essential oil.

uggested Use: Take 1 tablespoon daily mixed in 1 cup of water or juice one hour after meals (or medications) or before retiring.

ody System(s) Affected: CARDIOVASCULAR SYSTEM, MUSCLES and BONES, NERVOUS SYSTEM.

Mineral Essence

Over 60 organic, ionic trace minerals perfectly blended with Royal Jelly and Essential Oils o enhance bio-availability, provide anti-microbial protection, and significantly improve xygenation to the cells. Mineral Essence differs from other Colloidal Mineral products on the narket in that the ingredients are an ionic, electrolyte solution of minerals and trace minerals. The luids of the body are largely ionic solutions and every body process is dependent on ions. Calcium, potassium, sodium, chloride, and copper ions are some key ions that participate in the ody's electrical events. Potassium is the major positive ion inside the cell. Sodium is the major ositive ion found in the fluid outside the cell. Ionic chlorine is the most abundant negative ion. The minerals and trace minerals in an ionic solution like Mineral Essence are balanced and in ssociations such as ion pairs, which keep them from being reactive.

In contrast, colloidal minerals are a suspension of tiny non-soluble mineral and trace nineral particles in water. Most colloidal minerals are held in suspension by their tiny size and/or static electrical charge. Colloids do not dissolve into true solutions and are not capable of assing through a semipermeable membrane (such as a cell wall). True colloidal minerals uspended in a aqueous solution are not capable of conducting electricity and are not associated vith bio-electric activity in the body.

The physical opposite of a colloid is a crystalloid. The minerals from Utah's Inland Sea (the Great Salt Lake) as used in Mineral Essence are ionic and are electrolytes, thus capable of conducting electrical energy in the body. The full spectrum of minerals and trace minerals found Mineral Essence will form perfect crystals if all liquid was removed. When blended with essentia oils, Mineral Essence becomes the most bio-available mineral product on the market.

To demonstrate how blending trace minerals with essential oils increases their bio-availability, a group of volunteers consumed a teaspoon of liquid trace minerals without any essential oils. Each volunteer experienced diarrhea within 24 hours. Within days the same volunteers were given double the dosage of the same liquid trace minerals, but this time blended with essential oils. No diarrhea symptoms were experienced. This was due to the fact that the liquid trace minerals, blended with essential oils, were delivered more efficiently and utilized by th body's cells, or in other words made more bio-available.

In the July 1996 issue of Young Living Essential Edge, an article entitled "Sunburn Relie contained the following information. "Dr. Alex Schauss, a prominent mineral researcher, has discovered that burns are painful because certain trace minerals are depleted from the skin and surrounding tissue. If the trace minerals are replenished to the affected area, then the pain will subside almost immediately. . . . We have had many who have topically applied Mineral Essence directly on the sunburn or burn and received instant pain relief as the healing process began. . . ."

The minerals shown in the table below are in descending order according to the best testin information available. Several independent lab results for Mineral Essence were compared for thi approximation.

Comments: Some people may wonder if it is safe to consume trace minerals that have trace elements of mercury, arsenic, lead, etc., in such a product. Dr. Alex Schauss explains tha our bodies possess the same chemical makeup as sea water. In fact, sea water has been used many times for blood transfusions when plasma was not available. Products created in nature, like sea water, have many elements. Some of these elements, if separated and taken in larger quantities, can be dangerous to our health. When these same elements are synergistically blended by the Creator, we have a totally different product than the sum of the individual elements. Dr. Schauss suggests we consume sea water for its mineral content each day, for sea water provides the perfect balance of trace mineral intake that our body needs for optimum health.

Oxygen	Bismuth	Holmium
Hydrogen	Selenium	Lutetium
Chloride	Cesium	Rhenium
Magnesium	Molybdenum	Samarium
Sulfur	**Xenon	Terbium
Potassium	Lead	Thulium
Sodium	Arsenic	Ytterbium
Boron	Tungsten	Platinum
Lithium	Thorium	Dysprosium
Calcium	Tin	Erbium
Carbon	Thallium	Neodymium
Silicon	Mercury	Praseodymium
Phosphorus	Titanium	Yttrium
Fluorine	Hafnium	Zirconium
Nitrogen	Gold	Cerium
**Argon	Barium	Cobalt
Iron	Lanthanum	Niobium
Zinc	Cadmium	Gallium
Bromine	Uranium	Rubidium
Manganese	**Helium	Tantalum
Copper	Silver	Germanium
Chromium	Strontium	Aluminum
**Krypton	Iodine	Vanadium
Tellurium	Scandium	**Radon
Nickel	Beryllium	***Noble gases never tested for or not found, but are present in sea water according to CRC Press.*
**Neon	Europium	
Antimony	Gadolinium	

ngredients: Purified water (for diluting the minerals and liquefying the blend), ionic trace minerals (as listed in the previous chart), and essential oils (as shown below) in a base of royal jelly and honey.

ssential Oils:

Cinnamon Bark—is a powerful purifier and a powerful oxygenator; it enhances the action and the activity of the other oils; anti-fungal, anti-bacterial, and antiviral.

Peppermint—enhances the effect of other oils; cooling and soothing; aids digestion.

Lemon—helps promote leukocyte formation; helps to dissolve cholesterol and fats.

uggested Use: Shake well before using. Take one to two droppers morning and night or as needed as a food supplement.

ody System(s) Affected: EMOTIONAL BALANCE, CARDIOVASCULAR, HORMONAL, IMMUNE, and NERVOUS SYSTEMS, MUSCLES and BONES.

ompanion Products: Bodygize, Master Formula His/Hers, KidScents Mighty Mist/Vites, Power Meal, Sulfurzyme, VitaGreen, Wolfberry Bar.

Companion Oils: Citrus Fresh, Envision, Gathering, Harmony, Valor.

ParaFree

With virtually everyone in the world having parasites of one form or another, there is a tremendous need for a product like this that utilizes the anti-parasitic properties of essential oils to help combat this worldwide problem.

Ingredients: Base oils of sesame seed and olive.

Essential Oils:

Black Cumin (*Nigella sativa*)—anti-parasitic, antispasmodic; enhances immune function

Thyme—anti-inflammatory; anti-fungal; antiseptic; anti-viral.

Clove—anti-parasitic.

Anise—anti-parasitic; anti-inflammatory; promoter of better digestion.

Nutmeg—supports adrenal glands; anti-inflammatory; stimulates immune function.

Fennel—anti-parasitic; supports digestive and pancreatic functions.

Vetiver—antiseptic; anti-inflammatory; calming; grounding; locally warming; muscular rheumatism; arthritis; anxiety, insomnia, depression, oily skin, acne.

Idaho Tansy—highly regarded for its worm-expelling properties.

Melaleuca—anti-fungal, antiseptic, anti-bacterial.

Laurel (*Laurus nobilis*)—antiseptic, anti-bacterial, anti-parasitic, anti-viral; diuretic; fungicide; digestive for stomach; purifier; loss of appetite.

Liquid form:

Suggested Use: Take two to four droppers three times daily for 21 consecutive days and rest for 7 days. Cycle may be repeated three times.

Soft Gel form:

Suggested Use: Five capsules two to three times daily. For best results take for 21 days and rest 7 days. Cycle may be repeated three times.

Better results may be obtained when using ParaFree with ComforTone and ICP to help break up and remove the plaque and incrustation from the system.

Body System(s) Affected: DIGESTIVE and IMMUNE SYSTEMS.

fety Data: Do not take during pregnancy. Many of the oils contained in this product are contraindicated for pregnancy.

mments: Since both forms of this product are to be used orally and contraindications do exist, one would be well advised to review the safety data in the APPENDIX of this book. For additional information, review the books, Essential Oil Safety—A Guide for Health Care Professionals by Robert Tisserand and Tony Balacs and Aromatherapy for Health Professionals by Shirley and Len Price.

PD 80/20

A dietary supplement which provides the nutrients necessary to support internal health and lily functions.

gredients: Pregnenolone and DHEA. Also includes rice flour and gelatin.

dy System(s) Affected: EMOTIONAL BALANCE, HORMONAL SYSTEM, MUSCLES and BONES.

mpanion Products: Essentialzyme, Royaldophilus, Sulfurzyme (capsules or powder), and VitaGreen.

mpanion Oils: Clary sage, Dragon Time, and fennel.

Polyzyme

A protein-digestive blend of active ingredients that aids digestion and enhances absorption nutrients. Polyzyme may provide relief of occasional symptoms such as fullness, pressure, ›ating, gas, pain, and/or minor cramping that may occur after eating.

gredients: Protease, phytase, peptidase, papain, bromelain, lipase, pure therapeutic-grade essential oils (as listed below), vegetable cellulose, rice bran, deionized water, and silica.

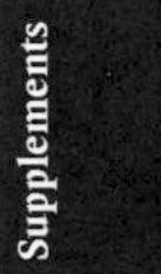

sential Oils:

Anise—may help calm and strengthen the digestive system.

Peppermint—is antispasmodic, and anti-inflammatory; soothing, cooling, and dilating to the system. It also enhances digestion and increases endurance.

Rosemary cineol—helps balance heart function, stimulates nerves, and decongests the liver.

Suggested Use: Take 2-3 capsules three times daily just prior to or with meals containing prote Can also be sprinkled on food or in beverages.

Body System(s) Affected: DIGESTIVE SYSTEM, MUSCLES and BONES.

Companion Products: ComforTone, JuvaTone, Sulfurzyme, Royaldophilus, and Power Meal.

Companion Oils: Di-Tone and JuvaFlex.

Warning: Do not give this product to children under 12 years of age except under the supervisio of a doctor. If symptoms persist, discontinue use of this product and consult your physician. Keep in a cool, dry place. Do not expose to excessive heat or direct sunlight If pregnant or under a doctor's care, consult your physician.

Power Meal

A complete vegetarian protein drink mix containing Chinese Wolfberry (high in protein and amino acids) and MSM with high-powered, immune-supporting, super-antioxidant propertie and Siberian ginseng. The Power Meal is designed as a high-protein, vitamin-rich meal replacement containing a large spectrum of vitamins, trace minerals, and amino acids. The Pow Meal provides the body with the tools to build lean muscle tissue while providing a vital source organic sulfur, which is an important facet of proper cellular metabolism and organ function.

Whether used as a meal replacement or a filling and nutritious snack, the Power Meal ca help serve as an excellent weight management tool. Free of fats, sugars, and synthetic ingredien Power Meal provides most of the building blocks the body requires for regeneration and maintenance.

The protein rich formula of Power Meal, when combined with exercise, can help the boc build lean muscle tissue that is the foundation of a lean physique and an important element to weight control. Because muscle burns 22 times as many calories as fat, the addition of muscle tissue can significantly accelerate metabolism and contribute to a more slender body. Because muscle tissue weighs more than adipose (fat) tissue, the addition of muscle mass to the body may not always be accompanied by weight loss–even though body fat may have dropped substantially

gredients: Rice protein concentrate, *Lycium barbarum* (Chinese wolfberry - Ningxia variety), rice bran, bee pollen, fructose, guar gum, calcium carbonate powder, lecithin (food for the brain), liquid vanilla flavoring, fructooligosaccharides, choline bitartrate, multi-enzyme complex (lipase (digests fats), mixed protease (digests proteins), phytase, and peptidase), silicon dioxide, magnesium oxide, potassium chloride, Eleuthero, methysulfonylmethane (MSM—regenerates nerve tissue; detoxifies liver), alpha lipoic acid, inositol, carotenoid complex (Lycopene 3%, astaxanthin, carocare betacarotene 7.5%, lutein 70%, zeaxanthin 50%, betain HCl), kelp extract, PABA (para-aminobenzoic acid), gingko biloba extract, L-carnitine tartrate (helps convert fatty acids into energy), ascorbic acid (vitamin C), zinc citrate, wolfberry polysaccharides, boron amino acid chelate (helps in the absorption and utilization of calcium), betatene, copper amino acid chelate, manganese citrate (antioxidant; regulates blood sugar levels; increases cellular energy), biotin (helps cell growth and fatty acid production), essential oils (as listed below), d-alpha tocopheryl succinate (vitamin E), niacin, ferrous citrate, calcium pantothenate (pantothenic acid), folic acid, vitamin D3, pyridoxine HCl (vitamin B6), selenium amino acid chelate (antioxidant, supports pancreas and heart functions), riboflavin (vitamin B2), thiamine HCl (vitamin B1), chromium nicotinate (helps body build enzymes and proteins, stabilizes blood sugar; helps build lean muscle tissue, and burns fat), and vitamin B12.

sential Oils:

Grapefruit—excellent for fluid retention and cellulite; diuretic, detoxifier, and stimulant of the lymphatic system; important as an antidepressant.

Orange—is rich in compounds noted for their stress-reducing effects.

Lemon—helps promote leukocyte formation; helps to dissolve cholesterol and fats.

Cypress—mucolytic, astringent, diuretic, lymphatic decongestant; reduces cellulite and strengthens connective tissue.

Anise—anti-parasitic; anti-inflammatory; promoter of better digestion.

Fennel—anti-parasitic; supports digestive and pancreatic functions.

Nutmeg—supports adrenal glands; anti-inflammatory; stimulates immune function.

)TE: The Canadian version of Power Meal contains all the same ingredients except creatine replaces L-carnitine.

ggested Use: Take 2 full scoops with 8 to 12 oz. of pure water or juice. Use as a meal alternative or dietary supplement. For added flavor, mix one serving (2 scoops) with rice or almond milk *(the authors enjoy mixing this with Rice Dream - a brown rice beverage).* For children under 12, use 1 scoop (½ serving).

dy System(s) Affected: CARDIOVASCULAR, DIGESTIVE, and IMMUNE SYSTEMS, MUSCLES and BONES.

Precautions: If pregnant or under a doctor's care, consult your physician. Keep in a cool, dry place. Do not expose to sunlight.

Companion Products: Be-Fit, Bodygize, Master Formula His/Hers, ComforTone, Essential Manna, Essentialzyme, ICP, Thyromin, VitaGreen, Wolfberry Bars.

Companion Oils: Abundance, Citrus Fresh, EndoFlex, Envision, Live with Passion, Magnify Your Purpose.

ProGen

All-vegetable and herbal support for the male glandular system. The *Pygeum africanum* has been used for years to prevent prostate atrophy and malfunction while saw palmetto is widely used for protecting the prostate from enlargement. This formula should help protect men from prostate cancer and promote better glandular function. The oils used to flavor enhance this formula have been reported in Europe to also help support and prevent degeneration.

Ingredients: *Dioscorea villosa* root (wild yam), *Pygeum africanum* bark, saw palmetto (*Serona serrulata*), alpha glutaric acid, L-glutathione (sulfur-bearing antioxidant for the liver), zinc aspartate, L-carnitine (helps lower cholestrol; supports the heart), L-alanine, L-arginine, magnesium citrate, Eleuthero, blessed thistle, marshmallow, sesame oil, dimethylglycine (supports heart muscle and tissue), and essential oils (as shown below).

Essential Oils:

Sage—contains estriol and has estrogen-like properties; may help improve estrogen and progesterone-testosterone balance.

Fennel—diuretic; may break up fluids and toxins, and cleanse the tissues.

Lavender—sedative; balances body systems; promotes a general sense of well being.

Myrtle—is a Decongestant of the respiratory system. It may help improve oxygenation and work as an expectorant in discharging mucus.

Yarrow—is a powerful decongestant of the prostate and a hormone balancer.

Peppermint—purifying and stimulating to the conscious mind; anti-inflammatory; helps with nerve regeneration. It also enhances digestion and increases endurance.

Suggested Use: Take four capsules daily (two with breakfast and two with lunch).

Body System(s) Affected: HORMONAL SYSTEM.

ompanion Products: Be-Fit, Exodus, Master Formula His, Protec tincture, Power Meal, Sulfurzyme, VitaGreen.

ompanion Oils: Exodus, Live with Passion, Magnify Your Purpose, Mister, Valor.

Royaldophilus

Acidophilus is a friendly bacteria that prevails in our intestines to keep harmful bacteria in ıeck. Excessive use of antibiotics and drugs, chlorinated water, and junk and processed foods duce the number of friendly bacteria in our intestines. When the acidophilus population is duced, yeast infection (candidiasis) occurs. Currently about 70% of females and 30% of males ıve yeast infections. The **New England Journal of Medicine** published a research article ıowing that acidophilus can prevent and even cure yeast infection.

Acidophilus has many benefits which include the following: the best natural digestive aid; orrects lactose intolerance; helps bad breath; helps acne; reduces cholesterol; inhibits candida bicans and prevents yeast infection.

Acidophilus can stand room temperatures for weeks, but it is recommended that it should refrigerated prior to opening the bottle and kept refrigerated at under 40 degrees F. It is unwise freeze acidophilus as this may affect its viability. (This information was taken in part from *ealthy and Natural Journal*).

Acidophilus works with the enzymes to digest our food. It also aids the growth of testinal flora. When we have a good enzyme base, acidophilus will complement enzyme oduction. It is extremely important for acidophilus to implant on the intestinal wall for the turning of intestinal flora. Lactobacillus and bifidus cultures derived from milk is the only true idophilus that the human body recognizes and accepts. The problem with lactose intolerance is at the pasteurization of the milk before being cultured kills the enzymes. The whole milk idophilus used in Royaldophilus provides greater culture and inhibits allergy reaction. After veral months of study, it was found that Plantain increases the culturing and bio-availability of e intestinal flora. Plantain also reduces digestive problems and is very smooth to irritable bowel oblems where intestinal flora is absent. This formulation of the **lactobacillus and bifidus ures combined with plantain** has proven to be superior to all forms of acidophilus.

ngredients: Plantain, lemon pectin, magnesium stearate, lactobacillus and bifidus cultures (250 million per capsule), and gelatin.

uggested Use: Take one to two capsules for maintenance. Under heavy stress or when traveling, it may be necessary to double or triple the amount. Best taken on an empty stomach.

Body System(s) Affected: DIGESTIVE and IMMUNE SYSTEMS.

Companion Products: ComforTone, Essentialzyme, ICP, VitaGreen.

Companion Oils: Di-Tone, Forgiveness, JuvaFlex, Harmony, Release, Thieves.

Stevia Extract

This product, the whole leaf stevia extract from Paraguay, is a dietary supplement which may effectively regulate blood sugar. It is a helpful aid to people who have diabetes and hypoglycemia. After hypoglycemics ingest Stevia, blood sugar rises and their energy levels and mental activities increase rapidly. It may also lower elevated blood pressure while not affecting normal blood pressure.

It may inhibit the growth and reproduction of some bacteria and other infectious organisms, including the bacteria that causes tooth decay and periodontal (gum) disease. Individuals using Stevia have reported a lower incidence of colds and flu. Individuals who have tried using Stevia as a mouthwash or added to toothpaste have seen significant improvements in t treatment of periodontal disease.

It is a wonderful aid in weight loss and weight management because it contains no calorie and research indicates that it significantly increases glucose tolerance and inhibits glucose absorption. People who ingest Stevia daily often report a decrease in their desire for sweets and fatty foods. It may also improve digestion and gastrointestinal function, soothe upset stomachs a help speed recovery from minor illnesses.

When applied to the skin, it effectively softens the skin and smooths out wrinkles while helping to heal various skin blemishes, acne, seborrhea, dermatitis, and eczema. People have reported that when Stevia is used on cuts and wounds, there is more rapid healing without scarrin **(Information obtained from United American Industries, Inc.)**

Suggested Use: Use three to six drops, or as desired, for supplementing food and/or beverages.

Body System(s) Affected: CARDIOVASCULAR, DIGESTIVE, and IMMUNE SYSTEMS.

Companion Products: Essentialzyme, Mineral Essence, Thyromin, VitaGreen.

Companion Oils: JuvaFlex, Thieves.

Stevia Select

This is a powdered form of the popular Stevia leaf extract (refer to Stevia Extract for more :ormation on the benefits of Stevia). It is combined with fructooligosaccharides (FOS) which ve a naturally sweet taste as well. FOS is one of the best documented nutrients for promoting : growth of the lactobacillus and bifidus cultures. FOS has been clinically shown to do the llowing: Increase calcium and magnesium absorption; lower blood glucose, LDL, and cholesterol vels; inhibit production of the reductase enzymes that contribute to cancer. FOS may also help wer blood pressure and support or increase cardiovascular health. Stevia Select has been used some individuals as a sugar substitute for many recipes. It may also work well as a sweetener r hot breakfast cereals.

ggested Use: Add to any meal or beverage.

dy System(s) Affected: CARDIOVASCULAR, DIGESTIVE, and IMMUNE SYSTEMS.

mpanion Products: Essentialzyme, Mineral Essence, Power Meal, Stevia, Thyromin, VitaGreen.

mpanion Oils: JuvaFlex, Thieves.

Sulfurzyme

An unique combination of Methylsulfonalmethane (MSM), the protein-building compound ınd in breast milk, and Lyceum Barbarum (the Chinese Wolfberry Powder) that together create a ld new concept in reviving the immune system, supporting almost every major body function, d forestalling an array of degenerative conditions. Of particular importance is MSM's ability to ualize water pressure inside of the cells—a considerable benefit for those plagued with bursitis, hritis, and tendinitis. It also activates enzymes, helps the body assimilate vitamins, and tabolizes carbohydrates.

Sulfurzyme may help reduce the following signs of sulfur deficiency: Poor nail and hair owth, falling hair, eczema, dermatitis, poor muscle tone, acne/pimples, gout, rheumatism, hritis, weakening of nervous system (MS, Parkinson's, Leu Gehrig's, and Alzheimer's disease), nstipation, impairment of mental faculties, lowered libido.

Supplements

gredients: MSM (Methylsulfonalmethane) and wolfberry powder *(Refer to the Wolfberry Bar at the end of this section for more information on the benefits of the Chinese Wolfberry)*, and gelatin.

Comments: Sulfur metabolism requires nutritional balance. It takes calcium to metabolize sulf magnesium to metabolize calcium, potassium to metabolize magnesium, phosphorus to metabolize potassium, etc. The list goes on! That is why wolfberry is contained in this product; it contains all of the necessary components for sulfur to be metabolized.

Capsule form:

Suggested Use: Five capsules two to three times daily.

Powder form:

Suggested Use: Mix ½ tsp. with juice or Bodygize, two times daily, one hour before or after meals.

Body System(s) Affected: IMMUNE and NERVOUS SYSTEMS, MUSCLES and BONES, SKIN.

Companion Products: ArthroTune, ComforTone, Essentialzyme, ICP, Master Formula, Ortho Ease and Ortho Sport Massage Oils, Power Meal, Ultra Young.

Companion Oils: En-R-Gee, Envision, Magnify Your Purpose, PanAway, Valor.

Super B

A B-complex is necessary for the delivery of the essential nutrients needed to support th body's cells, particularly under times of stress when assimilation is most difficult. Although research has shown that megadoses of B vitamins are not healthy, it has been noted that the diets many Americans do not provide the recommended amount of B vitamins, which are essential for normal functions of immune response. B vitamins included in this formula are B1, B2, B3, B6 a B12 (no essential oils are present in this formula). When all of these B vitamins are combined in the stomach it causes instant fermentation resulting in stomach upset. To alleviate this problem, this product utilizes a synergistic suspension isolation to provide the release of specific vitamins when necessary so that they can all work together in their separate stages of isolation. This product was designed to help build the body. **Natural antioxidant**.

Ingredients: Dicalcium phosphate, niacin, selenium, magnesium oxide, zinc, thiamine (vitamin B1), riboflavin (vitamin B2), vitamin B6, PABA, biotin, vitamin B12, folic acid, cellulo magnesium stearate, and stearic acid.

Suggested Use: One half to one tablet daily, preferably with a meal and not on an empty stoma

Body System(s) Affected: CARDIOVASCULAR and NERVOUS SYSTEMS, MUSCLES and BONES.

Safety Data: If taken on an empty stomach, one may experience a niacin flush.

Comments: If a niacin flush occurs, try one drop of peppermint in 20 drops of V-6 Mixing Oil for a full body massage. This may help the body cool down quickly.

Frequency: Approximately 63 MHz.

Super C

Research has shown that physical stress, alcohol, smoking and medication can lower the blood levels of this essential vitamin. When citrus fruits are not readily available, diets may not contain enough vitamin C. Super C is properly balanced with rutin, bioflavonoids, and minerals to work synergistically, balancing the electrolytes and increasing the absorption rate of the vitamin C. Without bioflavonoids, vitamin C has a hard time getting inside the cell and without proper electrolyte balance and minerals, it will not stay there for long. The essential oils contained in this product not only enhance the flavor, but they all have high levels of bioflavonoid activity. This product was designed to help build up the body.

Ingredients: Vitamin C (ascorbic acid), cellulose, citrus bioflavonoids, calcium, potassium, stearic acid, rutin, magnesium stearate, zinc, manganese, cayenne, dicalcium phosphate, and essential oils (as listed below) in a Synergistic Suspension Isolation.

Essential Oils:

Orange—is rich in compounds noted for their stress-reducing effects.

Mandarin—good for skin problems, stretch marks, nervous tension, and restlessness.

Lemon—helps promote leukocyte formation; helps to dissolve cholesterol and fats.

Grapefruit—excellent for fluid retention and cellulite; diuretic, detoxifier, and stimulant of the lymphatic system; important as an antidepressant.

Lime—helps remove dead skin cells; tightens skin and connective tissue.

Suggested Use: For reinforcing immune strength, two tablets daily. For maintenance, one tablet daily. Best taken before meals.

Body System(s) Affected: IMMUNE and RESPIRATORY SYSTEMS.

Companion Products: Exodus, ImmuGel, ImmuneTune, Rehemogen, VitaGreen.

Companion Oils: Citrus Fresh, Exodus II, ImmuPower, Motivation, Thieves, Valor.

Frequency: Approximately 80 MHz.

Super C Chewable

The vitamin C provided in this unique product is enhanced by that of the acerola cherry, tropical fruit that contains up to 4.5% vitamin C. The addition of citrus bioflavonoids increases vitamin C's support of the immune system while increasing capillary and connective tissue strength. Now you can have one of nature's most powerful antioxidants in a natural, delicious, chewable form.

Ingredients: Vitamin C (ascorbic acid), acerola cherry (*Malphighia glabra*) fruit extract, citrus bioflavonoids from lemon (*Citrus limon*), essential oils (as shown below), fructose, silico dioxide and vegetable-grade lubricant (sugar cane and palm oil).

Essential Oils:

Lemon—helps promote leukocyte formation; helps to dissolve cholesterol and fats.
Orange—is rich in compounds noted for their stress-reducing effects.

Suggested Use: Take 1 tablet 3 times daily as needed.

Body System(s) Affected: MUSCLE and BONE, IMMUNE SYSTEM.

Precautions: A study was published in 2002 suggesting that the acerola cherry can cause an allergic reaction similar to that caused by latex. If you have experienced such a reaction latex, you may want to choose a different vitamin C supplement.

Super Cal

Formulated with calcium, potassium, and magnesium citrate (which is easier for the body to utilize) specifically for proper electrolyte balance, hormonal balance, and muscle and bone development. **Natural antioxidant**. This product is ideal for those on a vegetarian diet or diets that are restricted in calories or high in carbonated beverages. It was designed to help build the body. *Refer to the chart shown under MegaCal in this same section for a comparison of SuperCal to MegaCal and Coral Sea.*

Ingredients: Calcium citrate, magnesium citrate, potassium citrate, zinc citrate, stearic acid, boron, essential oils (as shown below), cellulose, gelatin, and stearic acid in a Synergistic Suspension Isolation, which allows nutrients to be assimilated independently.

Essential Oils:

Marjoram—powerful muscle relaxant and anti-inflammatory; relaxing and soothing to cartilage tissue.

Lemongrass—helps repair connective tissue; when combined with marjoram, it helps stimulate the agents in the tissue to rejuvenate and reconnect.

Myrtle—is a Decongestant of the respiratory system. It may help improve oxygenation and work as an expectorant in discharging mucus.

May also contain wintergreen essential oil.

Suggested Use: One to two capsules before each meal.

Body System(s) Affected: EMOTIONAL BALANCE, CARDIOVASCULAR and NERVOUS SYSTEMS, MUSCLES and BONES.

Companion Products: ArthroTune, Essentialzyme, Ortho Ease and Ortho Sport Massage Oils, Power Meal, Sulfurzyme.

Companion Oils: Grounding, Harmony, PanAway, Valor.

Frequency: Approximately 78 MHz.

ThermaBurn

These easy-to-swallow capsules contain ingredients like HCA, chromium polynicotinate, and L-carnitine to help burn fat and build muscle while curbing the appetite. The addition of yerba maté extract helps boost energy and mental alertness.

Ingredients: Hydroxycitric acid, theobromine, L-carnitine, dl-methionine, licorice root extract, yerba maté extract, guarana seed extract, boron citrate, inositol hexaniacinate, essential oils (as shown below), and chromium polynicotinate.

Essential Oils:

Fleabane (*Conyza canadensis*)—is a rare essential oil studied by Daniel Pénoël, M.D. for its ability to stimulate the pancreas and liver and counteract retarded puberty. It is a mood enhancer and promoter of hGH.

Myrtle—is a Decongestant of the respiratory system. It may help improve oxygenation and work as an expectorant in discharging mucus.

Nutmeg—supports adrenal glands; anti-inflammatory; stimulates immune function.

Peppermint—purifying and stimulating to the conscious mind; anti-inflammatory; helps with nerve regeneration. It also enhances digestion and increases endurance.

Spearmint—may balance and increase metabolism; helps burn up fats and toxins in the body; aids digestion.

May also contain frankincense essential oil.

Suggested Use: Take one to two capsules two hours before or after meals. Individual needs may vary.

Body System(s) Affected: MUSCLES and BONES.

Companion Products: Master His/Hers, Thyromin, VitaGreen (enhances effect of Thyromin; take together for greater effect).

Companion Oils: En-R-Gee.

ThermaMist

A neutraceutical spray with ingredients formulated to quickly enter the blood stream and help curb appetite, raise metabolism, and boost energy levels. Similar to the ThermaBurn capsules described above, this spray adds guarana leaf and schizandra for their respective abilities to provide energy and speed the breakdown of fats in the liver.

Ingredients: Niacin (vitamin B3), guarana leaf extract (provides energy; suppresses appetite), yerba maté extract (caffeine-free and non-addictive; combats fatigue, increases endurance, and promotes health), yohimbe extract, schizandra (antioxidant; speeds breakdown of fats in liver), hydroxycitric acid (helps block the synthesis of fat and enhances fat burning), 5-HTP (5-hydroxytryptophan), stevia, chromium polynicotinate (helps regulate energy production and enhances muscle building; acts as transport agent to carry cholesterol from blood to liver for processing), and essential oils (as shown below). Includes distilled water, vegetable glycerin, phosphatidylcholine complex, ionic trace minerals, omega 3, 6, and 9 essential fatty acids complex, natural flavors, and grapefruit extract.

Essential Oils:

Grapefruit—excellent for fluid retention and cellulite; diuretic, detoxifier, and stimulant of the lymphatic system; important as an antidepressant.

Peppermint—purifying and stimulating to the conscious mind; anti-inflammatory; helps with nerve regeneration. It also enhances digestion and increases endurance.

Spearmint—may balance and increase metabolism; helps burn up fats and toxins in the body; aids digestion.

ggested Use: Spray three sprays into buccal cavity of mouth, three times a day or whenever "cravings" occur. Individual needs may vary. For additional benefits, take a deep diaphragmatic breath after each spray. ***Those with high blood pressure may need to check with a physician before using this product.***

ody System(s) Affected: DIGESTIVE SYSTEM, MUSCLES and BONES.

ompanion Products: Be-Fit, Power Meal, Thyromin, VitaGreen (enhances effect of Thyromin; take together for greater effect).

Thyromin

For nourishing the thyroid, balancing metabolism, and reducing fatigue, this product is a mbination of specially selected glandular nutrients, herbs, amino acids, and essential oils. All e grade A quality and are perfectly balanced to bring about the most beneficial, biological and tritional support to the thyroid. This product was not only designed to help build up the body, t to help lay a solid foundation for the healthy functioning of the many organs, tissues, and cells hich are effected by the thyroid. **Natural antioxidant**.

gredients: Vitamin E (d alpha tocopheryl acid succinate), iodine (derived from kelp), potassium (citrate), CoQ10, L-cysteine, L-cystine, carrageenan, bovine adrenal and pituitary extracts, parsley powder, magnesium stearate, and essential oils (as shown below).

ssential Oils:

Peppermint—purifying and stimulating to the conscious mind; anti-inflammatory; helps with nerve regeneration. It also enhances digestion and increases endurance.

Spearmint—may balance and increase metabolism; helps burn up fats and toxins in the body; aids digestion.

Myrtle—is a Decongestant of the respiratory system. It may help improve oxygenation and work as an expectorant in discharging mucus.

Myrrh—anti-inflammatory and antiseptic; helps to decongest the prostate gland.

ggested Use: One to two capsules daily, immediately before going to sleep.

Body System(s) Affected: HORMONAL SYSTEM.

Companion Products: Essentialzyme, FemiGen, JuvaTone, Mineral Essence, Ultra Young, VitaGreen (enhances effect of Thyromin; take together for greater effect).

Companion Oils: EndoFlex, Clarity, En-R-Gee, JuvaFlex, Magnify Your Purpose.

Frequency: Approximately 52 MHz.

Comments: Thyromin can replace thyroid medication. If currently using thyroid medication, work with your health care professional before starting Thyromin to ensure that the thyro medication is properly regulated/reduced. For those that are not on thyroid medication, b wonder if their thyroid is working properly, here is a simple way to find out. Take your **basal cell temperature** with a mercury thermometer upon awakening first thing in the morning, even before you go to the bathroom or get out of bed. Put the thermometer und your arm pit and rest for 10 minutes. If it reads below 97.6° F (36.5° C) then your thyro is low (hypothyroidism) and Thyromin may help. Start out with one capsule each night a bedtime and check your temperature in a couple of days. If it is not up to 97.6° F, add o more capsule, *but take it in the morning*. Continue adding more capsules and checking your basal cell temperature until it reads 97.6° F. *Alternate the additional capsules between morning and evening so that half of the number of capsules taken each day are immediately before bed and the other half are in the morning after rising*. Follow the directions on the bottle.

Ultra Young

This new spray neutriceutical utilizes a unique nutrient delivery system through **oral mucosa absorption** (directly into the bloodstream through the dense network of blood vessels lining the mucus membrane inside the mouth). The advantages of this type of delivery system are protection from rapid first-pass metabolism by the liver and up to ten times the amount of nutrien being delivered to the system compared to the pill or capsule form of the same ingredients. Ultra Young is **not** a human growth hormone (hGH or somatotrophin) supplement. This unique produc is formulated in such a way as to allow the body to use the hGH it produces naturally. Also, because low blood sugar levels are the key to hGH conversion and assimilation at the cellular lev Ultra Young contains Chinese wolfberry extract for its insulin–like action. *(Refer to the Wolfber Bar at the end of this section for more information on the benefits of the Chinese Wolfberry.)*

Ingredients: Vitamin A, natural vitamin E, *Vicia faba* extract, L-arginine, niacin, zinc complex, L-ornithine, pyroglutamate, L-glutamine, L-glycine, GABA (gamma amino butyric acid), grapeseed extract, L-lysine, wolfberry extract, *Ginkgo biloba*, stevia, vitamin B6 , selenium, and essential oils (as shown below), in a base of deionized water, vegetable glycerine, alcohol, hydrolyzed vegetable protein, natural raspberry flavor, ionic trace minerals, potassium sorbate, mono-, poly-, and oligo-saccharides, and extracts of Siberian ginseng, bee pollen, inosine, ginger, and octocosanol.

ssential Oils:

Sandalwood—helps strengthen the cardiovascular and lymphatic systems as well as increasing oxygen levels around the pineal and pituitary glands.

Fleabane (*Conyza canadensis*)—is a rare essential oil studied by Daniel Pénoël, M.D. for its ability to stimulate the pancreas and liver and counteract retarded puberty. It is a mood enhancer and promoter of hGH.

otal mgs per Serving: 405.2

uggested Use: Three sprays, three times a day for six consecutive days; no sprays on the seventh day. (This gives the body the opportunity to continue to generate its own supply of hGH.) Vial contains approximately 30 servings (on average, 9 sprays per day). Shake gently before using.

structions on Use: Spray Ultra Young directly on inside cheeks and on roof of mouth. Avoid swallowing for one to two minutes. Spray upon waking, between meals, and just before retiring. Avoid spraying on the tongue because this generates saliva, promotes swallowing, and reduces its effectiveness. (Comment: It is most effective when given time to penetrate the mucus membranes of mouth and directly enter the blood stream.) Ultra Young is best used two to four hours before or after meals with no snacking in between because high blood sugar levels reduce its effectiveness.

ody System(s) Affected: HORMONAL and IMMUNE SYSTEMS.

ompanion Supplements: AD&E, Be-Fit, Essential Manna, JuvaTone, Mineral Essence, Power Meal, Sulferzyme, Thyromin, VitaGreen, Wolfberry Bars.

ompanion Oils: Frankincense, lavender, Abundance, En-R-Gee, EndoFlex, Envision, Joy, JuvaFlex, Live with Passion, Magnify Your Purpose, Release, Valor.

Ultra Young +

This product contains the same ingredients as Ultra Young with the addition of DHEA (*dehydroepiandrosterone*). DHEA is produced in the adrenal gland and is a precursor to many important hormones. Like growth hormone, DHEA production steadily declines after the age of 20.

More Information on the Human Growth Hormone (hGH)

Benefits:

1. Reverses aging of the thymus gland, a part of our immune system.
2. Dramatically raises levels of cytokines, interleukin 1 & 2, and tumor necrosis factor, all of which play a central role in the human immune system.
3. Improves fat-to-lean ratios.
4. Reverses heart disease.
5. Boosts bone formation.
6. Firms and tightens skin by activating the production of skin proteins, collagen, a elastin.
7. Increases energy.
8. Lifts depression.
9. Restores deep sleep.

Supplementation is not enough: Taking a growth hormone (hGH) supplement is not the answer since research shows that most people continue to produce ample amounts of the human growth hormone well into their advanced years. The problem is not a lack of hGH, but t inability of the liver to convert it to IGF-1. IGF-1 is responsible for actually carrying ou the actions of the chemical message sent by hGH. Without a properly functioning liver, IGF-1 conversion does not take place and hGH has a limited effect in the body. This is why Ultra Young contains ingredients that dramatically facilitate the conversion of hGH IGF-1 in the liver; ingredients such as amino acids, the essential oil of *Conyza canadensi* zinc, vitamin B6, Chinese Wolfberry extract and more.

Ultra Young contains the anterior pituitary peptide isolate because it is a combination of all hormones secreted by the pituitary gland. Although hGH is the most important, the other hormones must be supplemented to help buffer and activate the effects of hGH. Without them, the body is being stimulated on only one level, a one-sided approach that i inherently abnormal.

Tips for maximizing Ultra Young's benefits:

1. Exercise. Rigorous exercises like running or weight lifting increase hGH levels.

2. Fasting. Extended periods (4 to 8 hours or more) of low blood sugar increase hGH levels and cell receptivity to hGH.
3. Thyroid, pancreas and liver support. For Ultra Young to work at its best, the liver needs to be supported and the thyroid and pancreas need to be functioning normally. For best results, take one to two Thyromin and two to four JuvaTone a day with Ultra Young.
4. Use lavender and frankincense. These oils are principle ingredients in supplements that support the pituitary. Because essential oils have the same lipid structure as the cell membrane, they have an unmatched ability to penetrate cell walls and transport hormones into the cells.

VitaGreen

High protein, high energy chlorophyll formula that helps the body maintain a high energy level. VitaGreen contains ingredients that may aid in cleansing the blood and supporting the immune system. Barley grass and spirulina have been reported to help balance blood sugar levels, alleviating that tired, run down feeling. High in chlorophyll, VitaGreen may support the thyroid, the digestive system, and strengthen and stimulate muscle development. According to European research, the essential oils in this formula may enhance immune function. Flavor enhanced with essential oils. **Natural antioxidant**.

Ingredients: Bee pollen, barley juice concentrate, spirulina, choline bitartrate, ginseng, alfalfa juice concentrate, Pacific kelp, L-arginine, L-cystine, L-tyrosine, essential oils (as shown below), and gelatin.

Essential Oils:

Lemon—helps promote leukocyte formation; helps to dissolve cholesterol and fats.

Lemongrass—helps repair connective tissue; when combined with marjoram, it helps stimulate the agents in the tissue to rejuvenate and reconnect.

Melissa—is a powerful anti-viral agent, yet is very gentle and very delicate because of the nature of the plant; has the ability to work with and enhance the gentle aspects of the human body; anti-inflammatory and energizing.

Rosemary cineol—helps balance heart function, stimulates nerves, and decongests the liver.

Suggested Use: For slow metabolism, take three to six capsules daily. For fast metabolism, take four to eight capsules daily. Best taken before meals.

Body System(s) Affected: CARDIOVASCULAR, DIGESTIVE, IMMUNE, and NERVOUS SYSTEMS, MUSCLES and BONES.

Companion Products: Be-Fit, JuvaTone, Power Meal, Sulfurzyme, Thyromin, Wolfberry Bars.

Companion Oils: Abundance, Awaken, En-R-Gee, Envision, JuvaFlex, Live with Passion, Magnify Your Purpose, Motivation, Release, Valor.

Frequency: Approximately 76 MHz.

Comments: Before putting oils in VitaGreen there was 42 percent blood absorption in 24 hours. After adding essential oils to VitaGreen, blood absorption increased to 64 percent in 30 minutes and 86 percent in an hour. The conclusion was that the cells were now receiving nutrients that they had previously not been able to assimilate. Therefore, VitaGreen is excellent for promoting pH (Alkaline/Acid) balance and for regulating blood sugar levels. (For more details, refer to page 105 of D. Gary Young's Aromatherapy—The Essential Beginning.)

WheyFit

This whey-based fitness drink is formulated with ingredients that provide three sources of protein (MF/UF whey, egg whites, and non-GMO soy) for building muscle and increasing strength. These high-quality sources of protein are combined with a digestion-promoting enzyme to ensure proper absorption. Blueberry and strawberry powders were added to provide natural antioxidants and FOS (fructooligosaccharides) was added as a sweetener and also for its ability to improve the absorption of calcium and magnesium.

Ingredients: MF/UF whey protein, egg whites, and non-GMO soy protein (none of which contain lactose); lecithin, fructooligosaccharides (FOS - low-glycemic sweetener; improves blood sugar control), stevia, blueberry powder (strong antioxidant compounds), strawberry powder (antioxidant; contains ellagic acid which slows growth of abnormal cells), blueberry flavor (liquid), natural flavors, vanilla extract, zinc citrate, sodium selenate, magnesium citrate, citric acid, essential oil (as shown below), and an enzyme complex blend, which includes amylase, celluase, lactase, lipase, and neutral protease.

Essential Oils:

Lemon—helps promote leukocyte formation; helps to dissolve cholesterol and fats; contains antioxidant compounds which helps strengthen immune function.

ıggested Use: Take one heaping scoop daily. Mix with water or, for added flavor, mix with rice milk or almond milk.

ody System(s) Affected: MUSCLES and BONES.

ompanion Products: AminoTech, Be-Fit, Power Meal, Sulfurzyme, ThermaBurn, ThermaMist, Wolfberry Bars.

Wolfberry Bar
(Almond)

A revolutionary breakthrough in nutrition made with the rare Chinese Wolfberry, naranth, and antioxidant essential oils. This is a high-protein bar, rich in the essential amino :ids and branched-chain amino acids necessary for building lean muscle and supporting normal ımune function. The **Wolfberry** is high in the branched-chain amino acid L-leucine. When etabolized, L-leucine produces a muscle-building compound in the body called HMB (beta-ydroxy beta-methylbutyrate). In one double-blind study by the American College of Sports ledicine, weight trainers that used HMB gained triple the strength and lean body mass compared those who did not use HMB. **Amaranth** is a high-protein grain (over 16% protein by weight) ontaining large amounts of another essential amino acid called L-lysine. In fact, amaranth has vice the L-lysine of wheat, three times that of maize and almost as much as that found in milk. oth L-leucine (found in the Wolfberry) and L-lysine (from the amaranth) work together nergistically to build muscle. Moreover, **essential oils** high in phenolpropanes may activate the nino acid conversion of L-leucine in the body.

ıgredients: Rice Syrup, honey, wolfberries, almond powder (almond bars **do not** contain peanuts or peanut powder), coconut, whole grain puffed amaranth, soy protein isolate, almonds, citric acid, vitamin C, cinnamon, natural flavors, and essential oils (as shown below).

ssential Oils:

Cinnamon Bark—is a powerful purifier and a powerful oxygenator; it enhances the action and the activity of the other oils; anti-fungal, anti-bacterial, and antiviral.

Orange—is rich in compounds noted for their stress-reducing effects.

uggested Use: Use as a meal alternative or a high-energy snack.

ody System(s) Affected: DIGESTIVE and IMMUNE SYSTEMS, MUSCLES and BONES.

Companion Products: Be-Fit, ComforTone, Essential Manna, Essentialzyme, ICP, Master Formula His/Hers, KidScents Mighty Mist/Vites, Thyromin, VitaGreen.

Companion Oils: Abundance, Citrus Fresh, EndoFlex, Envision, Live with Passion, Magnify Your Purpose.

Wolfberry Crisp Bar

A delicious, nutritious whole-food bar, made with the Chinese Wolfberry and other nutrient packed, natural ingredients. With over 15 grams of protein per serving, this bar makes a ideal meal replacement.

Ingredients: Soy/whey protein, almond butter, agave nectar (*Agave salmiana/angustifolia*), Ningxia wolfberry, pumpkin seeds (*Curcubita pepo*), xylitol, cashews (*Anacardium occidentale*), walnuts (*Juglans regia*), vanilla bean extract (*Vanilla planifolia*), and a natural banana flavor.

Suggested Use: Take 1 bar a day or as a meal alternative or a high-energy snack.

Body System(s) Affected: DIGESTIVE and IMMUNE SYSTEMS, MUSCLES and BONES.

Companion Products: Be-Fit, Berry Young Juice, ComforTone, Essential Manna, Essentialzym ICP, JuvaPower, JuvaSpice, Master Formula His/Hers, KidScents Mighty Mist/Vites, Thyromin, VitaGreen.

Companion Oils: Abundance, Citrus Fresh, EndoFlex, Envision, Juva Cleanse, Live with Passion, Magnify Your Purpose.

Benefits of the Chinese Wolfberry

A group of research scientists from Natural Science University in Beijing, China discovered a village in Inner Mongolia. Some of the people of the village were 120 or 130 years old and had no signs of cancer, arthritis, aids, or lupus. They lived predominately on the wolfberr and the vegetables from their gardens. This prompted research into the amazing benefits of the wolfberry. The wolfberry is over 12% protein by itself, has 21 amino acids (6 times higher in proportion than bee pollen). It also contains a complete profile of over 80 trace minerals, carbohydrates, and minimum fats.

ssibly Support the Immune System: According to scientific research in China, the Wolfberry contains compounds known as *lycium polysaccharides*, which have been studied for their effects on immune function. One study involving cancer patients found that the Wolfberry triggered an increase in both *lymphocyte transformation rate* and *white blood cell count* (measures of immune function). In another study, it was shown to increase *phagocytosis* (another index of immune function). Yet another study showed that the consumption of Wolfberry led to a strengthening of immunoglobulin A levels (a part of our immunity).

Powerful Antioxidant: One clinical study of individuals who consumed Wolfberry, *superoxide dismutase (SOD)* levels in the blood increased 48% while *hemoglobin* increased 12%. Even better, *lipid peroxide* levels dropped 65%.

ssibly Inhibit Tumor Growth: From July 1982 to January 1984, the Ningxia Institute of Drug Inspection conducted a clinical experiment using multi-index screening. They concluded: The fruits and pedicels of the wolfberry were effective in increasing white blood cells, protecting the liver, and relieving hypertension. The alcoholic extract of wolfberry fruits inhibited tumor growth in mice by 58%, and the protein of wolfberry displayed an insulin-like action that was effective in promoting fat decomposition and reducing blood sugar.

ssibly Reverse Aging: A clinical experiment by the Ningxia Institute of Drug Inspection (Register No. 870306, from October 1982 to May 1985) studied the effects of Wolfberry on the blood of aged volunteers. The results were published by the State Scientific and Technological Commission of China, and the authors concluded that the wolfberry caused the blood of older people to **noticeably revert to a younger state**.

reat Potential for High Performance Gains: Wolfberry has a high concentration of the branched-chain amino acid *L-leucine*. Inside the body, L-leucine is converted into a powerful compound called HMB (beta-hydroxy beta-methylbutyrate). According to Richard Passwater, Ph.D., a noted researcher in the field of health-maintenance, "HMB showed that it lowered total and LDL cholesterol levels in blood and helped strengthen the immune system while building muscles and burning body fat. This news is certainly of interest to body builders and other athletes, but it may also become of interest to cancer, AIDS, and muscular dystrophy patients.

APPLICATION NOTES AND EXPLANATIONS

1. *Aromatic* means diffuse, breathe, or inhale.
2. A superscripted "F" (i.e. FClary sage) means the oil has been used medicinally in France.
3. *Neat* means to apply the oil without diluting it with a pure vegetable oil.
4. If essential oils get into your eyes by accident or they burn a little, do not try to remove the oils with water. This will only drive the oils deeper into the tissue. It is best to dilute the essential oils with a pure vegetable oil.
5. The FDA has approved some essential oils for internal use and given them the following designations: GRAS (Generally Regarded As Safe for internal consumption), FA (Food Addictive), or FL (FLavoring agent). These designations are listed in the Single Oil Summary Information chart in the Appendix of this book under Safety Data.
6. Using some oils such as lemon, orange, grapefruit, mandarin, bergamot, angelica, etc. befo or during exposure to direct sunlight or UV rays (tanning beds, etc.) may cause a rash, pigmentation, or even severe burns. These oils are designated as photosensitive (PH) or extremely photosensitive (PH*) in the Single Oil or Blend Summary Information in the Appendix of this book. It is best to check the safety data for the oils to be used, then either dilute and test a small area or avoid their use altogether.
7. Caution should be used with oils such as Clary sage, sage, and fennel during pregnancy. These oils contain active constituents with hormone-like activity and could possibly stimul adverse reactions in the mother, although there are no recorded cases in humans.
8. Particular care should be taken when using cinnamon bark, lemongrass, oregano, and thym as they are some of the strongest and most caustic oils. It is best to dilute them with a pure vegetable oil.
9. Essential oils are not listed in a specific order (an attempt was made to list them alphabetically) so you will have to be intuitive on which one(s) to use. It is not necessary t use all of the oils listed. Try one oil at a time. If you do not see a change soon, try a different one. What one person needs may be different than another person. (Hint: Use Kinesiology to test yourself on the oils that are right for you.)
10. In this document, several homemade blends are suggested. However, it is done with great hesitancy. Some of the blends listed come from individuals who may not be experts in the field of essential oils and aromatherapy. Rather than mix the oils together, it may be better to **layer the oils**; that is, apply a drop or two of one oil, rub it in, and then apply another oi If dilution is necessary, a pure vegetable oil can be applied on top.

1. When someone is out of electrical balance, try the following:
   A. Place a drop or two of Harmony into one hand, then rub the palms of both hands together in a clockwise motion.
   B. Place one hand over the thymus (heart chakra) and the other hand over the navel.
   C. Take three deep breaths and switch hands, then take three more deep breaths.

   (Refer to ALLERGIES in this section for more information).
2. Less is often better; use one to three drops of oil and no more than six drops at a time. Stir and rub on in a clockwise direction.
3. When applying oils to **infants** and **small children**, dilute one to two drops pure essential oil with ½-1 teaspoon (tsp.) of a pure vegetable oil (V-6 Mixing Oil). If the oils are used in the bath, always use a bath gel base as a dispersing agent for the oils. See BABIES for more information about the recommended list of oils for babies and children.
4. The body absorbs oils the fastest through inhalation (breathing) and second fastest through application to the feet or ears. Testing on the thyroid, heart, and pancreas showed that the oils reached these organs in three seconds. Layering oils can increase the rate of **absorption**.
5. When an oil causes **discomfort** it is because it is pulling toxins, heavy metals, chemicals, poisons, parasites, and mucus from the system. Either stop applying the oils for a short time, to make sure your body isn't eliminating (detoxifying) too fast, or dilute the oils until the body catches up with the releasing. These toxins go back into the system if they cannot be released.
6. When the cell wall thickens, oxygen cannot get in. The life expectancy of a cell is 120 days (4 months). Cells also divide, making duplicate cells. If the cell is diseased, new diseased cells will be made. When we stop the mutation of the diseased cells (create healthy cells), we stop the disease. Essential oils have the ability to penetrate and carry nutrients through the cell wall to the nucleus and improve the health of the cell.
7. Each oil has a **frequency**, and each of our organs and body parts have a frequency. The frequency of an oil is attracted by a like frequency within the body. Lower oil frequencies become a sponge for negative energy. The frequency is what stays in the body to maintain the longer-lasting effects of the oil.

   Low frequencies can make **physical** changes in the body.

   Middle frequencies can make **emotional** changes in the body.

   High frequencies can make **spiritual** changes in the body.

   A. Average frequency of the human body during the day time is between 62 and 68 Megahertz (MHz).
      1) Bone frequency is 38 to 43 MHz.
      2) Frequencies from the neck down vary between 62 and 68 MHz.
   B. Spiritual frequencies range from 92 to 360 MHz.
8. *Use extreme caution when diffusing cinnamon bark* because it may burn the nostrils if you put your nose directly next to the nebulizer of the diffuser.
9. When traveling by air, you should always have your oils hand-checked. X-ray machines may interfere with the frequency of the oils.

20. Keep oils away from the light and heat, although they seem to do fine in temperatures up to 90 degrees. If stored properly, they can maintain their maximum potency for many years.
21. The following information will be useful to those who are familiar with the art and techniqu of blending. (*See the Science and Application section of Reference Guide for Essential Oils for more information.*)

    1st—The **Personifier** (1-5% of blend) oils have very sharp, strong and long-lasting fragrances. They also have dominant properties with strong therapeutic action.

    Oils in this classification may include: Angelica, birch, cardamom, German chamomile, cinnamon, cistus, Clary sage, clove, coriander, ginger, helichrysum, mandarin, neroli, nutmeg, orange, patchouli, peppermint, petitgrain, rose, spearmint, tangerine, tarragon, wintergreen, ylang, ylang

    2nd—The **Enhancer** (50-80% of blend) oil should be the predominant oil as it serves to enhance the properties of the other oils in the blend. Its fragrance is not as sharp as the personifiers and is usually of a shorter duration.

    Oils in this classification may include: Basil, bergamot, birch, Roman chamomile, Black cumin, cajeput, cedarwood, dill, eucalyptus, frankincense, galbanum, geranium, grapefruit, hyssop, jasmine, lavender, lemon, lemongrass, lime, marjoram, melaleuca (Tea Tree), melissa, myrtle, orange, oregano, palmarosa, patchouli, petitgrain, ravensara, rose, rosemary, sage, spruce, thyme, wintergreen

    3rd—The **Equalizer** (10-15% of blend) oils create balance and synergy among the oils contained in the blend. Their fragrance is also not as sharp as the personifier and is o a shorter duration.

    Oils in this classification may include: Basil, bergamot, cedarwood, Roman chamomile, cypress, fennel, fir, frankincense, geranium, ginger, hyssop, jasmin juniper, lavender, lemongrass, lime, marjoram, melaleuca (Tea Tree), melissa, myrrh, myrtle, neroli, oregano, pine, rose, rosewood, sandalwood, spruce, tarragon, thyme.

    4th—The **Modifier** (5-8% of blend) oils have a mild and short fragrance. These oils add harmony to the blend.

    Oils in this classification may include: Angelica, bergamot, cardamom, coriander, eucalyptus, fennel, grapefruit, hyssop, jasmine, lavender, lemon, mandarin, melissa, myrrh, neroli, petitgrain, rose, rosewood, sandalwood, tangerine, ylang ylang.

The Science and Application section of Reference Guide for Essential Oils contains more information on the art of blending. In that same section, another method of blending explains how to use "notes (top, middle, and base notes)" to help determine how different single oils are to be blended together. It also includes an odor intensity chart that further assists in the blending process. Refer to that section for more details and instructions on blending.

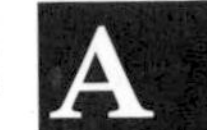

BANDONED: See EMOTIONS. Acceptance, Forgiveness, Valor.

BSCESS: See ANTI-FUNGAL, ANTI-BACTERIAL, FUNGUS: FUNGAL INFECTION or INFECTION. Bergamot, birch, elemi, frankincense, galbanum, lavender, melaleuca (Tea Tree), Melrose, myrrh, Purification, Roman chamomile, Thieves, thyme, wintergreen. To reduce swelling, pain, inflammation, and to draw out toxins, it may help to apply the oil(s) with a hot compress.

BLEND—Roman chamomile, lavender, and melaleuca (Tea Tree).

SUPPLEMENTS—ImmuGel, Royaldophilus, Super B. Put ImmuGel and Thieves on a rolled-up gauze and place over abscess to pull out the infection.

DENTAL—Helichrysum, Purification, Roman chamomile. Apply using a hot compress on face. It may also help to apply one drop of oil to a cotton ball and apply directly to the abscess. Put ImmuGel and Thieves on a rolled-up gauze and place over abscess to pull out the infection.

> *I had an abscess tooth. The dentist and the specialist he referred me to insisted I have a root canal. I used 3 to 4 drops of Thieves in a glass of water to gargle with. Then I used a mixture of half Thieves and half olive oil and rubbed this on both sides of my gums on the infected area. I then used the Dentarome Plus toothpaste. It has been 2 months and my mouth is fine.*
>
> ***-Submitted by K. Ernst (July 2004)***

BLEND #1—Use clove, birch/wintergreen, and helichrysum to help with infection.

MOUTH—[F]Lavender.

****COMMENTS—Some sources recommend a non-toxic diet and an increase in liquid intake.*

BSENT MINDED: See MEMORY. Basil, Brain Power, cardamom, Clarity, frankincense, lemongrass, M-Grain, peppermint, rosemary, sandalwood.

SUPPLEMENTS—Mineral Essence, Power Meal, Sulfurzyme, Ultra Young, VitaGreen.

BUNDANCE: Abundance, Acceptance, bergamot, cinnamon bark, cypress, Harmony, Gathering.

ATTRACTS—Abundance, cinnamon bark.

MONEY—Ginger, patchouli.

****COMMENTS—One waitress demonstrated her luck when she wore Abundance and Harmony together; she received a whopping $120.00 tip! Who knows, it may work for you too!*

BUSE: Acceptance, Brain Power, Citrus Fresh, Christmas Spirit, geranium, Forgiveness, Grounding, Harmony, Hope, Humility, Inner Child, Joy, lavender, melissa, Peace & Calming, Release, 3 Wise Men, sandalwood, SARA (releases memory and trauma of sexual or ritual abuse), Surrender, Trauma Life, Valor, ylang ylang. Apply l drop of the oils desired on each Chakra to allow blocked emotions to come out.

SUPPLEMENTS—Power Meal, Super B, Super C / Super C Chewable.

BY FATHER—Forgiveness, lavender, Sacred Mountain (empowers self).

BY MOTHER—Forgiveness, geranium, lavender.

****COMMENTS—Refer to the page on Auricular Emotional Therapy in the Basic Information section of this book for the points where oils can be applied.*

FEELINGS OF REVENGE—Forgiveness (around navel), Present Time (on thymus), Surrender (on sternum over heart).

PROTECTION or BALANCE—Harmony (over thymus; on energy centers/chakras), Whi Angelica (on shoulders).

SEXUAL/RITUAL—Forgiveness (around navel), Harmony, Joy, Present Time, Release (liver Vita Flex point on feet; under nose), sage, SARA (over area of abuse), 3 Wise Men, Trauma Life, Valor, and White Angelica.

ESPOUSAL—Acceptance, Envision, Forgiveness, Joy, Release, Trauma Life, Valor.

SUICIDAL—Brain Power, Hope (on rim of ears), melissa, Present Time.

ACCIDENTS: See EMOTIONS. Trauma Life.

ACHES/PAINS: Blue cypress, Idaho balsam fir, PanAway, Relieve It, sage lavender. Vetiver & valerian together make a powerful pain killer.

MASSAGE OILS—Ortho Ease or Ortho Sport (stronger). *These massage oils help seal in and enhance the effectiveness of the single oils or oil blends.*

SUPPLEMENTS—Sulfurzyme contains MSM which has been shown to be very effective in controlling pain, especially in the joints and tissues.

BONE—All the tree oils–**Birch**, cedarwood, cypress, fir, helichrysum, juniper, PanAway, peppermint, sandalwood, spruce, **wintergreen**.

SUPPLEMENTS—Coral Sea (highly bio-available calcium, contains 58 trace minerals), Super Cal, ArthroTune (1 capsule twice a day).

CHRONIC—Basil, birch, clove, cypress, cedarwood, elemi, fir, helichrysum, Idaho tansy, ginger, juniper, PanAway (add 1-2 drops birch for extra strength), peppermint, rosemary cineol, Relieve It, sandalwood, spruce, valerian, wintergreen.

BLEND—Equal parts of birch/wintergreen, elemi, and Idaho tansy.

MASSAGE OILS—Ortho Ease or Ortho Sport (stronger).

SUPPLEMENTS—Coral Sea (highly bio-available calcium, contains 58 trace minerals), Super Cal, ArthroTune (1 capsule twice a day).

GENERAL—Aroma Siez, birch, Blue cypress, frankincense, ginger, helichrysum, Idaho balsam fir, lavender, marjoram, PanAway, Relieve It, Roman chamomile, rosemary, sage lavender, **White fir** (pain from inflammation), wintergreen.

GROWING—Massage with birch/wintergreen, cypress, peppermint, wait 5 minutes and apply PanAway, then seal with Ortho Ease.

MASSAGE OILS—Ortho Ease.

SUPPLEMENTS—Coral Sea (highly bio-available calcium, contains 58 trace minerals). Sulfurzyme, Super Cal, 1 ArthroTune twice a day.

JOINTS—Birch (discomfort), Idaho balsam fir, nutmeg, Roman chamomile (inflamed), spruce, wintergreen.

MUSCLE—Aroma Siez, [F]birch, basil, [F]clove, ginger, helichrysum, Idaho balsam fir, lavender, lemongrass (especially good for ligaments), marjoram, nutmeg, oregano, PanAway, peppermint, Relieve It, Roman chamomile, rosemary verbenon, sage lavender, spearmint, spruce (torn muscles), thyme, vetiver, **White fir** (pain from inflammation), wintergreen.

TISSUE—Helichrysum, PanAway, Relieve It or Balsam fir (good for deep tissue pain).

IDOSIS: See ALKALINE and pH BALANCE. Lemon, peppermint.

ACID-FORMING FOODS—Avoid meat, dairy products, whole wheat or rye bread, coffee, tea, wine, beer, root beer, cider, yeast products, soy sauce, cold cereals, potato chips, etc.

SUPPLEMENTS—AlkaLime (acid-neutralizing mineral), Bodygize, Exodus (may increase oxygen), Mineral Essence, Power Meal, Royaldophilus, VitaGreen (for alkaline/acid balance).

****COMMENTS—Cancer and candida need an acid condition in order to thrive and spread. In acidic conditions, the oils will take longer to work and won't last as long. When a person does not like the smell of an oil it is usually because of an acidic condition. THE BODY CAN ONLY HEAL IN AN ALKALINE STATE.*

__Acidosis__ is a condition of over-acidity in the blood and body tissues. When the body loses its alkaline reserve, pleomorphic virus, bacteria, yeast, and fungus take over and cause degenerative diseases such as, diabetes, cancer, aids, arteriosclerosis, arthritis, osteoporosis, chronic fatigue, etc.

__Symptoms of acidosis__ may include: frequent sighing, insomnia, water retention, recessed eyes, rheumatoid arthritis, migraine headaches, abnormally low blood pressure, and alternating constipation and diarrhea.

__Causes of acidosis__ may include: improper diet, kidney, liver, and adrenal disorders, emotional disturbances, fever, and an excess of niacin, vitamin C, and aspirin.

__Oxygen reduces the acidity of the blood.__ All essential oils contain oxygen. We like to flavor our water with 1-2 drops of lemon or peppermint oil. Lemon has the ability to counteract acidity in the body. The citric acid found in lemons is neutralized during digestion, giving off carbonates and bicarbonates of potassium and calcium, which helps maintain the alkalinity of the system.

ACNE: See HORMONAL IMBALANCE, SCARRING, SKIN, and STRESS. Bergamot, cedarwood, Clarity (on temples), Clary sage, clove, eucalyptus, *Eucalyptus radiata*, frankincense, Gentle Baby, geranium, [F]German chamomile, [F]juniper, [F]lavender, lemon, lemongrass, marjoram, melaleuca (Tea Tree), Melrose, my patchouli, petitgrain, Purification, Raven, ravensara, RC, rosemary, [F]rosewo sage, sage lavender, sandalwood, Sensation, spearmint, thyme, vetiver, yarro Apply one of the above oils on location or try putting about 10 drops of an o into a small spray bottle and mist your face several times a day.

PERSONAL CARE—
Prenolone/Prenolone+, Progessence, Rose Ointment, Sensation Massage Oil.

SUPPLEMENTS—
ComforTone, ICP, Essentialzyme, JuvaTone, and Sulfurzyme. Cleansing the colon may help (see CLEANSING).

ADULT ONSET—
Prenolone/Prenolone+, Progessence if the acne stems from a hormonal imbalance.

CELLULAR REGENERATIVE—
Palmarosa, rosewood.

> ***Acne** is often a result of seborrhea (an overproduction of fat from the sebaceous glands), which can oftentimes be traced back to a hormonal imbalance. Stress is another reason for increased sebum production. Consequently, it may be of help to use oils that balance the hormones and reduce stress.*
>
> *Essential oil treatments combined with a good diet (lots o vegetables and lots of water), exercise, and increased lymphatic and circulatory flow, will allow the toxic waste to leave the body as the oxygen and nutrients reach the skin in greater proportions.*
>
> *One of the best ways to release toxins through the skin is to sweat. Chamomile, hyssop, juniper, lavender, rosemary, and thyme contain sudorific properties and may facilitate the sweating process. The anti-bacterial and anti-inflammatory oils may assist in the healing process.*

HEALING—Use anti-bacterial and anti-inflammatory oils like geranium, melaleuca (Tea Tree), Melrose, and rosewood.

INFECTIOUS—Clove.

MENSTRUAL—Premenstrual or mid-menstrual cycle acne may be helped by balancing hormones.

PERSONAL CARE—Prenolone/Prenolone+, Progessence.

SUPPLEMENTS—CortiStop (Women's), FemiGen, Super B.

TOXIN RELEASE—Use sudorific oils like chamomile, hyssop, juniper, lavender, rosem and thyme to help promote sweating.

ACNE ROSACEA: See ROSACEA.

ADD: See ATTENTION DEFICIT DISORDER.

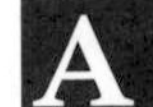

DDICTIONS: Acceptance, bergamot (helps with over indulgences), calamus (tobacco), JuvaFlex, Peace & Calming, Purification.

SUPPLEMENTS—JuvaTone, Mineral Essence, Super C / Super C Chewable.

The following recipe has worked for individuals who are trying to break addictions:

RECIPE #1—Use JuvaPower, JuvaTone, ComforTone, JuvaFlex and Acceptance together.

ALCOHOL—(to stop drinking) Purification, Peace & Calming. Do not use Clary sage and alcohol together; it may result in nightmares. *For professional assistance, contact the local chapter of Alcoholics Anonymous.*

COFFEE/TOBACCO—Bergamot, calamus. Apply to stomach, abdomen, liver area, and bottom of feet.

DRUGS—Basil, bergamot, birch, eucalyptus, fennel, grapefruit (withdrawal), lavender, marjoram, nutmeg, orange, Peace & Calming, Purification, Roman chamomile, sandalwood, wintergreen. Apply to Vita Flex points on feet.

SUPPLEMENTS—Super C / Super C Chewable (at least 250 mg per day).

SMOKING—Use the above recipe. Applying either clove or Thieves to the tongue before lighting up helps remove the desire to smoke. Calamus may also help.

****COMMENTS—One individual used JuvaTone to break a habit of smoking 2 ½ packs of cigarettes a day for 20 years. It only took him three to five days!*

SUGAR—Dill, Purification, Peace & Calming. Apply to Vita Flex points on feet. Place dill on wrists to help remove addiction to sweets.

SUPPLEMENTS–Allerzyme (aids the digestion of sugars, starches, fats, and proteins), Cleansing Trio (ComforTone, Essentialzyme, and ICP).

WITHDRAWAL—Dill, grapefruit, lavender, marjoram, nutmeg, orange, sandalwood. Apply to temples and diffuse. Applying dill to the wrists helps reduce the sweating that often accompanies withdrawal.

DDISON'S DISEASE: See ADRENAL GLANDS. En-R-Gee, EndoFlex, Joy, nutmeg (increases energy; supports adrenal glands),sage (combine with nutmeg).

> ***Addison's Disease*** *is an autoimmune disease where the body's own immune cells attack the adrenal glands and either severely limit or completely shut down the production of the adrenal cortex hormones. Extreme fluid and mineral loss are the life-threatening results.*

SUPPLEMENTS—ImmuPro, Master Formula His/Hers, Mineral Essence (help supplement mineral loss), **Sulfurzyme** (shown to slow or reverse autoimmune diseases), Super B, VitaGreen.

DENITIS: See LYMPHATIC SYSTEM. Garlic, onion, pine, rosemary, sage.

> ***Adenitis*** *is an acute or chronic inflammation of the lymph glands or nodes. Drink a lot of water to help remove the toxins from the body.*

ADRENAL GLANDS: See ENDOCRINE SYSTEM, LUPUS, THYROID. EndoFlex, En-R-Gee, Forgiveness, Joy, nutmeg (increases energy; supports adrenal glands).

BLEND—Add 3 drops clove, 4 nutmeg, and 6 rosemary to 1 tsp. V-6 Mixing Oil. Apply 4-5 drops of this mixture to kidney areas and cover with hot compress. Also apply 1-2 drops of mixture to Vita Flex kidney points on the feet and wor in with fingers using Vita Flex technique.

STIMULANT—[F]Basil, clove, geranium, pine, rosemary, [F]sage.

STRENGTHEN—Spruce (Black), peppermint.

UNDERACTIVE ADRENALS—See ADDISON'S DISEASE.

SUPPLEMENTS—Thyromin (1-4 tablets daily. *See Suggested Use under Thyromin in the Supplements section of the Reference Guide for Essential Oils.*) Also Master Formula His/Hers, Mineral Essence, Super B, and VitaGreen.

*The **adrenal glands** are made up of an inner part (medulla) and an outer part (cortex). The outer portion (or cortex) produces critical steroid hormones, including glucocorticoids and aldosterone. These hormones directly affect blood pressure and mineral content. They also help regulate the conversion of carbohydrates into energy. Nutmeg displays similar properties and is contained in EndoFlex.*

When the adrenal glands are working properly, it is easier to correct low thyroid function.

AFTERSHAVE: See SKIN. Valor. Awaken can be used instead of aftershave lotion. Try adding Awaken to Sandalwood Moisture Creme, Satin Hand & Body Lotion, Sensation Hand & Body Lotion, or Genesis Hand & Body Lotion as an aftershave.

PERSONAL CARE–Genesis Hand & Body Lotion, KidScents Lotion (soothes and rehydrates the skin- smells great too), Prenolone/Prenolone+, Rose Ointment, Sandalwood Moisture Creme, Satin Hand & Body Lotion, Sensation Hand & Body Lotion.

AGENT ORANGE POISONING: JuvaFlex (over liver with hot compress), EndoFlex (over adrenal glands/kidneys).

BATH—in 1 cup Epsom salts and 4 oz. of food grade hydrogen peroxide.

SUPPLEMENTS—ComforTone, Essentialzyme, ICP, ImmuneTune, ImmuPro, Thyromin.

RECIPE #1—3 drops EndoFlex on throat, feet (under big toes and kidney Vita Flex point). Also across the back over the kidneys. After 90 days, start the Cleansing Trio (ComforTone, Essentialzyme, and ICP) and continue for one year.

***Agent Orange** is a toxic herbicide that was used to defoliate areas of the forest during the Vietnam War.*

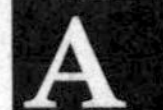

RECIPE #2—3 ImmuneTune four times a day, 2 Thyromin at bedtime. After 90 days, start on Cleansing Trio (ComforTone, Essentialzyme, and ICP) and continue for one year.

GING: See WRINKLES. Carrot, frankincense, Longevity (take as a dietary supplement to help prevent premature aging), rosehip, rosewood, sandalwood.

SUPPLEMENTS—Berry Young Juice (a delicious blend of highly antioxidant fruit juices - measures higher on the ORAC (oxygen radical absorbance capacity) scale than even Tahitian Noni Juice), Longevity Capsules.

MOISTURIZERS—

PERSONAL CARE—Boswellia Wrinkle Creme, Satin Facial Scrub - Mint, Prenolone/Prenolone+, Progessence, Rose Ointment, Sandalwood Moisture Creme, Sensation Hand & Body Lotion, Wolfberry Eye Creme.

SUPPLEMENTS— Essentialzyme, Mineral Essence (antioxidant), Wolfberry Bar *(Refer to the Wolfberry Bar in the Supplements section of the Reference Guide for Essential Oils for more information on the benefits of the Chinese Wolfberry).*

GITATION: [F]Bergamot, cedarwood, Chivalry, Clary sage, Forgiveness, frankincense, geranium, Harmony, Joy, juniper, lavender, marjoram, myrrh, Peace & Calming, rose, rosewood, sandalwood, Transformation, Trauma Life (calms), Valor, ylang ylang.

IDS: Brain Power, cistus, cumin (supports immune system; inhibits HIV virus), Exodus II, helichrysum, ImmuPower, lemon, nutmeg, Thieves, Valor. Apply to Thymus and bottom of feet.

SUPPLEMENTS—Cleansing Trio (ComforTone, Essentialzyme, and ICP), Exodus, ImmuGel, ImmuneTune, ImmuPro, Mineral Essence, Power Meal (contains wolfberry which is an immune stimulator), Super B, Super C / Super C Chewable, Thyromin, Ultra Young, VitaGreen.

****COMMENTS—Refer to The chapter entitled "How to Use - The Personal Usage Reference" in the Essential Oils Desk Reference under "AIDS" for specific oil blend and supplement recommendations.*

Personal Guide

AIRBORNE BACTERIA: Cinnamon bark, fir, Idaho balsam fir, Mountain savory, oregano, Purification, and Thieves.

Diffusing essential oils in the home or work place is one of the best ways to purify our environment. The anti-viral, anti-bacterial, and antiseptic properties of the oils, along with the negative ions and oxygenating molecules that are released when essential oils are diffused, all help to reduce chemicals, bacteria, and metallics in the air.

Cinnamon bark, Mountain savory, oregano, and Thieves. were all tested by Weber State University and were shown to kill 100% of the airborne bacteria present. This was all done by diffusing the oils into the atmosphere. (KID-Radio with Lance Richardson and Dr. Gary Young, N.D., Aromatologist, March 5, 1996)

AIR POLLUTION: Abundance, Christmas Spirit, cypress, eucalyptus, fir, grapefruit, ImmuPower, lavender, lemon (sterilize air), lime, Purification, rosemary, Thieves.

DISINFECTANTS—Birch, citronella, clove, eucalyptus, grapefruit, [F]lemon, peppermint, Purification, sage, spruce, wintergreen.

ALCOHOLISM: See ADDICTIONS. Fennel, juniper, and rosemary (Alternative Medicine—A Definitive Guide, p. 492). Can also use Acceptance, elemi, Forgiveness, helichrysum, Joy, JuvaFlex, lavender, Motivation, orange, Roman chamomile, rosemary verbenon, Transformation, Surrender.

SUPPLEMENTS—Mineral Essence, Power Meal, Thyromin. Work on cleaning out the colon and liver with the Cleansing Trio, JuvaPower/JuvaSpice, and JuvaTone or the Master Cleanser (see CLEANSING).

ALERTNESS: Basil, Citrus Fresh, Clarity, lemon, peppermint, rosemary. Apply to temples an bottom of feet.

ALKALINE: See ACIDOSIS, pH BALANCE.

__Alkaline__ refers to a substance or solution that has a pH of 7.0 or above. The optimum pH for our blood and body tissues is about 7.2 (The use of saliva and urine test strips will show a much lower pH level due to the protein present in the solution. Saliva and urine tests from a healthy body should be about 6.6 to 6.8).

The body heals best when it is slightly alkaline. To keep the blood and body tissue at an optimum pH, avoid acid-forming food. See ACIDOSIS. Make sure your food intake is 80 percent alkaline and drink plenty of water.

ALKALI-FORMING FOODS—Dark green and yellow vegetables, sprouted grains, legumes, seeds, nuts, essential fats (omega 3 and 6), and low sugar fruits like avocados and lemons.

PERSONAL CARE—Genesis Hand & Body Lotion balances pH on the skin.

SUPPLEMENTS—AlkaLime, JuvaPower (contains many acid-binding foods), Mineral Essence, Power Meal (pre-digested protein), Royaldophilus (replaces

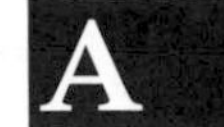

intestinal flora), Stevia Select (with FOS to help rebuild and protect friendly intestinal flora), VitaGreen (helps normalize blood pH levels).

KALOSIS: See pH BALANCE. Anise, Di-Tone, ginger, tarragon.

SUPPLEMENTS—Bodygize, Essentialzyme, Mineral Essence, Power Meal (pre-digested protein), Royaldophilus (replaces intestinal flora), Sulfurzyme, VitaGreen (helps normalize blood pH levels).

> ***Alkalosis** refers to a condition where the blood and intestinal tract becomes excessively alkaline. Slight alkalinity is important for a healthy body but excessive alkalinity can cause depression, fatigue, and sickness.*

ONE (Feeling): See EMOTIONS. Acceptance, Valor.

LERGIES: Elemi (rashes), eucalyptus, Harmony, [F]lavender, ledum, *Melaleuca ericifolia*, *Melaleuca quinquenervia*, melissa (skin and respiratory), [F]patchouli, peppermint, ImmuPower, Raven, RC, Roman chamomile, spikenard. Apply to sinuses, bottom of feet, and diffuse.

****COMMENTS—According to the Essential Oils Desk Reference, ". . . rub three drops [Harmony] on sternum, breathing deeply." (EDR-June 2002)*

SUPPLEMENTS—AlkaLime, ComforTone, Coral Sea (highly bio-available calcium, contains 58 trace minerals), ICP fiber beverage (beneficial when there is an allergy to psyllium), ImmuneTune, ImmuPro, Mineral Essence, Super C / Super C Chewable, Super Cal.

COUGHING—Purification (diffuse).

HAY FEVER—See HAY FEVER.

PSYCHOLOGICAL ALLERGIES (in the mind)—Put Harmony on feet, neck, navel, or in your shoes for one to five days.

> *If you have a reaction to the oils, it is only a reaction to all of the chemicals you have been dumping into your body throughout the years. The oils are merely reacting with the toxins in the sub-dermal tissues and beginning their removal.* ***Cleanse the body!***

TO OILS—Put one drop of the oil, to which there is an allergy reaction, on a cotton ball and place it in a shoe. Add a drop each day until the allergy to that particular oil is gone. Since allergies often indicate an electrical imbalance, try the following:

A. Place a drop or two of Harmony into one hand, then rub the palms of both hands together in a clockwise motion.

B. Place one hand over the thymus (heart chakra) and the other hand over the navel.

C. Take three deep breaths and switch hands, then take three more deep breaths.

Harmony helps open the energy meridians and balance the bio-electrical field of the body.

The following recipes have been used for allergies:

RECIPE #1—Apply 1 drop of peppermint on the base of the neck two times a day. Tap the thymus (located just below the notch in the neck) with pointer and in fingers (energy fingers). Diffuse peppermint. For some individuals, the use peppermint oil has resulted in no more allergy shots!

RECIPE #2—Apply 1 drop of RC and Raven on the base of the neck two times a day. Tap on thymus, massage chest and back with 5 Raven, 5 RC, and 2 tsp V-6 Mixing Oil. Diffuse RC and Raven.

RECIPE #3—For allergy rashes and skin sensitivity, Dr. Gary Young applies 3 lavender, 6 Roman chamomile, 2 myrrh, and 1 peppermint on location.

ALOPECIA AREATA: (Inflammatory hair-loss disease) See HAIR: LOSS.

ALUMINUM TOXICITY: See ATTENTION DEFICIT DISORDER. Juva Cleanse.

SUPPLEMENTS—Chelex helps remove aluminum from the body.

> ***Aluminum toxicity** may contribute to the cause of rickets, colic, kidney and liver dysfunction, speech and memory problems, osteoporosis, and Alzheimer's disease.*

ALZHEIMER'S DISEASE: See BRAIN, MEMORY, PINEAL GLAND, PITUITARY GLAND.

SUPPLEMENTS—Chelex, Cleansing Trio (ComforTone, Essentialzyme, and ICP), JuvaTone, Power Meal, Sulfurzyme.

***COMMENTS—*The gingko biloba that is found in Power Meal has been shown to help improve memory loss, brain function, depression, cerebral and peripheral circulation, oxygenation, and blood flow.*

> *Autopsies have revealed that victims of **Alzheimer's disease** have four times the normal amount of aluminum in the nerve cells of their brain.*
>
> ***Prevention:** Use glass, iron, or stainless steel cookware. Avoid products containing aluminum, bentonite, or dihydroxyaluminum. Some of these products are: aluminum cookware, foil, antacids, baking powders, buffered aspirin, most city water, antiperspirants, deodorants, beer, bleached flour, table salt, tobacco smoke, cream of tartar, Parmesan and grated cheeses, aluminum salts, douches, and canned goods.*

BLOOD-BRAIN BARRIER—Studies have shown that sesquiterpenes can pass the blood brain barrier. Oils that are high in sesquiterpenes include cedarwood, vetiver, sandalwood, Black pepper, patchouli, myrrh, ginger, German chamomile, spikenard, galbanum, and frankincense. Some essential oil blends containing some of these oils include: 3 Wise Men, Acceptance, Brain Power, Forgiveness, Gathering, Harmony, Inspiration, Into the Future, Transformation, and Trauma Life. Apply to temples, bottom of feet, and diffuse.

***COMMENTS—*Oils that pass through the blood-brain barrier cannot carry unwanted substances with them.*

BRAIN FUNCTION—Clarity.

EMOTIONS—Acceptance, cypress, Peace & Calming, 3 Wise Men (crown).

MINO ACIDS: Lavender.

SUPPLEMENTS—Bodygize, Cleansing Trio (ComforTone, Essentialzyme, and ICP), Exodus, FemiGen, JuvaTone, ImmuGel, Master Formula His/Hers, KidScents Mighty Mist/Vites, Mineral Essence, Power Meal, Thyromin.

***Amino acids** have the ability to neutralize and help eliminate free radicals in the system.*

MNESIA: See MEMORY. Basil, clove, rosemary.

NALGESIC: Bergamot, birch, clove, eucalyptus, geranium, helichrysum, lavender, lemongrass, marjoram, melaleuca, oregano, PanAway, peppermint, Roman chamomile, rosemary, wintergreen.

****COMMENT—See the "single oil property chart" in the APPENDIX of this book for additional analgesic oils and their strengths.*

NEMIA: Carrot, ImmuPower, Juva Cleanse, lavender, [F]lemon. Apply to bottom of feet and stomach.

FOOD—Flavor water with a drop of lemon. Can also use an H2Oils packet of lemon to infuse the drinking water with lemon oil.

SUPPLEMENTS—Rehemogen tincture (10 drops twice a day) and JuvaTone together help raise blood cell count.

NESTHESIA: See ANALGESIC. Clove, helichrysum, PanAway.

****COMMENTS—One individual applied helichrysum every 15 minutes during gum surgery and there was no bleeding and no pain. No other anesthetic was used.*

NEURYSM: See BLOOD. Aroma Life (chelates plaque), cypress (strengthens the capillary walls and increases circulation), frankincense, helichrysum, Idaho tansy. Apply to temples, heart, Vita Flex heart points, and diffuse.

BLEND—5 frankincense, 1 helichrysum, and 1 cypress. DIFFUSE.

HERBS—Cayenne pepper, Garlic, Hawthorn Berry.

MASSAGE OIL—Cel-Lite Magic dilates blood vessels for better circulation.

SUPPLEMENTS—Cleansing Trio (ComforTone, Essentialzyme, and ICP), Sulfurzyme, Super C / Super C Chewable.

TINCTURES—HRT.

NGER: See LIVER. Australian Blue, Bergamot, cedarwood, cypress, Forgiveness, frankincense, geranium, German chamomile, Grounding, Joy, Harmony, helichrysum, Hope, Humility, Inspiration, lavender, lemon, mandarin, marjora melissa, myrrh (soothes), myrtle, orange, Peace & Calming, petitgrain, Presen Time, Release, Roman chamomile, rose, Sacred Mountain, sandalwood, Surrender, Trauma Life, Valor, ylang ylang.

****COMMENTS—Refer to the Emotional Release part of the Science and Application section of the Reference Guide for Essential Oils.*

CALMS ANGER—Australian Blue, Inspiration, Peace & Calming, spruce, Trauma Life.

CLEANSING AFTER ARGUMENT and PHYSICAL FIGHTING—Eucalyptus.

CLEANSE THE LIVER—(Anger is stored in the liver) JuvaFlex, [F]geranium (cleanses and detoxifies the liver), grapefruit (liver disorders).

DISPELS ANGER—Ylang ylang.

FOR COMMUNICATION WITHOUT ANGER—Roman chamomile.

LESSENS ANGER—Myrrh.

OVERCOME—Bergamot, [F]cedarwood, Release, Roman chamomile.

RELEASES LOCKED UP ANGER and FRUSTRATION—Roman or German chamomil Release (together with JuvaFlex), Sacred Mountain, sandalwood, Surrender, Transformation, Valor.

SUPPLEMENTS—JuvaTone, Thyromin, Super B.

BLEND—4 drops lavender, 3 geranium, 3 rosewood, 3 rosemary, 2 tangerine, 1 spearmint, 2 Idaho tansy, 1 German chamomile, and 1 oz. V-6 Mixing Oil. Apply to back of neck, wrist, and heart.

ANGINA: Aroma Life, [F]ginger, laurel, [F]orange (for false angina). Apply to heart and Vita Flex heart point.

TINCTURES—HRT.

***Angina pectoris** is a severe spasmodic pain in the chest that is due to an insufficient supply of blood to the heart.*

ANIMALS: Only a 1-2 drops of oil is all that is necessary on animals as they respond much mo quickly to the oils than do humans. V-6 Mixing Oil can be added to extend oil over larger areas and to heavily dilute the essential oil for use on smaller animals, especially cats.

PERSONAL CARE—Animal Scents Pet Shampoo, Animal Scents Pet Ointment. Other alkaline shampoos without chemicals are good for animals.

SUPPLEMENTS—BLM (added to their food, can help speed the healing of bones), Power Meal and Sulfurzyme.

BLEEDING—Geranium, helichrysum.

BONES (Pain)—Birch/wintergreen, lemongrass, PanAway, spruce.

MASSAGE OILS—Ortho Ease or Ortho Sport.

SUPPLEMENTS—BLM (added to their food, can help speed the healing of bones), Power Meal and Sulfurzyme.

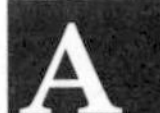

CALM—Citrus Fresh, lavender, Peace & Calming, Roman chamomile (for horses, add to feed), Trauma Life. Dilute well for cats.

CANCER—

SKIN—Frankincense and cumin.

CATS—Valerie Worwood says that you can treat a cat like you would a child (see BABIES). Dilute oils heavily with V-6 Mixing Oil. Avoid melaleuca.

COMMENTS—Cat physiology is so different from other animals and from humans that oils should be used with extreme caution on cats. In fact, melaleuca (or Tea Tree oil) should never be used on a cat as death can result. Some cases exist where a blend of oils containing melaleuca have killed cats.

COLDS and COUGHS—Eucalyptus, melaleuca (not for cats). Apply on fur or stomach.

COWS—For scours, use 5 drops Di-Tone on stomach (can mix with V-6 Mixing Oil to cover larger area) and repeat 2 hours later.

CUTS and SORES—Melrose (not on cats). 1 drop on location. Work in with finger.

DOGS—There was a dog that walked with its head down and its tail between its legs.

I have a large brown tabby cat that was limping bad so I took him to the vet. The vet said he had a knee injury (he compared it to a football player's injured knee-"Cruciate Ligament Rupture") and said it would need surgery. He wanted me to bring my cat back in a week to see his son (who is also a vet) to make arrangements for the surgery. Later, using V6 as my carrier oil and a couple drops of lavender oil, I rubbed my cat from the bottom of the paw up to his hip area. The next day I could see an improvement, and by the time I took him back to the vet he was walking on his leg with only a slight limp. The vet said he would heal nicely on his own and there would be no need for surgery. Today he walks, runs and is even now jumping with no problems.

-Submitted by M. Rynicki (July 2004)

One Saturday in February, my husband woke me up by yelling from the living room for me to bring my oils and any oil books I had at hand to him immediately. Our dog, Buddy, (a mutt from the pound, age approx. 7+ years) was lying on the floor and all of his muscles were completely seized up and tensed to the point where we couldn't move any part of his body. I had most of my oils in my large case and the Higley reference guide at my side. I put 4 or 5 drops of lavender oil in my husband's hand and he put that on Buddy's paws, ears and all over his back and legs, anywhere he was tense that we could reach. We followed the lavender with Peace & Calming, Valor and frankincense applied the same way. Those four were the oils I was drawn to by instinct. We massaged him and continued to stroke and pet him during and after the application of oils and after about 10 minutes he was able to get up and go to the door to go outside and run around. In between applying oils I looked up the info on animals as well as the info on seizures and strokes (we weren't sure what kind of episode he was having), just to make sure my instincts were near to on target (which they were). We had plans to travel about an hour out of town to visit with family, and kept Buddy with us the whole day just to be sure he was ok. When I tell this story to other people they tell me about how their dog(s) had seizures and had to be put on steroids and eventually put down because of the seizures. I am very thankful for Young Living and the oils that allowed me to go the natural route for the care of our dog.

-Submitted by A. Cornn
Machesney Park, Illinois (July 2004)

Valor was put on its feet and 3 Wise Men and Joy on its crown. The next day its head was up and it was happy.

ANXIETY / NERVOUSNESS— Lavender, Peace & Calming, valerian, Valor. Rub 1-2 drops between hands and apply to muzzle, between toes, on top of feet to smell when nose is down, and on edge of ears.

ARTHRITIS—A blend of rosemary, lavender, and ginger diluted with V-6 Mixing Oil. Ortho Ease Massage Oil can also be applied to arthritic areas. Add Sulfurzyme (powder) or Vitamin C to their food.

BONE INJURY— Birch/wintergreen and Ortho Ease Massage Oil on injury. Sulfurzyme and BLM in food.

CHEWING ON FURNITURE—Mineral Essence (helps satisfy mineral deficiency).

DIGESTION—Essentialzyme.

HEART PROBLEMS—Myrtle, ravensara, and Thieves on back using Raindrop Technique with warm wet pack. Peppermint on paws. HRT Tincture can also be added to food.

LIMPING—4 ArthroTune per day for two weeks, then 3 per day until healed. Use 2 per day for maintenance.

PAIN and STRESS—Do Raindrop Technique (*the video "Essential Tips for Happy, Healthy Pets" demonstrates this technique on a dog and a horse*). This technique helps relieve stress on the back, shoulders, and legs as well as raise immune function and protect against illness.

SLEEP—Lavender (on paws), Peace & Calming (on stomach).

STROKE—Brain Power (on head), frankincense (on brain stem/back of neck), Valor (on each paw).

TICKS and BUG BITES—Purification. 1 drop directly on live tick. Can also be applied to untreated tick wound and worked in with finger.

TRAVEL SICKNESS—Peppermint. Dilute with V-6 Mixing Oil and rub on stomach. Also helps calm stomachaches.

I went to visit my son in Ft. Lauderdale, FL...and was also happy to see his dog, Luna, who I've known for 7 years since she was a puppy. I could tell she was in pain, as she was not as active as usual and was limping. My son, Jason, told me that she is part German Shepherd-a breed that is prone to hip dysplasia. It broke my heart to see her in such pain. Jason had been giving her various vitamins and other supplements for several months, without much success. I myself have had success with Sulfurzyme for an arthritic knee, and asked if he would like to try that for Luna. We began to give her 1/4 tsp. twice a day with her meals. Within two days, we began to see a change. My son was amazed ! As the two weeks passed while I was visiting, we saw a huge change. She was running like her old self, and you could sense that the pain was almost (if not totally) gone. Within a month, Jason told me that she was now even jumping up on furniture, which she was unable to do when we started with the Sulfurzyme. That was 18 months ago, and Luna is still taking Sulfurzyme...and still doing great !

-Submitted by Linda Griffith
Dixon, New Mexico (July 2004)

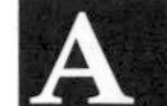

TRAUMATIZED—Trauma Life. Rub 1-2 drops between hands and cup over nose and mouth for dog to inhale.

EARACHE—1 drop Melrose or a blend of 1 drop melaleuca (Tea Tree), 1 lavender, and 1 Roman chamomile diluted in V-6 Mixing oil. Put in ear and rub around the ear.

EAR INFECTIONS—ImmuPower, Purification (helps ward off insects too). Dip cotton swab in oil and apply to inside and front of ear.

FLEAS—Citronella, eucalyptus, lemongrass, Melrose, pine. Add 1-2 drops of oil to shampoo.

BLEND—Combine eucalyptus, orange, citronella, and cedarwood. Add blend to distilled water in a spray bottle, shake well, and mist over entire animal.

HORSES—

ANXIETY/NERVOUSNESS—Peace & Calming. Rub 1-2 drops between hands and apply to nose, on front of chest, knees, and tongue.

FLIES—Idaho Tansy Floral Water. Spray over animal to keep flies and other insects away.

HOOF ROT—Blend of Roman chamomile, thyme, and melissa in V-6 Mixing Oil.

INFECTION—Melrose, Thieves.

INJURIES—Do Raindrop Technique (*the video "Essential Tips for Happy, Healthy Pets" demonstrates this technique on a dog and a horse*). When a frisky race horse took a fall and was unable to walk, application of the oils using the Raindrop Technique brought the horse out of it in a matter of days.

LEG FRACTURES—Ginger and V-6 Mixing Oil. Wrap the leg with a hot compress. Massage leg after the fracture is healed with a blend of rosemary and thyme with V-6 Mixing Oil. This may strengthen the ligaments and prevent calcification.

MUSCLE TISSUE/LIGAMENTS—Equal parts lemongrass and lavender on location and wrap to help regenerate torn muscle tissue.

*I have a 21-year-old gelding who was diagnosed with "**kidney colic**" back in January. He would be down one day, up the next, down the next, up for several days, down again, etc. He would show all the general signs of colic but was also wanting to urinate frequently, passing little or nothing. This went on for about four weeks, and the vet thought he probably was trying to pass kidney stones. Since it was happening so often, I was wanting something to give him for the pain instead of using Banamine so much. I had used marjoram, clary sage and lavender successfully on an intestinal colic, so I tried them, but they just didn't work as well on the kidneys. So I tried JuvaFlex, and the results were dramatic! Four drops over each kidney, with or without a warm compress, would get him up and back to eating and drinking in 10-20 minutes. The pain-killing effects would last from 2-4 hours and seemed to be cumulative. After I had done this for two separate "episodes," the symptoms went away completely. I don't know if the stones dissolved or he passed them, but he's been pain free for six months.*

-Submitted by Jan Early
Tallahassee, Florida (July 2004)

WOUNDS—Helichrysum, Melrose, and Rose Ointment.

SADDLE SORES—Melrose and Rose Ointment.

INFECTION—Di-Tone and ImmuPower on the paws.

PARASITES—Cedarwood, lavender, Di-Tone. Rub on paws to release parasites.

SUPPLEMENTS—ParaFree.

SNAKE BITES (Venomous Wounds)—Do Raindrop Technique (*the video "Essential Tips for Happy, Healthy Pets" demonstrates this technique on a dog and a horse*).

One couple had a horse that got kicked in the flank, creating a large wound. The Vet treated the wound and gave her some medication. Unfortunately, the wound became reinfected and worsened to the point that the horse almost died. The Vet came over and reopened the wound and flushed out nearly two gallons of blood clots. However, the Vet had no medication with him and would not be able to deliver any more for a couple of days. So, the wife put 15 drops of Thieves in about 1/4 cup of olive oil and while the husband held open the horse's mouth, she poured the oil down its throat. This was repeated three or four times and within just a few days, the horse was fully recovered.

ANOREXIA: Angelica, Christmas Spirt, Citrus Fresh, coriander, grapefruit, Purification, Melrose, [F]tarragon, Valor. Apply to stomach and bottom of feet. It may also help to diffuse anti-depressant oils.

****COMMENTS—Some studies have shown that people suffering from anorexia have a tendency to have lower levels of zinc.*

SUPPLEMENTS—Mineral Essence.

ANTI-DEPRESSANTS— Acceptance, basil, bergamot, Clary sage, lavender, neroli, Roman chamomile, ylang ylang.

ANTHRAX: [F]Thyme.

***Anthrax** is an infectious, fatal animal disease found in cows and sheep. It can be transmitted to human beings through contact with contaminated animal substances, such as hair, feces, or hides. It may also be used in biological warfare and is transmitted as spores through the air. It is characterized by ulcerative skin lesions.*

ANTI-BACTERIAL: [F]Basil, bergamot, cassia, Canadian Red cedar, cedarwood, citronella, Christmas Spirit, Citrus Fresh, [F]cinnamon bark, Clary sage, [F]clove, [F]cypress, eucalyptus, Evergreen Essence, fir, geranium, grapefruit, Idaho tansy, juniper, lavender, lemon, marjoram, melaleuca, *Melaleuca ericifolia*, Mountain savory, neroli, [F]oregano, palmarosa, petitgrain, pine, Purification, ravensara, RC, Roman chamomile, [F]rosemary, [F]rosewood, Sacred Mountain, [F]spearmint, tarragon, Thieves (annihilates bacteria), [F]thyme, valerian, Western Red cedar

****COMMENTS—All oils are anti-bacterial; see the "single oil property chart" in the APPENDIX of this book for additional anti-bacterial oils and their strengths*

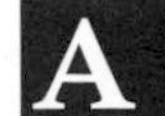

ESSENTIAL WATERS (HYDROSOLS)— Mountain Essence. Spray into air directly on area of concern, or diffuse using the Essential Mist Diffuser.

AIRBORNE—See AIRBORNE BACTERIA. Cinnamon bark, fir, Mountain savory, oregano, Purification, Thieves.

CLEANSING—Purification.

INFECTION—Nutmeg (fights).

PREVENTS GROWTH OF—Melrose.

Research at Weber State University has shown that out of 67 oils tested, 66 of them were powerful anti-bacterial agents. Oregano, cinnamon bark, Mountain savory, ravensara, and peppermint were all more powerful as anti-bacterial agents than Penicillin or Ampicillin. Thieves was shown to be 60 percent higher in activity against bacteria, germs, and anti-microbial action than either Ampicillin or Penicillin! (KID-Radio with Lance Richardson and Dr. Gary Young, N.D., Aromatologist, March 5, 1996)

NTI-CANCEROUS: Clove, frankincense, ImmuPower, ledum (may be more powerful than frankincense).

SUPPLEMENTS—Exodus, Power Meal, Sulfurzyme.

NTI-CATARRHAL: Black pepper, [F]cypress, elemi, eucalyptus, [F]fir, frankincense, ginger, [F]helichrysum (discharges mucus), hyssop (opens respiratory system and discharges toxins and mucous), jasmine, onycha (benzoin), RC, Raven, ravensara, and rosemary. Apply on lung area, feet, around nose, Vita Flex lung points, and diffuse.

****COMMENTS—See the "single oil property chart" in the APPENDIX of this book for additional anti-catarrhal oils and their strengths.*

NTI-COAGULANT: Angelica, cassia, [F]helichrysum, lavender, tangerine, tarragon. Apply on location, bottom of feet, and diffuse.

NTI-DEPRESSANT: See DEPRESSION. Elemi, [F]frankincense, lavender, onycha (combine with rose for massage). Apply to bottom of feet, heart, and diffuse.

SUPPLEMENTS—Essential Omegas

****COMMENTS—See the "single oil property chart" in the APPENDIX of this book for additional anti-depressant oils and their strengths.*

RECOVERY FROM COMMERCIAL ANTI-DEPRESSANTS LIKE PROZAC—Brain Power, Clarity, Joy, Peace & Calming, and Valor all help repair brain damage from the commercial drugs that inhibit serotonin metabolism. They also stimulate the pineal gland which normally metabolizes 50% of the serotonin in the body. The liver and pancreas are extremely toxic. Cleanse with JuvaPower, Juva Cleanse, and/or JuvaFlex. Coriander, dill and Thieves help regulate the blood sugar. Frankincense helps prevent cancer (risk of breast cancer increases by 7x with use of Paxil). Balsam fir helps to decrease the cortisol levels. Also focus on strengthening the smooth muscle tissues (especially heart and intestines) as they are contracted by the drugs.

SUPPLEMENTS—Carbozyme (to help control blood sugar levels), CortiStop (Men's or Women's), Essential Omegas, JuvaPower/JuvaSpice, Power Meal.

ANTI-FUNGAL: Abundance, [F]cinnamon bark, [F]clove, geranium, ImmuPower, juniper, lavender lemon, lemongrass, mandarin, [F]melaleuca, *Melaleuca ericifolia*, Mountain savory, [F]oregano, palmarosa, [F]rosewood, sage, [F]spearmint, [F]thyme. Apply to bottom of feet, on location, and diffuse.

****COMMENTS—See the "single oil property chart" in the APPENDIX of this book for additional anti-fungal oils and their strengths.*

BLEND—2 myrrh and 2 lavender. Rub on location.

SUPPLEMENTS—AlkaLime, Essentialzyme, ICP, ImmuGel.

ANTI-HEMORRHAGING: See HEMORRHAGING. Helichrysum, rose.

ANTI-INFECTIOUS: [F]Basil, cassia, [F]cinnamon bark, clove, [F]cypress, davana, elemi, eucalyptus hyssop, Idaho tansy, [F]lavender, marjoram, melaleuca, *Melaleuca ericifolia*, myrrh, [F]patchouli, petitgrain, [F]pine, [F]ravensara, rose, [F]rosemary, [F]rosewood, Purification, Roman chamomile, spearmint, spikenard, [F]spruce, tarragon, [F]thyme. Apply on location and bottom of feet.

****COMMENTS—See the "single oil property chart" in the APPENDIX of this book for additional anti-infectious oils and their strengths.*

SUPPLEMENTS—ImmuGel, Super C / Super C Chewable.

ANTI-INFLAMMATORY: [F]Birch, Black pepper, Blue cypress, calamus (gastrointestinal), citronella, coriander, cypress, eucalyptus, [F]German chamomile, helichrysum, hyssop (of the pulmonary), [F]lavender, lemongrass, melaleuca, [F]myrrh, onycha (benzoin), [F]patchouli, peppermint, petitgrain, ravensara, [F]Roman chamomile, spearmint, spikenard, [F]spruce, tangerine, [F]tarragon, wintergreen. Apply on location.

****COMMENTS—See the "single oil property chart" in the APPENDIX of this book for additional anti-inflammatory oils and their strengths.*

ANTI-PARASITIC: [F]Cinnamon bark, clove, Di-Tone, fennel, ginger, hyssop, lemon, lemongras melaleuca, Mountain savory, oregano, [F]Roman chamomile, rosemary, rosewoo spearmint, spikenard, tarragon. Apply to stomach, liver, intestines, and Vita Flex points on feet.

****COMMENTS—See the "single oil property chart" in the APPENDIX of this book for additional anti-parasitic oils and their strengths.*

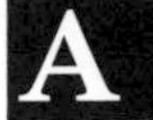

SUPPLEMENTS—Cleansing Trio (ComforTone, Essentialzyme, and ICP), ImmuneTune, ParaFree.

ANTI-RHEUMATIC: Birch, eucalyptus, juniper, onycha (benzoin), oregano, rosemary, thyme, wintergreen.

****COMMENTS—See the "single oil property chart" in the APPENDIX of this book for additional anti-rheumatic oils and their strengths.*

ANTI-SEXUAL: [F]Marjoram (helps balance sexual desires).

ANTI-TUMORAL: Clove, [F]frankincense, ImmuPower, ledum (may be more powerful than frankincense).

ANTI-VIRAL: Abundance, bergamot, [F]cinnamon bark, Clary sage, [F]clove, Cumincense (available through Creer Labs 801-465-5423), *Eucalyptus radiata*, galbanum, geranium, hyssop, Idaho tansy, ImmuPower, juniper, lavender, lemon, [F]melaleuca, melissa, Mountain savory, myrrh, [F]oregano, palmarosa, pine, RC, [F]ravensara, [F]rosewood, sandalwood, tarragon, Thieves, [F]thyme.

****COMMENTS—See the "single oil property chart" in the APPENDIX of this book for additional anti-viral oils and their strengths. Dr. J. C. Lapraz found that viruses cannot live in the presence of cinnamon oil. However, because of its high phenol content, it must be diluted before being applied to the skin.*

SUPPLEMENTS—ParaFree.

ANTIBIOTIC: Bergamot, cinnamon bark, clove, eucalyptus, frankincense, hyssop, lavender, lemon, melaleuca, Melrose, myrtle, nutmeg, oregano, patchouli, Purification, ravensara, Roman chamomile, Thieves, thyme. Apply on location, liver area, bottom of feet, and diffuse.

> *Dr. Terry Friedmann, MD would often recommend the following **Essential Oil Antibiotic Regimen**: In a "00" capsule put 12 drops of Thieves, 6 drops of oregano, and 2 drops of frankincense. Ingest one capsule every 4 hours for 3 days, then every 8 hours for 4 days.*

ANTIHISTAMINE: Lavender, Roman chamomile. Apply to sinuses, Vita Flex points, and diffuse.

ANTIMICROBIAL: Abundance, cinnamon bark, cypress, helichrysum, jasmine, lavender, lemongrass, *Melaleuca ericifolia* (powerful), melissa (shown in lab tests to be effective against *Streptococcus haemolytica*), myrrh, palmarosa, pine, rosemary, rosewood, sage, thyme.

****COMMENTS—See the "single oil property chart" in the APPENDIX of this book for additional antimicrobial oils and their strengths.*

ESSENTIAL WATERS (HYDROSOLS)—Idaho Tansy, Melissa. Spray into air directly on area of concern, or diffuse using the Essential Mist Diffuser.

SUPPLEMENTS—ImmuGel.

ANTIOXIDANTS: Cinnamon bark, Di-Tone, Exodus II, frankincense, helichrysum, hyssop, ImmuPower, JuvaFlex, melaleuca, Longevity (take as a dietary supplement to promote longevity), melaleuca, Melrose, onycha (benzoin), oregano, PanAway, Purification, ravensara, RC, Relieve It, Roman chamomile, Thieves, thyme.

> ***Antioxidants** create an unfriendly environment for free radicals. They prevent all mutations, work as free radical scavengers, prevent fungus, prevent oxidation in the cells, and help to oxygenate the cells.*

SUPPLEMENTS—ArthroTune, Berry Young Juice {a delicious blend of highly antioxidant fruit juices - measures higher on the ORAC (oxygen radical absorbent capacity) scale than even Tahitian Noni Juice}, Essentialzyme, Exodus, ImmuGel, ImmuneTune, JuvaTone, CardiaCare (with *Rhododendron caucasicum*), Longevity Capsules (highest known ORAC score), Master Formula His/Hers, Mineral Essence, Super C / Super C Chewable, Super B, VitaGreen, Wolfberry Bar (*Refer to the Wolfberry Bar in the Supplements section of the Reference Guide for Essential Oils for more information on the benefits of the Chinese Wolfberry*).

TINCTURES—AD&E

ANTISEPTIC: Bergamot, Canadian Red cedar, [F]cedarwood, cinnamon bark, citronella, clove, cumin, Di-Tone (all oils in this blend are antiseptic), elemi, eucalyptus, Evergreen Essence, fennel, [F]fir, frankincense, Idaho balsam fir, lavender, lemon, mandarin, marjoram, melaleuca, Melrose, Mountain savory, mugwort, [F]myrtle (skin), [F]nutmeg (intestinal), orange, onycha (benzoin), [F]oregano, [F]patchouli, [F]peppermint, [F]pine (pulmonary, urinary, hepatic), Purification, ravensara, Roman chamomile, rosemary cineol, rosemary verbenon, [F]sage, [F]sandalwood, [F]spearmint, [F]thyme, thyme linalol, Western Red cedar, ylang ylang. Apply on location.

ESSENTIAL WATERS (HYDROSOLS)—Eucalyptus, Western Red Cedar, Thyme. Spray directly onto area of concern.

****COMMENTS—Most oils can be used as antiseptics. See the "single oil property chart" in the APPENDIX of this book for additional antiseptic oils and their strengths.*

PERSONAL CARE—Rose Ointment (apply over oils to increase antiseptic properties and extend effectiveness).

SUPPLEMENTS—ImmuGel, Super C / Super C Chewable.
TINCTURES—AD&E.

NTISPASMODIC: Anise, [F]**basil**, calamus, citronella, cumin, fennel, [F]German chamomile, helichrysum, [F]lavender, mandarin, [F]marjoram, mugwort [F]peppermint, petitgrain, [F]Roman chamomile (relaxes spastic muscles of the colon wall), [F]rosemary, [F]sage, spearmint, spikenard, [F]spruce, tarragon, valerian, ylang ylang.

****COMMENTS—See the "single oil property chart" in the APPENDIX of this book for additional antispasmodic oils.*

NXIETY: Basil, bergamot, cedarwood, Clary sage, cypress, Evergreen Essence, frankincense, geranium, hyssop, jasmine, juniper, lavender, lemon, lime, marjoram, melissa, onycha (combine with rose for massage), patchouli, pine, Release, Roman chamomile, rose, sandalwood, Surrender, tangerine, tsuga (grounding), [F]ylang ylang.

ATHY: Frankincense, geranium, Harmony, Highest Potential, Hope, jasmine, Joy, marjoram, orange, peppermint, rose, rosemary, rosewood, sandalwood, 3 Wise Men, Transformation, thyme, Valor, White Angelica, ylang ylang.

PHRODISIAC: Cinnamon bark, Clary sage, ginger, jasmine, Lady Sclareol, patchouli, rose, [F]sandalwood, Sensation, neroli, ylang ylang.

BATH & SHOWER GELS—Sensation Bath & Shower Gel.
MASSAGE OILS—Sensation Massage Oil.
PERSONAL CARE—Sensation Hand & Body Lotion.

*Many books of aromatherapy tout the **aphrodisiac** qualities of a number of oils. Perhaps an aphrodisiac to one individual may not be to another. The most important factor is to find an oil that brings balance to the mind and body. A balanced individual is more likely to extend love.*

PNEA: Brain Power, Clarity (diffuse), Raven, RC, Valor (on feet).
SUPPLEMENTS—Super B, Thyromin, VitaGreen.
RECIPE #1—Try 3 VitaGreen twice per day, 1 Super B three times per day with meals, and 1 Thyromin before bed.

Apnea is the cessation of breathing. During sleep, periods of apnea can occur for a few seconds before breathing resumes. May be due to irregular heartbeats, high blood pressure, obesity, or damage to the area of the brain responsible for controlling respiration.

PPETITE-LOSS OF: [F]Bergamot, calamus, cardamom, ginger, hyssop, lemon, myrrh, [F]nutmeg, orange, spearmint. Apply to stomach, bottom of feet, and diffuse.
SUPPLEMENTS—ComforTone, Essentialzyme.

APPETITE SUPPRESSANT:
SUPPLEMENTS—ThermaBurn (tablets), ThermaMist (oral spray).

ARGUMENTATIVE: Acceptance, cedarwood, Chivalry, eucalyptus, frankincense, Harmony, Hope, Humility, jasmine, Joy, orange, Peace & Calming, Roman chamomile, thyme, Transformation, Trauma Life, Valor, ylang ylang.

ARMS-FLABBY: Cypress, fennel, juniper, lavender.

ARTERIAL VASODILATOR: Aroma Life, [F]marjoram. Apply to carotid arteries in neck, ov heart, Vita Flex points on feet.

ARTERIAL WALLS: Aroma Life (strengthens).

ARTERIES: (blocked after surgery), Aroma Life, lavender, Melrose.
MASSAGE OIL (body)—Cel-Lite Magic and drink Chamomile Tea.
SUPPLEMENTS—Cleansing Trio (ComforTone, Essentialzyme, and ICP).

ARTERIOSCLEROSIS: See BLOOD. Aroma Life, birch, [F]cedarwood, ginger, juniper, lemo (increase white and red blood cells), rosemary, thyme, wintergreen. Apply to heart and Vita Flex points on feet.
BLOOD CLOTS—(See BLOOD) Balsam fir, grapefruit, helichrysum.
SUPPLEMENTS—In addition to Vitamins E and C, all supplements containing essential oils should help increase the supply of oxygen in the blood stream. Rehemogen (tincture) together with JuvaTone may help build blood and hemoglobin platelets (raise cell count). ImmuneTune is good for building whi blood cells.

ARTHRITIS: See ACIDOSIS. Aroma Life, Aroma Siez, basil, birch (drains toxins that cause pain), cedarwood, clove, [F]cypress, eucalyptus, fir (has cortisone-like action), ginger, Harmony (with Valor), helichrysum, hyssop, Idaho balsam fir, Idaho tansy, ImmuPower, lavender, [F]marjoram, Melrose, nutmeg, onycha (benzoin), PanAway, Peace & Calming, peppermint, pine, Purification, Roman chamomi [F]rosemary, sage lavender, [F]spruce, Valor, white fir (has cortisone-like action), wintergreen (drains toxins that cause pain). Apply oils on location and diffuse
BLEND #1—Combine 1 oz. Ortho Ease with 25 drops birch/wintergreen, 12 cypres 9 Roman chamomile, and 3 juniper. Massage on location.
BLEND #2—Combine Ortho Ease with birch/wintergreen alone and apply on locati
BLEND #3—Birch/wintergreen with PanAway.
MASSAGE OILS—Ortho Ease.

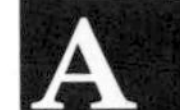

PERSONAL CARE—Prenolone/Prenolone+, Progessence, Regenolone.

SUPPLEMENTS— AlkaLime, ArthroTune, BLM, CardiaCare (with *Rhododendron caucasicum* which inhibits the enzyme hyaluronidase), Coral Sea (highly bio-available calcium, contains 58 trace minerals), Mineral Essence, Power Meal (contains wolfberry), Sulfurzyme (contains wolfberry), Super C / Super C Chewable, Super Cal, Thyromin (improves thyroid function and energy levels), VitaGreen.

ARTHRITIC PAIN—Birch, ginger, PanAway, spruce, wintergreen.

OSTEOARTHRITIS—Basil, birch, eucalyptus, lavender, lemon, marjoram, thyme, wintergreen.

Detoxify with cypress, fennel, and lemon. Massage affected joints with rosemary, chamomile, juniper and lavender (Alternative Medicine—A Definitive Guide, p. 537).

RHEUMATOID—Angelica, [F]birch, [F]bergamot, Black pepper, cajeput, cinnamon bark, coriander, [F]cypress, eucalyptus, fennel, fir, galbanum, geranium, [F]ginger, hyssop, Idaho balsam fir, juniper, lavender, [F]lemon, [F]marjoram, [F]nutmeg, oregano (chronic), PanAway, Peace & Calming, peppermint, [F]pine, Roman chamomile, rosemary, [F]spruce, tarragon, thyme, wintergreen.

PERSONAL CARE—Prenolone/Prenolone+, Progessence, Regenolone.

BLEND #4—Combine 2 oz. of Ortho Ease with 7 drops birch/wintergreen, 6 ginger, 19 eucalyptus, 6 juniper, 8 marjoram, and 3 peppermint. Rub on location.

SHAMED: See EMOTIONS. Acceptance, Forgiveness, Valor.

SSAULT: See EMOTIONS. Trauma Life.

SSIMILATING FOOD:

SUPPLEMENTS—Enzyme products: Allerzyme (aids the digestion of sugars, starches, fats, and proteins), Carbozyme (aids in the digestion of carbohydrates), Detoxzyme (helps maintain and support a healthy intestinal environment), Essentialzyme, Fiberzyme (aids the digestion of fiber and enhances the absorption of nutrients), Lipozyme (aids the digestion of fats) Polyzyme (aids the digestion of protein and helps reduce swelling and discomfort). Also Power Meal (pre-digested protein) and Super B.

STHMA: See RESPIRATORY SYSTEM. Cajeput, calamus, Clary sage, cypress, [F]eucalyptus, Evergreen Essence, fir, [F]frankincense (on crown), hyssop, laurel, lavender, [F]lemon, [F]marjoram, myrrh, myrtle, onycha (benzoin), [F]oregano, [F]peppermint, [F]pine, Raven (diffuse), ravensara, RC (some people use RC or Raven instead of inhaler), rose, rosemary, [F]sage, sage lavender, [F]thyme, tsuga (opens respiratory tract). Avoid steam inhalation. Apply topically over lungs and throat. Drop on pillow or diffuse. May insert RC and Raven with 1 tsp. V-6 Mixing Oil in rectum, OR Raven rectally with RC on chest and back; reverse each night.

BLEND #1—Combine 10 drops cedarwood, 10 eucalyptus, 2 Roman chamomile, ar 2 oz. water. Put on hanky and inhale. Can also be used to gargle.

BLEND #2—Combine 10 drops Raven, 5 hyssop, and 2 tsp. V-6 Mixing Oil. Massage on spine and chest.

PERSONAL CARE—Prenolone/Prenolone+.

SUPPLEMENTS—ImmuneTune (drainage), Super C / Super C Chewable, Thyromi

****COMMENTS—Do a colon and liver cleanse with either the MASTER CLEANSER (se CLEANSING) or the Cleansing Trio supplements (ComforTone, ICP, Essentialzyme) and JuvaTone.*

ATTACK—RC or Raven. Just smelling from bottle has stopped attacks.

RECIPE #1—3 Wise Men on crown, Raven on throat, RC on lungs, Thieves on fee ImmuPower on spine. May insert RC and Raven with V-6 Mixing Oil in rectum, OR Raven rectally with RC on chest and back; reverse each night.

RECIPE #2—Inhale or diffuse bergamot, eucalyptus, hyssop, lavender, or marjorar Try frankincense for calming. (Alternative Medicine—The Definitive Guide, p 824).

RECIPE #3—Apply frankincense to the crown, RC on the throat and chest and Rav on the back. Then, inhale the aroma of the oils from your hands.

ASTRINGENT: Lemon, onycha (benzoin).

ATHLETES FOOT: Cajeput, cypress, *Eucalyptus citriodora*, geranium, lavender, [F]melaleuca, myrrh, thyme.

BLEND—Combine 2 oz. of Genesis Hand & Body Lotion with 10 drops thyme, 10 lavender, and 10 melaleuca. Rub on feet.

ATTENTION DEFICIT DISORDER (ADD): See HYPERACTIVITY. Ledum.

BLEND—Lavender with basil (on crown), Harmony, or Peace & Calming; Basil wit Clarity; Frankincense with Valor. Apply 1-3 drops of any of these blends on t bottom of the feet and on the spine; diffuse.

MASSAGE, BATH, DIFFUSE—Citrus Fresh, lavender.

SUPPLEMENTS—Allerzyme (aids the digestion of sugars, starches, fats, and protiens), Chelex, Essential Omegas (absolutely necessary), Mineral Essence.

CHELATING AGENT—Helichrysum.

SLEEPING—Diffuse either Peace & Calming or Gentle Baby.

****COMMENTS—Avoid sweeteners such as sugar and corn syrup. Eliminate caffeine a food additives from diet. Individuals who have ADD often have high aluminum toxicity. Chelex may help remove aluminum from the body.*

AURA: Awaken, Joy, Sacred Mountain, White Angelica.
INCREASE AURA AROUND BODY—White Angelica (use with Awaken and Sacred Mountain).
PROTECTION OF—White Angelica.
STRENGTHEN—White Angelica.

AUTISM:
REDUCE ANXIETY/FEAR—Bergamot, geranium, and Clary sage. Layer or dilute in V-6 Mixing Oil for a massage.
STIMULATE THE SENSES—Basil, lemon, peppermint, and rosemary. Layer or dilute in V-6 Mixing Oil for a massage.
****COMMENTS—Make sure that no negativity exists when the oils are used because the autistic child will make those associations when the oil is used again.*

AUTO-IMMUNE SYSTEM: For diseases, see GRAVES DISEASE, HASHIMOTO'S DISEASE, and LUPUS. Cistus, ImmuPower.
SUPPLEMENTS—ImmuPro, Sulfurzyme (helps mitigate effects of autoimmune diseases), Thyromin, VitaGreen.

AVOIDANCE: See EMOTIONS. Magnify Your Calling, Motivation.

AWAKE:
JET LAG—Eucalyptus, geranium, grapefruit, lavender, lemongrass, peppermint.
STAYING AWAKE WHILE DRIVING—Clarity and En-R-Gee together.

AWAKEN THE MIND, SPIRIT: Awaken, myrrh.

AWAKEN THE PAST: Cypress.

AWARENESS:
GREATER AWARENESS OF ONES POTENTIAL—Believe, Into the Future, White Angelica.
INCREASES SENSORY SYSTEM—Awaken, birch, wintergreen.
OPENS SENSORY SYSTEM—Birch, peppermint, wintergreen.
REVITALIZES—Lemongrass.
SELF—Acceptance, Believe.
SPIRITUAL—Believe, Frankincense, Inspiration (enhances spiritual mood), myrrh, 3 Wise Men.

BABIES/CHILDREN:

FORMULA—Bodygize. Mix 1/3 scoop in 10 oz. distilled water or Rice Dream.

PERSONAL CARE— KidScents Bath Gel, KidScents Lotion, KidScents Shampoo, KidScents Tender Tush, KidScents Toothpaste, Rose Ointment.

SUPPLEMENTS—KidScents Mighty Mist (vitamin spray), KidScents Mighty Vites (chewable tablets), KidScents MightyZyme (chewable enzymes).

BONDING—Gentle Baby (one drop gently rubbed on baby's feet and another drop or two brushed over mom's hair and aura–open palms skimming body surface, head to foot).

COLIC—[F]Bergamot, ginger, mandarin, [F]marjoram, Roman chamomile, rosemary, or ylang ylang.

BLEND #1—Combine 2 Tbs. Almond oil with 1 drop Roman chamomile, 1 drop lavender, and 1 drop geranium. Mix and apply to stomach and back.

****COMMENTS—Burping the baby, and keeping the abdomen warm with a warm water bottle will often bring relief.*

COMMON COLD—Cedarwood, lemon, *Melaleuca ericifolia*, rosemary, rose, sandalwood or thyme.

BLEND #2—Combine 2 Tbs. V-6 Mixing Oil with 2 drops melaleuca (Tea Tree), 1 lemon, and 1 rose otto. Massage a little of the blend on neck and chest.

CONSTIPATION—Ginger, mandarin, orange, or rosemary. Dilute one of the oils and massage stomach and feet.

CRADLE CAP REMEDY—

BLEND #3—Combine 2 Tbs. Almond oil with 1 drop lemon and 1 geranium or with drop cedarwood and 1 sandalwood. Mix and apply a small amount on head.

CROUP—Marjoram, ravensara, rosewood, sandalwood, or thyme. Dilute for massage; diffuse. Bundle the baby up and take outside to breathe cold air.

CRYING—Cypress, frankincense, geranium, lavender, Roman chamomile, rose otto, or ylang ylang. Dilute for massage or diffuse.

DIAPER RASH—Lavender (dilute and apply).

BLEND #4—Combine 1 drop Roman chamomile and 1 lavender with V-6 Mixing Oil or Genesis Hand & Body Lotion. Apply.

PERSONAL CARE—KidScents Tender Tush (formulated specifically for diaper rash), Rose Ointment.

DIGESTION (sluggish)—Lemon or orange. Dilute and massage feet and stomach.

DRY SKIN—Rosewood or sandalwood. Dilute and apply.

EARACHE—Lavender, melaleuca (Tea Tree), *Melaleuca ericifolia*, Roman chamomile, or thyme (sweet). Put a diluted drop of oil on a cotton ball and place in the ear; rub a little bit of diluted oil behind the ear.

BLEND #5—Combine 2 Tbs. V-6 Mixing Oil with 2 drops lavender, 1 Roman chamomile, and 1 melaleuca (Tea Tree). Put a drop on a cotton ball and put in ear, rub behind the ear and on the ear Vita Flex feet points.

OTHER—Garlic oil works great too, but it is stinky!

FEVER—Lavender. Dilute in V-6 Mixing Oil and massage baby (back of neck, feet, behind ears, etc.). Peppermint (diffuse only).

FLU—Cypress, lemon, *Melaleuca ericifolia*. Dilute 1 drop of each in 1 Tbs. Bath Gel Base for a bath; diffuse.

HICCOUGHS—Mandarin. Diffuse.

JAUNDICE—Geranium, lemon, lime, mandarin, or rosemary. Dilute and apply on the liver area and on the liver Vita Flex feet points.

PREMATURE—Since premature babies have very thin and sensitive skin, it is best to avoid the use of essential oils.

RASHES—Lavender, Roman chamomile, rose otto, or sandalwood. Dilute and apply.

TEETH GRINDING—Lavender (rub on feet), Peace & Calming (on feet or diffuse).

TEETHING—German chamomile, ginger, lavender, marjoram, or melaleuca (Tea Tree). Dilute and apply.

TONSILLITIS—Ginger, lavender, lemon, or melaleuca (Tea

*When using essential oils on babies and children, it is **always** best to **dilute 1-2 drops of pure essential oil with ½-1 tsp. V-6 Mixing Oil**. If the oils are used in the bath, always use a bath gel base as a dispersing agent for the oils.*

***Keep the oils out of children's reach.** If an oil is ever ingested, give the child an oil-soluble liquid such as milk, cream, or half & half. Then call your local poison control center or seek emergency medical attention. A few drops of pure essential oil shouldn't be life-threatening, but for your protection, it is best to take these precautions.*

*In Shirley Price's book, Aromatherapy for Babies and Children, she mentions **twenty oils that are safe for children**. Nineteen of them are oils with the same botanical names as those mentioned in this book. These oils are:*

Bergamot (Citrus bergamia)*
Cedarwood (Cedrus atlantica)**
Chamomile, Roman (Chamaemelum nobile),
Cypress (Cupressus sempervirens)
Frankincense (Boswellia carteri)
Geranium (Pelargonium graveolens)
Ginger (Zingiber officinale)
Lavender (Lavandula angustifolia)
Lemon (Citrus limon)*
Mandarin (Citrus reticulata)*
Marjoram (Origanum majorana)
Melaleuca-Tea Tree (Melaleuca alternifolia)
Orange (Citrus aurantium)*
Rose Otto (Rosa damascena)
Rosemary (Rosmarinus officinalis)**
Rosewood (Aniba rosaeodora)
Sandalwood (Santalum album)
Thyme (Thymus vulgaris CT linalol)
Ylang Ylang (Cananga odorata)

**These oils are photosensitive; always dilute. To prevent a rash or pigmentation of the skin, do not use citrus oils when exposed to direct sunlight.*

***These oils should never be used undiluted on babies and children.*

***Caution:** Do not use synthetic or adulterated oils. Do not use oils with different botanical names until the safety data has been thoroughly reviewed.*

Tree), Roman chamomile. Dilute and apply.

THRUSH—Geranium, lavender, lemon, melaleuca (Tea Tree), *Melaleuca ericifolia*, rosewood, or thyme. Dilute and apply.

BLEND—2 Tbsp. garlic oil, 8 drops lavender, 8 drops *Melaleuca ericifolia*, 1 ml. (1 softgel) Vitamin E oil. Apply to nipples just before nursing, or with a clean finger into baby's mouth. Also try Animal Scents Pet Ointment.

****COMMENTS—Besides Gentle Baby listed under bonding, no other commercial blend are listed in this section because many of them contain oils that are not recommended for babies. The author's admit, however, that they have used many of the commercial blends mentioned in this book on their babies and children with great success and no side effects. We are careful, however, to use only a couple drops at a time, diluted in V-6 Mixing Oil, and only for external application. Also, we do not continue applications for any extended period of time.*

BACK: Basil, birch, Black pepper, cypress, EndoFlex, eucalyptus, geranium, ginger, juniper, lavender, oregano, peppermint, PanAway, Relieve It, Roman chamomile, rosemary, sage, tangerine, thyme (for virus in spine), Valor (aligns; a chiropractor in a bottle), wintergreen.

I was about 8 1/2 hours into a 10 hour roundtrip drive and my back started to seize up. I have an old muscle injury and I knew I was in trouble. I had my oils on the seat next to me and grabbed my PanAway at a stoplight and poured it in my hand. I was in a hurry. I had planned on putting on about 5 drops, but the oil was warm and I think I ended up with about 20 in my hand. Rather than waste it, I put it all on my lower back and sat back in my seat. Within a few minutes my spine did a complete correction starting at the base and going up to the back of my head. I felt each click as it ran up my spine. Needless to say, my back no longer hurt and I had no stiffness when I finally got out of the car!

-Submitted by Andrea Safford
Warrenton, Virginia (July 2004)

SUPPLEMENTS—BLM

CALCIFIED (spine)—Geranium, PanAway, rosemary.

MASSAGE OILS—Ortho Ease and PanAway (on spine).

DETERIORATING DISCS—Do RAINDROP THERAPY with just the application of the oils, none of the working along the spine.

HERNIATED DISCS—Cypress (strengthens blood capillary walls, improves circulation, powerful anti-inflammatory), PanAway, Relieve It, (massage up disc area three times to help with pain), pepper, peppermint (a compress is good too). Valor (: drops) on location may help relieve pressure. Do RAINDROP THERAPY wit just the application of the oils, none of the working along the spine.

MASSAGE OILS—Ortho Ease.

SUPPLEMENTS—BLM, Super C / Super C Chewable.

LOW BACK PAINS—

RECIPE #1—Rub Valor on top and bottom of feet, Di-Tone on colon, Ortho Ease up the back. Massage cypress up the disc area three times. Cypress strengthens blood capillary walls, improves circulation, and is a powerful anti-inflammatory. Use helichrysum to increase circulation, decongest, and to reduce inflammation and pain. Use peppermint to stimulate the nerves (may need to dilute with Ortho Ease). Layer basil, Aroma Siez, Relieve It, and spruce.

SUPPLEMENTS—BLM

MUSCULAR FATIGUE—Clary sage, lavender, marjoram, rosemary.

PAIN—

BLEND #1—5 to 10 drops each rosemary, marjoram, sage **OR**

BLEND #2—5 to 10 drops each of lavender, eucalyptus, ginger **OR**

BLEND #3—5 to 10 drops each of peppermint, rosemary, basil.

RECIPE #2—Apply PanAway and Valor on the shoulders. If the individual being worked on is laying on their stomach, the person applying the oils to the shoulders should cross their arms so the electrical frequency is not broken (right to right etc.). Apply the following oils **up** the spine, one at a time, using a probe on each vertebra if possible, stroke with fingers, feathering gently in 4" strokes three times for each oil: Peppermint (excites the back), cypress (anti-inflammatory), Aroma Siez, Relieve It, and spruce. Follow the procedure with a hot compress. The blends above have also been used with success. Follow the same stroking procedure and dilute the blends with a little V-6 Mixing Oil for a massage.

SUPPLEMENTS—ArthroTune, BLM.

ACTERIA: See ANTI-BACTERIAL.

ALANCE: Acceptance, Aroma Siez, Awaken, cedarwood, frankincense (balances electrical field), Harmony, Mister, Roman chamomile, Valor, ylang ylang.

BALANCE MALE/FEMALE ENERGIES—Acceptance, ylang ylang.

CHAKRAS—Harmony, Valor.

EMOTIONAL—Envision.

ELECTRICAL ENERGIES—Frankincense, Harmony, Valor. Start by applying 3-6 drops Valor on the bottom of each foot. Some may be applied to the neck and shoulders if desired. When working on someone else, place the palms of the hands on the bottom of each foot (left hand to left foot and right hand to right foot) and hold for 5 to 15 minutes. If working on yourself, perform the Cook's Hookup by lifting the right foot and placing the right ankle on top of the left knee in cross-legged fashion. Next place the left hand on the right ankle and cup the front of the ankle with the fingers. Then cross the right hand over the left and with the right hand grasp the heel of the right foot (with thumb around the back and fingers cupping the bottom of the heel). Hold this for 5 to 15 minutes.

The balancing of the electrical energies can be felt by either a pulse in the han and feet or a warming sensation.

FEELING OF—Envision, spruce.

HARMONIC BALANCE TO ENERGY CENTER—Acceptance, Harmony.

SUPPLEMENTS—Bodygize, Master Formula His/Hers.

BALDNESS: See HAIR. Cedarwood, lavender, rosemary, sage. Apply 2-3 drops of each oil c location and on bottom of feet before bedtime and/or in the morning after washing with Lavender Volume products shown below.

PERSONAL CARE—Lavender Volume Shampoo and Lavender Volume Conditione together.

SUPPLEMENTS—Sulfurzyme may help if the hair is falling due to a sulfur deficiency.

BATH: While tub is filling, add oils to the water; oils will be drawn to your skin quickly from t top of the water, so use gentle oils like: Lavender, Roman chamomile, rosewoc sage, ylang ylang, etc. For the most benefit, add 5-10 drops of your favorite essential oil to one-half ounce Bath and Shower Gel Base.

BATH & SHOWER GELS—Evening Peace, Relaxation, and Sensation Bath and Shower Gels as well as Lavender Rosewood, Sacred Mountain, and Peppermi Cedarwood Moisturizing Soaps are all wonderfully soothing in the evening. Morning Start Bath and Shower Gel as well as Lemon Sandalwood and Thiev Cleansing Soaps are all terrific ways to jump-start your day.

AQUA ESSENCE BATH PACKS—Finally, some of the most popular essential oil blends have been combined with the latest hydro-diffusion technology to create the perfect solution for adding oils to your bath water. Just place a packet in t tub while hot water is being added and the oils are perfectly dispersed into the water. The packets contain 10 ml of oil and are reusable. Packets can be ordered with either Joy, Valor, Peace & Calming, or Sacred Mountain.

BED WETTING: See BLADDER. Before bedtime, rub the abdomen with a couple drops of cypress mixed with V-6 Mixing Oil.

BELCHING: Di-Tone. Apply to stomach and on Vita Flex points.

BEREAVEMENT: Basil, cypress.

BETRAYED (Feeling): See EMOTIONS. Acceptance, Forgiveness, Transformation, Valor.

BIRTHING: See PREGNANCY.

ITES: See also INSECT. Basil, cinnamon bark, garlic, lavender, lemon, sage, thyme (all have antitoxic and anti-venomous properties).

ALLERGIC—Purification.

BEES AND HORNETS—Remove the stinger, apply a cold compress of Roman chamomile to area for several hours or as long as possible. Then, apply 1 drop of Roman chamomile three times a day for two days. Idaho tansy may also work.

GNATS AND MIDGES—Lavender, or 3 drops thyme in 1 tsp. cider vinegar or lemon juice. Apply to bites to stop irritation.

INSECT—Cajeput, patchouli.

MOSQUITO—Helichrysum, lavender.

SNAKE—Basil, patchouli.

SPIDERS, BROWN RECLUSE, BEE STINGS, ANTS, FIRE ANTS—**Basil** (neutralizes), cinnamon bark, lavender, lemon, lemongrass, peppermint, Purification, thyme.

SPIDERS—3 drops lavender and 2 drops Roman chamomile in 1 tsp. alcohol. Mix well in clockwise motion and apply to area three times a day.

TICKS—After getting the tick out, apply 1 drop lavender every 5 minutes for 30 minutes. How to remove:

- Do not apply mineral oil, Vaseline, or anything else to remove the tick as this may cause it to inject the spirochetes into the wound.
- Be sure to remove the entire tick. Get as close to the mouth as possible and firmly tug on the tick until it releases its grip. Don't twist. If available, use a magnifying glass to make sure that you have removed the entire tick.
- Save the tick in a jar and label it with the date, where you were bitten on your body, and the location or address where you were bitten for proper identification by your doctor, especially if you develop any symptoms.
- Do not handle the tick.
- Wash hands immediately.
- Check the site of the bite occasionally to see if any rash develops. If it does, seek medical advice promptly.

WASPS (are alkaline)—1 drop basil, 2 Roman chamomile, 2 lavender, and 1 tsp. cider vinegar. Mix in clockwise motion and put on area three times a day.

ITTERNESS: See EMOTIONS. Acceptance, Forgiveness, Roman chamomile, Valor.

LADDER: Apply EndoFlex over kidneys as a hot compress.

BED WETTING AND INCONTINENCE—Before bed rub cypress on abdomen.

TINCTURES—Take K&B morning, noon, and night.

INFECTION—See CYSTITIS. Cedarwood, Inspiration, onycha (benzoin), and sandalwood (for 1st stages of bladder infection), [F]lemongrass, or 1 drop Thieves in 8 oz. juice or water and drink three times a day.

SUPPLEMENTS—ImmuGel, K&B.

****COMMENTS—One individual who had bladder infection took 1 tsp. ImmuGel every two hours. They were over the infection in two days.*

HANGING DOWN—Valor on feet, 3 drops ravensara and 1 drop lavender on calves, (bladder should pull up).

BLAME: See EMOTIONS. Acceptance, Forgiveness, Valor.

BLISTER: (on lips from sun): Lavender (Apply as often as needed. It should take fever out and return lip to normal).

BLOATING: Di-Tone. Apply to stomach, Vita Flex points, and diffuse.

SUPPLEMENTS—ComforTone.

BLOCKED (Emotionally): See EMOTIONS.

BLOOD: Red blood cells carry oxygen throughout the body.

BLOOD TYPES—Different blood types have different dominating glands.

TYPE A: more prone to be alkaline pH balanced. Natural vegetarians. Type A child living in a home of type O parent is affected by parents' programing or conditioning or visa versa. They have problems with their thyroid, may have tendency to gain weight, and need exercise.

TYPE AB: may want to be a vegetarian some days, but not on others. Can go either way like A or O types. They may be affected by either the A or O parent. AB types haven't decided whether to be an A or B type. They may even need more protein than O types.

TYPE B: down the middle, more balanced. Takes them about 3 years to convert to being a vegetarian.

TYPE O: more prone to acidic condition in blood. AlkaLime is an acid-neutralizing mineral formulation and may help preserve the body's proper pH balance. Big eaters and may need to take more supplements because they are not assimilating the nutrients. If they are not assimilating their food, they eat and get full quick and one hour later they are hungry again. They get more gas because they lack enzyme secretion. They may need ESSENTIALZYME for the enzymes. They eat more, digest less, but don't gain weight. May take 8 years to totally convert to vegetarian diet. Need more protein; BODYGIZE, VITAGREEN and POWER MEAL are mainstays for O types as they are high protein and high energy formulas; nuts and seeds are good too. Nutrients in purest form reduces the need to eat. They have a harder time structuring their diet and they get cold because of poor circulation. If an O type is slender, has high energy, is compulsive in behavior, and/or is a hard worker, they may need as many as 16 VitaGreen and 10 Master Formula His/Hers per day.

BLOOD PRESSURE—

HIGH (hypertension)—Aroma Life, Fbirch, Clary sage, clove, goldenrod, Flavender, lemon, Fmarjoram (regulates), nutmeg, Fspearmint, wintergreen, Fylang ylang (arterial; put in hand, rub palms together, cup over nose, and breathe deeply for 5 minutes and/or put on feet). Place oils on heart points on left arm, hand, foot, and over heart. Can also smell from palms of hands, diffuse, or place a few drops on a cotton ball and put in a vent.

****COMMENTS—Refer to The chapter entitled "How to Use - The Personal Usage Reference" in the Essential Oils Desk Reference under "Blood Pressure, High" for specific product recommendations.*

> ***OILS TO AVOID IF HYPERTENSIVE***
>
> ***Single oils:*** *Hyssop, rosemary, sage, thyme, and possibly peppermint.*
>
> **This list is a compilation of the safety data contained in aromatherapy books written by the following authors: Ann Berwick, Julia Lawless, Shirley & Len Price, Jeanne Rose, Robert Tisserand, and Tony Balacs.*

BATH—3 ylang ylang and 3 marjoram in bath water. Bathe in the evening twice a week.

BLEND #1—5 geranium, 8 lemongrass, 3 lavender, and 1 oz. V-6 Mixing Oil. Rub over heart and heart Vita Flex points on left foot and hand.

BLEND #2—10 ylang ylang, 5 marjoram, 5 cypress, and 1 oz. V-6 Mixing Oil. Rub over heart and heart Vita Flex points on left foot and hand.

TINCTURES—HRT (1-2 droppers two to three times per day).

LOW—Aroma Life, hyssop (raises), pine, Frosemary, ylang ylang.

SUPPLEMENTS—CardiaCare (with *Rhododendron caucasicum* which helps to normalize blood pressure).

BLOOD PROTEIN—Bodygize, VitaGreen.

BLEEDING (STOPS)—Aroma Life, cistus, geranium (will increase bleeding first to eliminate toxins, then stop it), helichrysum, onycha (benzoin), Cayenne pepper, rose.

BROKEN BLOOD VESSELS—Grapefruit, helichrysum.

****COMMENTS—One woman had some blood vessels break in her brain which effected her short-term memory, concentration, focus, and emotions. She used the oils of Clarity, basil, rosemary, peppermint, and cardamom. Not only did her blood vessels heal, but her concentration, awareness, focus, and self-esteem increased.*

BUILD—Rehemogen (tincture) together with JuvaTone and Juva Cleanse may help build blood and hemoglobin platelets (raise cell count). ImmuneTune is good for building white blood cells.

CHOLESTEROL—Helichrysum (regulates).

CLEANSING—[F]Helichrysum, Juva Cleanse, Roman chamomile. Apply on bottom of fee

SUPPLEMENTS—VitaGreen.

TINCTURES—Rehemogen (purifier).

CLOTS—Balsam fir (reduces pressure), grapefruit, helichrysum (anti-coagulant). Balsar fir, helichrysum, and cistus together (both topically and internally 3-4 times p day) help to dissolve blood clots.

HEMORRHAGING—See FEMALE PROBLEMS. Cistus, helichrysum, rose, Cayenne pepper.

LOW BLOOD SUGAR—Cinnamon bark, clove, Thieves (balances blood sugar), thyme.

SUPPLEMENTS—AlkaLime, VitaGreen (balances blood sugar), Mineral Essence.

TINCTURES—Sugar-Up (balances blood sugar; available through Creer Labs 801-465-5423).

STIMULATES—[F]Lemon (helps with the formation of red and white blood cells).

VESSELS—Aroma Life, cypress (strengthens the capillary walls, and increases circulatic lemongrass (vasodilator).

SUPPLEMENTS—Cel-Lite Magic dilates blood vessels for better circulation.

BODY SYSTEMS:

CARDIOVASCULAR SYSTEM: See CARDIOVASCULAR SYSTEM. Aroma Life, clove, cypress, goldenrod, helichrysum, marjoram, onycha (benzoin), rosemar tsuga (opens and dilates for better oxygen exchange), ylang ylang.

SUPPLEMENTS—CardiaCare (contains ingredients that have been scientifically tested for their abilities to support and strengthen the cardiovascular system), Coral Sea (highly bio-available calcium, contains 58 trace minerals), ICP, Mineral Essence, Super B, Super Cal.

TINCTURE—HRT.

DIGESTIVE SYSTEM: See DIGESTIVE SYSTEM. Clove, Di-Tone (acid stomach; aid secretion of digestive enzymes), [F]fennel (sluggish), ginger, laurel, myrtle, [F]peppermint, rosemary, spearmint, tarragon (nervous and sluggish). Add the oil(s) to your food, rub on stomach, or apply as a compress over abdomen.

SUPPLEMENTS—Essential Manna, Essentialzyme (digestive enzymes; take before meals for acid stomach), ParaFree, Royaldophilus, Stevia Select.

EMOTIONAL BALANCE: See EMOTIONS. Australian Blue, Forgiveness, frankincens geranium, Grounding, Harmony, Hope, Idaho balsam fir, Inner Child, Joy, juniper, lavender, onycha (combine with rose for massage), orange, Present Time, Release, Roman chamomile, sage lavender, sandalwood, SARA, 3 Wise Men, Transformation, Trauma Life, Valor, vetiver, White Angelica.

HORMONAL SYSTEM: See HORMONAL SYSTEM. Clary sage, EndoFlex, fennel, goldenrod, Mister, myrrh, myrtle, peppermint, sage, sage lavender, ylang ylang The most common places to apply oils for hormonal balance are the Vita Flex points on ankles, lower back, thyroid, liver, kidneys, gland areas, the center of the body and along both sides of the spine, and the clavicle area. Diffusing them may also help.

MASSAGE OILS—Dragon Time.

PERSONAL CARE—Prenolone/Prenolone+, Progessence.

SUPPLEMENTS—CortiStop (Men's and Women's), FemiGen (female), ProGen (male), Thyromin, Ultra Young+.

TINCTURES—Estro.

IMMUNE SYSTEM: See IMMUNE SYSTEM. Clove, Exodus II, frankincense, ImmuPower, ledum (supports), lemon, Mountain savory, rosemary (supports), Thieves (enhances; massage on feet and body), thyme (supports immunological functions).

SUPPLEMENTS—Essential Manna, Exodus, ImmuneTune, ImmuPro, Super B, Super C / Super C Chewable, Ultra Young (may help raise levels of cytokines, interleukin 1 & 2, and tumor necrosis factor).

MUSCLES and BONES: See individual listings for BONES and MUSCLES. Aroma Siez, basil, birch, cypress, Idaho balsam fir, lavender, lemongrass, marjoram, oregano, peppermint, sage lavender, thyme, Valor, wintergreen.

MASSAGE OILS—Ortho Ease or Ortho Sport Massage Oils.

SUPPLEMENTS—Be-Fit, BLM, Coral Sea (highly bio-available calcium, contains 58 trace minerals), Essential Manna, Mineral Essence, Power Meal, Sulfurzyme, Super C Chewable, Super Cal, WheyFit.

NERVOUS SYSTEM: See NERVOUS SYSTEM. Brain Power, cedarwood (nervous tension), ginger, Idaho balsam fir, lavender, Peace & Calming, **peppermint** (soothes and strengthens), rosemary, sage lavender, vetiver.

PERSONAL CARE—NeuroGen, Regenolone (nerve regeneration).

SUPPLEMENTS—Mineral Essence, Sulfurzyme, Super B.

RESPIRATORY SYSTEM: See RESPIRATORY SYSTEM. [F]Eucalyptus (general stimulant and strengthens), *Eucalyptus radiata*, ledum (supports), melaleuca, [F]myrtle, [F]peppermint (aids), pine (dilates and opens bronchial tract), RC, Raven (all respiratory problems), ravensara, rosemary verbenon, sage lavender, tsuga (dilates and opens respiratory tract).

ESSENTIAL WATERS (HYDROSOLS)—Canadian Red Cedar (supportive), Eucalyptus (calming), Mountain Essence (enhances respiratory action). Spray into air, onto chest, or diffuse using the Essential Mist Diffuser.

SUPPLEMENTS—ImmuGel, Super C / Super C Chewable.

SKIN: See SKIN. Frankincense, Gentle Baby (youthful skin), geranium, German chamomile (inflamed skin), lavender, ledum (all types of problems), Melrose, myrrh (chapped and cracked), onycha (chapped and cracked), patchouli (chapped; tightens loose skin and prevents wrinkles), rosewood (elasticity and candida), sage lavender, Valor, vetiver, Western Red cedar.

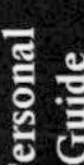

BAR SOAPS—Lavender Rosewood Moisturizing Soap, Lemon Sandalwood Cleans Soap, Peppermint Cedarwood Moisturizing Soap, Sacred Mountain Moisturizing Soap for oily skin, Thieves Cleansing Soap.

PERSONAL CARE—AromaGuard Deodorants, Boswellia Wrinkle Creme, ClaraDerm, Genesis Hand & Body Lotion (hydrates, heals, and nurtures the skin), Satin Facial Scrub - Mint (eliminates layers of dead skin cells and slow down premature aging of the skin), Orange Blossom Facial Wash combined with Sandalwood Toner and Sandalwood Moisture Creme (cleans, tones, and moisturizes dry or prematurely aging skin), Prenolone , Progessence, Regenolone (helps moisturize and regenerate tissues), Rose Ointment (for ski conditions and chapped skin), Satin Hand & Body Lotion (moisturizes skin leaving it feeling soft, silky, and smooth).

SUPPLEMENTS FOR SKIN—Sulfurzyme.

TINCTURES—AD&E.

BALANCING—Harmony, Joy, lavender, spruce, Valor.

CONTROLLING—Cedarwood.

ODORS—Purification (obnoxious odors), sage.

STRENGTHEN VITAL CENTERS—Oregano.

SUPPORT—Fir, ledum, Valor.

BOILS: Bergamot, Clary sage, frankincense, galbanum, Gentle Baby, lavender, lemon, lemongrass, melaleuca, Melrose, Purification, Raven, ravensara, RC, Roman chamomile.

PERSONAL CARE—Rose Ointment.

I have suffered large boils on the tops of my legs for abou 30 years and nobody could help me get rid of them. Last fall I counted 12 boils. I started using Lavender and did the Master Cleanser, lemonade cleanse. On the third day, my boils opened and ran freely. This was in January of this year. Now I only occasionally get them and they are many times smaller than before. I know if I continue the regimen, they will eventually leave altogether.

-Submitted by K. Ernst (July 2004

****COMMENTS—One individual put lemon oil on a sore that looked like a boil. The n day it turned black, puss came out and it got smaller and finally disappeare*

BONDING: See EMOTIONS. Gentle Baby.

****COMMENTS—Use Release or other oils listed under Emotional Release in the Scie and Application section of the Reference Guide for Essential Oils to help release emotional connections to one who has passed on. Also, to help children create good bonds with others, tell them about the person when working with the oils.*

BONES: All the tree oils, **birch**, cedarwood, cypress, fir, juniper, lavender, lemongrass, marjoram, PanAway (bone pain), peppermint, Relieve It, sandalwood, spruce, wintergreen.

SUPPLEMENTS—Be-Fit, BLM, Coral Sea (highly bio-available calcium, contains 58 trace minerals), Essential Manna, Mineral Essence, Power Meal, Sulfurzyme, Super Cal.

BONE SPURS—Birch/wintergreen, cypress, marjoram, RC (dissolves). Rub on location.

One lady had a heel spur flare up one evening, so she took a bath with birch and cypress before retiring. The next morning, the pain was a little better. She then put 6 drops birch, 6 drops cypress, and on top of that, 5 drops RC on a cotton pad and applied it to her heel. In 10 minutes all pain was gone and even after four days, the pain had not returned.

BROKEN HEAL—Birch/wintergreen and cypress (before bed), helichrysum, oregano and Valor (in morning).

BLEND—9 drops birch/wintergreen, 8 drops each of spruce, White fir, and helichrysum, 7 drops clove (good when inflammation is causing the pain).

MASSAGE OILS—3 droppers full of Ortho Ease mixed with lavender, lemongrass, and PanAway. Ortho Sport with juniper, lemongrass, and marjoram (apply over broken bones).

SUPPLEMENTS—BLM or 4 Super Cal and 14 ArthroTune for three weeks, then cut in half.

BRUISED—Helichrysum, Relieve It, and PanAway.

CARTILAGE—Sandalwood (regenerates), White fir (pain from inflammation).

DEGENERATION—Ortho Ease then peppermint.

SUPPLEMENTS—Super C / Super C Chewable.

DEVELOPMENT—

SUPPLEMENTS—Super C / Super C Chewable, Ultra Young (may help boost bone formation).

PAIN—**Birch**, PanAway, White fir, wintergreen.

ROTATOR CUFF (Sore)—See SHOULDER. **Birch/wintergreen** (bone), lemongrass (torn or pulled ligaments), PanAway, peppermint (nerves), Relieve It, spruce, White fir (inflammation).

BOREDOM: Awaken, Believe, cedarwood, cypress, Dream Catcher, fir, frankincense, Gathering, juniper, lavender, Motivation, pepper, Roman chamomile, rosemary, sandalwood, spruce, thyme, Valor, ylang ylang.

BOWEL:

IRRITABLE BOWEL SYNDROME—Di-Tone and peppermint. Take 2 drops of each in distilled water 1-2 times per day. Idaho tansy and Juva Cleanse (can also be taken as a dietary supplement) may also help. Dilute 1-2 drops with V-6 Mixing Oil and apply over abdomen with a hot compress.

SUPPLEMENTS—ComforTone, JuvaPower/JuvaSpice, JuvaTone, ICP (fiber beverage), Royaldophilus, Stevia Select (with FOS).

NORMAL FUNCTION OF—

SUPPLEMENTS—ComforTone, ICP (fiber beverage for normal function of bowels)

PARALYSIS—ComforTone.

****COMMENTS—One women was paralyzed by surgery and had to have 2 colonic a day. She took ComforTone and then she was able to have natural bowel movements.*

BOXED IN (Feeling): Peace & Calming, Valor.

BRAIN: Aroma Life, Blue cypress (improves circulation), Clary sage (opens brain, euphoria), cypress, geranium, lemongrass, spearmint, Transformation.

ACTIVATES RIGHT BRAIN—Bergamot, birch, geranium, grapefruit, helichrysum, Roman chamomile, wintergreen.

BROKEN BLOOD VESSELS— See BLOOD.

CEREBRAL (BRAIN)—[F]Nutmeg.

INJURY—Frankincense, Valor. Massage on brain stem and diffuse.

*The **blood-brain barrier** is the barrier membrane between the circulating blood and the brain that prevents certain damaging substances from reaching brain tissue and cerebrospinal fluid. The American Medical Association (AMA) determined that if they could find an agent that would pass the blood-brain barrier, they would be able to heal **Alzheimer's, Lou Gehrig's, Multiple Sclerosis, and Parkinson's disease**. In June of 1994, it was documented by the Medical University of Berlin, Germany and Vienna, Austria that **sesquiterpenes have the ability to go beyond the blood-brain barrier**. **High levels of sesquiterpenes** are found in the essential oils of cedarwood, vetiver, sandalwood, Black pepper, patchouli, myrrh, ginger, vitex, German chamomile, spikenard, galbanum, and frankincense. Some blends containing these oils include: 3 Wise Men, Acceptance, Brain Power Forgiveness, Gathering, Harmony, Inspiration, Into the Future, and Trauma Life (refer to Single Oil Chart in the Appendix for other blends that contain these oils).*

INTEGRATION—Clary sage, cypress, geranium, helichrysum (increases neurotransmitter activity), lemongrass, spearmint, Valor.

NEUROLOGICAL INJURY (break down of Myelin sheath)—Peppermint, lemongrass, frankincense, Valor. Massage on brain stem and spine; diffuse.

FOOD—Omega 3 fatty acids found in Flax Seed Oil and Sesame Oil (taken internally). Can also try Essential Omegas supplement.

OXYGENATE—3 drops each of helichrysum and sandalwood once or twice a day on the back of neck, temples, and behind ears down to jaw. Also Blue cypress.

TUMOR—See CANCER. Frankincense, Valor. Massage on brain stem and diffuse.

REAST: Clary sage, cypress, elemi (inflammation), fennel, geranium, lemongrass, sage, spearmint, vetiver.

PERSONAL CARE—ClaraDerm, Prenolone/Prenolone+/Progessence (for tenderness and swelling).

ENLARGE AND FIRM—Clary sage, fennel, sage, SclarEssence.

BLEND—Equal parts vetiver, geranium, ylang ylang.

PERSONAL CARE—Sandalwood Toner (to tone and tighten skin)

LACTATION—See PREGNANCY.

MASTITIS (breast infection)—Citrus Fresh (with lavender), Exodus II, lavender, tangerine.

BLEND—Equal amounts of lavender and tangerine. Dilute with some V-6 Mixing Oil and apply to breasts and under arms twice a day.

SUPPLEMENTS—Exodus, ImmuGel.

MILK PRODUCTION—See PREGNANCY.

SORE NIPPLES—Roman chamomile.

PERSONAL CARE—Animal Scents Pet Ointment

STRETCH MARKS—Gentle Baby.

REATH(ING): Cinnamon bark, Exodus II, frankincense, ginger, hyssop, juniper, marjoram, nutmeg, Roman chamomile, rosemary, thyme. Raven or RC may work instead of an inhaler.

HYPERPNEA (Abnormal rapid breathing)—[F]Ylang ylang.

OXYGEN—Cedarwood, frankincense, sandalwood, all Essential Oils.

PERSONAL CARE—Satin Facial Scrub - Mint (deep cleansing that dispenses nutrients and oxygen). Mix with Orange Blossom Facial Wash for a milder cleanse.

SUPPLEMENTS—Exodus.

SHORTNESS OF—Aroma Life.

BLEND #1—For shortness of breath due to overexertion (lots of work, no sleep, etc.) add 10 drops each of eucalyptus and peppermint to a basin of lukewarm water. Soak some cloths in this water and wring them out leaving them fairly moist. Then wrap the joints (ankles, knees, wrists, elbows, and neck) with the cloths. While relaxing and allowing the compresses to cool the joints, have another person do Vita Flex on the points for the Pineal Gland and Adrenal Glands on the feet.

RONCHITIS: See RESPIRATORY SYSTEM. Abundance, basil, bergamot, birch, cajeput, [F]cedarwood, [F]Clary sage, clove, [F]cypress, elemi, *Eucalyptus radiata*, [F]fir (obstructions of Bronchi), frankincense, ginger, ImmuPower, lavender, ledum, lemon, [F]marjoram, [F]melaleuca, *Melaleuca ericifolia*, [F]myrtle, myrrh, nutmeg, onycha (benzoin), [F]peppermint, [F]pine, RC, Raven, ravensara, Roman chamomile, rose, [F]rosemary, sage lavender, sandalwood, [F]spearmint, Thieves (drops in drinking water, also put on chest & feet, may need to dilute with V-6 Mixing Oil), [F]thyme, tsuga (opens respiratory tract), wintergreen. Diffuse the oils or rub on chest (dilute with V-6 Mixing Oil if necessary).

BLEND #1—10 cedarwood, 10 eucalyptus, 2 Roman chamomile, and 2 oz. water. P on hanky and inhale. Blend can also be added to water for gargle.

BLEND #2—Clove, cinnamon bark, melissa, and lavender (Alternative Medicine—The Definitive Guide, p. 55).

****COMMENTS—Refer to the chapter entitled "How to Use - The Personal Usage Reference" in the Essential Oils Desk Reference under "Bronchitis" for specific oil blend and supplement recommendations.*

CHRONIC—Elemi, eucalyptus, laurel, [F]ravensara, [F]sage, [F]sandalwood, [F]oregano.

CHILDREN—Eucalyptus, lavender, melaleuca, *Melaleuca ericifolia*, Roman chamomile, rosemary, thyme (CT linalol).

SUPPLEMENTS—ImmuneTune, ImmuGel.

CLEAR MUCUS—Bergamot, sandalwood, and thyme (Alternative Medicine—The Definitive Guide, p. 824). Onycha (benzoin) may also help.

****COMMENTS—Diffusing the oils is a great way to handle a respiratory problem*

According to Dr. Daniel Pénoël, bronchitis can be broken down into three separate areas, each of which should be considered separately. Following are the three areas and specific blends recommended by Dr. Pénoël:

Inflamation—Mix equal portions of *Eucalyptus citriodora* and lemongrass. Apply 3-6 drops per foot to the sinus and lung Vita Flex points. Add to V-6 Mixing Oil and apply over the chest.

Infection—Mix 1 tsp. melaleuca, 25 drops palmarosa or geranium, 3 drops peppermint, 1 drop thyme. Apply 3-6 drops per foot to the sinus and lung Vita Flex points. Add to V-6 Mixing Oil and apply over the chest.

Accumulation of Fluids (mucus)—Mix 25 drops each of *Eucalyptus dives*, peppermint, dill. Apply 3-6 drops per foot to the sinus and lung Vita Flex points.

BRUISES: Angelica, fennel, geranium, helichrysum, hyssop, lavender, Melrose, PanAway, Thieves. Apply on location.

****COMMENTS—Refer to the chapter entitled "How to Use - The Personal Usage Reference" in the Essential Oils Desk Reference under "Bruising" for some excellent blend recipes and supplement recommendations.*

BUGGED (Feeling): See EMOTIONS. Acceptance, Forgiveness, Peace & Calming, Valor.

BUGS (Repel): See BITES and INSECT. Lemon (kills bugs), Purification. Diffuse.

BITES (All spiders, Brown Recluse, bee stings, ants, fire ants)—Basil, cinnamon bark, lavender, lemon, lemongrass, peppermint, Purification, thyme.

INSECT—Patchouli.

REPELLANT—Sunsation Suntan Oil; ACCELERATES TANNING in addition to repelling bugs. Idaho tansy may also work as a mosquito repellant. Also, Idaho Tansy Floral Water (used to keep flies away from horses while shoeing).

SNAKE—Patchouli.

LEMIA: Grapefruit. Apply to stomach and bottom of feet.

MPS: Frankincense, Melrose, PanAway, Peace & Calming.

NIONS: See BURSITIS. Aroma Siez, carrot, cypress, German chamomile, juniper, M-Grain.

> ***Bunions** are from bursitis located at the base of a toe.*

BLEND—6 drops eucalyptus, 3 lemon, 4 ravensara, and 1 birch/wintergreen in 1 oz. V-6 Mixing Oil. Apply a couple drops of this blend directly on area of concern as often as desired.

RDENS: See EMOTIONS. Acceptance, Hope, Release, Transformation, Valor.

RNS: Eucalyptus, geranium, helichrysum, Idaho tansy, [F]lavender (cell renewal), melaleuca (Tea Tree), peppermint, ravensara (healing), Roman chamomile, rosehip, tamanu (mix with helichrysum).

PERSONAL CARE—LavaDerm Cooling Mist (soothing and cooling for all burns), Satin Hand & Body Lotion (moisturizes and promotes healing).

SUPPLEMENT—Mineral Essence (can be taken internally and applied topically).

> *Dr. Alex Schauss, a prominent mineral researcher, has discovered that **burns** are painful because certain trace minerals are depleted from the skin and surrounding tissue. If the trace minerals are replenished to the affected area, then the pain will subside almost immediately. Many people have received instant pain relief when Mineral Essence was either taken internally or topically applied on the sunburn or burn.*

BLEND #1—Put 3 drops of lavender in some Satin Hand & Body Lotion and apply. This is effective for pain, healing, peeling, and sunburns.

BLEND #2—10 German chamomile, 5 Roman chamomile, and 10 lavender. Mix together and add 1 drop to each square inch of burn after it has been soaked in ice water. If you don't have the chamomile, lavender will do great. Can top with LavaDerm Cooling Mist to keep skin cool and moist.

CLEANSING—Melrose.

INFECTED—Purification.

PAIN—Blend #1 (above), Mineral Essence (apply topically).

HEALING—See SCARRING. Rosehip. Blend #1 (above), ravensara or geranium mixed with helichrysum.

PEELING—Blend #1, Blend #2 (both shown above).

SUNBURN—See SUNBURN. Australian Blue, [F]Melaleuca (Tea Tree), tamanu (mix wi helichrysum), Mineral Essence (applied topically), Blend #1 (above).

PERSONAL CARE—LavaDerm Cooling Mist, Lavender Floral Water or Lavender Essential Water, Satin Hand & Body Lotion.

BLEND #3—Put 10 drops of lavender in 4 oz. spray bottle of distilled water. Shak well then spray on location. This is effective for pain and healing.

SUN SCREEN—[F]Helichrysum, tamanu, Sunsation Suntan Oil (helps filter out the ultraviolet rays without blocking the absorption of vitamin D, which is important to skin and bone development. It also accelerates tanning).

> *René-Maurice Gattefossé, Ph.D., a French cosmetic chemist who coined the phrase "Aromatherapy," severely burned his hand in a laboratory accident. The continual application of lavender oil soothed the pain, nullified the effects of gas gangrene, and healed his hand without a scar.*

BURSITIS: Aroma Siez, cajeput, cypress, ginger, hyssop, juniper, onycha (benzoin), PanAway, Roman chamomile.

BLEND—Apply 6 drops of marjoram on shoulders and arms; wait 6 minutes. Then apply 3 drops of birch/wintergreen; wait 6 minutes. Then apply 3 drops of cypress.

MASSAGE OILS—Ortho Ease, Ortho Sport.

SUPPLEMENTS—BLM

> ***Bursitis** is a chronic inflammation of the fluid-filled sac that is located close to the joints. It is caused by infection, injury, or diseases like arthritis and gout. Sinc it can be very tender and painful, it may restrict the ability to move freely.*

CALCIUM: See HORMONAL IMBALANCE.

SUPPLEMENTS—Allerzyme (aids the digestion of sugars, starches, fats, and proteins), Coral Sea (highly bio-available, contains 58 trace minerals), Super Cal, Mineral Essence,

> *According to Dr. John R. Lee, processed foods, carbonated soft drinks, caffeine, and high protein, sugar and salt consumption all contribute to increased calcium deficiency in the human body (Burton Goldberg Group, Alt. Med., The Definitive Guide, pp 773-4). Sulfur cannot be metabolized if there is a calcium deficiency. This can cause poor nail and hair growth, falling hair, eczema, dermatitis, poor muscle tone, acne, pimples, gout, rheumatism, arthritis, and a weakening of the nervous system.*

Polyzyme (aids the digestion of protein and helps reduce swelling and discomfort).

B C

ALLOUSES: Carrot, Melrose and oregano (callouses on feet), peppermint, Roman chamomile.

ALMING: Bergamot, [F]cedarwood, Citrus Fresh, Clary sage (aromatic), Gentle Baby, jasmine, lavender, *Melaleuca ericifolia*, myrrh, onycha (benzoin), Peace & Calming, Release, Surrender, tangerine, Trauma Life, Western Red cedar, ylang ylang.

ANCER: See CHEMICALS, RADIATION. Di-Tone (rub on feet and stomach), ImmuPower (put on throat and all over feet, three times a day), Melrose (cancer sores, fights infection), clove, frankincense (diffuse), Juva Cleanse, rose, sage, [F]tarragon (anti-cancerous). Since it is very important to maintain a positive attitude while healing, it may be helpful to address the emotions using Acceptance, Believe, Envision, Forgiveness, Gathering, Gratitude, Hope, Joy, Live with Passion, and/or ravensara (*refer to the emotional therapies in the Science and Application section of the Reference Guide for Essential Oils*). One of the most common emotions cancer patients have to deal with is anger or a pattern of resentment. Others are fear, judgement, and doubt. Doubt limits God and restricts His ability to work miracles in our lives. Praying for all those with cancer can help release these emotions. Also, work on recognizing why cancer was chosen.

When the cell wall thickens, oxygen cannot get in. The life expectancy of a cell is 120 days (4 months). Cells also divide, making duplicate cells. If the cell is diseased, new diseased cells will be made. When we stop the mutation of the diseased cells (create healthy cells), we stop the disease. Essential oils have the ability to penetrate and carry nutrients through the cell wall to the nucleus and improve the health of the cell.

****COMMENTS—Refer to The chapter entitled "How to Use - The Personal Usage Reference" in the Essential Oils Desk Reference under "Cancer" for some excellent blend recipes, supplement recommendations, and cleansing and maintenance programs for many different kinds of cancer.*

*****IMPORTANT NOTICE: HEALTHCARE PROFESSIONALS ARE EMPHATIC ABOUT AVOIDING HEAVY MASSAGE WHEN WORKING WITH CANCER PATIENTS. LIGHT MASSAGE MAY BE USED, BUT NEVER OVER THE TRAUMA AREA. ALSO, THE INFORMATION IN THIS SECTION SHOULD NOT BE PERCEIVED AS A CURE FOR CANCER. ALWAYS CONSULT WITH YOUR HEALTHCARE PROFESSIONAL.**

SUPPLEMENTS—AlkaLime (acid-neutralizing mineral formulation), Bodygize (especially good for cancer), Cleansing Trio (ComforTone, Essentialzyme, and

ICP), ImmuneTune, ImmuPro, Power Meal, Super C / Super C Chewable, VitaGreen, Wolfberry Bar (*Refer to the Wolfberry Bar in the Supplements section of the Reference Guide for Essential Oils for more information on th benefits of the Chinese Wolfberry*).

> *There must be an acid condition in the body for cancer to thrive and spread. See pH Balance. VitaGreen and Power Meal contain predigested proteins and help the body move towards an alkaline balance. AlkaLime combats yeast and fungus overgrowth and helps preserve the body's proper pH balance.*
>
> *Cancer cells also have a very low frequency.*

****COMMENTS—One lady, who was receiving Chemo treatments for cancer of the spleen, used Di-Tone to promote elimination through the colon. Her doctors wondered why her Chemo treatments had not made her sick. When she felt any discomfort (light nausea or cramps in descending colon), she rubbed four to six drops of Di-Tone on her abdomen and within 10 minutes, all discomfort stopped.*

The following are recipes that some individuals have used successfully:

RECIPE #1—For the first month, supplement with the following: 6 VitaGreen thre times a day, 6 Super C / Super C Chewable three times a day, and 4 ImmuneTune three times a day. After remission, apply ImmuPower on the spi three times a day. Do a *light* full body massage with 6 clove and 15 frankincense in 1 oz. V-6 Mixing Oil.

RECIPE #2—Supplement with the following: Cleansing Trio (ComforTone, Essentialzyme, and ICP), 12 Super C / Super C Chewable, 15 ImmuneTune, and 9 VitaGreen. Drink ½ gallon of carrot juice each day. Eliminate white flour, white sugar and red meat from the diet. Rub Thieves on the feet and do *light* full body massage with frankincense.

RECIPE #3—Supplement with the following: 1 Master Formula His/Hers, 2 VitaGreen, 6 Super C / Super C Chewable, and 1 ImmuneTune. Do a *light* fu body massage with frankincense, clove, and V-6 Mixing Oil. Apply ImmuPower to the spine and feet twice a day.

BONE—Frankincense on neat, all supplements. The following is a recipe that has been us on some individuals with bone cancer:

RECIPE #1—ImmuneTune (antioxidant) and Cleansing Trio (ComforTone, Essentialzyme, and ICP) for a week, then JuvaTone was added for six days, th Super B was added morning and evening. Other vitamin supplements includec Super C / Super C Chewable, Mega Cal, and Super Cal. All processed foods were eliminated and a strict Vegetarian Diet was followed, including 8 glasses water each day. Birch was applied on location for pain. Frankincense and lavender were applied on the feet.

BRAIN TUMOR—The following are recipes that some individuals have used successfully

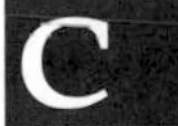

RECIPE #1—*Light* massage daily on spine with 1 oz. V-6 Mixing Oil, 15 drops frankincense, 6 drops clove. Rub brain stem with ImmuPower. Diffuse 15 drops frankincense, 6 drops clove for ½ hour three times a day.

RECIPE #2—Diffuse frankincense 24 hours a day and massage the brain stem with frankincense.

Frankincense contains sesquiterpenes which allow it to go beyond the blood brain barrier. Sesquiterpenes are also found in many of the emotional blends. ImmuPower builds the immune system. Clove is anti-parasitic and anti-tumoral.

BREAST—Frankincense and clove.

Often, there is an emotional issue of self-worth that must be dealt with as well.

CERVICAL—Clove, cypress, frankincense, geranium, lavender, lemon.

COLON—

SUPPLEMENTS—ICP (fiber beverage that helps prevent), CardiaCare (with *Rhododendron caucasicum* which inhibits the enzyme hyaluronidase), Coral Sea (highly bio-available, contains 58 trace minerals), Super Cal (studies have shown that taking calcium supplements at night helps protect the colon from polyps and cancer).

DIET—fast 21 days (See FASTING or CLEANSING) then have soup. See DIET.

HEART—HRT

LIVER—Frankincense (hot compress over liver), JuvaFlex, Juva Cleanse, and/or myrrh may help with liver congestion and function.

SUPPLEMENTS—JuvaTone was formulated to fight cancer in the liver.

One woman had ***cancer of the heart*** *which literally ate a hole in the heart. She took the tincture HRT and the tissue of her heart regenerated and the cancer disappeared!*

JuvaTone *and* ***Rehemogen*** *build blood and hemoglobin platelets One individual had total* ***liver regeneration*** *by using JuvaTone, Rehemogen, and JuvaFlex.*

LUNG—Frankincense (rub on chest or add 15 drops to 1 tsp. V-6 Mixing Oil for nightly retention enema), lavender.

BLEND #1—15 drops frankincense, 5 drops clove, 6 drops ravensara, 4 drops myrrh, and 2 drops sage. This blend can be mixed with 1 tsp. V-6 Mixing Oil if it is too strong. It is best when inserted into rectum.

LYMPHOMA—(nodes or small tumors) in neck and groin. Cleanse liver.

BLEND #2—10 drops frankincense, 5 drops myrrh, and 3 drops sage. Mix with small amount of V-6 Mixing Oil and apply daily over nodes or tumor areas and rectally. Every other day apply frankincense neat.

LYMPHOMA STAGE 4 (bone marrow)—extreme fatigue; eat vegetables and fruits, "NO MEAT". ImmuPower on the spine.

SUPPLEMENTS— Royaldophilus, Bodygize morning and night, Cleansing Trio (ComforTone, Essentialzyme, and ICP), 4 ImmuneTune three times a day (for one month or until remission), 6 Super C / Super C Chewable three times a day,

6 VitaGreen three times a day. After remission, continue one more month then reduce amounts for maintenance.

MELANOMA (skin cancer)—See CORNS, WARTS. Frankincense and lavender.

OVARIAN—ImmuPower on spine three times a day.

BLEND #3—15 drops frankincense, 6 drops geranium, 5 drops myrrh, ½ tsp. V-6 Mixing Oil; alternate one night in vagina (tampon to retain), next in rectum.

SUPPLEMENTS—Bodygize three times a day, ImmuneTune six times a day, 6 FemiGen a day, 8 Super C / Super C Chewable a day. Those with "A" type blood should take 8 VitaGreen day while those with "O" type blood should take 12 or more a day; VitaGreen a mainstay, it is a predigested protein and helps maintain an alkaline balance.

> *Aloha! I have been using essential oil for many years, resulting in many amazingly wonderful results. One of the best took place when a dear friend, was being consumed by cancer. She was in stage 4 for 4 years- amazing in itself. RC and frankincense were used the most. When she was put into the hospice, with only days left, the oils were still used and she remained in the hospice for another year and a half. Others at the hospice got sick with colds and flu, including the workers, but my friend never got any of the passing bugs...amazing to say the least but a true testimonial to the anti-viral and antibiotic effects of the oils.*
>
> ***-Submitted by Yvonne Vnuk-Nielsen***
> ***Kailua, Hawaii (July 2004)***

PROSTATE—Anise (blend with frankincense, fennel, ImmuPower, Mister, sage, and/or yarrow). Apply to posterior scrotum, ankles, lower back, and bottom of feet. Juva Cleanse taken as a dietary supplement can also help.

PERSONAL CARE—Protec was designed to accompany the nightlong retention enema. It helps buffer the prostate from inflammation, enlargement, and tumor activity.

SUPPLEMENTS—3 droppers of Male-Pro Tincture four times a day (available through Creer Labs 801-465-5423).

The following is a recipe that has been used on Prostate Cancer:

RECIPE #1—Diffuse ImmuPower. Do a spinal massage and Vita Flex on the feet with ImmuPower. Blend 5 frankincense, 15 Mister, and 2 tsp. V-6 Mixing Oil together OR 15 ImmuPower with 2 tsp. V-6 Mixing Oil; insert and retain in the rectum throughout the night.

CASE HISTORY #1—71 year old man had prostate cancer and bone metastasis. After three weeks of using frankincense, sage, myrrh, and cumin in rectal implants, he was free of cancer.

THROAT—Frankincense, lavender.

UTERINE—Geranium, ImmuPower.

BLEND #4—2 to 5 drops cedarwood OR 2 to 5 drops lemon OR 2 to 5 drops myrrh in 1 tsp. V-6 Mixing Oil.

C

ANDIDA: See ACIDOSIS, ALKALINE, BLOOD, DIET, FOOD, THYROID, pH BALANCE. Di-Tone, cinnamon bark, clove, EndoFlex, [F]eucalyptus, ImmuPower, melaleuca (dilute with V-6 Mixing Oil for body massage), *Melaleuca quinquenervia*, Melrose (+ rosemary), Mountain savory (dilute with V-6 Mixing Oil; can be hot), oregano, palmarosa (skin), peppermint (aromatic), rosemary, [F]rosewood, [F]spearmint, [F]spruce, tarragon (prevents fermentation), Thieves. Rub on stomach area and feet or over abdomen with a hot compress.

> ***Candida** is caused by the fermentation of yeast and sugar, antibiotics, thyroid shut down, stress, chlorinated water, etc. When there is candida there is usually hypoglycemia and hypothyroidism. It is usually a digestive problem; putrefaction in the system causes candida overgrowth. Candida is a natural fungus in the stomach; we need some, but it becomes a problem when there is an overgrowth. Yeast is not the problem but the fermentation of it. The fermentation exists because of a mineral imbalance and an enzyme imbalance in the digestive system. The enzymes needed for digestion are secreted by the thyroid, so it is necessary to support both the thyroid and the digestive system. Also, maintaining a slightly alkaline state in the blood and body can help to slow the overgrowth of candida.*

SUPPLEMENTS—Allerzyme (aids the digestion of sugars, starches, fats, proteins), AlkaLime (combats yeast and fungus overgrowth and preserves the body's proper pH balance), Bodygize, ComforTone, Detoxzyme (helps maintain and support a healthy intestinal environment), Essentialzyme (increases digestion), ImmuGel (½ tsp. per day cleared up candida in the brain in one week for one individual), ICP, Mineral Essence, ParaFree, Polyzyme (aids the digestion of protein and helps reduce swelling and discomfort), Power Meal (vegetable protein), Royaldophilus (prevents overgrowth), Stevia Select (with FOS; repopulates intestines with good flora), Super C / Super C Chewable, Thyromin (to help the thyroid), VitaGreen (balances the alkaline/acid condition in the body, and provides chlorophyll and oxygen).

TINCTURES—Anti-Cana (creates unfriendly environment for the candida; available through Creer Labs 801-465-5423).

DIGESTIVE CANDIDA—Di-Tone (hot compresses over abdomen; in a retention enema at night), ImmuPower, Thieves.

VAGINAL CANDIDA—[F]Bergamot, [F]melaleuca, [F]myrrh.

BLEND—2 Tbsp. garlic oil, 8 drops lavender, 8 drops melaleuca, 1 ml. (1 softgel) Vitamin E oil. Apply to irritated area.

ANKERS: See ACIDOSIS. Australian Blue, Chamomile (both German and Roman), Envision, hyssop, laurel, melaleuca, Melrose, myrrh, oregano, sage lavender, Thieves.

BLEND #1—Sage with clove and lavender.

BLEND #2—Sage with Thieves.

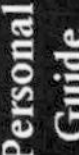

SUPPLEMENTS—AlkaLime (combats yeast and fungus overgrowth and preserves the body's proper pH balance), ImmuneTune, ImmuPro, Mineral Essence, VitaGreen.

Canker sores *are occasionally associated with Crohn's disease, which affects the bowels. Deficiencies of iron, vitamin B12, and folic acid have been linked to this disease in some people. Stress and allergies are usually the cause of open sores in the mouth. To avoid getting canker sores, it is important to have a body chemistry that is balanced in minerals, acidity, and alkalinity (Prescription for Nutritional Healing, p. 126).*

CAPILLARIES:

BROKEN—Cypress, geranium, hyssop, lime (soothes), Roman chamomile.

BLEND—Apply 1 lavender and 1 Roman chamomile.

CARBUNCLES: Melaleuca.

CARDIOTONIC: See HEART.

CARDIOVASCULAR SYSTEM: See HEART. Anise, Aroma Life, clove, cypress, fleabane (dilates), goldenrod, helichrysum, marjoram, onycha (benzoin), rosemary, tsug (opens and dilates for better oxygen exchange), ylang ylang.

SUPPLEMENTS—CardiaCare (contains ingredients that have been scientifically tested for their abilities to support and strengthen the cardiovascular system), Coral Sea (highly bio-available calcium, contains 58 trave minerals), ICP, Mineral Essence, Super B, Super Cal.

TINCTURE—HRT

CARPAL TUNNEL SYNDROME:

Carpal Tunnel Syndrome *is a condition where inflamed carpal ligaments at the wrist press upon the median nerve. Indications include tingling or numbness in the palm or thumb and first three fingers of the hand, weak grip, or impaired finger movement.*

Basil, cypress, eucalyptus, lavender, lemongrass, marjoram, oregano. Apply oils on location and either use massage or Vita Flex to work them in. First start with basil and marjoram on the shoulder to help release any energy blockages. Then lemongrass on wrist and oregano on the rotator cup in the shoulder. Next apply marjoram and cypress on the wrist and then cypress on the neck and down to the shoulder. Lastly, apply peppermint from the shoulder down the arm to the wrist then ou to the tips of each finger.

****COMMENTS—Make sure it is carpal tunnel syndrome because many people that thi they have carpal tunnel syndrome (one report says up to 90%) really have problems with muscles in the neck and shoulder that create similar symptom*

MASSAGE OILS—Ortho Ease or Ortho Sport. Massage into neck, shoulder, and wrist.

PERSONAL CARE—Prenolone/Prenolone+ / Progessence (on shoulder and wrist).

SUPPLEMENTS—ArthroTune, BLM, Coral Sea (highly bio-available calcium, contains 58 trace minerals), Mineral Essence, Sulfurzyme, Super Cal.

CATARACTS: See EYES.

CATARRH (mucus): See ANTI-CATARRHAL. Cajeput, cistus, dill, ginger, hyssop (opens respiratory system to discharge mucus), jasmine, myrrh, onycha (benzoin).

CAVITIES: See TEETH.

CELIBACY (vow not to marry): Marjoram (aromatic).

CELLS: All Essential Oils restore cells to original state. Need to change the RNA and DNA to change the habit.

DNA—cell chemistry.

SUPPLEMENTS—Super B, Thyromin, Body Balancing Trio (Bodygize, Master Formula His/Hers, VitaGreen).

FREQUENCY—Rose (enhances frequency of every cell, which brings balance and harmony to body).

LIVER—Helichrysum (stimulates cell function).

OXYGENATION—Black pepper.

REGULATING—Clary sage (removes negative programming).

RNA—cell memory.

STIMULATES—Abundance.

CELLULITE: See WEIGHT. Basil, [F]cedarwood, cumin, cypress, fennel, geranium, [F]grapefruit, juniper, lavender, lemon, lime, orange, oregano, patchouli, [F]rosemary, rosewood, sage, spikenard (increases metabolism to burn fat), tangerine (dissolves), thyme. *Refer to The chapter entitled "How to Use - The Personal Usage Reference" in the Essential Oils Desk Reference under "Cellulite" for some excellent blend recipes and recommendations.*

> *Try flavoring 1 gallon of water with 5 drops grapefruit and 5 drops lemon. Adjust to taste and drink. This may also improve energy levels. The new H2Oils packets can now be used to more easily and effectively flavor drinking water with lemon and grapefruit oils.*

SUPPLEMENTS—Allerzyme (aids the digestion of sugars, starches, fats, and proteins), Lipozyme (aids the digestion of fats), Power Meal (eat for breakfast).

ATTACKS FAT AND CELLULITE—Basil, grapefruit, lavender, lemongrass, rosemary, sage, thyme.

MASSAGE OILS—Cel-Lite Magic (add grapefruit to increase activity and dissolve cellulite even faster).

CHAKRAS (Energy Centers): (*Refer to the chart at the end of the Science and Application section of the Reference Guide for Essential Oils.*) Harmony (apply 1 drop or each chakra to open the energy centers and balance the electrical field of the chakras, starting at the base chakra located on the coccyx at the end of the spinal column and working up), lavender (brings harmony to chakras), rosema (opens chakras), sandalwood (affects each chakra differently).

UNITES HEAD AND HEART—Helichrysum.

ANGELIC CHAKRA (#8)—Located above the crown of the head. Angelica, neroli.

CROWN CHAKRA (#7)—3 Wise Men (to replace void with good/positives), angelica (links 7-8, 7-1), basil, cistus, frankincense (links 1-7), lavender, myrrh, onycha ravensara, rose, rosemary, rosewood (links 7-1), sandalwood (links 7-1), spikenard, spruce.

BALANCE—Highest Potential

OPEN—Forgiveness, Harmony.

BROW CHAKRA (3rd EYE - #6)—Acceptance, Awaken, and Dream Catcher (rub on lobe of ear to increase vision and spiritual vision); cedar leaf (Western Red), cedarwood, Clary sage, frankincense, Harmony, helichrysum, juniper, mugwor peppermint, pine, rose, rosemary, spruce, thymes, Transformation, tsuga.

OPEN—Frankincense, Harmony.

THROAT CHAKRA (#5)—Carrot seed, chamomile (Roman and German), cypress, frankincense, geranium, lavender, rose geranium, sandalwood, spearmint, spruce.

OPEN—Harmony.

HEART CHAKRA (#4)—Bergamot, carrot seed, cinnamon bark, frankincense, helichrysum, hyssop, inula, laurel, lavandin, lavender, marjoram, melissa, nero onycha, oregano, pepper (Black), rose, sage, sandalwood, spikenard, tansy.

OPENS A CLOSED HEART—Bergamot, Harmony.

SOLAR PLEXUS CHAKRA (#3)—Calamus, cardamon, carrot seed, cedarwood, cinnamo bark, citronella, fennel, ginger, juniper, lemon, lemongrass, melissa, pepper (Black), peppermint, rosemary, spikenard, thymes (all), valerian, vetiver, ylang ylang.

OPEN—Harmony.

SACRAL CHAKRA (SEX/NAVEL - #2)—Cassia, cinnamon bark, Clary sage, coriander, cypress, geranium, rose geranium, jasmine, myrrh, niaouli, patchouli, petitgrair pine, rose, sandalwood, tangerine, vetiver, ylang ylang.

BALANCE—Acceptance (balances Sacral Chakra which stores denial and sexual abuse), sage.

OPEN—Harmony.

BASE CHAKRA (ROOT - #1)—cardamon, carrot seed, cedar leaf (Western Red), cedarwood, clove, frankincense, ginger, laurel, myrrh, onycha, patchouli, pepper (Black), peppermint, sandalwood, vetiver.

OPEN—Harmony.

CHANGE (Personal): See EMOTIONS. Forgiveness, Into the Future, Joy, Magnify Your Calling, Sacred Mountain, 3 Wise Men, Transformation.

CHARLEY HORSE: See MUSCLE SPASMS. Aroma Siez, basil.

PERSONAL CARE—Prenolone/Prenolone+, Progessence.

CHEEKS: Jasmine.

BLEND—5 Aroma Siez, 3 birch/wintergreen, and 3 spruce. Work oils between hands in a clockwise motion and pat on cheeks. Cup hands over nose and inhale.

CHELATION: See METALS. Aroma Life, cardamom, helichrysum (powerful chelator and anti-coagulant). Drink lots of distilled water.

Traditional intravenous chelation therapy can cause scar tissue on the vascular walls. These oils, supplements, and tinctures provide a more natural approach to chelation. They may take longer to achieve the same results, but with minimal side effects.

MASSAGE OILS—Cel-Lite Magic.

SUPPLEMENTS—Cleansing Trio (ComforTone, Essentialzyme, and ICP), VitaGreen (use with cardamom to enhance effects of Chelex tincture).

****COMMENTS—The apple pectin that is contained in ICP helps remove unwanted metals and toxins from the body.*

TINCTURES—AD&E, Chelex, and Rehemogen for natural cleansing.

CHEMICALS: See METALS. [F]Helichrysum.

SUPPLEMENTS—Chelex.

CHICKEN POX: See CHILDHOOD DISEASES.

CHIGGERS: See INSECT. Lavender.

CHILD BIRTH: See PREGNANCY.

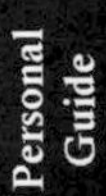

CHILDHOOD DISEASES:

CHICKEN POX (2 weeks)—(shingles) sleep is very good. See SHINGLES. Australian Blue, Bergamot, eucalyptus, lavender, melaleuca (Tea Tree), Roman chamomile, sage lavender.

BATH—(relieves the itching) 2 drops lavender, 1 cup bicarbonate of soda, and 1 cup soda in bath and soak.

BLEND #1—5 to 10 drops each of German chamomile and lavender to one ounce Calamine lotion. Mix and apply twice a day all over body.

BLEND #2—10 drops lavender, 10 Roman chamomile, and 4 oz. Calamine lotion. Mix and apply twice a day all over body.

BLEND #3—Add enough ravensara to some Green clay (from health food store) to form a paste that can be dabbed on the pox to relieve itching.

DIFFUSE—an anti-viral oil (such as lemon) and apply the same oil all over the body twice a day. See BABIES/CHILDREN.

MEASLES—[F]Eucalyptus, German chamomile, lavender, melaleuca. Spray or vaporize the room.

GERMAN (3 day)—use anti-viral oils. See ANTI-VIRAL.

RUBELLA—sponge down with one of these oils: Chamomile (Roman or German), lavender, melaleuca.

MUMPS—Lavender, lemon, melaleuca.

WHOOPING COUGH—Basil, cinnamon bark (diffuse or dilute well; avoid for children), Clary sage, cypress, grapefruit, hyssop, lavender, [F]oregano, thyme.

CHILDREN: See BABIES, HYPERACTIVE CHILDREN, CHILDHOOD DISEASES.

PERSONAL CARE—KidScents Bath Gel, KidScents Lotion, KidScents Shampoo, KidScents Tender Tush, KidScents Toothpaste.

SUPPLEMENTS—KidScents Mighty Mist (vitamin spray), KidScents Mighty Vites (chewable vitamin tablets), KidScents MightyZyme (chewable enzymes).

HYPERACTIVE—Citrus Fresh, Peace & Calming, Trauma Life. Diffuse.

CHILLS: Ginger, onycha (benzoin), sage lavender. Apply on bottom of feet and on solar plexus.

CHLOROPHYLL:

SUPPLEMENTS—VitaGreen.

CHOLERA: Clove, [F]ravensara, [F]rosemary.

CHOLESTEROL: [F]Clary sage, [F]helichrysum (regulates). Apply on Vita Flex points, over heart and along arms.

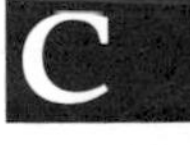

IOREA: See SAINT VITUS DANCE.

IRONIC FATIGUE: See ACIDOSIS, HORMONAL IMBALANCE. Basil, Clarity, Di-Tone, ImmuPower, lavender, lemongrass, peppermint, rosemary, Thieves, Transformation. (Note: Basil and peppermint are a good combination together). Combine any of the above with the Raindrop Technique.

SUPPLEMENTS—AlkaLime (acid-neutralizing mineral), Body Balancing Trio (Bodygize, Master Formula His/Hers, VitaGreen), Cleansing Trio (ComforTone, Essentialzyme, and ICP), Coral Sea (highly bio-available calcium), ImmuneTune, ImmuPro, Mineral Essence, Power Meal, Royaldophilus, and Super Cal.

> ***Chronic Fatigue** is often caused by the Epstein Barr virus. It may also be a result of chemical and metal toxicity, or conditions of high acidity.*
>
> *Women who are pregnant seldom have Chronic Fatigue Syndrome because of the higher amounts of natural progesterone being produced.*

PERSONAL CARE—Prenolone/Prenolone+, Progessence.

Dr. Friedmann uses the following recipe on his patients:

***RECIPE #1*—**1) Use the Cleansing Trio (ComforTone, Essentialzyme, and ICP) to detoxify. 2) Build the body and tissues with Mineral Essence and Master Formula His/Hers. 3) Build the immune system with ImmuPower and ImmuneTune or ImmuPro.

GARETTES:

PURIFY AIR—Purification.

QUIT SMOKING—See ADDICTIONS. Peace & Calming, Purification.

SUPPLEMENTS—JuvaPower/JuvaSpice, JuvaTone.

RCULATION: Aroma Life, basil, birch, cinnamon bark, Citrus Fresh, Clary sage, cumin, [F]**cypress**, geranium, helichrysum, hyssop, Juva Cleanse, nutmeg, onycha (benzoin), oregano, peppermint, Peace & Calming, RC, rosemary, sage lavender, thyme, wintergreen. Use in a bath, massage, or a compress.

CAPILLARY—**Cypress** (strengthens the capillary walls, and increases circulation), oregano, thyme.

PROMOTES HEALTHY—Onycha (benzoin), PanAway.

MASSAGE OILS—Cel-Lite Magic dilates the blood vessels for better circulation; may add grapefruit or cypress to enhance. Also Ortho Ease and Ortho Sport.

SUPPLEMENTS—Cleansing Trio (ComforTone, ICP, Essentialzyme), JuvaTone, Thyromin.

****COMMENTS—Constipation affects circulation. Improving the circulation in the colon and liver improves the circulation in the blood.*

CIRCULATORY SYSTEM: See also CARDIOVASCULAR SYSTEM. Aroma Life, Clary sage, cypress, En-R-Gee, helichrysum, PanAway.

STIMULANT—[F]Nutmeg, onycha (benzoin), pine.

SUPPORT—Goldenrod.

CIRRHOSIS: See LIVER.

CLARITY OF THOUGHTS: Clarity, rosemary, Transformation.

CLEANSING: Di-Tone when cramping, fennel, hyssop, juniper, melaleuca (aromatic), Melrose, Release (over liver), 3 Wise Men when trauma, put on liver to let emotions go.

> ***Cleansing** may help to prevent disease, improve immune function, and make the body stronger. It may also cause an emotional cleansing! DRINK LOTS OF WATER!! Any age child can go on a cleanse. Dr. Gary Young suggests that you spend two days cleansing for every year old you are. He recommends that you take ICP and Essentialzyme five days a week and fast once a week on distilled water and lemon juice.*

CUTS—Elemi, lavender, Melrose.

BODY CLEANSE—

SUPPLEMENTS—Cleansing Trio (ComforTone, Essentialzyme, and ICP). The oil contained in the Cleansing Trio will push heavy metals into the system; use Sacred Mountain and Peace & Calming to balance the system. If colon is blocked, start with ComforTone to open it. JuvaTone is the final stage of cleansing and can be taken as often as four times a day.

TINCTURES—Rehemogen supports the body during a cleanse.

MASTER CLEANSER or LEMONADE DIET—2 Tbs. fresh lemon or lime juice (approx. ½ lemon), 2 Tbs. of grade C maple syrup (grades A & B are not as rich in nutrients but can be used if grade C is not available). 1/10 tsp. cayenne pepper or to taste (cayenne is a thermal warmer and dilates the blood vessels; also has vitamin A). Combine above ingredients in a 10 oz. glass of distilled water. N substitute sugars. In the case of diabetes, use black strap molasses instead of the maple syrup. Drink between three quarts and a gallon of this lemonade ea

> *Lemon converts to alkaline in the body. Lemons can be harmful to teeth only when in water that is not distilled because there can be a reaction with the minerals in the water. Toxins are eliminated from the bowels and bladder. Drink 6 to 12 glasses of the lemonade drink daily. When you get hungry, just drink another glass of lemonade. No other food or vitamins should be taken; the lemonade is already a food in liquid form. An herbal laxative tea may be used to help elimination. More details can be found in the book by Stanley Burroughs, Healing for the Age of Enlightenment. It will take 30 days on lemon to change the chemistry in the body. We have to change the DNA and RNA (memory or belief system) to change a habit. Then, do 30 days on carrot juice.*

C

day with an herbal laxative tea first thing in the morning and just before retiring for the night. Refer to the book Healing for the Age of Enlightenment for more specific details including suggestions and specific instructions for how coming off the cleanse.

LOSED MINDED: Awaken, Inspiration.

LOTHES: Canadian Red cedar. This oil will leave a stain so place a few drops on a cotton ball and put it in a plastic sack. Leave the sack open so the odor of the oil can do its work without it staining any clothes. Place the bag in a closet or storage box.

CKROACHES:

BLEND—Combine 10 peppermint and 5 cypress in ½ cup of water and spray.

OFFEE (stop drinking): (*See case study on the body's frequency reaction to coffee in the Science and Application section of the Reference Guide for Essential Oils*). Peace & Calming, Purification.

SUPPLEMENTS—JuvaTone.

OLDS: Angelica, Australian Blue, basil, Blue cypress (aches & pains), cajeput, eucalyptus (in hot water, breathe deep), Exodus II, fir (aches and pains), ginger, Idaho tansy, lavender, ledum, [F]lemon, [F]melaleuca, myrtle, onycha (benzoin), orange, oregano, peppermint (relieves nasal congestion), pine, Raven, ravensara, RC (put a few drops in a box of tissue), [F]rosemary, sage lavender, Thieves, thyme. Apply Raven to the back and RC to the chest with Thieves on the feet. Next application rotate Raven and RC. Other oils can be diffused or applied to the forehead, temples, back of neck, and chest. *Refer to The chapter entitled "How to Use - The Personal Usage Reference" in the Essential Oils Desk Reference under "Colds and Flu" for some excellent recipes and supplement recommendations.*

BLEND—Mix 6 RC and 2 ravensara. Apply to the chest, neck, throat, and sinus area. Diffuse or put 4 drops in a half cup of hot water, then place nose and mouth into cup (not in the water) and breathe deeply.

It seems that because we live in the South there is a lot of "stuffy noses" in the spring and fall. When I have a client in my business complaining of these types of symptoms, I offer them some oils to sniff for relief. I offer a drop of peppermint first then a drop of RC blend. Then, if they have used the word "infection", I offer a drop of Thieves blend. I offer one drop of each in the palm of their hand, one at a time. Then I show them how to stir 3 times and cup their hands over the nose and deeply inhale each oil. They are always amazed at the immediate relief.

-Submitted by Pam Jones
Benton, Arkansas (July 2004)

Personal Guide

SUPPLEMENTS—Exodus, ImmuGel, Thieves Lozenges.

****COMMENTS—Dr. Pénoël recommends applying a trace of melaleuca alternifolia to the tip of the tongue and swallowing. This works best when done immediatel upon noticing a sore throat. Repeat every minute until the throat feels better Then apply it behind the ears and down under the jaw line. After repeating this a few times (every 5-10 minutes), massage a couple drops on the back of the neck to relieve any blockage.*

COLD SORES: See HERPES SIMPLEX. Australian Blue, Bergamot, Blue cypress. geranium lavender, lemon, melaleuca (Tea Tree), Melrose (fights infection), RC, Roman chamomile, Thieves.

COLIC: See BABIES. Angelica, bergamot, cardamom, carrot with fennel, coriander, cumin, di ginger, marjoram, melissa, Mountain savory, orange, pepper, peppermint, Roman chamomile, spearmint.

COLITIS: Anise, calamus (viral), clove (bacterial), [F]helichrysum (viral), [F]tarragon, [F]thyme (whe there is infection). Redmond clay (from Redmond Minerals 1-800-367-7258) helps clean fecal matter out of pockets in the colon.

SUPPLEMENTS—AlkaLime, Cleansing Trio (ComforTone, Essentialzyme, and ICI

COLON: See COLITIS and DIVERTICULITIS. Calamus may help reduce inflammation. Di-Tone and peppermint. Take 2 drops of each in distilled water 1-2 times per da Use Redmond clay (from Redmond Minerals 1-800-367-7258) to remove feca matter from pockets in the colon. Also Release topically with compress.

SUPPLEMENTS—Cleansing Trio (ComforTone, Essentialzyme, and ICP), JuvaPower/JuvaSpice, Royaldolphilus, Stevia Select. *Refer to the Supplemen section of the Reference Guide for Essential Oils for specific usages.*

Polyps are tumors that arise from the bowel surface and protrude into the inside of the colon. Most polyps eventually transform into malignant cancer tumors.

POLYPS—See POLYPS. Cleanse the colon! Stanley Burroughs' Master Cleanse is an ideal cleansing program which affects the entire body. However, if fecal matter is not being eliminated from t colon 2-3 times per day, it may be necessary to start with ComforTone first un bowel movements are more frequent. Then toxins released during the Master Cleanse can be quickly eliminated from the body. (*See Master Cleanser unde CLEANSING*)

SUPPLEMENTS—Cleansing Trio (ComforTone, Essentialzyme, and ICP). *Refer to the Supplements section of the Reference Guide for Essential Oils.*

PROLAPSED COLON—not assimilating; use Essentialzyme.

C

****COMMENTS—Stanley Burroughs recommends performing a colon lift and describes the procedure for doing so in his book Healing for the Age of Enlightenment on pages 55 to 59.*

SPASTIC—has no parasiticidal action.

SUPPLEMENTS—ComforTone then ICP (fiber beverage).

COMA: Awaken, Black pepper, cypress, frankincense, Hope, peppermint, sandalwood, Surrender, Trauma Life, Valor. Massage on brain stem, mastoids (behind ears), temples, and bottom of feet.

SUPPLEMENTS—Mineral Essence, Ultra Young.

COMFORTING: Gentle Baby.

COMPASSION: Helichrysum.

COMPLEXION: See SKIN. Apply oils to face, neck and intestines.

DULL—Jasmine, orange.

OILY—Bergamot, orange.

CONCENTRATION (POOR): Awaken, basil, Brain Power, cedarwood, Clarity, cypress, Dream Catcher, eucalyptus, Gathering, juniper, lavender, lemon, myrrh, orange, peppermint, rosemary, sandalwood, 3 Wise Men, ylang ylang.

CONCUSSION: Cypress. Rub on brain stem and bottom of feet.

****COMMENTS—One woman had a concussion with headaches and hallucinations. By applying cypress over her brain stem, her headaches left for good.*

CONFIDENCE: Jasmine, Live with Passion, sandalwood (self), Transformation, Valor.

CONFUSION: Awaken, basil, Brain Power, cedarwood, Clarity, cypress, fir, frankincense, Gathering, geranium, ginger, Harmony, jasmine, juniper, marjoram, peppermint, Present Time, rose, rosemary, rosewood, sandalwood, spruce, thyme, Transformation, Valor, ylang ylang.

CONGESTION: Di-Tone, cedarwood, coriander, cypress, *Eucalyptus radiata*, Exodus II, fennel, ginger, myrtle (excellent for children), Raven, RC, rosemary. To help discharge mucus, rub oil(s) on chest, neck, back, feet, and diffuse.

MASSAGE OILS—Cel-Lite Magic.

SUPPLEMENTS—Cleansing Trio (ComforTone, ICP, Essentialzyme).

CONJUNCTIVITIS: *Eucalyptus radiata*, jasmine, Mixta chamomile.

CONSCIOUSNESS: Lavender. Diffusing these oils is a great way to affect consciousness.
OPEN—Rosemary.
PURIFYING—Peppermint.
STIMULATING—Peppermint, Transformation.

CONSTIPATION: See ACIDOSIS.

Poor bowel function may be caused by enzyme deficiency, low fiber, poor bowel tone, not enough liquid in diet, stress, incorrect pH balance, and/or bad diet.

Anise, Black pepper, Di-Tone, fennel, ginger, juniper, [F]marjoram, [F]orange, patchouli, rose, rosemary, sandalwood, tangerine, tarragon. Massage clockwise around abdomen and on Vita Flex points (feet & shins).
SUPPLEMENTS—AlkaLime, ComforTone, Essentialzyme, ICP (fiber beverage), Sulfurzyme, and lots of water. If there is a chronic history of constipation, use ComforTone until the system is open, then start ICP.
BLEND #1—Mix together 6 drops of [F]orange, tangerine, and spearmint and rub on lower stomach and colon.
BLEND #2—15 cedarwood, 10 lemon, 5 peppermint, and 2 oz. V-6 Mixing Oil. Massage over lower abdomen three times a day clockwise and take supplements
CHILDREN—fruit juices or lots of water. Geranium, patchouli, Roman chamomile, rosemary, tangerine.

CONTAGIOUS DISEASES: [F]Ginger.

CONTROL:
OF YOUR LIFE—Cedarwood, Dream Catcher, Envision.
SELF—Motivation, Roman chamomile (aromatic).

CONVULSIONS: See SEIZURE. Brain Power, Clary sage, lavender, neroli, Roman chamomile, Valor.
SUPPLEMENTS—KidScents Mighty Mist/Vites, Mineral Essence, Ultra Young.

COOLING OILS: Angelica, Citrus oils, eucalyptus, lavender, melaleuca, Mountain savory, peppermint, Roman chamomile, spruce. Other oils that are high in aldehydes and esters can produce a cooling effect.

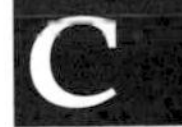

'ORNS: See WARTS. Carrot, Citrus Fresh, clove, grapefruit, lemon, myrrh, peppermint, Roman chamomile, tangerine. Apply 1 drop of oil directly on corn.

Stanley Burroughs touts clove oil as being wonderful for corns, skin cancer, and warts. He suggests using your finger to apply a small amount of clove oil directly on warts or corns. After a short time, use an emery stick to scrape off the top of the wart or corn and apply the oil again. Repeat several times daily until wart or corn disappears. The same technique can be used for skin cancer. (Healing for the Age of Enlightenment, p. 104.)

'ORTISONE: Birch, EndoFlex, lavender, Relieve It, Roman chamomile, [F]spruce (is like cortisone), wintergreen.

BLEND—Combine 3 drops Roman chamomile, 3 lavender, 5 spruce, and 1 birch/wintergreen and apply as a natural cortisone.

SUPPLEMENTS—ProGen and Thyromin, together with EndoFlex are beneficial for both men and women. The three items together may also help the body produce its own cortisone.

'OUGHS: Angelica, cajeput, cardamom, **cedarwood**, elemi (unproductive), [F]eucalyptus, fir, **frankincense**, ginger, jasmine, juniper, [F]melaleuca, [F]myrtle (helps remove mucus from lungs), myrrh, onycha (benzoin), peppermint, pine, myrrh, RC, ravensara, Roman chamomile, sage lavender, sandalwood, thyme.

ESSENTIAL WATERS (HYDROSOLS)—Clary Sage (gentle enough for smaller children - spray on chest or in air). Can also diffuse using Essential Mist Diffuser.

SUPPLEMENTS—Thieves Lozenges.

ALLERGY—Purification (diffuse).

SEVERE—Elemi, frankincense.

BLEND #1—3 drops fir, 3 lemon, 2 ravensara, 1 thyme.

Diffusing the oils is one of the best ways to handle a cough. It may also help to rub the oils on the throat and chest area.

BLEND #2—15 drops Raven, 15 RC, 5 lemon, and 10 Peace & Calming. Rub on chest, throat, and neck. Can also be diffused.

SMOKERS—Myrtle.

'OURAGE: Clove (aromatic), fennel (aromatic), ginger, Live with Passion, Valor (gives).

'RADLE CAP: See BABIES.

'RAMPS: See DIGESTIVE SYSTEM, HORMONAL IMBALANCE, MENSTRUATION, MUSCLES, PMS. Aroma Siez, basil, [F]birch, Blue cypress (abdominal), Clary sage, [F]cypress, Exodus II, galbanum, ginger, [F]lavender, rosemary, [F]marjoram, wintergreen.

MASSAGE OILS—Relaxation.

LEG CRAMPS—Aroma Siez, basil, German chamomile, lavender, marjoram, rosemary, vetiver.

MASSAGE OILS—Ortho Ease, Ortho Sport, Relaxation.

PERSONAL CARE—Prenolone/Prenolone+, Progessence.

SUPPLEMENTS—ArthroTune, BLM, Coral Sea (highly bio-available calcium, contains 58 trace minerals), Mineral Essence, Super Cal.

MENSTRUAL CRAMPS—See DYSMENORRHEA.

PERSONAL CARE—Prenolone/Prenolone+, Progessence.

SUPPLEMENTS—Exodus, FemiGen. Lady Flash, Lady Love (available through Creer Labs 801-465-5423).

RECIPE #1—Take 2 FemiGen three times a day, 10 days before period. Start again two days after cycle. May take up to 6 tablets three times a day. Lady Flash and Lady Love may be applied to the ovaries, pelvis, ankles, bottom of the feet or as a hot compress.

STOMACH CRAMPS—Di-Tone.

CREATES SACRED SPACE: Sacred Mountain.

CROHN'S DISEASE: Basil, calamus, Di-Tone, peppermint. Do Raindrop Technique on spine with ImmuPower.

SUPPLEMENTS—AlkaLime, Bodygize, Cleansing Trio (ComforTone, ICP, and Essentialzyme), ImmuGel, Mineral Essence, Power Meal, Royaldophilus, **Sulfurzyme**, VitaGreen.

****COMMENTS—Refer to The chapter entitled "How to Use - The Personal Usage Reference" in the Essential Oils Desk Reference under "Crohn's Disease" for a specific regimen of supplements.*

CROWN CHAKRA: (See CHAKRAS for more extensive list)

OPEN—3 Wise Men (releases and fills the void).

CUSHING'S DISEASE: See ADRENAL GLANDS. Basil, Forgiveness, ImmuPower, Joy, lemon, Thieves.

SUPPLEMENTS—Exodus, ImmuneTune, ImmuPro.

CUTS: See TISSUE. Cypress, elemi (infected), helichrysum, lavender, melaleuca, Melrose (rejuvenates tissue), onycha (benzoin), pine, ravensara, Relieve It, Roman chamomile (healing), rosewood, sage lavender, Thieves.

C

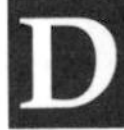

YSTIC FIBROSIS: Alternate with Thieves, RC, lavender, and myrtle. Apply to brain stem (back of neck), temples, chest, bottom of feet, and diffuse. Raven is stronger and can replace myrtle for helping to remove mucus accumulation in the lungs. EndoFlex and helichrysum can also be used with benefit.

BLEND—(Staphylococcus) oregano, thyme, and Melrose (up the spine using the Raindrop Technique), then 10 drops lemon, 5 drops melaleuca, and 3 drops frankincense (rub on feet, chest, and diffuse) OR 10 Raven and 5 hyssop.

SUPPLEMENTS—Essentialzyme, Master Formula His/Hers, VitaGreen, all vitamins.

YSTITIS (Bladder Infection): Basil, bergamot, cajeput, cedarwood, cinnamon bark, clove, eucalyptus, fennel, frankincense, [F]German chamomile, hyssop, juniper, lavender, marjoram, oregano, pine, sage, sandalwood, [F]spearmint, rosewood, [F]thyme. Massage or bathe with one of these oils.

TINCTURE—K&B.

ANDRUFF: Cedarwood, [F]lavender, melaleuca (Tea Tree), patchouli, [F]rosemary, sage, sage lavender, valerian.

PERSONAL CARE—Lavender Volume Shampoo and Lavender Volume Conditioner.

AY DREAMING: Awaken, cedarwood, Clarity, Dream Catcher, eucalyptus, Gathering, ginger, Harmony, helichrysum, Highest Potential, lavender, lemon, myrrh, peppermint, Present Time, rose, rosemary, rosewood, Sacred Mountain, sandalwood, spruce, 3 Wise Men, thyme, Valor, ylang ylang.

EATH (of Loved One): See EMOTIONS: LOSS. Trauma Life.

EBILITY: Cardamom, cumin (nervous), [F]nutmeg sage lavender.

ECONGESTANT: Any of the citrus oils, [F]cypress, [F]German chamomile, juniper, melaleuca, patchouli.

EFEATED: See EMOTIONS.

EGENERATIVE DISEASE: See pH BALANCE. Citrus Fresh, Exodus II, frankincense, lavender, lemon, orange, Purification, tangerine, and Transformation are excellent to diffuse in the room. Not only do these oils purify the air, but they help deliver needed oxygen to the starving cells. All other essential oils and supplements are beneficial for providing oxygen and nutrients to the cells of the body. See specific ailments.

SUPPLEMENT—Power Meal.

****COMMENTS*—***A lack of nutrients at the cellular level causes degenerative disease.*** *The general health condition of the body will improve if the necessary nutrients ar received by the body at the cellular level. Toxins change the pH of the cell wall, which significantly reduces the ability of the cell to assimilate nutrients and oxyge. This process is the beginning of cellular starvation, which leads to degenerative disease. Then, we are hosts to viral and bacterial invasions due to our weakened c compromised immune system. Essential Oils are antimicrobial and help our immu system fight off the ravages of disease. They also have the ability to deliver nutrie to our nutritionally depleted cells. When essential oils are blended with the prope nutrients that the body requires, the essential oils act as the delivery system to take the nutrients directly into the cell and through the compromised cell wall, which ha had the pH altered due to chemical toxins in the body. This process allows the bo to rebuild and regain its healthful condition and allows the body's immune system normalize. In addition, essential oils have the highest oxygenating molecules of ar know substance. So, they deliver oxygen to the cells which helps in the regeneratio process. (Young Living Essential Edge Newsletter — July 1996).*

DEHYDRATION: ImmuneTune, Mineral Essence.

****COMMENTS—An 18-month old infant was saved from dying of dehydration when it was given ½ capsule of ImmuneTune in applesauce.*

DELIVERY: See PREGNANCY.

DENIAL: Roman chamomile, sage.

OVERCOME—Abundance, Acceptance, Awaken, Transformation.

DENTAL INFECTION: Clove and frankincense, helichrysum, melaleuca, myrrh, Thieves. Apply to jaws and gums. It may be necessary to dilute Thieves with V-6 Mixing Oil.

PERSONAL CARE—Dentarome/Dentarome Plus Toothpaste (contains Thieves), Fresh Essence Mouthwash (contains Thieves), KidScents Toothpaste (for children).

DEODORANT: Acceptance, Aroma Siez, bergamot, citronella, cypress, Dragon Time, Dream Catcher, EndoFlex, eucalyptus, geranium, Harmony, Joy, lavender, melaleuca, Mister, myrtle, Peace & Calming, RC, Release, White Angelica. Apply oils neat to the skin or dilute with some V-6 Mixing Oil or Massage Oil Base for application under the arms. Also, 2-3 drops of an oil can be added to 4 oz. of unscented talcum powder and 2 oz. of baking soda. Mix this well and apply under the arms, on the feet, or on other areas of the body.

BATH & SHOWER GELS—Dragon Time, Evening Peace, Morning Start.

MASSAGE OILS—Dragon Time, Relaxation.

PERSONAL CARE—AromaGuard Deodorants, Satin Hand & Body Lotion, Sandalwood Moisture Cream. Add a couple drops of one of the oils listed above for additional fragrance.

EODORIZING: Clary sage, myrrh, [F]myrtle, peppermint, Purification, sage, thyme.

EPLETION: Cypress.

EPRESSION: See DIET. Acceptance, basil, [F]bergamot (aromatic), calamus, Clary sage, EndoFlex (apply often while taking Mineral Essence and Thyromin supplements), [F]frankincense, Gathering, Gentle Baby (on solar plexus), geranium, ginger, grapefruit, Harmony, Highest Potential, Hope (on ears, especially for emotional clearing), Inspiration, jasmine, Joy (5 drops in palm of non-dominant hand, stir clockwise three times with dominant hand, then apply over heart and breathe in deeply), juniper (over heart), lavender (aromatic), M-Grain, neroli, onycha (benzoin), PanAway, Live with Passion, patchouli, Peace & Calming (back of neck), pepper (on crown for spirit protection), ravensara (lifts emotions), Release, Roman chamomile, [F]rosemary (nervous), [F]rosewood, sage (relieves depression), sandalwood, Sensation, tangerine, Trauma Life, Valor (helps balance energies), [F]ylang ylang.

> ***Depression** can be caused by a calcium deficiency. Stay away from carbonated soft drinks, specifically cola drinks that are high in phosphorus; they leech calcium from the body. Eating heavy protein at night does not give the body enough time to digest the food before going to sleep. The undigested food then ferments which robs the system of needed oxygen and heightens the sense of depression.*

BATH AND SHOWER GELS—Sensation Bath & Shower Gel, Lemon Sandalwood or Thieves Cleansing Soaps.

MASSAGE OILS—Sensation Massage Oil.

PERSONAL CARE—Prenolone/Prenolone+, Progessence, Sensation Moisturizing Cream.

SUPPLEMENTS—Coral Sea (highly bio-available, contains 58 trace minerals), Essential Omegas, Mineral Essence, Thyromin, Ultra Young (helps lift depression).

BLEND #1—Combine 1-2 drops each of frankincense, 3 Wise Men, and Hope in the palm of your hand, rub hands together clockwise, cup hands over nose and mouth, and breathe deeply.

ANTI-DEPRESSANT—Abundance, Awaken, bergamot, Christmas Spirit, Citrus Fresh, Dream Catcher, frankincense, geranium, jasmine, Joy, lavender, lemon, melissa, Motivation, neroli, orange, onycha (benzoin), Peace & Calming, ravensara, Roman chamomile, rose, Sacred Mountain, sandalwood, 3 Wise Men, Valor.

IMMUNE DEPRESSION—[F]Spruce.

BATH AND SHOWER GELS—Morning Start Bath & Shower Gel, Thieves Cleansir Soap.

BLEND—5 bergamot, 5 lavender, diffuse.

SUPPLEMENTS—ImmuGel, ImmuPro.

SEDATIVES—Bergamot, cedarwood, Clary sage, cypress, frankincense, geranium, hysso jasmine, juniper, lavender, marjoram, *Melaleuca ericifolia*, melissa, neroli, onycha (benzoin), patchouli, Roman chamomile, rose, sandalwood, ylang ylan Use intuition as to which one may be best for the given situation. In addition, check the safety data for each of the oils in the APPENDIX of this book.

SUICIDAL DEPRESSION—Put Valor then Inspiration on feet and hold feet for a few minutes until relaxed; this may start to release a past negative memory, start crying, etc. If not, rub Present Time over thymus then a drop of Inner Child o their thumb and have them suck the thumb, pushing the pad of the thumb to th roof of the mouth. Once the emotional release starts, put Grounding on the ba of neck and sternum, then put Release on the crown of the head and wait for a while, allowing then to deal with the release. After the emotional release has subsided, rub Joy over the heart and Hope on the ears. After waking up the ne morning, apply a couple drops of Gentle Baby on solar plexus and over the heart. Magnify Your Calling may also be helpful to wear as a perfume/cologn

SUPPLEMENTS—Essential Omegas, Thyromin.

CLEANSING THE FLESH AND BLOOD OF EVIL DEITIES—Cedarwood and myrrh.

BIBLE—"Breaking the lineage of iniquity," The ancient Egyptians believed that if they didn't clear the body and mind of negative influences before dying, they could not progress into the next life and return to this world to take up the body they had left in the tomb (resurrection).

DEPROGRAMMING: Forgiveness, Inner Child, Release, SARA, Trauma Life.

DERMATITIS: Bergamot, chamomile (Roman and German), geranium, [F]helichrysum, hyssop, [F]juniper, lavender, *Melaleuca ericifolia*, onycha (benzoin), [F]patchouli, pine, sag lavender, [F]thyme.

SUPPLEMENTS—Essentialzyme, JuvaPower/JuvaSpice, Sulfurzyme.

****COMMENTS—Dermatitis may indicate a sulfur deficiency.*

DESPAIR: Acceptance, Believe, cedarwood, Clary sage, fir, Forgiveness, frankincense, Gathering, geranium, Gratitude, Grounding, Harmony, Hope, Joy, lavender, lemon, lemongrass, orange, peppermint, rosemary, sandalwood, spearmint, spruce, thyme, Transformation, Valor, ylang ylang.

:SPONDENCY: Bergamot, Chivalry, Clary sage, cypress, Gathering, geranium, ginger, Harmony, Hope, Inner Child, Inspiration, Joy, orange, Peace & Calming, Present Time, rose, rosewood, sandalwood, Transformation, Trauma Life, Valor, and ylang ylang.

:TOXIFICATION: [F]Helichrysum, [F]juniper (detoxifier), JuvaFlex. Apply oils to liver area, intestines, and Vita Flex points on feet.

SUPPLEMENTS—JuvaTone, Cleansing Trio (ComforTone, Essentialzyme, and ICP).

ABETES: Coriander (normalizes glucose levels), cypress, dill (helps lower glucose levels by normalizing insulin levels and supporting pancreas function), [F]eucalyptus, fennel, [F]geranium, ginger, hyssop, juniper, lavender, [F]pine, [F]rosemary, Thieves, [F]ylang ylang. Apply on back, chest, feet, and over pancreas. Diffuse.

BLEND #1—8 clove, 8 cinnamon bark, 15 rosemary, 10 thyme in 2 oz. of V-6 Mixing Oil. Put on feet and over pancreas.

BLEND #2—5 cinnamon bark and 5 cypress. Rub on feet and pancreas.

> ***Caution:** Diabetics should not use angelica Watch insulin intake carefully, may have to cut down. Keep physician informed!*

SUPPLEMENTS—Bodygize, Carbozyme (helps control blood sugar levels—can use as much as 2 capsules twice per day), Cleansing Trio (ComforTone, Essentialzyme, and ICP), ImmuneTune, ImmuPro, Mineral Essence, Power Meal, Stevia, Sulfurzyme (take in morning with Vitamin C before breakfast and at bed time), VitaGreen.

****COMMENTS—Seven-year old girl took 6 VitaGreen a day (balances blood sugar), Bodygize three times a day, and ImmuneTune.*

PANCREAS SUPPORT—Cinnamon bark, fennel, geranium.

SORES (diabetic)—Do the Raindrop Technique and put Valor on Vita Flex points. Also lavender, Melrose.

:APER RASH: [F]Lavender.

PERSONAL CARE—KidScents Tender Tush (formulated specifically for diaper rash), Rose Ointment.

IARRHEA: See ACIDOSIS. Cardamom, cistus, cumin, [F]geranium, [F]ginger, [F]melaleuca, [F]myrrh, myrtle, [F]peppermint, [F]sandalwood (obstinate), spearmint (not for babies).

SUPPLEMENTS—AlkaLime, Essentialzyme, and Royaldophilus.

ANTI-SPASMODIC—Cypress, eucalyptus, Roman chamomile.

CHILDREN—Geranium, ginger, Roman chamomile, sandalwood.

CHRONIC—Neroli, [F]nutmeg, [F]orange, Di-Tone (apply over stomach, colon, and VF points).

STRESS-INDUCED—Lavender.

DIET: See BLOOD, FASTING, FOOD, and CLEANSING. Diet is extremely important whe trying to correct cancer, hypoglycemia, candida, etc. First, cleanse the body, drink a lot of distilled water, stay away from sugars and meats, eat vegetable protein in the mornings, carbohydrates and starches for lunch, and fruit in the evening. Hydrochloric acid and pepsin are secreted in the morning to help dig protein.

SUPPLEMENTS—Enzyme products: Allerzyme (aids the digestion of sugars, starches, fats, and proteins), Carbozyme (aids the digestion of carbohydrates) Detoxzyme (helps maintain and support a healthy intestinal environment), Fiberzyme (aids the digestion of fiber and enhances the absorption of nutrient, Polyzyme (aids the digestion of protein and helps reduce swelling and discomfort), and Lipozyme (aids the digestion of fats).

POST-DIET SAGGY SKIN: Combine 8 drops each of sage, pine, lemongrass, and 1 oz. 6 Mixing Oil. Rub on areas.

> ***Digestive problems*** *may indicate a mineral deficiency. Use Mineral Essence. Royaldophilus is necessary when you are detoxifying or on any type of prescription drug; you must feed the intestinal tract. If you have digestion problems, take Royaldophilus or Stevia Select (with FOS) to stop the fermentation process.*

DIGESTIVE SYSTEM: See also INTESTINAL PROBLEMS. Anise (accelerates), basil, bergamot, Black pepper, cardamom (nervous), cinnamon bark, [F]Clary sage (weak), clove, coriander (spasms), cumin (spasms and indigestion), Di-Tone (acid stomach; aids the secretion of digestive enzymes), [F]fennel (sluggish ginger, [F]grapefruit, juniper, JuvaFlex (supports and detoxifies), laurel, lemon (indigestion), [F]lemongrass (purifier), mandarin (tonic), [F]marjoram (stimulates), myrrh, myrtle, neroli, [F]nutmeg (for sluggish digestion; eases), orange (indigestion), [F]patchouli (stimulant), [F]peppermint, rosemary, [F]sage (sluggish), spearmint, tangerine (nervous and sluggish), tarragon (nervous and sluggish). Add the oil(s) to your food, rub on stomach, or apply as a compress over abdomen.

DIFFUSION—See NEGATIVE IONS for oils that produce negative ions when diffused to help stimulate the digestive system.

ESSENTIAL WATERS (HYDROSOLS)—Peppermint or Spearmint. Spray into air, directly on abdomen, or diffuse using the Essential Mist Diffuser.

SUPPLEMENTS—AlkaLime (combats yeast and fungus overgrowth and preserves t body's proper pH balance), Berry Young Juice (helps with the reduction of fre radicals), Body Balancing Trio (Bodygize, Master Formula His/Hers, VitaGreen), ComforTone, Essential Manna , Essentialzyme (enzymes help bui the digestive system; take before meals for acid stomach), ICP (helps speed fo through digestive system; lower incidence of fermentation), Mineral Essence, ParaFree, Royaldophilus (3 times per week to support digestive function),

Stevia Select, Sulfurzyme. Other enzyme products include: Allerzyme (aids the digestion of sugars, starches, fats, and proteins), Carbozyme (aids the digestion of carbohydrates), Detoxzyme (helps maintain and support a healthy intestinal environment), Fiberzyme (aids the digestion of fiber and enhances the absorption of nutrients), Polyzyme (aids the digestion of protein and helps reduce swelling and discomfort), and Lipozyme (aids the digestion of fats).

D

PHTHERIA: Frankincense, goldenrod.

SAPPOINTMENT: Clary sage, Dream Catcher, eucalyptus, fir, frankincense, Gathering, geranium, ginger, Grounding, Harmony, Hope, Joy, juniper, lavender, orange, Present Time, spruce, thyme, Valor, ylang ylang.

SCOURAGEMENT: Bergamot, cedarwood, Dream Catcher, frankincense, geranium, Hope, Joy, juniper, lavender, lemon, orange, rosewood, Sacred Mountain, sandalwood, spruce, Valor.

SINFECTANT: Grapefruit, [F]lemon, Purification, [F]sage.

BLEND—Add the following number of drops to a bowl of water: 10 lavender (2), 20 thyme (4), 5 eucalyptus (1), 5 oregano (1). If using the larger portions, add to a large bowl of water. If using the numbers in the parentheses, add the oils to a small bowl of water. Use blend to disinfect small areas.

URETIC: Cardamom, [F]cedarwood, cypress, EndoFlex, fennel, grapefruit (all citrus oils), juniper, [F]lavender, lemon, [F]lemongrass, marjoram, mugwort, onycha (benzoin), orange, oregano, [F]rosemary, [F]sage, **tangerine**, valerian. Apply oil(s) to kidney area on back, bottom of feet, and on location.

ALLEVIATES FLUIDS—Cypress, fennel, **tangerine**.

BLEND—1 fennel, 2 cypress, 5 tangerine, apply from the top of the foot to the knee.

VERTICULITIS: Use Redmond clay (1-800-367-7258) to get help remove fecal matter from the pockets. Rub abdomen with cinnamon bark and V-6 Mixing Oil. Anise or lavender may also help. Calamus may help with earlier stages of diverticulitis.

Diverticula, sac-like herniations through the muscular wall of the large intestine (colon), are caused by increased pressure in the bowel from constipation. The existence of these sacs that are filled with trapped fecal sludge is called ***diverticulosis****. When they become infected, the rotting feces erodes the surrounding mucousa and blood vessels and bleeding, rupturing, and infection begins. This is known as* ***diverticulitis****.*

Personal Guide

SUPPLEMENTS— ComforTone to open blocked colon (use daily, increasing dosag by one until bowels are eliminating waste 2-4 times per day), then ICP (fiber beverage) to cleanse colon, and Essentialzyme for digestive enzyme support. JuvaPower/JuvaSpice may also help.

DIZZINESS: Tangerine.

DNA: Chamomile strengthens positive imprinting in DNA.

UNLOCK EMOTIONAL TRAUMA IN DNA—Acceptance, 3 Wise Men (instructs DNA to open for discharge of negative trauma), sandalwood (unlocks negative programing in DNA and enhances the positive programming in the DNA cell create a feeling of security and protection).

DOWN SYNDROME: Clarity, Valor. Apply to bottom of feet and diffuse.

SUPPLEMENTS—Master Formula His/Hers, Mineral Essence.

DREAM STATE: Dream Catcher dissipates negative thoughts and helps one hold onto dream until they become reality.

INFLUENCES—Clary sage (aromatic) enhances vivid dream recall. Transformation.

PROTECTION FROM NEGATIVE DREAMS (that might steal your vision)—Dream Catcher helps one achieve dreams.

DROWNING IN OWN NEGATIVITY: Grapefruit (prevent, aromatic), Transformation.

DRUGS: See ADDICTIONS.

DYING: Awaken, Lazarus (available through Creer Labs 801-465-5423), Transformation.

DYSENTERY: Black pepper, cajeput, cistus, clove (amoebic), cypress, eucalyptus, lemon, melissa, [F]myrrh, Roman chamomile. Apply on abdomen and bottom of feet.

SUPPLEMENTS—JuvaPower/JuvaSpice

DYSPEPSIA (IMPAIRED DIGESTION): Cardamom, coriander, cumin, tarragon, goldenrod [F]grapefruit, laurel, myrrh, [F]orange (nervous), [F]thyme. Apply to stomach, intestines, and Vita Flex points on feet.

SUPPLEMENTS—Essentialzyme.

EARS: Cumin (deafness following a bad viral flu infection), elemi, eucalyptus, geranium, **helichrysum** (improves certain hearing losses), Idaho tansy, juniper, marjoram

Melrose (fights infection and for earache), Purification, valerian (combine with helichrysum for added pain relief), Valor, vitex.

ISTRUCTIONS TO INCREASE AND RESTORE HEARING—

1. Rub Valor on bottom of feet, especially 2 smallest toes and smallest fingers.
2. For each ear, layer 2 drops of **helichrysum, Purification, juniper,** and **peppermint** (in that order), around the inside (not deep) and back of ear, on the mastoid bone (behind ear), along the bottom of the skull around to the back of the head, and down the brain stem.
3. Then do the following ear adjustment.
    1. Pull one ear **up** then the other ear up 10 times each side; 20 times total.
    2. Pull one ear **back** then the other, 5 times each side; 10 times total.
    3. Pull one ear **down** then the other, 5 times each side; 10 times total.
    4. Pull one ear **forward** then the other, 5 times each side; 10 times total.
    5. Then one quick pull with finger in each direction. Up, back, down, forward.
4. Rub **geranium** all around back and front of ear.
5. (Optional) Rub 2 drops **ravensara** around base of both ears.

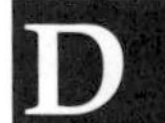

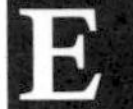

EARACHE—1 drop of either basil, **Melrose**, or ImmuPower. Can also try 1 drop each of helichrysum and valerian together. Put the drop in your hand and soak a small piece of cotton (small enough to fit snugly in the ear) in the oil. Place the piece of cotton in the ear and apply the left over oil on both the front and back of the ear with a finger.

SUPPLEMENTS—JuvaPower/JuvaSpice.

EARACHE IN ANIMALS—(Not cats) 1 drop Melrose on cotton swab then around in well of ear. **Do not put oils directly into ear canal**.

HEARING IN A TUNNEL—Purification, ravensara.

INFECTION—ImmuPower, melaleuca, Melrose (inside well of ear, down and around ear on the outside and under chin). Purification inside well of ear, *Melaleuca ericifolia* and lavender all around outside of ear.

> ***Ear infections** can be caused by food allergies!*
>
> ***Caution:** When working on the ears, do not put the oils directly into the ear canal. Apply only 1-2 drops of oil to the ear by rubbing on the inside, outside, and on the mastoid bone directly behind the ear.*

INFLAMMATION—Eucalyptus.

PIMPLES (in ears)—ImmuPower.

TINNITUS (ringing in the ears, block in eustachian tube)—**Helichrysum** (rub on inside and out of ears), juniper.

EATING DISORDERS:

ANOREXIA—Citrus Fresh, coriander, grapefruit.

BULIMIA—Citrus Fresh, grapefruit.

OVEREATING—Ginger, lemon, peppermint, spearmint.

ECZEMA: Bergamot, eucalyptus, geranium, [F]German chamomile, [F]helichrysum, [F]juniper, lavender, *Melaleuca ericifolia*, melissa, [F]patchouli, [F]rosewood, sage, sage lavender.

SUPPLEMENTS—JuvaPower/JuvaSpice, Sulfurzyme.

****COMMENTS—Eczema may indicate a sulfur deficiency.*

DRY—Bergamot, geranium, [F]German chamomile, hyssop, rosemary.

WET—[F]German chamomile, hyssop, juniper, lavender, myrrh.

EDEMA: See HORMONAL IMBALANCE. [F]Cypress (alleviates fluids), fennel (breaks up fluids), juniper, geranium, [F]grapefruit, ledum, [F]lemongrass, rosemary, **tangerin** (alleviates fluids). *Drink water every 3 hours.*

BLEND—1 fennel, 2 cypress, 5 tangerine. Apply from the top of the foot to the knee

ANKLES—5 cypress, 3 juniper, and 10 tangerine or use equal parts of cypress and tangerine. Apply from ankles to knees and on Vita Flex bladder points on feet.

DIURETIC—[F]Cedarwood, cypress, EndoFlex, fennel, grapefruit, juniper, [F]lavender, lemon [F]lemongrass, onycha (benzoin), orange, oregano, [F]rosemary, [F]sage.

****COMMENTS—For water retention in the legs, Dr. Friedmann rubs tangerine, cypres and juniper on inside of ankle(s) and leg(s) and on the kidney and heart Vita Flex points. He also has his patients inhale the oils as they are rubbed on.*

ELBOW: See TENNIS ELBOW.

ELECTRICAL PROBLEMS IN THE BODY: See BALANCE for methods of balancing the electrical energies of the body. Frankincense, Harmony, Valor.

ELECTROLYTES:

BALANCING—Citrus Fresh (increases absorption of Vitamin C).

SUPPLEMENTS—Super C / Super C Chewable, Mineral Essence.

EMERGENCY OILS: The following oils are recommended by Dr. Daniel Pénoël as ones that everyone should have with them for any emergency:

Melaleuca (Alternifolia)—Colds, coughs, cuts, sore throat, sunburn, wounds.

Ravensara—Powerful antiviral, antiseptic. Respiratory problems, viral infections, wounds.

Peppermint—Analgesic (topical pain reliever) for bumps and bruises. Also for fever, headache, indigestion, motion sickness, nausea, nerve problems, spastic colon, vomiting.

Basil—Earache, fainting, headaches, spasms (can substitute fennel), poisonous insect or snake bites, malaria.

Lavender—Burns (mix with melaleuca), leg cramps, herpes, heart irregularities, hives, insect bites and bee stings, sprains, sunstroke. *If in doubt, use lavender!*

Geranium—Bleeding (increases to eliminate toxins, then stops; can substitute cistus), diarrhea, liver, regenerates tissue and nerves, shingles.

Helichrysum—Bruises, bleeding (stops on contact), hearing, pain, reduce scarring, regenerate tissue.

****COMMENTS: Dr. Pénoël also recommends including Melaleuca ericifolia because it is more suited to children then Melaleuca alternifolia, and also elemi because it has similar properties to frankincense and myrrh but is less expensive.*

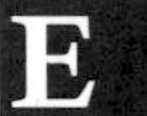

> *For **EMOTIONS**, see other topics such as: ABUSE, AGITATION, ANGER, APATHY, ARGUMENTATIVE, BOREDOM, CONFUSION, DAYDREAMING, DESPAIR, DESPONDENCY, DISAPPOINTMENT, DISCOURAGEMENT, FEAR, FORGETFULNESS, FRUSTRATION, GRIEF/SORROW, GUILT, IRRITABILITY, JEALOUSLY, MOOD SWINGS, OBSESSIVENESS, PANIC, POOR CONCENTRATION, RESENTMENT, RESTLESSNESS, and SHOCK.*
>
> *For more information on using essential oils to help release stored emotions, read Releasing Emotional Patterns using Essential Oils by Carolyn Mein.*
>
> *For some exciting information about how emotions and feelings affect one's physical health, you may want to read Karol K. Truman's books, Feelings Buried Alive Never Die . . . and Healing Feeling from Your Heart.*

MOTIONS: *See EMOTIONAL RELEASE in the Science and Application section at the beginning of the Reference Guide for Essential Oils. Refer to the Auricular Emotional Therapy chart in the Basic Information section of this book for points on the ears where the oils can be applied.* Acceptance, Aroma Siez, Awaken (supports spiritual emotions), Citrus Fresh and spruce (on the chest and breathe in Sacred Mountain), cypress (aromatic, healing), Envision (support and balance), Gathering (to help with feelings and thoughts), geranium (women), German chamomile (stability), goldenrod (relaxing and calming), Gratitude, Humility and Forgiveness (to help with forgiveness), Idaho balsam fir (balancing), lavender (men), melissa (supports mind and body), Live with Passion (balancing, uplifting, strengthening, and stabilizing), ravensara (lifts emotions), Release (soothing), rose (brings balance and harmony to the body), sage lavender (improves mood), Surrender (calming and balancing), 3 Wise Men,

Personal Guide

Transformation, Trauma Life, valerian (helps replace emotions), White Angelica (balances and protects), White lotus.

BLEND—Layer the oils listed below. Wait 10 minutes between each oil to allow the emotions to be released more gently. The individual releasing the emotions should shut their eyes and should have no sounds, music, or candles in the roo to distract them. They need to shut down their senses to get into their subconscious deep seated emotions. Breathe synergistically with their breathi

1. Rub Valor on feet. If there are 2 helpers, have one person hold the individual's feet (your right hand to their right foot, left to left; cross arr if necessary) during the entire procedure. Be sure not to break the energ
2. Rub Peace & Calming on navel, feet, and on the forehead (from left to right).
3. Put Harmony on each chakra in clockwise direction, on wrists, shoulder and inside ankles.
4. Put 3 Wise Men on crown.

BATH AND SHOWER GELS—Evening Peace or Sensation Bath & Shower Gel, Sacred Mountain, Lavender Rosewood, or Peppermint Cedarwood Moisturizi Soaps.

MASSAGE OILS—Relaxation or Sensation Massage Oil.

PERSONAL CARE—Prenolone/Prenolone+, Progessence, Sensation Hand & Body Lotion.

******APPLICATION***—*The oils listed here under Emotions can either be diffused, worn a perfume/cologne, applied behind ears and across forehead, applied directly the ears as specified, or applied to locations as listed in the Emotional Relea part of the Science and Application section of the Reference Guide for Essential Oils.*

ACCEPTANCE (Self-Acceptance)—Acceptance, Forgiveness, Joy, and Transformation. Layer oils on the specific ear point (*refer to the Auricular Emotional Therapy chart in the Basic Information section of this book for location of the HEART point to use for Acceptance*).

ANGER and HATE—Joy (apply to pituitary Vita Flex points on feet and hands as well), Release, and Valor. Layer oils on the specific ear point (*refer to the Auricular Emotional Therapy chart in the Basic Information section of this book for location of the point to use for Anger & Hate*). Other oils that may be useful include Acceptance, Forgiveness, helichrysum (with deep-seated anger for strength to forgive), and Humility.

BALANCE—Forgiveness, frankincense, geranium, Grounding, Harmony, Hope, Inner Child, Joy, juniper, lavender, orange, Present Time, Release, Roman chamomi sandalwood, SARA, 3 Wise Men, Trauma Life, Valor, vetiver, White Angelic

PERSONAL CARE—Prenolone/Prenolone+, Progessence.

BLOCKS—Cypress, frankincense, Harmony, helichrysum, Release (over liver), sandalwood, spearmint, spikenard, spruce, 3 Wise Men, Trauma Life, and Valor help to release emotional blocks. Acceptance can help one accept the change.

BURDENED (Bearing Burdens of the World)—Release and Valor. Layer oils on the specific ear point (*refer to the Auricular Emotional Therapy chart in the Basic Information section of this book for the location of the point to use for Bearing Burdens of the World*). Acceptance may also be good to use.

CHILDHOOD ISSUES—SARA. Apply to the HEART point on the ears.

FEAR (relating to Childhood Issues)—Gentle Baby, Highest Potential, Inner Child, SARA. Apply to the FEAR point on the ears.

FATHER or MOTHER—Gentle Baby and/or Inner Child. Apply to the FATHER or MOTHER point on the ears (*refer to the Auricular Emotional Therapy chart in the Basic Information section of this book for the location of the HEART, FEAR, FATHER, or MOTHER points to use for Childhood Issues*).

The emotions of the mind are the most elusive part of the human body. People are extremely handicapped emotionally and are continually looking for ways to clear these negative emotions. Many of the emotional blends referred to in this book were created from the research of the ancient Egyptian rituals of clearing emotions. They were created with the intent of helping people overcome the trauma of emotional and physical abuse enabling them to progress and achieve their goals and dreams. The Egyptians took three days and three nights to clear emotions. In order to create a very peaceful setting, they would put the person in a room with 10 to 12-inch thick walls of solid cement and close the door so there would be no sight or sound.

CLEARING—Forgiveness, Grounding, Harmony (use Hope when emotional clearing), Inner Child, Joy, juniper, Present Time, Release (massage a couple drops on both ears for a general clearing), SARA, 3 Wise Men, Valor, White Angelica. *For some simple instructions on how to do emotional clearing, refer to the page on Emotional Release in the Science and Application section of the* Reference Guide for Essential Oils. *Another good reference for information on clearing negative emotions is the book, "Releasing Emotional Patterns" by Carolyn L. Mein, D.C.*

COLDNESS (Emotional)—Myrrh, ylang ylang.

CONFIDENCE—Chivalry, Envision, Highest Potential, jasmine (euphoria), Live with Passion.

DEFEATED—Acceptance, cypress, fir, Forgiveness, Inspiration, Joy, juniper, spruce, 3 Wise Men, Valor.

DEPRESSION—Most of the single oils and blends help with depression as they tend to lift by raising one's frequency. Some of the best include Christmas Spirit, Citrus Fresh, Gentle Baby, Highest Potential, Hope, Joy, Peace & Calming, Valor, and White Angelica. Use whichever blend(s) work best for you. Layer oils on the specific ear point (*refer to the Auricular Emotional Therapy chart in the Basic*

Information section of this book for the location of the point to use for Depression). Other oils that may be good to use include Humility, Inner Chi lavender, SARA, and Transformation.

SUPPLEMENTS—Essential Omegas.

EMOTIONAL TRAUMA—Sandalwood, Trauma Life.

EXPRESSION (Self-Expression)—Motivation and Valor (for courage to speak out). Joy may be added to encourage enjoying life to its fullest. Apply to the SELF-EXPRESSION point on the ears. Take deep breaths to help express oneself.

EXCESSIVE—Surrender. Apply to the SELF-EXPRESSION point on the ears.

FOCUSED—Release, then Acceptance or Gathering. Layer oils on the SELF-EXPRESSION point on the ears.

LOST IDENTITY—Inner Child. Apply to the SELF-EXPRESSION point on the ears (*refer to the Auricular Emotional Therapy chart in the Basic Informati section of this book for the location of the SELF-EXPRESSION point*).

EYES—See EYES for oils that help with eyesight.

VISION OF GOALS—Believe, Dream Catcher, Acceptance, 3 Wise Men. Layer o the EYES & VISION point on the ears (*refer to the Auricular Emotional Therapy chart in the Basic Information section of this book for the location the EYES & VISION point*). Envision and Into the Future may also help.

FATHER—Lavender. Apply to the FATHER point on the ears. Another oil that may be helpful to layer on top of lavender is helichrysum, especially when deep-seate anger is present.

CHILDHOOD ISSUES—Gentle Baby or Inner Child. Apply to the FATHER poir on the ears.

MALE ABUSE—Helichrysum and lavender. Layer oils on the FATHER point on ears.

SEXUAL ABUSE—Lavender, Release, and ylang ylang. Layer oils on the FATHI point on the ears. SARA may also be helpful (*refer to the Auricular Emotion Therapy chart in the Basic Information section of this book for the location the FATHER point to use for Father related issues*).

FEAR—Valor, Release, and Joy. Layer on the FEAR point on the ears. Acceptance Harmony, and Highest Potential may also be helpful.

CHILDHOOD ISSUES—Gentle Baby, Inner Child, or SARA. Apply to the FEAR point on the ears.

FUTURE—Into the Future. Apply to the FEAR point on the ears (*refer to the Auricular Emotional Therapy chart in the Basic Information section of this book for the location of the FEAR point*).

FEMALE ISSUES—See MOTHER.

GRIEF—Bergamot. Apply to the HEART point on the ears (*refer to the Auricular Emotional Therapy chart in the Science and Application section for the location of the HEART point to use for Grief*). Another oil that may be helpful is tangerine (when diffused, increases optimism and releases emotional stress).

HEART (Broken or Heavy Heart)—Refer to both GRIEF and LOSS as well. Acceptance, Forgiveness, and Joy. Layer oils on the HEART point on the ears (*refer to the Auricular Emotional Therapy chart in the Science and Application section for the location of the point to use for Heart*). Release, Transformation, and Valor may also be good to use.

LOSS (Eases the Feeling)—Joy, Sensation, tangerine (stability).

MALE ISSUES—See FATHER.

MIND (Open)—3 Wise Men. Apply to the OPEN THE MIND point on the ears as well as the crown of the head and the navel (*refer to the Auricular Emotional Therapy chart in the Basic Information section of this book for the location of the OPEN THE MIND point*). Acceptance, Believe, Clarity, frankincense, Gathering, Magnify Your Purpose, Motivation, Release, sandalwood, and Transformation may also be helpful.

MOTHER—Geranium. Apply to the MOTHER point on the ears. Inner Child and SARA may also be helpful.

ABANDONMENT—Geranium, Acceptance, and Forgiveness. Layer oils on the MOTHER point on the ears.

SEXUAL ABUSE—Geranium and ylang ylang. Layer oils on the MOTHER point on the ears (*refer to the Auricular Emotional Therapy chart in the Basic Information section of this book for the location of the MOTHER point to use for Mother related issues*).

OVERWHELMED—Acceptance and Hope. Layer on the OVERWHELMED point on the ears (*refer to the Auricular Emotional Therapy chart in the Science and Application section for the location of the OVERWHELMED point*). Grounding and Valor may also be helpful.

PITY (Self-Pity)—Acceptance. Apply to the SELF-PITY point on the ears. Forgiveness and Joy may also be helpful.

COURAGE (to move beyond feeling)—Release then Valor. Layer on the SELF-PITY point on the ears.

PAINFUL—Can feel like heaviness in the chest. PanAway. Apply to the SELF-PITY point on the ears (*refer to the Auricular Emotional Therapy chart in the Basic Information section of this book to locate the SELF-PITY point*).

PROTECTION FROM NEGATIVE EMOTIONS—Magnify Your Purpose (empowering and uplifting), grapefruit, Highest Potential, 3 Wise Men (release), White Angelica. Apply oils to the forehead and over the heart.

REJECTION—Forgiveness and Acceptance. Layer on the REJECTION point on the ears. Grounding and Valor may also be helpful.

FROM FATHER—Use lavender first then Forgiveness and Acceptance. Layer on the REJECTION point on the ears.

FROM MOTHER—Use geranium first then Forgiveness and Acceptance. Layer o the REJECTION point on the ears (*refer to the Auricular Emotional Therap chart in the Science and Application section for the location of the REJECTION point*).

RELEASE—[F]Roman chamomile.

STRESS—Believe, Clary sage, Evergreen Essence, Live with Passion, Surrender.

SUICIDAL—Gathering, Hope, Joy, Live with Passion, Release, Trauma Life.

SYMPATHY & GUILT—Joy and Inspiration. Layer on the SYMPATHY & GUILT poi on the ears (*refer to the Auricular Emotional Therapy chart in the Basic Information section of this book for the location of the SYMPATHY & GUIL point*). Release, PanAway, and/or Acceptance may also be helpful.

UPLIFTING—Valor (on feet), birch, Dream Catcher, En-R-Gee, Gratitude, Highest Potential, lemon, orange, Transformation, wintergreen.

VISION—See EYES.

EMPHYSEMA: Eucalyptus, Exodus II, Raven (Hot compress on chest). May use Raven rectally, RC on chest and back. Reverse each night. Thieves on feet, ImmuPower on spine.

SUPPLEMENTS—Exodus.

****COMMENTS—Dr. Terry Friedmann used Exodus on a 68-year-old male who had emphysema. He was on oxygen 24 hours a day. He gave him four per day f one week. When the man came back in, Dr. Friedmann used an oxymeter to test his concentration of blood oxygen. His concentration of blood oxygen, without his oxygen tank, was higher after taking Exodus than it was when he just had his oxygen tank.*

EMPOWERMENT: Magnify Your Purpose, Sacred Mountain, Transformation.

ENDOCRINE SYSTEM: See ADRENAL CORTEX, THYROID, PITUITARY, LUPUS, etc. Black pepper, cinnamon bark, dill, EndoFlex, [F]rosemary, sage lavender.

PERSONAL CARE—Prenolone/ Prenolone+, Progessence.

SUPPLEMENTS—Thyromin and FemiGen (women) or ProGen (men), Power Meal (pre-digested protein). ThermaMist may also help.

The adrenal glands, pituitary gland, thyroid gland, parathyroid glands, thymus gland, pineal gland, pancreas, ovaries, and testes are all a part of the endocrine system. The endocrine glands secrete hormones, transmitted via the bloodstream, which are responsible for regulating growth, metabolism, enzyme activity, and reproduction. Essential oils may either act as hormones or stimulate the endocrine glands to produce hormones. This production of hormones has a regulating effect on the body.

NDOMETRIOSIS: See HORMONAL IMBALANCE. Clary sage, cypress, eucalyptus, geranium, Melrose (hot compress on abdomen), nutmeg, Thieves (on feet).

Endometriosis is the growth of endometrial tissue in abnormal locations as on ovaries or peritoneal (abdominal) cavity.

PERSONAL CARE—Prenolone/ Prenolone+, Progessence, ClaraDerm (spray).

SUPPLEMENTS—Cleansing Trio (ComforTone, Essentialzyme, and ICP), Super C / Super C Chewable, FemiGen.

RECIPE #1—Combine bergamot, lavender, and Clary sage and use with a hot compress over the abdomen or add 2 drops of each to 1 Tbsp. V-6 Mixing Oil and insert into the vagina. Use a tampon to retain overnight. This may help rebuild the normal tissue.

NDURANCE:

PHYSICAL—Balsam fir (inhale from hands), En-R-Gee (on feet), peppermint (cooling)

SUPPLEMENTS—Be-Fit, CardiaCare (with *Rhododendron caucasicum* which has been shown clinically to enhance physical endurance by increasing blood supply to the muscles and brain), Power Meal, WheyFit.

NERGY: Abundance, Awaken, basil (when squandering energy), Black pepper, Clarity, cypress, En-R-Gee, Envision (balances), eucalyptus (builds), [F]fir, Hope, Joy, juniper, lemon, lemongrass, Motivation, myrtle (supports adrenal glands to increase energy), nutmeg (increases), orange (aromatic), peppermint, rosemary, thyme (aromatic; gives energy in times of physical weakness and stress), Valor (balances), White Angelica.

BATH AND SHOWER GELS—Morning Start Bath & Shower Gel or Lemon Sandalwood Cleansing Soap gives you a fresh start with a surge of energy.

ESSENTIAL WATERS (HYDROSOLS)—Basil, Mountain Essence, Peppermint, Thyme. Spray into air or directly on face (don't spray directly in eyes or ears) or diffuse using the Essential Mist Diffuser.

SUPPLEMENTS—VitaGreen (gives energy), Master Formula His/Hers (Multi-Vitamin), Mineral Essence, Thyromin, Super B.

ELECTRICAL ENERGY (frequency)—Forgiveness (high frequency), rose.

INCREASE—Brain Power, Clarity, En-R-Gee, eucalyptus, grapefruit, peppermint, rosemary.

DIFFUSION—See POSITIVE IONS for oils that produce positive ions when diffused to help increase energy.

SUPPLEMENTS—Ultra Young.

INTEGRATES ENERGY FOR EQUAL DISTRIBUTION—Patchouli.

MAGNETIC—Abundance, Joy (enhances and attracts magnetic energy of prosperity and joy around the body).
NEGATIVE—White Angelica (frequency protects against bombardment of), ginger, junipe (clears negative energy).
PHYSICAL—Bergamot, cinnamon bark (aromatic), lemon (aromatic), patchouli (aromatic
SEXUAL ENERGY—Lady Sclareol, Ylang ylang (aromatic; influences).

ENERGY CENTERS: See CHAKRAS.

ENLIGHTENING: Helichrysum.

ENTERITIS: Cajeput.

ENZYMES: Fresh carrot juice has one of the largest concentrations of enzymes. Drink 8 oz. pe day. Add apple and lemon to help with detoxification.
SUPPLEMENTS—Enzyme products: Allerzyme (aids the digestion of sugars, starches, fats, and proteins), Carbozyme (aids the digestion of carbohydrates), Detoxzyme (helps maintain and support a healthy intestinal environment), Fiberzyme (aids the digestion of fiber and enhances the absorption of nutrients) Polyzyme (aids the digestion of protein and helps reduce swelling and discomfort), and Lipozyme (aids the digestion of fats). Also KidScents MightyZyme (chewable, just for kids!).

EPILEPSY: See SEIZURE. Brain Power, Clary sage. Apply to back of neck and brain Vita Flex points on bottom of feet.
SUPPLEMENTS—Cleansing Trio (ComforTone, Essentialzyme, ICP), JuvaPower/JuvaSpice.

OILS TO AVOID IF EPILEPTIC

There are several oils that should not be used if prone to epilepsy. Please see the APPENDIX for safety data on the oils and products mentioned in this book. For further contraindication information, please consult the following books:

Essential Oil Safety—A Guide for Health Care Professionals by Robert Tisserand and Tony Balacs and Aromatherapy for Health Professionals by Shirley and Len Price.

EPSTEIN BARR: See CHRONIC FATIGUE, HYPOGLYCEMIA. Eucalyptus, ImmuPower, Thieves. Do RAINDROP TECHNIQUE on spine with the addition of ImmuPower.
SUPPLEMENTS—AlkaLime, ComforTone, Essentialzyme, Exodus, ICP, ImmuGel, ImmuneTune, ImmuPro, JuvaPower/JuvaSpice, JuvaTone, Mineral Essence, Super C / Super C Chewable, Thyromin, VitaGreen.

QUILIBRIUM: Surrender (emotional), ylang ylang.
NERVE—Petitgrain.

SSENTIAL OILS: Essential oils function as a catalyst to deliver nutrients to starving cells.
SENSITIVE TO SKIN (caustic, high in phenols, may need to dilute)—Cinnamon bark, clove, fennel, grapefruit, lemon, nutmeg, orange, oregano, peppermint. Test the oil first in a small, sensitive area. If irritation occurs, dilute with 1 drop of above oil to 20 drops lavender or mix with V-6 Mixing Oil.

E

STROGEN: Clary sage, SclarEssence, and Mister help the body produce estrogen. Anise (increases).
****COMMENTS—Some sugar sweeteners block estrogen. Honey goes into blood stream quickly, which affects the pancreas and the production of estrogen.*
PERSONAL CARE—Prenolone/Prenolone+ (pregnenolone is master hormone; used to balance estrogen and progesterone, whichever is needed).
SUPPLEMENTS—2 FemiGen three times a day, ten days before period. Start again two days after cycle. May take up to 6 tablets three times a day. CortiStop (Women's) can also help increase estrogen levels by lowering cortisol levels.
TINCTURE—1 dropper of Estro three times a day in water.

UPHORIA: Clary sage (aromatic), jasmine.

XHAUSTION: First, work with one or more of the following nervous system oils to calm and relax: Bergamot, Clary sage, coriander, cumin, elemi, frankincense, lavender, pine, sage lavender. Secondly, use basil, ginger, grapefruit, lavender, lemon, Roman chamomile, rosemary, sandalwood, or Transformation.

XPECTORANT: Black pepper, elemi, eucalyptus, frankincense, helichrysum, [F]marjoram, mugwort, pine, [F]ravensara. Apply oils to throat, lungs, and diffuse.

XPRESSION (Self Expression): Helichrysum, Into the Future, Joy (when unable to express physically), Motivation, Raven, RC, Transformation, Valor.

YES: Thieves on feet (especially 2 big toes), M-Grain on thumb prints, layer Mister, Dragon Time and EndoFlex on Vita Flex points, ankles, and pelvis. Carrot is good around eye

NEVER PUT OILS DIRECTLY IN THE EYES!

Be careful when applying oils near the eyes. Be sure to have some V-6 Mixing Oil handy for additional dilution if irritation occurs. Never use water to wash off an oil that irritates.

Personal Guide

area, cypress (also helps circulation), fennel, frankincense, German chamomile lavender, lemon, lemongrass (improves eyesight).

BASE OILS (good blends of)—Almond or hazelnut.

SUPPLEMENTS—Essential Manna, Power Meal, Sulfurzyme, Wolfberry Bars.

TINCTURES—Add AD&E drops for all eye problems.

****COMMENTS—Refer to The chapter entitled "How to Use - The Personal Usage Reference" in the Essential Oils Desk Reference under "Eye Disorders" for additional recipe, oil, and supplement recommendations.*

EYE DROP RECIPE—Combine 5 parts distilled water, 2 parts honey, and 1 part apple cider vinegar (do not use white vinegar). Mix together and store in a bottle. Does not need to be refrigerated. This special eye drop formula is fou in Stanley Burroughs' book, *Healing for the Age of Enlightenment* and has proven over the years to be superior to most commercial eye drops. These drc have been successful for helping to clear glaucoma, cataracts, spots, film, and growths of various kinds. Apply drops one at a time to each eye several times day until condition has cleared.

CATARACTS—

BLEND #1—8 lemongrass, 6 cypress, and 3 eucalyptus. Apply around the eye area two times a day. Don't get in the eyes.

DRY-ITCHY—Melaleuca (in humidifier).

EYE LID DROP (or DROOPING EYELIDS)—

BLEND #2—Aroma Life, 1 helichrysum, 5 lavender.

BLEND #3—Helichrysum and peppermint (don't get in the eyes).

MASSAGE OILS—Cel-Lite-Magic (around eyes).

SUPPLEMENTS—3 VitaGreen four times a day. After massaging Vita Flex points eat 2 whole oranges a day with the white still on the orange. It is very importa to eat all the white you can plus Super C / Super C Chewable, ComforTone, a ICP (fiber beverage) after meals.

VITA FLEX POINTS—Fingers, toes, and around the eyes.

IMPROVE VISION—Dragon Time, EndoFlex, frankincense, juniper, lemongrass, Mister, M-Grain, Thieves. Apply oils to feet, Vita Flex eye points, thumbs, ankles, pelvis, eye area (not in eyes), eyebrows. *According to Dr. Mercola, just about any oil can be used if it is consistently rubbed aroun each eye for several minutes twice a day. This must be continued for at leas*

I have had glaucoma for several years and have had my eye drop prescription changed numerous times because of rising pressure. I used a mixture of one third clove, one third lemon, and one third olive oil and rubbed it on my face above and below my eyes. The last time I was at the doctor, my pressure was 14. It was the lowest pressure I have had since I was diagnosed.

-Submitted by K. Ernst (July 2004)

weeks before any improvement can be seen. He recommends using ***frankincense and lavender.***

BLEND #4—10 lemongrass, 5 cypress, 3 *Eucalyptus radiata*, in 1 oz. V-6 Mixing Oil. Apply around eyes morning and night to improve eyesight. Can also be applied to Vita Flex eye points on fingers and toes, and also on the ears *(refer to the Auricular Emotional Therapy chart in the Basic Information section of this book for the Eyes and Vision point on the ears).*

BLEND #5—5 lemongrass, 3 cypress, 2 eucalyptus, in 1 oz. of V-6 Mixing Oil. Apply as a blend or layer the oils on the eye area (not in eyes).

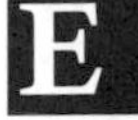

TINCTURES—AD&E to take the pressure off the liver and intestines and to improve the vision.

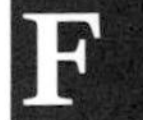

****COMMENTS—One individual, who was not able to see color and had no peripheral vision, rubbed frankincense on his eyelids and just above his eyebrows. Soon thereafter he was able to see color and his peripheral vision returned.*

IRIS, INFLAMMATION OF—Eucalyptus.

RETINA (Bleeding)—

BLEND #6—5 tangerine, 5 orange, and 5 grapefruit. Mix and apply 2 drops on fingers and toes. Massage Vita Flex points two times a day or more. Diffuse and let vapor mist around eye. Rub Cel-Lite Magic around the eyes too. Then, eat two whole oranges a day with the white still on the orange. Eat all of the white you can.

SUPPLEMENTS—Super C / Super C Chewable.

RETINA (Strengthen)—Cypress, lavender, lemongrass, helichrysum, juniper, peppermint, sandalwood. Apply oil(s) around eye area.

BLEND #7—5 juniper, 3 lemongrass, 3 cypress. Rub on brain stem twice a day.

SPIRITUAL EYES (3rd eye, brow chakra)—Acceptance, Awaken, Dream Catcher. Rub oil on ear lobe to increase both physical and spiritual vision.

SWOLLEN EYES—Cypress and helichrysum. Lavender (antiseptic) is also safe around eyes. If swollen eyes are due to allergies, try putting peppermint on the back of the neck.

ACIAL OILS: Refer to the Personal Care section of the Reference Guide for Essential Oils for many other beneficial skin care products.

BROKEN CAPILLARIES—Cypress, geranium, hyssop, Roman chamomile.

DEHYDRATED—Geranium, lavender.

DISTURBED—Clary sage, geranium, hyssop, juniper, lavender, lemon, patchouli, Roman chamomile, sandalwood.

DRY—Geranium, German chamomile, hyssop, lemon, patchouli, rosemary, sandalwood.

ENERGIZING—Bergamot, lemon.

HYDRATED—Cypress, fennel, geranium, hyssop, lavender, lemon, patchouli, sandalwood.

NORMAL—Geranium, lavender, lemon, Roman chamomile, sandalwood.
OILY—Cypress, frankincense, geranium, jasmine, juniper, lavender, lemon, marjoram, orange, patchouli, Roman chamomile, rosemary.
REVITALIZING—Cypress, fennel, lemon.
SENSITIVE—Geranium, German chamomile, lavender.

FAINTING: See SHOCK. Nutmeg. Hold one of the following under the nose: Basil, Black pepper, Brain Power, Clarity, lavender, neroli, peppermint, rosemary, spearmint, Trauma Life.

FAITH: Hope (increases), Transformation (for anchoring and stabilizing new-found faith).

FASTING: Fasting is the avoidance of solid foods altogether, while liquid consumption ranges between nothing (complete avoidance of all liquids as well) to fresh juices with just water being somewhere in the middle. **Complete avoidance fasting (no food or liquid) should only be done when feeling good**, while fasting on fres juices can be very healing when sick. The Master Cleanser Lemonade fast (se CLEANSING) is one of the most beneficial juice fasts. While it takes 30 days on this cleanse to change the chemistry in the body (such as eliminating the nee or desire for animal proteins), very effective health results can be achieved afte only 10 days. To enhance the effectiveness of the change in body chemistry, th 30-day lemon juice fast can be followed by a carrot juice fast for another 30 days. Bodygize and VitaGreen may be taken two times a day for two weeks bu should then be stopped so changes can be made at the cellular level; protein prevents this change. When a mother fasts, the breast fed baby gets the benefi as well (the mammary glands filter the toxins so they are not harmful to the baby).

FAT: See CELLULITE, DIET and WEIGHT.

BATH (ATTACK FAT)—Add 6 drops of blend to the bath water and soak in tub.

BLEND—8 grapefruit, 5 cypress, 4 lavender, 4 basil, and 3 juniper.

> *Ultra Young may help stimulate the pituitary for increased production of the human growth hormone. This hormone is one of the most powerful side-effect-free agents for rejuvenating the body, restoring lean body mass, and reducing fat.*

SUPPLEMENT—Allerzyme (aids the digestion of sugars, starches, fats, and proteins Lipozyme (aids the digestion of fats), ThermaMist (blocks fat synthesis and regulates appetite with HCA, spray before meals or when cravings occur), Power Meal (eat for breakfast as a meal replacement), Ultra Young (improves fat-to-lean ratios by stimulating production of the human growth hormone).

****COMMENTS—Eat more grapefruit to dissolve fat faster.*

FATHER (Problems with): Acceptance, lavender, Valor. Apply to ears (*refer to the Auricular Emotional Therapy chart in the Basic Information section of this book*).

FATIGUE: Clove, En-R-Gee, pine, [F]ravensara (muscle), [F]rosemary (nervous), [F]thyme (general).

MENTAL—Basil, Clarity, lemongrass, Peace & Calming. Basil and lemongrass together are a good combination. Apply on temples, back of neck, feet and diffuse.

OVERCOMING—Thyme or En-R-Gee on spine, wait a few minutes, then Awaken all over the back and spine; OR En-R-Gee on feet and Awaken on temples and cheeks.

PHYSICAL—See ENERGY. Clarity, Peace & Calming. Apply on liver, feet, diffuse, and as a body massage.

SUPPLEMENTS—AlkaLime (acid-neutralizing mineral formulation), Berrygize Nutrition Bars, ImmuGel, Power Meal, Sulfurzyme, Thyromin, VitaGreen.

FATTY DEPOSITS: See CELLULITE and WEIGHT.

DISSOLVE—

SUPPLEMENTS—Allerzyme (aids the digestion of sugars, starches, fats, and proteins), Body Balancing Trio (Bodygize, Master Formula His/Hers, VitaGreen), Lipozyme (aids the digestion of fats), Power Meal.

FEAR: Bergamot, Clary sage, cypress, fir, geranium, Highest Potential, Hope, juniper, marjoram, Motivation (releases emotional and physical fears), myrrh, orange, Present Time, Roman chamomile, rose, sandalwood, spruce, Valor, White Angelica, ylang ylang.

Fear causes the blood vessels to tighten, restricting the amount of oxygen and nutrients that can reach the cells.

FEET: Fennel, lavender, lemon, pine (excessive sweating), Roman chamomile.

CALLOUSES—

CLUB FOOT—Massage with one of the following—Ginger (see below), lavender, Roman chamomile, rosemary (see below).

CORNS—See CORNS.

NOT TO BE USED ON BABIES EXCEPT FOR CLUB FOOT—Ginger, rosemary.

ODOR—Mix 1 Tbs. baking powder with 2 drops of sage and put in a plastic bag. Shake and eliminate lumps with a rolling pin and put in shoes. Rub calamus of feet.

FEMALE PROBLEMS: See HORMONAL IMBALANCE, INFERTILITY, MENOPAUSE, MENSTRUATION, OVARIES, PMS, PREGNANCY, UTERUS, ETC. Anise, Mister (during time of month when you are out of sorts), Clary sage, Sacred Mountain (female balance).

SUPPLEMENTS—Body Balancing Trio Hers (Bodygize, Master Formula Hers, VitaGreen), FemiGen, Prenolone/Prenolone+, Progessence.

ABNORMAL PAP SMEARS—

RECIPE #1—Add 10 drops ImmuPower and 5 drops frankincense to 1 Tbsp. V-6 Mixing Oil and insert into vagina. Use tampon to retain overnight. Take Master Formula Hers to support nutrient levels and ImmuneTune to support the body. May continue daily for as long as necessary.

BALANCE FEMALE HORMONES—Bergamot, sage lavender, ylang ylang.

BATH AND SHOWER GELS—Dragon Time Bath & Shower Gel for that time of month which leaves women with lower back pain, stress, and sleeping difficulties. Pour 1 tsp. to 1 oz. of the gel in water while filling your tub.

SUPPLEMENTS—Three times a day one week before cycle starts, take 2 droppers full of F.H.S. (available through Creer Labs 801-465-5423) in water after starting. One week after the cycle, take Master Formula Hers four times a day and 6 VitaGreen a day. CortiStop (Women's) can also help reduce cortisol levels and balance hormones.

HEMORRHAGING—See HEMORRHAGING.

MASSAGE OILS—Combine 10 helichrysum with 1 tsp. V-6 Mixing Oil and massage around ankles, lower back, and stomach.

INFECTION—[F]Bergamot (general), frankincense, and Melrose (may mix and insert in vagina at night; may alternate with the blend below).

BLEND #1— 8 juniper, 8 melaleuca, and 8 Purification. Put in water and douche OR 3 drops of each in 1 tsp. V-6 Mixing Oil and insert at night using a tampon to retain.

BLEND #2—8 juniper, 8 lavender, and 8 Melrose. Alternate with Blend #1 and follow same instructions.

INFERTILITY (FEMALE)—See FERTILITY. Clary sage, cypress, fennel, geranium, melissa, nutmeg, Roman chamomile, SclarEssence, thyme. Before the cycle, rub 10 drops Dragon Time around ankles, lower back, and lower stomach. During the cycle, rub 4 drops basil in the same places as before.

PERSONAL CARE—Prenolone/Prenolone+, Progessence.

SUPPLEMENTS—Essential Manna, FemiGen, Master Formula Hers, VitaGreen.

OVARIES—See OVARIES.

PMS—See PMS.

MASSAGE OILS—Dragon Time.

PERSONAL CARE—Prenolone/Prenolone+, Progessence.

SUPPLEMENTS—Berrygize Nutrition Bars, Body Balancing Trio Hers (Bodygize, Master Formula Hers, VitaGreen), Essential Omegas, FemiGen.

POSTPARTUM DEPRESSION— Basil, Clary sage, Gentle Baby, Harmony, Joy, nutmeg (see the safety data in the APPENDIX of this book), Peace & Calming, Valor, White Angelica.

PERSONAL CARE—Prenolone/Prenolone+, Progessence.

SUPPLEMENTS—Essential Omegas.

Some women have had wonderful results with the following recipe:

Natural Progesterone or Pregnenolone may help prevent postpartum depression. *Just before a woman has a baby her body produces about 400 mg of progesterone each day to help hold the placenta in place. When the baby is born, the production of progesterone falls dramatically. The body's inability to produce high doses of progesterone can help induce postpartum depression.*

RECIPE #1—Valor first (2-5 drops on each foot and hold to balance energies), Harmony (use finger to dab small amount on each energy center (chakra)), Joy (apply a drop between and just above the breasts), and White Angelica (on the crown of the head and over the top of the shoulders).

REPRODUCTIVE SYSTEM—FemiGen (may help build and balance the reproductive system and maintain better hormonal balance for developmental years all the way through menopause).

ERTILITY: Bergamot, Clary sage, Dragon Time, fennel, geranium, melissa, Mister, sage, SclarEssence (taken as a dietary supplement to help raise estradiol and testosterone levels), Sensation, yarrow. Apply on reproductive Vita Flex areas on feet, particularly around front of ankle, in line with ankle bone, on each side of ankle under ankle bone, and up along the Achilles tendon. Women: on lower back and on lower abdomen near pubic bone. Can also dilute with V-6 Mixing Oil and use as vaginal retention implant. Men: on lower abdomen near pubic bone, on area between scrotum and rectum, and as a rectal implant (diluted with V-6 Mixing Oil).

PERSONAL CARE—Prenolone/Prenolone+, Progessence, Protec (as rectal or vaginal implant).

SUPPLEMENTS—AlkaLime, Essential Manna, Ultra Young, VitaGreen. FemiGen (women) and ProGen (men).

****COMMENTS—An accumulation of petrochemicals in the body can cause sterility in both men and women. Do the MASTER CLEANSER (See CLEANSING) for 10 to 20 days consecutively. After coming off the cleanse, focus on alkaline-ash foods. When the body is acidic, it can be hard to conceive.*

EVER: Basil, bergamot, clove (taken internally), [F]eucalyptus, fennel (breaks up), fir, ginger, ImmuPower (rub on spine), lavender, ledum, [F]lemon or lime (reduces–1 or 2 drops in rice milk or water and sip slowly), melaleuca, [F]peppermint (reduces–1 or 2 drops in rice milk or water and sip slowly), rosemary cineol, sage lavender, spearmint (not on babies). Peppermint can also be diffused in the room or applied to the bottom of feet.

PERSONAL CARE—Cinnamint Lip Balm.

SUPPLEMENTS—AlkaLime, ImmuGel, Mineral Essence, Super C / Super C Chewable.

TO COOL THE SYSTEM—Bergamot, Clove (internally), *Eucalyptus radiata*, peppermint (or Peppermint Floral Water).

My daughter, Haley, at age 18 was ill one Sunday, and later in the evening was feeling quite worse. When we checked, she had a fever of 105 degrees. I filled a gel capsule with 10 drops of Clove oil and had her take it with some water. In 1/2 an hour I checked her temperature again and it was down to 102. I gave her 5 more drops in another capsule and in another 1/2 hour, her fever was totally gone!!

-Submitted by Sally Donahue
Wilsonville, Oregon (July 2004)

TO INDUCE SWEATING—Basil, cypress, fennel, lavender, melaleuca, peppermint, Roman chamomile, rosemary.

FIBER: ICP is a fiber beverage, designed to bulk up in liquid and flush out the intestines.
SUPPLEMENTS—Cleansing Trio (ComforTone, Essentialzyme, and ICP).

FIBROCYSTS: See HORMONAL IMBALANCE.

FIBROIDS: See HORMONAL IMBALANCE. Cistus, EndoFlex, frankincense, helichrysum, Idaho tansy, lavender, oregano, pine, Valor. Put 3 drops of either oil in douch Also apply to Vita Flex points of feet.
MASSAGE OILS—Cel-Lite Magic.
PERSONAL CARE—Protec.
SUPPLEMENTS—AlkaLime, Essentialzyme, Power Meal, Thyromin, Ultra Young, VitaGreen.

FIBROMYALGIA: See ACIDOSIS, HORMONAL IMBALANCE. May need to detoxify the liver. ImmuPower; massage with PanAway adding birch/wintergreen & spruce for an additional cortisone response. It may be helpful to use some anti-inflammatory oils like birch, helichrysum, lavender, myrrh, patchouli, rosemary, rosewood, spruce, thyme, or wintergreen.

***Fibromyalgia** is a condition of high acid and generalized pain all over the body; tiny movement brings on pain; extra low pain threshold. Since there are very few positive findings, it is difficult to diagnose. Some sources say that natural progesterone may be beneficial.*

MASSAGE OILS—Ortho Ease or Ortho Sport (for full body), and do the Raindrop Technique.
SUPPLEMENTS— Allerzyme (aids the digestion of sugars, starches, fats, and proteins), AlkaLime (combat yeast and fungus overgrowth and preserve the body's proper pH balance), Bodygize (for vitamins and minerals), Coral Sea (highly bio-available calcium, contains 58 trace minerals), Essential Manna,

ImmuneTune (four days), JuvaTone, Mineral Essence, Power Meal, Royaldophilus, Stevia Select, **Sulfurzyme**, Super C / Super C Chewable, Super Cal (no more than 1 per day, because of the poor ability to utilize minerals), VitaGreen (to get alkaline balance).

****COMMENTS—Dr. Bernard Jensen suggested that people with fibromyalgia should eliminate all refined sugars from their diet. Refer to The chapter entitled "How to Use - The Personal Usage Reference" in the Essential Oils Desk Reference under "Fibromyalgia" for an excellent supplement regimen.*

BROSITIS: See HORMONAL IMBALANCE.

BLEND—Combine 2 cinnamon bark, 10 eucalyptus, 10 ginger, 6 nutmeg, 10 peppermint, and 3 rosemary with 2 Tbs. V-6 Mixing Oil and massage chest and back once a day.

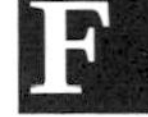

NGER:

MASHED—Geranium (for the bruising), helichrysum (to stop the bleeding), lavender (to help for all things), lemongrass (for tissue repair), and PanAway (for the pain).

.ATULENCE (gas): Angelica, anise, bergamot, cardamom, coriander, cumin, eucalyptus, fennel, [F]ginger, juniper, [F]lavender, myrrh, nutmeg, onycha (benzoin), peppermint, Roman chamomile, rosemary, spearmint (not for babies), [F]tarragon. Apply oil(s) to stomach, abdomen, and Vita Flex points of feet.

.U: Blue cypress (aches and pains), clove, ImmuPower, RC, Raven (apply to thymus area, Vita Flex points on feet, chest, back, and on any place where the flu has settled), *Eucalyptus radiata*, Exodus II, fir (aches and pains), goldenrod, ginger, Idaho tansy (on bottom of feet), lavender, ledum, [F]melaleuca, *Melaleuca ericifolia*, [F]myrtle, onycha (benzoin), orange, oregano, [F]peppermint,

One Sunday after church a friend commented that I looked "exhausted." I thought that strange because I had gotten a good night's sleep. I walked over to a meeting for a mission trip I would be participating in, and an hour later I started getting a headache and felt something happening to my throat. About 30 minutes later I knew I was coming down with the flu as the headache and sore throat intensified and I started feeling shaky. Fortunately I had peppermint, oregano and Thieves in my truck, and as soon as I got in, I rubbed several drops of oregano on my feet, rubbed Thieves on my neck and throat, and put several drops of peppermint in my water and started drinking it. By the time I got home the headache and sore throat had lessened. That evening and for the next several days I took by capsule a combination of lemon, Mountain savory and oregano three times a day. While I could tell my body was fighting an infection (as indicated by my desire to take naps), the oils completely stopped the flu in its tracks and the headache and sore throat never returned.

-Submitted by Kevin Dunn
Los Angeles, California (July 2004)

Personal Guide

pine, [F]rosemary, sage lavender, Thieves, thyme (apply to thymus point on feet and where flu has settled), tsuga.

****COMMENTS—According to the Essential Oils Desk Reference, "[Idaho] tansy shou be applied topically on stomach and bottom of feet." (EDR-June 2002; Ch. 2 Flu)* It may be best to dilute Idaho tansy first in one teaspoon V-6 Mixing Oil or Massage Oil before topical application.

BATH—2 Tbs. Evening Peace Bath & Shower Gel with drops of the following oils: birch/wintergreen, 20 eucalyptus, 5 frankincense, 3 helichrysum, 15 ravensara and 6 spruce. Mix together and put mixture under the faucet while running HOT bath water. SOAK until cool. Also consider using Thieves Cleansing Soap to wash hands with, especially during cold and flu season.

SUPPLEMENTS—Essentialzyme, Exodus, ImmuneTune, ImmuGel, Master Formu His/Hers, ParaFree, Super C / Super C Chewable.

FLUIDS: See EDEMA or DIURETIC.

FOCUS: Believe, Brain Power (during strenuous mental activity), Clarity, Gathering (for great focus), Highest Potential, Surrender (balancing; clears the mind).

SUPPLEMENTS—Sulfurzyme.

FOOD: See pH BALANCE. Use basil for soups and stuffing. Use cinnamon bark, clove, orange, tangerine, and thyme for flavorings.

The body secretes pepsin, protease and hydrochloric acid in the morning for the digestion of protein. If you eat fruit in the morning you have almost instant putrefaction (fermentation). Sub-acid fruits (like strawberries) are the only fruit that can be eaten with protein.

****COMMENTS—According to the Essential Oils Desk Reference, "They are so concentrated that only 1-2 drop of an essential oil is equivalent to a full bottle (1-2 oz. size) of dried herbs. . For a recipe that serves six to ten people, add 1 to 2 drops of an oil and stir after cooking and just before serving, so the oil does not evaporate." (EDR-June 2002; Ch. 4; Other Uses; Cooking) Refer to that same section in the Essential Oils Desk Reference for more ideas on cooking with essential oils.*

BREAKFAST—Proteins (meat, fish, eggs), mixed grains, sunflower seeds, nuts, Power Meal, and Bodygize. Fruit in the morning will cause candida overgrowth, hypoglycemia, and dysfunction of the thyroid gland. Take Essentialzyme or Polyzyme to help with the digestion, especially when animal protein has been eaten. Also, 8 oz. of carrot juice per day with apple and lemon helps detoxify the body and provides necessary enzymes.

LUNCH—Eat salads, complex carbohydrates like rice, beans, soup, steamed vegetables, bread (Jack Sprout Bread is good) that is toasted (reduces gluten content), bak potatoes, yams, squash, Bodygize.

AFTER 3:00 p.m.—Refrain from eating animal proteins. Bodygize and Power Meal are predigested proteins and can be eaten with fruit. Foods that are easier on the digestive system at night are fruit, soups, lightly steamed vegetables, and salads.

ASSIMILATION OF—

SUPPLEMENTS—Enzyme products: Allerzyme (aids the digestion of sugars, starches, fats, and proteins), Carbozyme (aids the digestion of carbohydrates), Detoxzyme (helps maintain and support a healthy intestinal environment), Essentialzyme (multiple enzyme product), Fiberzyme (aids the digestion of fiber and enhances the absorption of nutrients), Polyzyme (aids the digestion of protein and helps reduce swelling and discomfort), and Lipozyme (aids the digestion of fats).

FIBER—ICP (fiber beverage).

OIL—V-6 Mixing Oil (six different vegetable oils) is excellent for cooking and making salad dressings.

SUGAR SUBSTITUTE—Stevia, Stevia Select.

Buttered Basil Garlic Melt
1 loaf cheese bread or any artisan bread, cut into 1 inch slices
1/2 stick butter
1/2 teaspoon garlic powder
*4 drops **basil** essential oil*
Sliced mozzarella cheese

Melt butter then add garlic powder and stir well. Add basil oil, mix well. With a large unused paint brush, brush on butter mixture until saturated. Cover sliced bread with slices of cheese and bake at 350° until golden brown. Yummmmmie! Even my Baby loved it.

-Submitted by Jill Burk
Saginaw, Michigan (July 2004)

F

FOOD POISONING: Flavor a cup of water with 6 drops Di-Tone, swish around in mouth, and swallow. Exodus II, patchouli, rosemary cineol, tarragon, Thieves.

SUPPLEMENTS—Detoxzyme, Essentialzyme, Exodus.

FOREHEAD: Jasmine.

FORGETFULNESS: See MEMORY. Acceptance (over heart and liver), Brain Power (1 drop under tongue), cedarwood, Clarity, cypress, Dream Catcher, Highest Potential, Hope, fir, Gathering, geranium, juniper, marjoram, myrrh, orange, Present Time, Roman chamomile, rose, sandalwood, 3 Wise Men, rose, sage lavender Valor, White Angelica, ylang ylang. Wear as perfume/cologne or put a couple drops in hands, rub together, cup over nose and mouth, and breathe deeply.

SUPPLEMENTS—Essential Manna, Ultra Young/Ultra Young+, VitaGreen.

FORGIVE (and FORGET): Acceptance, Forgiveness, 3 Wise Men, Transformation, Valor, White Angelica.

FORMALDEHYDE: Purification (removes).

FORTIFYING: Cypress.

FRECKLES: Idaho tansy. Mix 2-3 drops with lotion and spread over face. Can be used two or three times per week.

FREE RADICALS:

ELIMINATE—

SUPPLEMENTS—Berry Young Juice, Chelex, and ImmuGel help eliminate and prevent the build up of free radicals.

FRIGIDITY: See LIBIDO, SEX STIMULANT. Chivalry, [F]Clary sage, jasmine, Lady Sclareol, nutmeg (overcome frigidity and impotence), rose, [F]ylang ylang (helps balance male/female energies).

SUPPLEMENTS—Prenolone/Prenolone+, Progessence.

FRUSTRATION: Acceptance, Clary sage, frankincense, Gathering, ginger, Hope, Humility, juniper, lavender, lemon, orange, peppermint, Present Time, Roman chamomile, spruce, 3 Wise Men, thyme, Valor, ylang ylang.

FUNGUS: Abundance, cajeput, clove, fennel, geranium, ImmuPower, lavender, lemongrass, melaleuca, Melrose, RC, Raven, Roman chamomile, rosemary verbenon, Thieves. Apply topically (dilution with V-6 Mixing Oil may be necessary depending on the oil) or add to bath water. Do the RAINDROP TECHNIQUE to help purge the body of pathogenic fungi that may exist along the spinal cord or in the lymphatic system. May also try the MASTER CLEANSER (See CLEANSING) to clean out the intestinal tract and re-alkalinize the body.

BLEND—2 myrrh, 2 lavender. Put on location.

SUPPLEMENTS—AlkaLime (designed to combat yeast and fungus overgrowth and preserve the body's proper pH balance), Essentialzyme, ImmuGel, Royaldophilus, Stevia Select (with FOS - combats overgrowth of bad bacteria), Super C / Super C Chewable, Thyromin, VitaGreen.

I had developed a ***fungus*** *on my big toenails. The fungus was bad enough that the white, thick toenail was making shoes painful. I went to a podiatric doctor. The doctor removed the inside edge of the left big toenail down to the nail bed. He then prescribed some medicine that was $80 a tube to get rid of the rest. It continued to get worse and was spreading all over the nails and was headed for the rest of the nail beds. I decided to use Animal Scents Ointment on my toes 3 times a day. Now my nails are normal and the thickness is gone.*

-Submitted by K. Ernst (July 2004)

****COMMENTS—Refer to The chapter entitled "How to Use - The Personal Usage Reference" in the <u>Essential Oils Desk Reference</u> under "Fungal Infections" for some excellent blends and tips for combating systemic fungal infections.*

FUNGAL INFECTIONS—*Eucalyptus citriodora*, geranium, melaleuca (Tea Tree), patchouli.

PREVENTS GROWTH OF—<u>Melrose</u> (two times a day for seven days), <u>Purification</u>.

ALLBLADDER: <u>Forgiveness</u>, [F]geranium, [F]German chamomile, juniper, <u>Juva Cleanse</u>, <u>JuvaFlex</u> (stimulates), lavender, <u>Release</u>, rosemary (supports), <u>Surrender</u> (over liver & pancreas). Apply over gallbladder area (can use a hot compress) and vita Flex points on feet. Also, 2 capsules <u>JuvaFlex</u> - AM, 2 <u>Juva Cleanse</u> - PM.

SUPPLEMENTS—Essentialzyme, Sulfurzyme (aids bile secretion and magnifies effects of vitamins).

INFECTION IN—[F]Helichrysum.

STONES—Geranium, grapefruit, juniper, <u>Juva Cleanse</u>, lime, [F]nutmeg, rosemary, wintergreen.

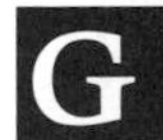

ANGRENE: Cistus, elemi, <u>Exodus II</u>, <u>ImmuPower</u>, lavender (used by Dr. Gattefossé to recover from gas gangrene), <u>Melrose</u>, Mountain savory, ravensara, <u>Thieves</u>, thyme.

SUPPLEMENTS—Exodus, ImmuGel, ImmuneTune, ImmuPro, Super C / Super C Chewable.

AS: See FLATULENCE. [F]Lavender, nutmeg, onycha (benzoin), tarragon. Apply to large intestine Vita Flex points on the feet.

ASTRITIS: (Inflammation of the stomach lining). See ANTI-INFLAMMATORY. Calamus, <u>Di-Tone</u>, fennel, laurel, peppermint, pine, sage, spikenard, tarragon, yarrow. Apply over stomach area with hot compress. One drop of oil in rice or almond milk taken as a dietary supplement (*NOTE: use only those oils approved for internal use by FDA. Look for GRAS or FA designations in "Single Oil Summary Information" in the Appendix*).

SUPPLEMENTS—AlkaLime, Cleansing Trio (ComforTone, Essentialzyme, and ICP), Mineral Essence, Royaldophilus.

ENERAL TONIC: Grapefruit, lemon, Mountain savory, [F]spruce.

ENITALS: [F]Clary sage.

ENTLENESS: Rosewood (aromatic).

GERMS: See BACTERIA.
AIRBORNE—Fir.
GERMICIDAL—[F]Lemon, RC.

GINGIVITIS: Forgiveness, Harmony, helichrysum, melaleuca, Melrose, myrrh, Present Time, rose, rosemary, [F]sage, Thieves. Apply on throat and gums.
PERSONAL CARE—Dentarome/Dentarome Plus Toothpaste (contains Thieves), Fresh Essence Mouthwash (contains Thieves), KidScents Toothpaste (for children).

GLANDULAR SYSTEM: [F]Sage, spearmint, spruce. Blue cypress may help stimulate the amygdala, pineal gland, pituitary gland, and hypothalamus.
SUPPLEMENTS—ProGen (male) or FemiGen (female) for glandular nutrients.

GLAUCOMA: See EYES.
SUPPLEMENTS—Essentialzyme (to help relieve stress on the pancreas, if congestec Sulfurzyme (to help regulate the fluid pressure in the eye), Super C / Super C Chewable, Super B.

GOITER: See ENDOCRINE SYSTEM, LYMPHATIC SYSTEM. Cleanse the lymphatic system. Balance the endocrine system with EndoFlex.

GOUT: Basil, birch, calamus, [F]fennel, geranium, hyssop, Juva Cleanse, JuvaFlex, [F]lemon, nutmeg, onycha (benzoin), PanAway, pine, thyme, wintergreen, yarrow. Cleanse with MASTER CLEANSER (See CLEANSING) and drink lots of fluids (water, juices, etc.).
MASSAGE OILS—Ortho Ease and Ortho Sport.
SUPPLEMENTS—ArthroTune, Cleansing Trio (ComforTone, Essentialzyme, and ICP), CardiaCare (with *Rhododendron caucasicum* which helps increase uric acid elimination), Cleansing Trio (ComforTone, Essentialzyme, and ICP), Cor Sea (highly bio-available calcium, contains 58 trace minerals), Essential Mann JuvaTone, Mineral Essence, Sulfurzyme, Super C / Super C Chewable, Super Cal, Thyromin, VitaGreen.
****COMMENTS—Refer to The chapter entitled "How to Use - The Personal Usage Reference" in the Essential Oils Desk Reference under "Gout" for some excellent blend recipes and supplement recommendations.*

GRAVES DISEASE: See THYROID: HYPERTHYROIDISM. Blue tansy, EndoFlex, lemongrass, myrrh, spruce.

SUPPLEMENTS—ImmuPro, Mineral Essence, Sulfurzyme (helps mitigate effects of autoimmune diseases), Thyromin, VitaGreen.

RIEF/SORROW: Bergamot (turns grief into joy), Clary sage, eucalyptus, Forgiveness, Gentle Baby (massage whole body), Hope, Joy (over the heart), juniper, lavender, Present Time, Release, Roman chamomile, Sacred Mountain (back of the neck), 3 Wise Men (rub on crown), Transformation, Valor (on the feet), White Angelica (on the forehead or shoulders).

ROUNDING: Fir, Grounding, Hope, Joy, patchouli, spruce, 3 Wise Men, tsuga.
FEELING OF—cypress (aromatic).

UILT: Acceptance, Awaken, cypress, Forgiveness, frankincense, Gathering, geranium, Harmony, Inner Child, Inspiration, juniper, lemon, marjoram, Peace & Calming, Present Time, Release, Roman chamomile, rose, sandalwood, spruce, thyme, Valor, White Angelica.

ULF WAR SYNDROME: Exodus II.

UM DISEASE: See GINGIVITIS. Forgiveness, Harmony, [F]melaleuca, Melrose (fights infection), myrrh, Present Time, tsuga.
PERSONAL CARE—Dentarome/Dentarome Plus Toothpaste (contains Thieves), Fresh Essence Mouthwash (contains Thieves).

UMS: See GINGIVITIS. Lavender, Melrose (fights infection), myrrh (infection), Roman chamomile, sage lavender (infection).
PERSONAL CARE—Dentarome/Dentarome Plus Toothpaste (contains Thieves), Fresh Essence Mouthwash (contains Thieves), KidScents Toothpaste (for children).
SURGERY ON GUMS—For one individual, helichrysum was applied with a Q-tip every 15 minutes to kill the pain. No other pain killer was used.

ABITS: See ADDICTIONS. Acceptance, lavender, Transformation.
****COMMENTS—To break bad habits, you need to change the DNA and RNA. sandalwood and frankincense help with this.*

AIR: *Refer to the Personal Care Products section of the Reference Guide for Essential Oils for a list of ingredients and more details on chemical-free shampoos and conditioners.*
TINCTURES—AD&E

******COMMENTS*—*Refer to The chapter entitled "How to Use - The Personal Usage Reference" in the* <u>*Essential Oils Desk Reference*</u> *under "Hair and Scalp Problems" for some excellent blend recipes.*

BEARD—Cypress, lavender, lemon, rosemary, thyme.

BODY—Cedarwood (gives the hair shaft more body, more strength, and more life), tamar

CHILDREN—Lavender Volume Shampoo with Lavender Volume Conditioner or KidSce Shampoo.

COLOR—(keep light) 1 Mixta chamomile, 1 lemon, and 1 quart of water. Rinse hair.

DAMAGED (perms, color-treated, bleached)—Tamanu.

PERSONAL CARE—Lemon Sage Clarifying Shampoo and Lemon Sage Clarifying Conditioner (leave on hair for about 10 minutes) together helps remove buildu of styling products and recondition hair. Rosewood Moisturizing Shampoo an Rosewood Moisturizing Conditioner (leave on hair for about 10 minutes) together may restore manageability and shiny, healthy look. Also KidScents Shampoo.

DANDRUFF—Basil, birch, Canadian Red cedar, cedarwood, cypress, [F]lavender, rosemar sage, thyme, wintergreen.

PERSONAL CARE—KidScents Shampoo, Lavender Volume Shampoo, Lavender Volume Conditioner.

DRY—Birch, geranium, lavender, rosemary, sandalwood, wintergreen.

PERSONAL CARE—Rosewood Moisturizing Shampoo and Rosewood Moisturizing Conditioner (leave on hair for about 10 minutes) together may restore manageability and shiny, healthy look.

ESTROGEN BALANCE—Clary sage in Lavender Volume Shampoo and Lavender Volu Conditioner help promote estrogen balance in the membrane tissue around the hair follicle. This serves to balance testosterone levels and prevent the thickening of the tissue around the follicle that results in hair loss.

BLEND #1—1 lavender, 6 patchouli in 2-5 oz. Rosewood Moisturizing Shampoo.

BLEND #2—Mix together 2 cinnamon bark, 4 cypress, 4 geranium, 2 juniper, 5 lavender, and 3 rosemary. Then put one drop of the blend into ¼ tsp of water and rub on bald area and entire scalp. A gentle night treatment.

PERSONAL CARE—Lavender Volume Shampoo and Lavender Volume Conditione with Clary sage (see ESTROGEN BALANCE above).

SUPPLEMENTS—ComforTone, Essentialzyme, Super B (for stress), Thyromin, VitaGreen.

FRAGILE HAIR—Birch, Clary sage, lavender, Roman chamomile, sandalwood, thyme, wintergreen.

PERSONAL CARE—KidScents Shampoo, Lavender Volume Shampoo and Lavende Volume Conditioner.

GREASY—Petitgrain.

GROWTH (stimulate)—Basil, Canadian Red cedar, cedarwood, cypress, geranium, ginger, grapefruit, hyssop, lavender, lemon, rosemary, sage, thyme, ylang ylang (promotes).

PERSONAL CARE—Lavender Volume Shampoo and Lavender Volume Conditioner.

SUPPLEMENTS—Sulfurzyme. A deficiency in sulfur can result in hair loss or poor hair growth.

ITCHING—Lavender and [F]peppermint (skin).

LOSS—Birch, Canadian Red cedar, [F]cedarwood, Clary sage, cypress, [F]lavender, laurel (after infection), lemon, Roman chamomile, [F]rosemary, sage, sage lavender, thyme, wintergreen, [F]ylang ylang.

In males, hair loss can often be blamed on heredity, hormones (high levels of testosterone), and aging. Other reasons for hair loss may include poor circulation, hypertension, acute illness, surgery, radiation, Scarlet Fever, Syphilis, stress, sudden weight loss, iron deficiency, diabetes, hypothyroidism, drugs, poor diet, and vitamin deficiency.

Avoid hair products that are not natural on the hair. Avoid chlorinated swimming pools or polluted seas. Chemical products may also leave a residue build-up which can cause hair loss. Correcting a hormonal imbalance or hypertension (dilate blood vessels and stimulate cell division) may help.

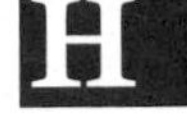

ALOPECIA AREATA (inflammatory hair loss disease) thyme (CT thymol), rosemary (CT cineol), lavender, cedarwood. Add any or all of these oils to jojoba and grapeseed carrier oils and massage into scalp daily.

PERSONAL CARE—Lavender Volume Shampoo and Lavender Volume Conditioner.

SUPPLEMENTS—Sulfurzyme, Super B, Thyromin.

****COMMENTS—Refer to The chapter entitled "How to Use - The Personal Usage Reference" in the Essential Oils Desk Reference under "Hair Loss" for some excellent blend recipes.*

SILKY AND SHINY—Tamanu.

PERSONAL CARE—KidScents Shampoo, Rosewood Moisturizing Shampoo and Rosewood Moisturizing Conditioner (leave on hair for about 10 minutes) together may help maintain manageability and shiny, healthy look.

SPLIT ENDS—

PERSONAL CARE—KidScents Shampoo, Rosewood Moisturizing Shampoo and Rosewood Moisturizing Conditioner (leave on hair for about 10 minutes) together may restore manageability and shiny, healthy look.

Don't you just love the feel of clean teeth and fresh breath! Try putting a drop of Thieves on your toothbrush instead of toothpaste. At first, it is a little warm, but it sure feels refreshing. If this doesn't work for you, try putting a drop on your toothpaste or put 10 drops of Thieves in a small spray bottle full of distilled water and mist in your mouth before brushing your teeth.

HALITOSIS: Cardamom, lavender, [F]nutmeg, [F]peppermint, Thieves.

SUPPLEMENTS—AlkaLime.

PERSONAL CARE— Dentarome/Dentarome Plus Toothpaste (contains Thieves), Fresh Essence Mouthwash (contains Thieves), KidScents Toothpaste (for children).

HANDS: Eucalyptus, geranium, lavender, lemon, patchouli, rosemary, sandalwood.

DRY—Geranium, patchouli, sandalwood.

PERSONAL CARE—Genesis Hand & Body Lotion, Rose Ointment, Sunsation Sunt Oil.

NEGLECTED—Geranium, lemon, patchouli.

TINGLING IN—Lemongrass in Genesis Hand & Body Lotion.

HANGOVERS: Fennel, grapefruit, lavender, lemon, rose, rosemary, sandalwood.

SUPPLEMENTS—Super C / Super C Chewable.

HAPPINESS: Christmas Spirit, Joy.

HARMONY IN BODY SYSTEMS: Acceptance, clove (aromatic), geranium (harmonizing), Harmony, Inspiration, Lady Sclareol (women), Roman chamomile.

MASSAGE OILS—Sensation Massage Oil creates an exotic arousal and increases sexual desire. The fragrance creates a peaceful and harmonious feeling that is helpful in easing relationship stress. Relaxation Massage Oil also creates a peaceful and harmonious feeling.

PERSONAL CARE—Sensation Hand & Body Lotion.

OF MIND AND BODY—Release.

HARSHNESS: Jasmine.

HASHIMOTO'S DISEASE: See THYROID: HYPERTHYROIDISM. Blue tansy, EndoFlex, lemongrass, myrrh, spruce.

SUPPLEMENTS—ImmuPro, Mineral Essence, Sulfurzyme (helps mitigate effects of autoimmune diseases), Thyromin, VitaGreen.

HATE: Acceptance, Forgiveness, Release.

HAY FEVER: Cajeput, eucalyptus, Juva Cleanse, lavender, Roman chamomile, rose.

HEADACHES: See MIGRAINE HEADACHES. Basil, Aroma Life (massage on

Clarity may cause headaches when chemicals or metals are in the brain. To break this blockage put Aroma Life or helichrysum on arteries in the neck.

arteries in neck), Aroma Siez, calamus, cardamom, Clarity, clove, cumin, eucalyptus, Dragon Time, frankincense, Gentle Baby, lavender, marjoram, Mister, M-Grain, [F]peppermint, Relieve It, [F]rosemary, sage lavender. Apply to temples, back of neck, forehead, and diffuse.

****COMMENTS—According to the Essential Oils Desk Reference, "For headaches, put one drop [Thieves] on tongue and push tongue against the roof of the mouth." (EDR-June 2002; Ch. 8; Thieves; Application) Also, Refer to The chapter entitled "How to Use - The Personal Usage Reference" in the Essential Oils Desk Reference under "Headaches" for some excellent blend recipes and supplement recommendations for several different types of headaches.*

ESSENTIAL WATERS (HYDROSOLS)—Clary Sage, Spearmint (cooling and soothing). Spray into air or directly on face (don't spray directly in eyes or ears) or diffuse using Essential Mist Diffuser.

COLD/FLU HEADACHES—Cumin.

EMOTIONAL HEADACHES—Joy.

MENSTRUAL MIGRAINES—See HORMONAL IMBALANCE. Sage lavender.

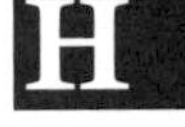

CHILDREN'S MIGRAINES—

BLEND—5 drops Mixta chamomile, 10 grapefruit, 5 peppermint, 3 rosemary, and 4 oz. V-6 Mixing Oil for children under seven and 2 oz. V-6 Mixing Oil for children over seven.

SUPPLEMENTS—KidScents MightyZyme (to help children digest their food).

MIGRAINE HEADACHES—(may be caused by problems in the colon. Cleanse the colon using supplements). Aroma Siez, [F]basil, birch, marjoram, M-Grain, PanAway, Peace & Calming, [F]peppermint, Relieve It, Release, Roman chamomile, spearmint, wintergreen, ylang ylang.

My husband has been bothered by migraine headaches for much of his adult life. Doctors have treated this condition with various medications - all with their own bag of side-effects. So one day I decided to have him try peppermint oil, a drop on each temple. To his amazement the headache was gone in seconds and the cooling feel of the peppermint gave him a feeling of energy and revitalization.

-Submitted by Kathleen Mueller, Menomonee Falls, WI (July 2004)

SUPPLEMENTS—AlkaLime (if caused from acidosis), Cleansing Trio (ComforTone, Essentialzyme, and ICP). Do not use ComforTone and JuvaTone together (*See ComforTone in Supplement section of the Reference Guide for Essential Oils*).

STRESS HEADACHES—M-Grain, Roman chamomile.

SUGAR HEADACHES—Thieves for low blood sugar headaches.

SUPPLEMENTS—Allerzyme (aids the digestion of sugars, starches, fats, and proteins), AlkaLime, Carbozyme, Mineral Essence.

Personal Guide

HEALING: Acceptance, Clary sage (aromatic), clove, cypress, eucalyptus (aromatic), frankincense, Humility, lemon (aromatic), melaleuca, PanAway, sage.

HEALTH: Abundance, lavender (aromatic), lemon (aromatic).

IMPROVE—

SUPPLEMENTS—Cleansing Trio (ComforTone, Essentialzyme, and ICP).

PROMOTES—Eucalyptus, juniper (aromatic).

HEARING: See EARS.

HEART: Aroma Life on heart and all Vita Flex heart points, Citrus Fresh, Clarity, cypress, Dragon Time, fleabane, Forgiveness, Gentle Baby, geranium, ginger, Harmony, Hope, hyssop, Joy, lavender, Mister, M-Grain, PanAway, Relieve It, rosemary, Valor on feet, White Angelica, ylang ylang (balances heart function). Apply oils to carotid arteries, heart, feet, under left ring finger, abc elbow, behind ring toe on left foot, and Vita Flex points on the feet.

> ***HEART PUMP FOR HEART STRESS***
>
> *Using your thumbs, apply pressure in an alternating "pumping" fashion between the following two heart points: (1) on the left hand at the lifeline under the ring finger; and (2) just inside the elbow. Also apply Aroma Life to the chest and the hand and heart points. And of course, GET HELP FAST!*

SUPPLEMENTS—Berrygize Nutrition Bars, CardiaCare, Mineral Essence, Power Meal, Sulfurzyme, Ultra Young (may help reverse heart disease), Wolfberry Bars.

TINCTURES—HRT and Rehemogen.

ANGINA—Aroma Life, [F]ginger, laurel, [F]orange (for false angina). Apply to heart and Vit Flex heart point.

TINCTURES—HRT.

ARRHYTHMIA—PanAway on heart and Relieve It on left foot Vita Flex heart point (rot each application). Goldenrod and lavender are also good. Research done by I Pénoël indicates that ylang ylang may be beneficial in preventing or correcting an irregularity in the force or rhythm of the heart.

TINCTURES—HRT.

BRINGS JOY TO HEART—Christmas Spirit, Citrus Fresh, Joy.

CARDIOTONIC—Lavender, thyme.

SUPPLEMENTS—CardiaCare (strengthens and supports).

CARDIOVASCULAR SYSTEMS—See CARDIOVASCULAR SYSTEM. Aroma Life (cardiac spasms), cinnamon bark (strengthens), cypress (strengthens the capillary walls and increases circulation), fennel, fleabane (dilates), Joy, [F]oran (cardiac spasms), palmarosa (supports), sandalwood (strengthens).

SUPPLEMENTS—CardiaCare (strengthens and supports).

TINCTURES—1-2 droppers of HRT two to three times per day.

CORONARY ARTERY—Prenolone/Prenolone+, Progessence.

****COMMENTS—Research has shown that natural progesterone protects the coronary artery from going into spasms. Provera, a synthetic progestin, offers no protection from coronary artery spasms. In fact, it promotes the spasm to the point of completely shutting off the flow of blood. This may explain the increase in heart attacks in women 5 to 10 years after menopause, many of whom are on synthetic progestin.*

SUPPLEMENTS—CardiaCare (contains Hawthorne Berry which helps dilate the coronary arteries and increase blood circulation to the heart).

HEART TISSUE—Marjoram has been found to help rejuvenate smooth muscle tissue of the heart.

TINCTURES—HRT.

****COMMENTS—One woman had cancer of the heart which literally ate a hole in her heart. She used HRT and the heart tissue regenerated itself and the cancer disappeared. One man had a heart attack and was awaiting a heart transplant, he used <u>Aroma Life</u>, <u>Valor</u>, and lavender topically and HRT orally. After four weeks of using the oils, he was told by his doctor that he was doing too well to have a heart transplant.*

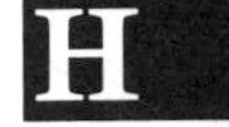

HYPERTENSION (high blood pressure)—See BLOOD.

LARGE VALVE—<u>Aroma Life</u> (shortness of breath).

TINCTURES—HRT.

PALPITATIONS (rapid and forceful contraction of the heart)—<u>Aroma Life</u>, lavender, melissa, [F]orange, peppermint, [F]ylang ylang.

SUPPLEMENTS—CardiaCare (strengthens and supports).

TINCTURES—HRT.

PROLAPSED MITRAL VALVE—Marjoram.

STIMULANT—Coriander, cumin.

STRENGTHENS HEART MUSCLE—Lavender, marjoram, peppermint, rose, rosemary (<u>Alternative Medicine—A Definitive Guide</u>, p. 722).

STRENGTHENING—Cinnamon bark.

SUPPLEMENTS—Berrygize Nutrition Bars, CardiaCare (strengthens and supports).

TACHYCARDIA (accelerated rhythm of the heartbeat)—Goldenrod, [F]lavender, orange, spikenard, ylang ylang.

SUPPLEMENTS—CardiaCare (strengthens and supports), Power Meal, Wolfberry Bars.

TINCTURES—HRT.

HEARTBURN: Cardamom, Di-Tone (over stomach and colon), Gentle Baby, [F]lemon, [F]peppermint (over thymus).

BLEND—2 lemon, 2 peppermint, 3 sandalwood, and ½ oz. V-6 Mixing Oil. Apply breast bone. Using palm of hand, massage in a clockwise motion applying pressure. Do Vita Flex on feet.

SUPPLEMENTS—AlkaLime, Essentialzyme, JuvaPower/JuvaSpice.

HEMATOMA (swelling or tumor filled with diffused blood): Aroma Life, German chamon [F]helichrysum.

HEMORRHAGING: Helichrysum, rose, ylang ylang. Massage around ankles, lower back, a stomach. Cayenne pepper may also help.

HEMORRHOIDS: Aroma Life, basil, [F]Clary sage, [F]cypress, frankincense, helichrysum, junip myrrh, [F]patchouli, [F]peppermint, [F]sandalwood. Put cypress and helichrysum inside on location.

HEPATITIS: Cinnamon bark, cypress, eucalyptus, JuvaFlex (over the liver), ImmuPower (on spine and liver), melaleuca, myrrh, oregano, patchouli, Release (on feet and liver), Roman chamomile, rosemary, thyme.

SUPPLEMENTS—Cleansing Trio (ComforTone, Essentialzyme, and ICP) for 1 w 4 Royaldophilus a day, Master Formula His/Hers, 1 VitaGreen a day, 4 Supe C / Super C Chewable three times a day, 1/4 tsp. ImmuGel three times a day. Add JuvaTone on the 3rd day.

****COMMENTS—Refer to The chapter entitled "How to Use - The Personal Usage Reference" in the Essential Oils Desk Reference under "Liver" subcategory "Hepatitis" for a specific daily program using supplements and blends.*

DETOXIFY LIVER—Ledum and JuvaTone together.

VIRAL—[F]Myrrh and JuvaFlex, ledum, [F]ravensara, [F]rosemary. Apply to spine, compress over liver area, and Vita Flex points on feet. Alternate oils.

SUPPLEMENTS—Super C / Super C Chewable.

HERNIA: Apply oil(s) on location, lower back, and Vita Flex points on feet.

HIATAL HERNIA—Basil, cypress, fennel, geranium, ginger, hyssop, lavender, pepperm rosemary, vitex. Drink water. Put the first two fingers of each hand just belo the sternum (under center of rib cage), press in firmly, and brush down quickl and firmly. This can also be done after raising up on toes and while dropping down on heels to more firmly emphasize the effect.

SUPPLEMENTS—Essentialzyme before meal, ComforTone, ICP (fiber beverage) after meal.

INCISIONAL HERNIA (usually caused by scar tissue failing to heal from an abdominal wound or incision)—Basil, geranium, ginger, helichrysum, lavender, lemon, lemongrass, melaleuca.

INGUINAL—Lavender, lemongrass.

ERPES SIMPLEX: Australian Blue, Blue cypress, bergamot with *Eucalyptus radiata*, eucalyptus, geranium, [F]lavender, lemon, melissa, [F]ravensara, rose.

Jean Valnet, M.D., a French physician, recommends a blend of lemon and geranium. Tisserand suggests eucalyptus and bergamot. Dr. Wabner says that a one-time application of either true rose oil or true melissa oil led to complete remission of herpes simplex lesions. Apply the oil directly on the lesions at the first sign of an outbreak. (Alternative Medicine—The Definitive Guide, p. 56).

ICCOUGHS: Sandalwood, [F]tarragon.

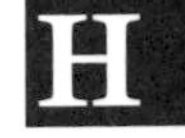

IGH BLOOD PRESSURE: See BLOOD.

IVES: See ACIDOSIS, pH BALANCE. Hives may be the result of too much acid in the blood or the result of a niacin flush (vitamin B3 taken on empty stomach). Patchouli (may relieve itching), peppermint, Roman chamomile.

SUPPLEMENTS—AlkaLime (combat yeast and fungus overgrowth and preserve the body's proper pH balance), Coral Sea (highly bio-available calcium, contains 58 trace minerals), Super Cal (may prevent), VitaGreen.

****COMMENTS—One woman broke out in hives over her entire body, she used peppermint oil diluted with V-6 Mixing Oil for a body massage. Almost instantly, her body cooled off and the hives diminished until gone.*

IODGKIN'S DISEASE: Clove. Apply to liver, kidney, and Vita Flex points on feet.

IOPE: Hope (restores).

IORMONAL IMBALANCE: Anise, SclarEssence, ylang ylang.

PERSONAL CARE— Prenolone/Prenolone+, Progessence.

SUPPLEMENTS—Exodus, FemiGen, Mineral Essence, Sulfurzyme (lowered libido).

IORMONAL SYSTEM: Acceptance, Aroma Life, Clarity, davana, Dragon Time, EndoFlex, fennel, goldenrod, Gentle Baby, Mister, M-Grain, myrrh, myrtle, peppermint, Relieve It, sandalwood, SclarEssence, [F]spearmint (hormone-like), ylang ylang. The most common places to apply oils for hormonal balance are the Vita Flex points on ankles, lower back, thyroid, liver, kidneys, gland areas, the center of the body and along both sides of the spine, and the clavicle area. It may also help to diffuse them.

ESSENTIAL WATERS (HYDROSOLS)—Clary Sage (contains natural scleral - helps stimulate production of estrogen). Spray into air of diffuse using Essential Mi Diffuser.

BALANCE—Bergamot, [F]Clary sage, clove (aromatic), EndoFlex, fennel, geranium, Legacy, Mister (creates greater balance), nutmeg, sage, ylang ylang.

MASSAGE OILS—Dragon Time.

PERSONAL CARE—Prenolone/Prenolone+, Progessence.

SUPPLEMENTS—Coral Sea (highly bio-available calcium, contains 58 trace minerals), CortiStop (Men's and Women's), Exodus, FemiGen (female), ProGen (male), Super B, Super Cal, Thyromin, Ultra Young+, VitaGreen.

TINCTURES—Estro.

> *A hormonal imbalance can cause many problems including, PMS, pre- and post-menopausal conditions, depression, endometriosis, fibromyalgia, fibrocysts, infertility, insomnia, irregular menstrual cycles, lowered libido, menstrual migraines, osteoporosis, ovarian cysts, unexplained first-trimester miscarriages, water retention, etc. Carbonated water can cause hormone deficiency. But, most often, it is a result of estrogen dominance; that is, not enough progesterone to balance out the amount of estrogen. Estrogen is manufactured in several places of the body, even after menopause, and is also found in much of our food, especially animal and dairy products. Progesterone is secreted by the corpus luteum, by the placenta, and in small amounts by the adrenal glands. If the ovaries are not functioning properly, have been removed, or if they have atrophied because of menopause or hysterectomy, the woman is undoubtedly estrogen dominant. Therefore, she is a candidate for the problems listed above. One successful approach for the above problems is NATURAL PROGESTERONE (obtained from the Wild Yam or SOY). Two good books to read about natural progesterone are What Your Doctor May Not Tell You About Premenopause and What Your Doctor May Not Tell You About Menopause. Both books were written by John R. Lee, MD.*

DISTURBANCES—

SUPPLEMENTS—ProGen (male) or FemiGen (female).

FEMALE—Lady Sclareol, Mister (for estrogen).

SUPPLEMENTS—CortiStop (Women's), FemiGen, Ultra Young+.

TINCTURES—Estro.

MALE—Mister.

SUPPLEMENTS—CortiStop (Men's), ProGen, Ultra Young+.

SEXUAL ENERGY—Goldenrod, Lady Sclareol, ylang ylang.

HOT FLASHES: See HORMONAL IMBALANCE. Bergamot (estrogen), Clary sage (estrogen), Dragon Time, EndoFlex, fennel, Mister (estrogen) works for womei in Canada, or [F]peppermint. Apply these oils on the ankles at the ovary and uterus Vita Flex points. If hypoglycemic, use Aroma Siez with M-Grain.

***COMMENTS*—Some women have had success using a drop of EndoFlex under their tongue three times a day. Be cautious as it contains nutmeg and an overdose could cause problems.*

PERSONAL CARE—Prenolone/Prenolone+, Progessence.

SUPPLEMENTS—CortiStop (Women's), FemiGen, Mineral Essence.

TINCTURES—AD&E.

OTHER—Lady Flash & Lady Love (available through Creer Labs 801-465-5423). Apply on ovaries, pelvis, ankles, bottom of feet.

OUSECLEANING: Put a few drops of oil on your dust cloth or put 10 drops in a spray bottle of water and mist.

BATHROOMS/KITCHENS—Fir, lemon, or spruce for cleaning and disinfecting.

CARPETS—Purification, lemon (has been used to remove black shoe polish)

DISHES—A couple of drops of Melrose or lemon in the dishwater make for sparkling dishes and a great smelling kitchen.

FURNITURE POLISH—Fir, lemon, or spruce work well for polishing furniture.

GUM/GREASE—Lemon oil is terrific for dissolving gum and grease.

LAUNDRY—Adding oils to the washer can increase the anti-bacterial benefits, provide greater hygiene, and the clothes come out with a fresh, clean smell.

MOLD/FUNGUS—Purification.

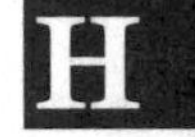

YPERACTIVITY: Citrus Fresh, lavender, Peace & Calming (gets them off Ritalin), Roman chamomile, Trauma Life (calming), Valor (sometimes works better than Peace & Calming). Apply to Vita Flex points on the feet and diffuse.

> ***Hyperactivity** may indicate a trace mineral deficiency. Get off Prozac and Ritalin and use Mineral Essence. It is interesting to note that 48 out of 49 death row inmates were tested and found to be deficient in the same trace minerals.*

SUPPLEMENTS—ComforTone, Essentialzyme, ICP, Mineral Essence, healthy diet.

YPERPNEA (abnormal rapid breathing): [F]Ylang ylang. Apply to lung area and Vita Flex points.

YPERTENSION (high blood pressure): See BLOOD.

YPOGLYCEMIA: See PROTEIN. Cinnamon bark, clove,

> *Protein deficiency causes **hypoglycemia**. Honey enters the blood stream faster than sugar and can cause hypoglycemia. When flu and virus enter the body and mix with problems of hypoglycemia, it can cause candida, Epstein barr virus, allergies, etc. There is a progressive deterioration from hypoglycemia. Signs of hypoglycemia are: headaches, fatigue, PMS, ornery, moody, weak, light headed, not hungry in the morning because body is still digesting its food from the night before.*

Feucalyptus, Gentle Baby, Gratitude (over pancreas and on VF points), Thieve thyme.

SUPPLEMENTS—Allerzyme (aids the digestion of sugars, starches, fats, and proteins), AlkaLime, Bodygize, Polyzyme (aids the digestion of protein and helps reduce swelling and discomfort), Power Meal, Stevia, Stevia Select, Sulfurzyme, VitaGreen, WheyFit (lactose-free protein from three sources; provides highest ranking protein for digestibility), Wolfberry Bars.

HYSTERIA: Lavender, melaleuca, neroli. Apply to heart, bottom of feet, and diffuse.

IMMUNE SYSTEM: Abundance, cistus, clove, cumin, Exodus II, frankincense, geranium, Idaho tansy, ImmuPower, lavender, ledum (supports), lemon, melaleuca, Mountain savory, Raven, ravensara, rosemary (supports), Thieves (enhances; massage on feet and body), thyme (immunological functions), White lotus.

SUPPLEMENTS—AlkaLime (designed to combat yeast and fungus overgrowth and preserve the body's proper pH balance), Body Balancing Trio (Bodygize, Master Formula His/Hers, VitaGreen), Cleansing Trio (ComforTone, Essentialzyme, and ICP), Essential Manna, Exodus, ImmuGel, ImmuneTune, ImmuPro, Mineral Essence, Power Meal, Super B, Super C / Super C Chewable, Thyromin, Ultra Young (may help raise levels of cytokines, interleukin 1 & 2, and tumor necrosis factor), VitaGreen, Wolfberry Bar (*Refe to the Wolfberry Bar in the Supplements section of the Reference Guide for Essential Oils for more information on the benefits of the Chinese Wolfberry*.

TINCTURES—AD&E.

STIMULATES—FCinnamon bark, Ffrankincense, ImmuPower, lavender (for immune system), Fmelaleuca, Mountain savory, Foregano, Thieves. Apply oil(s) to bottom of feet, along spine, under arms, dilute for massage, and diffuse for ½ hour at a time.

BOOSTING IMMUNE DEFENSE—Cumin, ledum.

IMPETIGO: Lavender, myrrh. Boil 4 ounces water, cool, add 5 to 10 drops lavender and wash. You may also use myrrh (cover for an hour). Do hot compress on site.

> ***Impetigo** is an infection of the outer layers of the skin. It is caused by an infected scratch or insect bite. It starts as tiny red spots, then it turns into blisters that can fill with pus. It is contagious to self and others. Approach the problem and handle it as it is noticed.*

ESSENTIAL WATERS (HYDROSOLS)—Lavender or Lavender Floral Water.

IMPOTENCY: FClary sage, Fclove, goldenrod, Fginger, jasmine, Mister, nutmeg, rose, Fsandalwood, SclarEssence (taken internally as a dietary supplement, helps to raise testosterone levels), ylang ylang.

SUPPLEMENTS—CortiStop (Men's - reduces the levels of cortisol and enhances the production of testosterone), ProGen.

PERSONAL CARE—Prenolone+

CONTINENCE: See BLADDER.

DIFFERENCE: Jasmine.

DIGESTION: Angelica, cumin, ginger, JuvaFlex, [F]lavender, [F]peppermint, nutmeg, valerian (nervous indigestion).

SUPPLEMENTS—AlkaLime, Cleansing Trio (ComforTone, Essentialzyme, and ICP).

FECTION: See ANTI-INFECTIOUS. [F]Bergamot, cajeput (urethra), [F]cinnamon bark, clove, [F]Clary sage, cypress, elemi (chest/bronchial infections), Idaho tansy, jasmine (bacterial infection), juniper, fennel, lavender, lemongrass, *Melaleuca quinquenervia* (viral), Melrose (prevents growth of all infections), myrrh (fungal infection), oregano, peppermint, [F]pine (severe), Raven, ravensara, rosemary (oral infection), Thieves, thyme (urinary infection).

FUNGICIDAL—Cedarwood.

INFECTED WOUNDS—Frankincense, melaleuca, patchouli.

BLEND (to draw infection out)—1 thyme. Apply hot compress twice daily. Mix together 3 lavender, 2 melaleuca, and 2 thyme with 1 tsp. V-6 Mixing Oil. After the infection and pus have been expelled, apply a little of the mixture twice daily on the infected area.

SUPPLEMENTS—Bodygize, ImmuGel, ImmuneTune, ImmuPro, Super C / Super C Chewable.

FECTIOUS DISEASE: Bergamot, cinnamon bark, clove, Exodus II, ginger, hyssop (viral infections), ImmuPower, juniper (viral infections), lemon, melaleuca, myrtle, Raven, RC, and thyme (bacterial infection).

****COMMENTS—Dr. Young uses Raven, RC, and ImmuPower together for infectious diseases.*

FERIORITY:

OVERCOMING—Peppermint, Transformation.

FERTILITY: See HORMONAL IMBALANCE. Anise, bergamot, Clary sage, cypress, Dragon Time (place on ankles, lower abdomen, and in vagina for women), fennel, geranium, melissa, Mister (for men, place in rectum, across lower back, around and under ankles), nutmeg, Roman chamomile, sage, thyme, yarrow, ylang ylang. Feed the thyroid.

SUPPLEMENTS—ProGen (male) or FemiGen (female), Prenolone/Prenolone+ / Progessence, and 1-3 VitaGreen three times a day.

INFLAMMATION: See ANTI-INFLAMMATORY. Birch, calamus (intestines and colon), clove, elemi (breast and uterus), frankincense, helichrysum, juniper, lavender myrrh, PanAway, Peace & Calming, Relieve It, Roman chamomile, spruce, wintergreen.

MASSAGE OILS—Ortho Sport.

****COMMENTS—Refer to The chapter entitled "How to Use - The Personal Usage Reference" in the Essential Oils Desk Reference under "Inflammation" for some excellent blend recipes.*

INFLUENZA: See FLU or COLDS.

INJURIES: See TISSUE, SCARRING. Balsam fir (with frankincense for pain), Melrose (regenerates tissue), helichrysum (reduces scarring and discoloration).

SPORT—Balsam fir, helichrysum, Melrose, PanAway.

MASSAGE OILS—Ortho Ease, Ortho Sport.

INNER KNOWING: Inner Child (reconnects you with your inner child), SARA.

INSANITY: Hope (ears), Release (liver), Relieve It.

INSECT:

BITES—See BITES. Cajeput, bergamot cajeput, Idaho tansy.

BLEND #1—Combine 3 drops Roman chamomile, 4 eucalyptus, 10 lavender, and 1 thyme with 1 Tbs. V-6 Mixing Oil.

****COMMENTS—Refer to The chapter entitled "How to Use - The Personal Usage Reference" in the Essential Oils Desk Reference under "Insect Bites" for some excellent blend recipes for*

Dr. Jean Valnet says that basil, cinnamon, garlic, lavender, lemon, onion, sage, savory, and thyme are effective against insect bites because of their antitoxic and anti-venomous properties.

My husband was bitten by a spider on his stomach. The bite swelled with a large blister and it itched terribly. I used lavender oil - about a drop - on the area. In about 4 hours my husband asked for another application of the "magic oil". My husband has an allergy and reacts to any type of a bite. In fact, he usually has to go to the Dr. and get shots and prescriptions.

-Submitted by Mary Rynicki (July 2004

bites/stings from different types of insects.

POISONS FROM BROWN RECLUSE SPIDER OR WASPS—Purification (removes poisons from the body).

INSECTICIDAL—Citronella.

ITCHING—Lavender.

PERSONAL CARE—Satin Hand & Body Lotion with lavender.

REPELLENT—Basil, bergamot, cedarwood, Purification.

FLORAL WATERS—Idaho Tansy (has been used with success as a fly and mosquito repellent on horses and other animals).

PERSONAL CARE—Sunsation Suntan Oil.

BLEND #2—Combine 5 lavender, 5 lemongrass, 3 peppermint, and 1 thyme and put on feet or add to cup of water and spray on.

BLEND #3—Clove, lemon, and orange.

BLEND #4—Put 5 lemon and 5 Purification in a little spray bottle of water and mist on your skin to protect yourself against insects, flies, and mosquitos.

> *My husband was stung by a wasp last year on the inside of the hand. He removed the stinger and asked me to put something on it. I put Purification on it, and the itching stopped. After his shower that evening, I put Purification on it again. The next morning, you couldn't see or even tell that he'd been stung. I've also put Purification on coworkers who have had mosquito/bug bites that itched. After the Purification went on the bites, the itching stopped.*
>
> ***-Submitted by Christie Krajewski Batesville, Arkansas (July 2004)***

PERSONAL CARE—Sunsation Suntan Oil helps filter out the ultraviolet rays without blocking the absorption of vitamin D, which is important to skin and bone development. ACCELERATES TANNING.

****COMMENTS—Dr. Friedmann came in contact with a person who had bugs growing on their face and scalp. Somehow they were subjected to a fungus to which the bugs were attracted. They established their nests, laid and hatched their eggs on her skin. She had been using many products and was only able to suppress the problem but not correct it. Dr. Friedmann applied Melrose, helichrysum, lavender, and ImmuPower on her Thymus. She stopped using all other chemicals and several weeks later the bugs were almost gone.*

ISOMNIA: Angelica, basil, [F]bergamot, Citrus Fresh, Clary sage, [F]cypress, [F]lavender, lemon, [F]marjoram, *Melaleuca ericifolia*, [F]myrtle (for hormone-related insomnia), neroli, nutmeg (small amount), [F]orange, Peace & Calming, petitgrain, [F]ravensara, Roman chamomile (small amount), rosemary, sandalwood, Surrender (behind the ears), valerian, [F]ylang ylang.

BLEND #1—Combine 6 Citrus Fresh with 6 lavender or 6 Peace & Calming. Apply blend to big toes, bottom of feet, 2 drops around navel, 3 drops on back of neck.

BLEND #2—2 drops Roman chamomile, 6 geranium, 3 lemon, and 4 sandalwood. Mix together and add 6 drops in your bath at bedtime and 5 drops with 2 tsp. 6 Mixing Oil for a massage after bath.

SUPPLEMENTS—ImmuPro.

****COMMENTS—Refer to The chapter entitled "How to Use - The Personal Usage Reference" in the Essential Oils Desk Reference under "Insomnia" for some excellent blend recipes.*

FOR CHILDREN—12 months to 5 years—lavender, Roman chamomile; 5 to 12 years—Clary sage, geranium, *Melaleuca ericifolia*, ylang ylang (infection).

INTESTINAL PROBLEMS: See ACIDOSIS, COLITIS, COLON, CONSTIPATION, DIGESTIVE SYSTEM, DIVERTICULITIS, PARASITES, etc. [F]Basil, cajeput, calamus (reduces inflammation and detoxifies), ginger, [F]marjoram, patchouli (aids in the digestion of toxic waste), rosemary, tarragon.

SUPPLEMENTS—AlkaLime, Cleansing Trio (ComforTone, Essentialzyme, and ICP), ParaFree, JuvaTone, Royaldophilus.

ANTISEPTIC—Nutmeg.

CRAMPS—Blue cypress, [F]Clary sage, Di-Tone.

FLORA—Royaldophilus.

PARASITES—[F]Bergamot, [F]clove, Di-Tone, [F]fennel, [F]lemon, peppermint, ravensara, [F]Roman chamomile.

SUPPLEMENTS—AlkaLime, Cleansing Trio (ComforTone, Essentialzyme, and ICP) and ParaFree assist in cleansing the intestinal tract of toxic debris and parasites which are hosts for many diseases.

SOOTHE—Spearmint.

SPASM—[F]Tarragon, [F]fennel.

INVIGORATING: Birch/wintergreen.

IN SUMMER—Eucalyptus, peppermint.

IONS:

INCREASE NEGATIVE IONS—Bergamot, citronella, lemongrass, orange.

INCREASE POSITIVE IONS—Cajeput, frankincense, helichrysum, juniper, *Melaleuca quinquenervia,* pine, ravensara, ylang ylang.

IRON: Important for learning. Raisins are good natural source.

SUPPLEMENTS—Master Formula Hers/His, KidScents Mighty Vites (chewable).

RRITABILITY: Forgiveness, Hope, Humility, Inspiration, lavender, myrrh, Present Time, Surrender, Valor. All single oils EXCEPT: Eucalyptus, pepper, peppermint, and rosemary.

SUPPLEMENTS—AlkaLime.

RRITABLE BOWEL SYNDROME: Calamus, Di-Tone, peppermint. Take 2 drops of each in distilled water 1-2 times per day. Anise and Juva Cleanse may also help.

SUPPLEMENTS—ComforTone, JuvaPower/JuvaSpice, JuvaTone, ICP (fiber beverage), Royaldophilus, Stevia Select (with FOS).

TCHING: Lavender, Peace & Calming (ears), peppermint (ears). Apply on location too.

BLEND—6 lavender and 3 rosemary with Satin Hand & Body Lotion.

PERSONAL CARE—Rose Ointment, Satin Hand & Body Lotion.

AUNDICE (liver disease): [F]Geranium, Juva Cleanse, lemon, rosemary, sage lavender.

EALOUSY: Bergamot, eucalyptus, Forgiveness, frankincense, Harmony, Humility, Joy, lemon, marjoram, orange, rose, rosemary, Sacred Mountain, sandalwood, thyme, Valor, White Angelica.

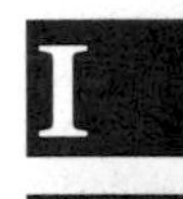

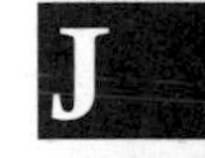

ET LAG: Brain Power, Clarity, En-R-Gee, eucalyptus, geranium, grapefruit, ImmuPower (for protection), lavender, lemongrass, peppermint, Present Time, Valor. Apply to temples, thymus, and bottom of feet. It is best not to eat heavy foods and to drink as much water as possible.

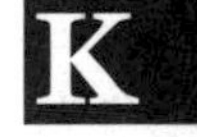

SUPPLEMENTS—Power Meal, Sulfurzyme, Super C / Super C Chewable.

OINTS: Birch (discomfort), cajeput (stiff), Douglas fir (calming to tired and overworked joints), Idaho balsam fir (pain from exercising), nutmeg, Roman chamomile (inflamed), spruce (aching), wintergreen.

****COMMENTS—Refer to The chapter entitled "How to Use - The Personal Usage Reference" in the Essential Oils Desk Reference under "Joint Stiffness and Pain" for some excellent blend recipes.*

OYOUS: Abundance, bergamot (turns grief to joy), Christmas Spirit, Citrus Fresh (brings joy to children), Joy, orange (aromatic).

IDNEYS: Aroma Life, calamus (reduces congestion after intoxication), Clary sage, EndoFlex, geranium, grapefruit, juniper (for better function of kidneys), JuvaFlex, ledum (strengthen), [F]lemongrass (combine with juniper for greater synergistic effect), Release. Apply over kidneys as a hot compress. Drink plenty of distilled water

(3-4 quarts each day). When kidneys start producing ammonia, it can go to th brain and people have died from that alone. Do the MASTER CLEANSER (See CLEANSING).

SUPPLEMENTS—VitaGreen (turns blood back to alkaline).

TINCTURES—K&B.

****COMMENTS—Refer to the chapter entitled "How to Use - The Personal Usage Reference" in the Essential Oils Desk Reference under "Kidney Disorders" for some excellent blend recipes and supplement recommendations.*

BLOCKAGE—

MASSAGE—Release and other oils on kidney points on feet twice a day.

SUPPLEMENTS—Cleansing Trio (ComforTone, Essentialzyme, and ICP), JuvaTon (First week: 2 tablets a day; Second week: 3 tablets a day for 90 days).

CAPILLARIES BEING ATTACKED IN KIDNEYS—

SUPPLEMENTS—Need to support the body and cleanse the blood with VitaGreen, Cleansing Trio (ComforTone, Essentialzyme, and ICP).

INFECTION IN—Rosemary. Apply to kidneys and Vita Flex points.

BLEND #1—Cypress, marjoram, and Thieves or JuvaFlex. Apply as a hot compres

FOOD—Drink one gallon of distilled water and 2 quarts cranberry juice in a day.

INFLAMMATION (Nephritis)—Aroma Life, juniper, JuvaFlex. Do a colon cleanse (see CLEANSING).

FOOD—Drink one gallon of distilled water and 2 quarts cranberry juice in a day.

SUPPLEMENTS—ImmuneTune, Power Meal, Super C / Super C Chewable, VitaGreen.

TINCTURES—K&B, Rehemogen.

****COMMENTS—Refer to the chapter entitled "How to Use - The Personal Usage Reference" in the Essential Oils Desk Reference under "Kidney Disorders" subcategory "Inflammation in the Kidneys (Nephritis)" for a very specific regimen of supplements and blends.*

MUSCLES THAT WON'T WORK IN THE KIDNEYS—Aroma Siez and EndoFlex.

BLEND #2—8 fennel and 10 juniper.

STONES—Eucalyptus, hyssop, juniper.

BLEND #3—10 juniper and 10 geranium. Apply as a hot compress over kidneys on a day.

SUPPLEMENTS—After being on the Cleansing Trio (ComforTone, Essentialzyme, and ICP) for 10 days, add ImmuneTune, and Super C / Super C Chewable.

PASS (without edges)—Drink 4 oz. distilled water with juice from ½ lemon every 3(minutes for 6 hours straight. Then take 2 Tbsp. extra light virgin olive oil witl the juice from 1 full lemon. Repeat daily until stone passes.

NEE CARTILAGE INJURY:

BLEND—8 clove, 12 ginger, 10 nutmeg with 2 oz. V-6 Mixing Oil. Massage three times a day. Apply ice for swelling and inflammation. Wrap knee and elevate when sitting. Use the ice method three times a day and alternate with a hot compress and the oils.

MASSAGE OILS—Ortho Ease, Ortho Sport.

PERSONAL CARE—Regenolone.

SUPPLEMENTS—BLM

ABOR: See PREGNANCY. Gentle Baby, jasmine (pain).

ACTATION (secretion of breast milk): See NURSING. [F]Fennel or basil (increase flow), peppermint with cold compress (decrease flow). Apply above the breasts on the lymph area and 2-3 drops on the spine, about breast level.

SUPPLEMENTS—PD 80/20, Prenolone/Prenolone+, Progessence.

ACTOSE INTOLERANCE: Lemongrass (reported to help eliminate lactic acid from fermentation of lactose in milk).

SUPPLEMENTS—Allerzyme, Essentialzyme, Power Meal, WheyFit.

ARYNGITIS: Jasmine, ledum, Melrose, onycha (benzoin), sage lavender, sandalwood.

DIFFUSE—Frankincense, lavender, sandalwood, thyme.

BLEND—Add one drop each of Melrose and lemon to 1 tsp. honey. Swish around in mouth for a couple of minutes to liquify then swallow.

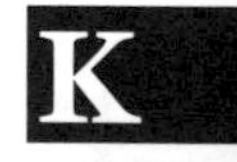

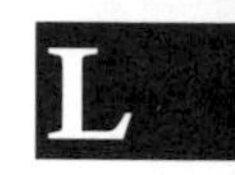

AUNDRY: Lemon, Purification.

****COMMENTS—Adding oils to the washer can increase the anti bacterial benefits, provide greater hygiene, and the clothes come out with a fresh, clean smell. A few drops of oil can also be placed on a washcloth and put in the dryer with laundry or added to a bottle of water, shook well, and sprayed into the dryer before drying the laundry.*

AXATIVE: Hyssop, jasmine, tangerine.

SUPPLEMENTS—Cleansing Trio (ComforTone, Essentialzyme, and ICP).

ETHARGY: Jasmine, Transformation.

BIDO (Low): See FRIGIDITY, SEX STIMULANT. Chivalry, Dragon Time, Joy, Mister, nutmeg, Live with Passion, rose, SclarEssence (take internally), Sensation, ylang ylang. Do the MASTER CLEANSER (See CLEANSING).

SUPPLEMENTS— PD 80/20, Prenolone/Prenolone+, Progessence, Sulfurzyme.

MEN—Additional oils include Black pepper, cinnamon, ginger, myrrh, and pine. See also PROSTATE.

PERSONAL CARE—Protec (combine with frankincense to decongest the prostate).

WOMEN—Additional oils include Clary sage, geranium, jasmine, and Lady Sclareol.

LICE: Eucalyptus, geranium, lavender, lemon, pine (repels), rosemary. Apply oil(s) to bottom feet and rub over scalp three times a day.

LIGAMENTS: See MUSCLES. **Lemongrass** (torn or pulled; combine with marjoram to stimulate torn ligaments).

ESSENTIAL WATERS (HYDROSOLS)—German Chamomile (relaxing and soothing Spray directly on area of concern.

SUPPLEMENTS—BLM

TORN—Birch, clove, helichrysum, marjoram, PanAway, wintergreen.

MASSAGE OILS—Ortho Sport.

LIPOMA: See TUMORS.

LIPS: German chamomile, lavender, lemon, melaleuca.

DRY LIPS—

BLEND—2 to 5 drops geranium and 2 to 5 drops lavender.

LISTLESSNESS: Jasmine.

LIVER: Acceptance, cypress, dill, Di-Tone, fleabane, [F]geranium (cleanses and detoxifies the liver), [F]German chamomile, goldenrod (supports liver function), grapefruit (li disorders), [F]helichrysum, JuvaFlex (detoxification), Juva Cleanse, ledum (powerful detoxifier), myrrh, Peace & Calming, ravensara, [F]sage (for liver problems), sage lavender (congestion), Release (apply to liver and Vita Flex points), Roman chamomile, 3 Wise Men (on crown).

SUPPLEMENTS—JuvaTone.

****COMMENTS—When the liver is toxic, it makes the mind lethargic and slows the emotions. For those who have liver problems, be careful about the oils used and the amounts. Ease into a liver cleanse!*

CIRRHOSIS OF LIVER—Frankincense, geranium, juniper, lavender, myrrh, Roman chamomile, rosemary, rose.

SUPPLEMENTS—Bodygize, JuvaTone, Super C / Super C Chewable.

CLEANSING—Carrot seed, helichrysum, geranium, German chamomile, JuvaFlex, Juva Cleanse, ledum (with JuvaTone), myrrh, sage lavender.

SUPPLEMENTS—Sulfurzyme may help detoxify the liver.

FUNCTION (improve)—JuvaFlex, goldenrod, and myrrh. Do a compress over the liver and alternate the oils on the liver Vita Flex points.

HEPATITIS—See HEPATITIS. JuvaFlex, **ravensara** (viral).

JAUNDICE (liver disease)—[F]Geranium, Juva Cleanse.

REGENERATION—

****COMMENTS—One individual had total liver regeneration using JuvaTone, Rehemogen, and JuvaFlex.*

SPOTS—Idaho Tansy Floral Water, Prenolone/Prenolone+, Progessence.

STIMULANT FOR LIVER CELL FUNCTION—[F]Helichrysum, ledum (combine with JuvaTone).

SUPPLEMENTS—Cleansing Trio (ComforTone, Essentialzyme, and ICP), JuvaTone (helps increase digestion in the liver).

ONGEVITY: Fennel (aromatic), Longevity (can be taken internally as dietary supplement).

SUPPLEMENTS—Berry Young Juice {a delicious blend of powerful antioxidant fruit juices - measures higher on the ORAC (oxygen radical absorbent capacity) scale than ever Tahitian Noni Juice}, CardiaCare (with *Rhododendron caucasicum*), Longevity Capsules.

OSS OF LOVED ONE: Basil, cedarwood, cypress (diffuse), fir, Forgiveness, jasmine, Joy, rose, spruce, Transformation, Valor, ylang ylang.

BATH & SHOWER GELS—Sensation Bath & Shower Gel.

MASSAGE OIL—Sensation Massage Oil.

PERSONAL CARE—Sensation Hand & Body Lotion.

OSS OF SMELL: Basil.

OVE: Forgiveness, Joy, juniper, Lady Sclareol, lavender, Sensation, ylang ylang.

BATH & SHOWER GELS—Sensation Bath & Shower Gel contains oils used by Cleopatra to enhance love and increase the desire to be close to that someone special.

MASSAGE OILS—Sensation Massage Oil.

PERSONAL CARE—Sensation Hand & Body Lotion.

ATTRACTS—Joy.

SELF LOVE—Joy.

OU GEHRIG'S DISEASE: See ALZHEIMER'S DISEASE, BRAIN, MULTIPLE SCLEROSIS, PARKINSON'S DISEASE, PINEAL GLAND, PITUITARY GLAND. Use the same oils as you would if you were handling Multiple

Sclerosis, Alzheimer's, and Parkinson's Disease. Drink steam distilled water. Acceptance (may help to oxygenate the pineal and pituitary glands), Clarity (fo brain function), cypress (circulation), Peace & Calming, Valor.

SUPPLEMENTS—Cleansing Trio (ComforTone, Essentialzyme, and ICP), JuvaPower/JuvaSpice, JuvaTone, Sulfurzyme.

LUMBAGO: See BACK PAIN. Sandalwood.

LUNGS: See RESPIRATORY SYSTEM. Aroma Life, Believe, [F]eucalyptus, Forgiveness, Joy, Raven (stronger than RC), RC (diffuse to open lungs and to send oxygen to red blood cells), frankincense (stimulates), hyssop (diffuse to clear lungs of mucus), ravensara. Apply on chest with hot compress or on Vita Flex lung points on the feet.

BLEND—Equal parts *Melaleuca ericifolia* and either RC or Raven (depending on strength desired). Add to 1 oz. V-6 Mixing Oil and insert into rectum for retention (at least 15 min. if not overnight). Rectal implant is one of the quickest ways to affect the lungs.

PULMONARY—Aroma Life, cypress, eucalyptus, pine (antiseptic), [F]sage, [F]sandalwood.

> *The pulmonary is the designated artery conveying blood from the right ventricle of the heart to the lungs or any of the veins conveying oxygenated blood from the lungs to the left atrium of the heart.*

LUPUS: See ADRENAL CORTEX, DIGESTIVE SYSTEM, ENDOCRINE SYSTEM IMMUNE SYSTEM, THYROID. Acceptance, clove, EndoFlex, ImmuPower (alone has cleared up Lupus), Joy, Present Time (key oil for Lupus), Thieves (every 2 hours on the feet), Valor (always use first on the feet for courage to overcome fear and build self esteem).

BATH—Put 30 drops EndoFlex in softened Bath Gel Base (to soften, put in small container and set in hot water) and shake 30 times. Bathe 30 minutes every day. Bath Gel Base cleanses the pores of the skin.

> ***Lupus*** *is a collagen break-down that may effect the skin, joints, and other systems of the body. It occurs because of thyroid and adrenal malfunction. The immune system cells malfunction and some of the good immune cells turn and destroy other good immune cells. This attack leads to an allergic reaction. The immune cells go crazy and attack whatever is convenient for them. The endocrine systems are usually affected and may shut down. In order to heal Lupus, it is necessary to cleanse the body, reduce the toxins, increase blood circulation, and nutritionally support the endocrine functions. When this happens, the adrenal glands can secrete the cortisone that is necessary for connective tissue repair and maintenance.*
>
> *To determine whether or not the thyroid needs help, you must monitor your basal cell temperature. Place a mercury thermometer under your arm pit and leave it there for 10 minutes. If your temperature is below 97.6º you need to work on the thyroid (See RECIPE #1).*

MASSAGE—Thieves (every 2 hours on feet).

PERSONAL CARE— Regenolone (may help reverse symptoms).

SUPPLEMENTS— ComforTone, ICP, and Essentialzyme (cleanses the body of toxins and supports the digestive function), Thyromin (is a main stay for Lupus as it feeds and regulates the thyroid), ImmuneTune (immune support), ImmuPro, Power Meal (pre-digested protein that contains wolfberry), and VitaGreen (high in chlorophyll; contains melissa which supports the connective tissue and the immune function). Carrot juice is also very supportive.

****COMMENTS—Refer to The chapter entitled "How to Use - The Personal Usage Reference" in the Essential Oils Desk Reference under "Lupus" for a specific daily regimen using supplements and blends.*

ADRENAL GLANDS—Nutmeg has adrenal cortex properties and is contained in EndoFlex. EndoFlex or Blend #1 can be applied over the adrenal gland area using a hot compress. Also, apply on and massage the Vita Flex points.

BLEND #1—3 drops clove (rub in), 5 drops nutmeg (rub in), 7 drops rosemary (rub in), and 20 drops V-6 Mixing Oil. Apply a hot compress.

BLEND #2—30 cypress, 30 lemongrass, and 30 EndoFlex in 4 oz. V-6 Mixing Oil. Massage whole body every day.

FLUID RETENTION (caused by steroids)—EndoFlex.

ENDOCRINE SYSTEM SUPPORT—See ENDOCRINE SYSTEM. EndoFlex.

The following is a recipe that has been used for individuals with Lupus:

RECIPE #1—If your basal cell temperature is below 97.6º F (36.5º C), you need to work on the thyroid. Take 2 Thyromin at bedtime. If your temperature doesn't come up in three days, you will need to increase the amount of Thyromin you are taking. Take 1 upon arising along with the 2 at bedtime. When your temperature gets back up to 97.6º F, stop taking the one in the morning. Gradually go off the 2 at night. Check regularly to see that your temperature continues to stay at 97.6° F. In addition, choose one of the following oils to work as tissue generators: Acceptance, Joy, Present Time, or Valor; apply to Vita Flex points and thyroid. To support the adrenal glands, use Blend #1. To determine the adrenal area, lay a yard stick across the back from elbow to elbow and go up 2". Apply ImmuPower on the spine and Vita Flex points. Finally, supplement with Super C / Super C Chewable, 2 Thyromin or more if needed, and ImmuneTune.

CASE HISTORY #1—After doing the following for two months, one individual was totally free from Lupus: Thyromin 2 caps morning, 2 evening until temperature stayed down for three days, then increased to 3 morning and 3 evening. Also, oils used included ImmuPower, and Valor among others.

CASE HISTORY #2—Nurse in a hospital in the east gave ImmuPower to a patient as she was leaving the hospital from another serious bout with Lupus. She had

Lupus for 22 years. She felt better very soon after she used ImmuPower. No symptoms of Lupus were found after eight days.

CASE HISTORY #3—After suffering from systemic lupus for some time, one lady decided there was nothing left to try from the doctors. She turned to the oils an started applying ImmuPower, EndoFlex, and Joy over her thymus and on her feet over the Vita Flex points for the pineal and pituitary glands. She also bega taking Thyromin supplements. After only a day and a half of applying EndoFlex to her toes, she began to have some feeling return. After a while (specific time unknown), the "butterfly" on her face disappeared and blood test returned "just fine".

THOUGHT PATTERNS AND EMOTIONS—Feelings experienced may be those you are not aware of or patterns you brought forward from your ancestors in th DNA. A feeling of giving up. Better to die than stand up for one's self. Anger and a need to be punished. Feelings of deep grief. Laughing on the outside, bu crying on the inside. Self destructive programming, an internal cannibalism, a loss of self worth. (Remember it may not have begun with you, we carry in ou cells the programming of our ancestors for 4 generations back). May feel one c more of the above. Reprogram your cells by claiming your power, loving and approving of yourself in every way (no judgment). You are free and safe; spea up for yourself freely and easily. Righteous judgment is seeing only the good w do; God's judgment. Visualize your body healed or healing. Learn the reason you chose this lesson and learn from it so you can get past it and be healed. Pu as little energy as possible into your affliction.

LYME DISEASE: Clarity (back of ears), Joy (over heart), RC (on chest and inhale), Sacred Mountain (on back of neck), Thieves (on feet and thymus), White Angelica (on forehead).

SUPPLEMENTS—Cleansing Trio (ComforTone, Essentialzyme, and ICP), ArthroTune.

LYMPHATIC SYSTEM: See IMMUNE SYSTEM. [F]Cypress (aromatic), Di-Tone, JuvaFlex (detoxifying), ledum (inflamed lymph nodes), [F]sage, sandalwood (supports), tangerine.

BALANCE AND LONGEVITY—Aroma Life, Mister.

BLEND—5 drops Roman chamomile, 5 lavender, and 5 orange in 2 Tbs. V-6 Mixing Oil. Apply a few drops of blend and massage.

CLEANSING—Lemon, lime.

ESSENTIAL WATERS (HYDROSOLS)—Idaho Tansy (supports cleansing). Spray into air, directly on area of concern, or diffuse using the Essential Mist Diffuse

DECONGESTANT FOR—Aroma Life, Citrus Fresh, cumin, [F]cypress, [F]grapefruit, helichrysum, lemongrass, myrtle, orange, rosemary, tangerine, thyme.

MASSAGE OILS—Cel-Lite Magic.

SUPPLEMENTS—Bodygize.

DRAINAGE OF—[F]Helichrysum, [F]lemongrass.

ELIMINATES WASTE THROUGH—[F]Lavender.

INCREASE FUNCTION OF—Lemon.

MASSAGE OILS—Cel-Lite Magic (stimulates lymph), Relaxation.

SUPPLEMENTS—Body Balancing Trio (Bodygize, Master Formula His/Hers, VitaGreen), ImmuGel, Power Meal.

ALARIA: Lemon with honey in water to prevent.

ALE: See AFTERSHAVE or SKIN. Awaken.

PERSONAL CARE—PD 80/20, Prenolone/Prenolone+, Satin Hand & Body Lotion (moisturizes skin leaving it soft, silky, and smooth), Sensation Hand & Body Lotion (moisturizes and protects skin with an alluring fragrance). KidScents Lotion makes a great aftershave as it soothes and rehydrates the skin.

GENITAL AREA—

INFECTION—Eucalyptus, lavender, melaleuca, oregano, patchouli.

INFLAMMATION—Hyssop, lavender, Roman chamomile.

SWELLING—Cypress, eucalyptus, hyssop, juniper, lavender, rosemary.

HORMONAL SYSTEM (male)—Mister (balances), SclarEssence (increases testosterone levels).

INFERTILITY (male)—Basil, cedarwood, Clary sage, sage , SclarEssence, thyme.

SUPPLEMENTS—Body Balancing Trio His (Bodygize, Master Formula His, VitaGreen).

JOCK ITCH—-Cypress, lavender, melaleuca, or patchouli. Put 2 drops of any one of these oils in 1 tsp. V-6 Mixing Oil and apply to area morning and night OR put 2 drops of any one of these oils in a small bowl of water and wash and dry area well.

SUPPLEMENTS—ProGen, Body Balancing Trio His (Bodygize, Master Formula His, VitaGreen).

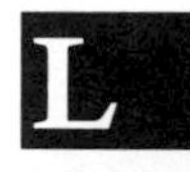

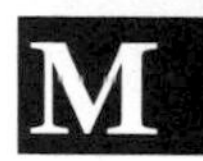

ASSAGE: Any of the different Massage Oils - Ortho Ease and Ortho Sport are excellent.

BLEND—5 drops Mixta chamomile, 5 lavender, 5 orange with 2 Tbs. V-6 Mixing Oil. Apply as a relaxing massage.

EASLES: See CHILDHOOD DISEASES. Eucalyptus.

EDICATION:

SUPPLEMENTS—Super C / Super C Chewable.

MEDITATION: Canadian Red cedar, Dream Catcher (also for sweat lodges), elemi (aromatic) Gratitude, Humility, Inspiration, myrrh (aromatic), Roman chamomile, sandalwood, Sacred Mountain, tsuga (uplifting and grounding).

MELANOMA: See CANCER.

OF SKIN—Frankincense and lavender.

MEMORY: See AMNESIA. Aroma Life, basil (for poor memory), bergamot, calamus, Clarit clove (memory deficiency), Dragon Time, En-R-Gee, Gentle Baby, ginger, grapefruit, Joy (of love), lavender, lemon (improves), lemongrass, Mister, Mountain savory (may bring back good memories), M-Grain, Relieve It, rose, rosemary, sage lavender. Wear as a perfume, apply to temples, and diffuse.

BLEND #1—Add a drop of lemongrass to 1-3 drops of Clarity. May be best to dilu with a few drops of V-6 Mixing Oil. Apply to forehead, temples, behind ears, and on back of neck. Cup hands over nose and mouth and breathe deeply.

BLEND #2—Add a drop of rosemary to 1-3 drops of M-Grain. Apply as described Blend #1.

IMPROVE—Clary sage (aromatic), [F]clove, lime, sage lavender.

BLEND #3—5 basil, 2 peppermint, 10 rosemary, and 1 oz. V-6 Mixing Oil.

RELEASES NEGATIVE—Forgiveness (has high frequencies), geranium (aromatic), 3 W Men.

RETENTION—Clarity.

STIMULATE—Calamus, rosemary (aromatic).

BLEND #4—2 drops Blue tansy, 2 Roman chamomile, 3 geranium, 4 lavender, 3 rosemary, 3 rosewood, 1 spearmint, 2 tangerine, and 1 oz. V-6 Mixing Oil. Apply a few drops of blend to back of neck, wrist, and heart.

MENOPAUSE: See HORMONAL IMBALANCE. Angelica, basil, bergamot, cardamom, Cl sage, [F]cypress, Dragon Time (add V-6 Mixing Oil and use in douche, enema, in rectum), EndoFlex (on throat, parathyroid, and thyroid), [F]fennel, geranium, jasmine, [F]lavender, Mister, neroli, nutmeg (balances hormones), [F]orange, Rom chamomile, rose, rosemary, [F]sage, SclarEssence, thyme. Apply oil(s) to feet, ankles, lower back, groin, and pelvis.

BATH & SHOWER GELS—Add 1 tsp. - 1 oz. Dragon Time Bath & Shower Gel to bath while filling tub with water. Soaking helps relieve lower back pain, stres and sleeping difficulties that are associated with a woman's cycle.

MASSAGE OILS—Dragon Time.

SUPPLEMENTS—CortiStop (Women's), FemiGen, PD 80/20, Prenolone/ Prenolone+, Progessence.

****COMMENTS—The possibility for heart attacks in women increase by 5 to 10% following menopause.*

PRE-MENOPAUSE—[F]Clary sage, EndoFlex, [F]fennel, lavender, Mister, nutmeg (balances hormones), sage lavender (helps raise hormone levels naturally), SclarEssence, tarragon.

ENSTRUATION: See HORMONAL IMBALANCE and PMS.

AMENORRHEA—[F]Basil, carrot, cistus, Clary sage, Dragon Time, fennel, hyssop, juniper, lavender, marjoram, myrrh, peppermint, Roman chamomile, rose, rosemary, sage, sage lavender.

> ***Amenorrhea*** *is the absence of menstruation. The oils listed are those which induce menstrual flow (emmenagogic).*
>
> ***Emmenagogue*** *is an agent that induces or hastens menstrual flow. Many of these oils should be avoided during pregnancy. Please see PREGNANCY for safety data.*

DYSMENORRHEA—Clary sage then basil, cypress, Dragon Time, EndoFlex, fennel, jasmine, juniper, lavender, marjoram, peppermint, Roman chamomile, rosemary, sage, sage lavender, [F]tarragon, yarrow.

> ***Dysmenorrhea*** *is painful menstruation. Apply one or more of these oils to the abdomen. It may also help to use a hot compress. Each of us have different body chemistries so if one oil doesn't work, try a different one.*
>
> ***Menorrhagia*** *is abnormally heavy or extended menstrual flow. It may also refer to irregular bleeding at any time. This situation may be a sign of a more serious condition so please see your doctor.*

BATH & SHOWER GELS—

Add 1 tsp. - 1 oz. Dragon Time Bath & Shower Gel to bath while filling tub with water. Soaking helps relieve lower back pain, stress, and sleeping difficulties that are associated with a woman's cycle.

GENERAL CARE—

BLEND—Before and during cycle, combine 10 drops Dragon Time with 4 basil and rub around ankles, lower back, and lower stomach.

MASSAGE OILS—Dragon Time (uncomfortable days and irregularity)

PERSONAL CARE—PD 80/20, Prenolone/Prenolone+, or Progessence may help to regulate the hormones

> *I have been using Young Living Essential Oils for a little over a year now. Since then, my health has improved somewhat. I decided to stop using birth control pills on Labor Day of 2003, due to being sick from them most of the time and wanting to try something else. I started putting EndoFlex on the bottom of my feet on the endocrine reflex areas. I also continued receiving colonics twice a month and eating cultured vegetables. Between the EndoFlex, colonics, and cultured vegetables, my* ***periods*** *have become more regular and less painful. A friend of mine who's also using EndoFlex on her feet has said that her* ***hot flashes*** *have stopped since she's been using EndoFlex.*
>
> ***-Submitted by Christie Krajewski***
> ***Batesville, Arkansas (July 2004)***

which should alleviate many of the problems associated with menstruation. Se HORMONAL IMBALANCE.

SUPPLEMENTS—Three times a day one week before cycle starts, take 2 droppers full of F.H.S. (available through Creer Labs 801-465-5423) in water. One we after the cycle, take Master Formula Hers four times a day and 6 VitaGreen a day. Also FemiGen (for PMS), Exodus.

IRREGULAR—Clary sage, fennel, lavender, melissa, [F]peppermint, Roman chamomile, ro [F]rosemary, [F]sage.

MENORRHAGIA—Cypress, geranium, Roman chamomile, rose.

SCANTY—Jasmine, lavender, melissa, peppermint. See oils listed under AMENORRHE

MENTAL: Brain Power (increases capacity and clarity by dissolving petrochemicals), [F]oregano (mental diseases), sage (strain, aromatic), vitex (unrest).

ACCURACY—Clarity, peppermint. Diffuse or inhale.

ALERTNESS—Clarity, En-R-Gee.

****COMMENTS—These oils are good for night driving.*

FATIGUE—Aroma Life, Awaken, [F]basil, cardamom, Clarity, Dragon Time, Gentle Baby, lemongrass, Mister, M-Grain, Relieve It, [F]rosemary, sage (diffuse), [F]ylang ylang. Basil and lemongrass together are a good combination.

IMPAIRMENT—Sulfurzyme.

RETARDATION—Can be due to a mineral deficiency. Essential Manna, KidScents Mighty Mist/Vites, Mineral Essence.

STRESS—Clary sage, Evergreen Essence, pine (aromatic), Surrender.

SUPPLEMENTS—ImmuPro.

METABOLISM:

BALANCE—Clove (aromatic), EndoFlex (increases), oregano, spearmint, Valor.

INCREASE (over all)—Spearmint, spikenard.

LIPID—Hyssop (regulates).

STRENGTHEN (vital centers)—Sage.

SUPPLEMENTS—Thyromin (regulates metabolism), ThermaBurn (tablets), ThermaMist (oral spray), Power Meal.

METALS: See CHELATION.

Helichrysum, Juva Cleanse (helps to remove metals from the body), Peace & Calming, Sacred Mountain, Valor.

Heavy metals in the system give off toxic gases and can create allergic symptoms and hormonal imbalances. For example, cadmium can create hyperactivity and learning disabilities in children. Cigarette smoke and caffeine all contain cadmium. Ridding the body of heavy metals is extremely important for proper immune function. Cast-iron cookware leaves heavy iron deposits in the body. Aluminum cookware leaves aluminum deposits in the body. Glass or Stainless Steel cookware is best.

SUPPLEMENTS—Chelex, Cleansing Trio (ComforTone, Essentialzyme, and ICP), JuvaTone.

PULL OUT—Drink steam distilled water. The absence of minerals in distilled water creates a vacuum-like action that pulls metals and toxins from the body.

BLEND #1—Combine 10 cypress, 10 juniper, 10 lemongrass with 1 oz. V-6 Mixing Oil and massage under arms, over kidneys, and on bottoms of feet.

BLEND #2—Add 2-4 drops Thieves and 1-3 drops helichrysum to a rolled gauze and place between cheek and gums to pull out dental mercury. Leave in one place during the night and throw away the gauze roll in the morning. Next night place a new gauze roll with oil in a different place. Continue in like manner until all areas have been affected. ***NOTE: Dilute with V-6 Mixing Oil for use on very sensitive gums or on children.***

MICE (REPEL): Purification.

MIGRAINE HEADACHES: See HEADACHES. Aroma Siez, [F]basil, cumin, [F]eucalyptus, German chamomile, grapefruit, lavender, M-Grain, [F]marjoram, [F]peppermint, spearmint, valerian.

SUPPLEMENTS—Cleansing Trio (ComforTone, Essentialzyme, and ICP).

MILDEW: Purification (put a few drops in a squirt bottle and spray into the air or directly onto a wall to neutralize mildew).

MIND: Basil (absent minded), Believe (stimulates), Surrender (clearing), Western Red cedar (powerful effects on subconscious and unconscious mind).

ESSENTIAL WATERS (HYDROSOLS)—Western Red Cedar. Spray into air or diffuse using the Essential Mist Diffuser.

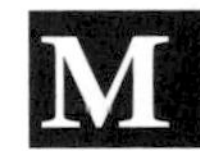

MINERALS (deficiency):

SUPPLEMENTS—Cleansing Trio (ComforTone, Essentialzyme, and ICP), Mineral Essence.

MISCARRIAGE: See PREGNANCY.

MOLD: Purification.

MOLES: Frankincense, geranium, lavender, Melrose.

I am not sure if this is an original idea. I used a combination of lavender and frankincense on a new ***mole*** *that grew in with a very crusty surface. By the time I was able to have an appointment with my doctor it had totally disappeared.*

-Submitted by Judi Arndt
Colorado Springs, Colorado (July 2004)

MOMENT:

BEING IN—Present Time.

MONO (MONONUCLEOSIS): ImmuPower, RC, Thieves.

BLEND—3 oregano, 3 Thieves, and 3 thyme. Rub on feet.

INFECTIOUS—[F]Ravensara.

SUPPLEMENTS—Build immune system. Cleansing Trio (ComforTone, Essentialzyme, and ICP), ImmuneTune, ImmuGel, ImmuPro, Power Meal, Super C / Super C Chewable.

MOOD SWINGS: See HORMONAL IMBALANCE. Can be due to a Vitamin B deficiency. Acceptance, bergamot, Clary sage, Dragon Time or Mister, fennel, Gathering, geranium, Harmony, jasmine, Joy, juniper, lavender, lemon, Peace & Calming, peppermint, Present Time, rose, rosemary, sage, sage lavender, sandalwood, spruce, Trauma Life, Valor, yarrow, ylang ylang.

SUPPLEMENTS—AlkaLime (may help if the mood swing is a result of over acidification), Super B.

MORNING SICKNESS: See PREGNANCY.

MOSQUITOS: See INSECT. Frequent mosquito bites could be due to a Vitamin B deficiency.

SUPPLEMENTS—Super B.

MOTHER (Problems with): Acceptance, geranium, Valor. Apply to ears (*refer to the Auricular Emotional Therapy chart in the Basic Information section of this book*).

MOTION SICKNESS: Di-Tone, ginger, M-Grain, nutmeg, [F]peppermint, spearmint. Apply to feet, temples, and wrists. Can also apply a drop or two of Di-Tone to the hand stir in a clockwise motion, apply behind both ears, rub hands together, cup over nose and mouth and breathe deeply.

****COMMENTS—According to the Essential Oils Desk Reference, "Mix 4 drops peppermint and 4 drops ginger in 1 ounce V-6 Mixing Oil or Massage Oil Base. Rub on chest and stomach before traveling." (EDR-June 2002; Ch. 28, Digestion Problems; Travel Sickness)*

MOTIVATION:

TO MOVE FORWARD—Envision (emotional support), Magnify Your Purpose (empowering and uplifting), Motivation, myrrh, Live with Passion.

SUPPLEMENTS—Sulfurzyme.

MUCUS: See ANTI-CATARRHAL. [F]Cypress, helichrysum (discharge), goldenrod (discharges respiratory mucus), hyssop (opens respiratory system and discharges toxins and mucus), mugwort (expels), onycha (benzoin), [F]rosemary.

MULTIPLE SCLEROSIS (M.S.): See MYELIN SHEATH. Aroma Siez, birch, Clarity, cypress, elemi, frankincense, geranium, helichrysum, Idaho tansy, juniper, oregano, Peace & Calming, peppermint, rosemary, sage, sandalwood, thyme, wintergreen. Do the Raindrop Technique.

> ***Multiple Sclerosis** is a chronic degenerative disorder of the central nervous system where the myelin sheath, which covers the nerves, is gradually destroyed throughout the brain and/or spinal cord. Eventually it causes muscular weakness, loss of coordination, speech and visual disturbances, and bladder and bowel problems. It may be caused by a virus or a defect in the immune system.*
>
> *According to D. Gary Young, progesterone is absolutely necessary in manufacturing, building, repairing, and rejuvenating the myelin sheath. Progesterone is naturally produced from pregnenolone.*

PERSONAL CARE—PD 80/20, Prenolone/Prenolone+, Progessence.

SUPPLEMENTS—ArthroTune, Bodygize, Cleansing Trio (ComforTone, Essentialzyme, and ICP), Essential Omegas, ImmuneTune, ImmuPro, JuvaPower/JuvaSpice, JuvaTone, Mineral Essence, Power Meal, Sulfurzyme, Super B, Super C / Super C Chewable, VitaGreen.

The following are recipes that have been used successfully:

RECIPE #1—Supplement with VitaGreen, Cleansing Trio (ComforTone, Essentialzyme, and ICP), ImmuneTune, and Super C / Super C Chewable. Blend 10 cardamom, 10 peppermint, and 10 rosemary with 1 oz. V-6 Mixing Oil for a full body massage. Finally, diffuse Acceptance and Awaken.

RECIPE #2—Supplement with 8 Super Cal, 2 Super B (after breakfast), 6 Super C / Super C Chewable, 6 VitaGreen four times a day, 4 ImmuneTune, Master Formula His/Hers, and ArthroTune. Apply juniper and peppermint, one at a time, on the spine. If the M.S. is in the neck, work up the spine. If it is in the legs, work down the spine. Do a cold compress and wait for 30 minutes. Remove the compress and repeat again.

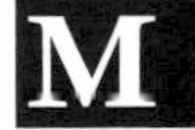

RECIPE #3—Take 2 droppers full of Mineral Essence morning and evening to conduct current to reconnect the nerve tissues. Take ½ Super B in the morning and evening with meals for the first week. Then increase the dosage. Use juniper, geranium, and peppermint on the bottom of the feet and up the legs and spine. Apply oils in the direction of the paralysis. Apply juniper and cypress on the base of the neck, then add Aroma Siez. Next do the Raindrop Technique on the spine using oregano and thyme. Use Peace & Calming and Clarity for brain function and cypress for circulation. Use the Cleansing Trio (ComforTone, Essentialzyme, and ICP) and JuvaTone. Also use ArthroTune and Super C / Super C Chewable for six days. Then start on Super B morning and evening,

Bodygize or meal, 6 VitaGreen four times a day, 4 ImmuneTune two times a day.

BLEND—6 juniper, 4 sandalwood, 2 peppermint, 12 geranium. Mix and massage in neck, spine, and bottom of feet.

****COMMENTS—Avoid hot baths, etc. Heat is the worst thing you can do. If anything, insulate the body with ice packs. Lowering the body temperature with cold packs helps to regenerate the myelin sheath. The person can be kept in the cold packs either for as long as they can stand it or until their body temperature drops 3 degrees. The body temperature must be monitored closely to avoid lowering it to far. This process can be repeated until the person can only stand being in the cold packs for 20 minutes. It is also best avoid diet foods, especially those that contain aspartame as it is known to cause MS, brain damage, and other problems.*

MUMPS: See CHILDHOOD DISEASES. Lavender, melaleuca.

MUSCLES: Aroma Siez, basil, birch, cypress, Idaho balsam fir, lavender, lemongrass, **marjoram**, peppermint, White fir, wintergreen.

ESSENTIAL WATERS (HYDROSOLS)—Basil (relaxing), German Chamomile (relaxing and soothing for sore muscles). Spray directly on area on concern.

MASSAGE OILS—Ortho Ease, Ortho Sport, Relaxation (these oils are great for all problems associated with muscles).

SUPPLEMENTS—AminoTech (enhances muscle building and body toning), Be-Fit (enhances strength and endurance), BLM, CardiaCare, Coral Sea (highly bio-available calcium, contains 58 trace minerals), Essential Manna, Mineral Essence, Power Meal, Sulfurzyme, Super Cal, WheyFit, Wolfberry Bar (*Refer to the Wolfberry Bar in the Supplements section of the Reference Guide for Essential Oils for more information on the benefits of the Chinese Wolfberry*).

****COMMENTS—One professional trainer for body builders used Be-Fit, Power Meal, and Wolfberry Bars to increase muscle mass and strength beyond anything he had previously achieved!*

ACHES AND PAINS—Aroma Siez, [F]birch, Blue cypress, [F]clove, Douglas fir, ginger, helichrysum, Idaho balsam fir, lavender, lemongrass (especially good for ligaments), **marjoram**, nutmeg, oregano, PanAway, peppermint, Relieve It, Roman chamomile, rosemary, spearmint, thyme, vetiver, White fir (with inflammation), wintergreen.

SUPPLEMENTS—Sulfurzyme.

****COMMENTS—Refer to The chapter entitled "How to Use - The Personal Usage Reference" in the Essential Oils Desk Reference under "Muscles" for some excellent blends to help with sore and tight muscles.*

ANTI-INFLAMMATORY—Basil, peppermint, White fir. See ANTI-INFLAMMATORY and INFLAMMATION for additional oils.

****COMMENTS—Refer to The chapter entitled "How to Use - The Personal Usage Reference" in the Essential Oils Desk Reference under "Muscles" for an excellent blend to help reduce inflammation.*

CARDIAC MUSCLE—Goldenrod, lavender, marjoram, neroli, peppermint, rose, rosemary.

SUPPLEMENTS—CardiaCare (strengthen and support).

CRAMPS/CHARLEY HORSES—Aroma Siez, basil, Clary sage, coriander, cypress, grapefruit, jasmine, lavender (aromatic), **marjoram**, pine, Roman chamomile, rosemary, thyme, vetiver.

SUPPLEMENTS—ArthroTune, BLM, Coral Sea (highly bio-available calcium, contains 58 trace minerals), Essential Manna, Mineral Essence, Sulfurzyme, Super Cal.

*Every fall when the weather is hot, then cold, then hot, then cold here in Florida, I get chest pains that my doctor has characterized as **charley horses** in the deep muscles of my chest. Unlike a leg or foot muscle, you can't massage these or walk to stretch them, so there was nothing to do but "endure" these annoying episodes, which sometimes lasted for two hours. One night I woke up with this chest pain, and as I lay there thinking about what I could do for it, I remembered the instant results I had had with Aroma Siez on other people's leg cramps. So I got up and rubbed a few drops of Aroma Siez on my chest, and the pain went away in about 10 minutes!*

-Submitted by Jan Early
Tallahassee, Florida (July 2004)

BLEND—Equal parts rosemary and Aroma Siez. Apply neat or mix with V-6 Mixing Oil and massage.

DEVELOPMENT—Birch/wintergreen (with spruce), PanAway.

SUPPLEMENTS—Be-Fit, Coral Sea (highly bio-available calcium, contains 58 trace minerals), Power Meal, Super Cal, VitaGreen (stimulates and strengthens).

FATIGUE—Aroma Siez, cypress, Douglas fir, eucalyptus, grapefruit, Idaho balsam fir, **marjoram**, peppermint, ravensara, rosemary, thyme.

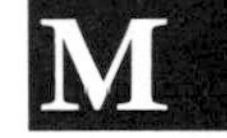

SUPPLEMENTS—ArthroTune, Coral Sea (highly bio-available calcium), Essential Manna (high in magnesium), Mineral Essence, Super Cal.

OVER-EXERCISED—Douglas fir, eucalyptus, **Idaho balsam fir**, ginger, lavender, thyme, White fir (with inflammation).

BATH—3 drops marjoram and 2 drops lemon in a tub of water. Soak.

BLEND—Equal parts of eucalyptus, peppermint, and ginger. Mix with V-6 Mixing Oil and massage.

RHEUMATISM (Muscular)—Rosemary, thyme.

SPRAINS—Black pepper, clove, eucalyptus, ginger, helichrysum, Idaho tansy, jasmine, lavender, lemongrass, **marjoram**, nutmeg, pine, rosemary, thyme, vetiver, White fir.

SPASMS—Aroma Siez, **basil**, Clary sage, cypress, lavender, jasmine, marjoram, PanAw peppermint, Roman chamomile.

MASSAGE OILS—Cel-Lite Magic, Ortho Ease.

SUPPLEMENTS—ArthroTune, Coral Sea (highly bio-available calcium), Super Ca

STIFFNESS—Aroma Siez, PanAway.

SUPPLEMENTS—ArthroTune.

SMOOTH MUSCLE—Bergamot, Black pepper, Clary sage, cypress, fennel, juniper, lavender, **marjoram**, melissa, neroli, peppermint, Roman chamomile, rosema sandalwood. Apply as a hot compress over the affected area.

****COMMENTS—Essential oils with high proportions of ester compounds are especially effective.*

TENSION (especially in shoulders and neck)—Aroma Siez, Douglas fir, helichrysum, juniper, lavender, **marjoram**, Relieve It, Roman chamomile, spruce.

BATH & SHOWER GELS—Evening Peace Bath & Shower Gel (relaxes tired, fatigued muscles and helps alleviate tension).

MASSAGE OILS—Ortho Ease and Ortho Sport.

TISSUE—

SUPPLEMENTS—Bodygize and Power Meal (contain a complete amino acid and vitamin profile and have a high level of predigested protein to maintain a goo food supply for muscle tissue), AminoTech (contains amino acids which help increase formation of lean muscle tissue and prevent muscle from being broke down), Be-Fit (contains ingredients necessary to build muscle mass), BLM, UltraYoung/UltraYoung+ (increase production of growth hormone which increases formation of lean muscle tissue), WheyFit.

****COMMENTS—Refer to The chapter entitled "How to Use - The Personal Usa Reference" in the Essential Oils Desk Reference under "Muscles" for some excellent blends to help improve circulation in the muscles and aid in the regeneration of muscle tissue.*

TONE—Basil, birch, Black pepper, cypress, ginger, grapefruit, juniper, lavender, lime, marjoram, orange, peppermint, petitgrain, pine, rosemary, thyme, wintergreen Apply before exercise.

SUPPLEMENTS—Be-Fit (promotes formation of muscle tissue), Sulfurzyme, WheyFit.

****COMMENTS—Poor muscle tone may indicate a sulfur deficiency.*

TORN MUSCLES—Helichrysum and spruce take pain away (use hot packs), ginger (circulation), **lemongrass**, Lemon myrtle.

MASSAGE OILS—Ortho Sport.

MUSCULAR DYSTROPHY: Aroma Siez, basil, eucalyptus, geranium, ginger, lavender, lem lemongrass, marjoram (combine with equal parts lemongrass), orange, pine, Relieve It, rosemary.

MASSAGE OILS—Ortho Ease, Ortho Sport.

SUPPLEMENTS—Essentialzyme, Mineral Essence, Power Meal, Sulfurzyme, Thyromin, Ultra Young, VitaGreen.

YELIN SHEATH: ImmuneTune, ImmuPro, ImmuPower, and **cold** compresses using peppermint, juniper, and geranium *(remember, **no heat**!)*.

AILS: Citrus Fresh, eucalyptus, frankincense, grapefruit, lavender, lemon (repeated use may help harden), lime, melaleuca, myrrh, oregano, patchouli, peppermint, ravensara, rosemary, thyme.

BLEND—Equal parts frankincense, lemon, and myrrh. Mix with a couple drops of Wheat Germ oil and apply 2-3 times per week.

SUPPLEMENTS—Coral Sea (highly bio-available calcium), Mineral Essence, Sulfurzyme (helps with growth and removal of ridges and cracks), Super Cal.

****COMMENTS—A deficiency in sulfur can cause poor nail growth.*

ARCOLEPSY: Brain Power

SUPPLEMENTS—Mineral Essence, Thyromin, Ultra Young, VitaGreen.

****COMMENTS—Establishing a routine of strict bedtimes and daytime naps may also help reduce the number of unexpected sleep attacks.*

Narcolepsy is a disorder that is characterized by sudden and uncontrollable drowsiness and attacks of sleep at unexpected and irregular intervals. It is frequently misdiagnosed as hypothyroidism (insufficient thyroid hormone), hypoglycemia (insufficient blood sugar), epilepsy, or multiple sclerosis. Proper diagnosis requires overnight monitoring with a device used to detect brain waves called an *electroencephalograph.*

ASAL: See NOSE.

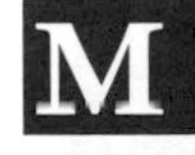

AUSEA: Calamus, cardamom, clove, Di-Tone (over stomach and colon), ginger, juniper, [F]lavender, M-Grain, nutmeg, [F]peppermint (aromatic), rosewood, spearmint, tarragon. Apply behind ears and on Vita Flex points.

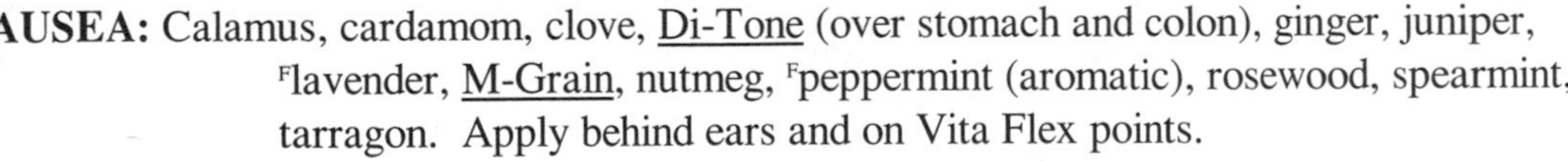

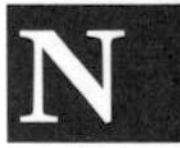

BLEND—2 lavender, 2 spearmint, and 2 drops of another oil for your type of nausea. Mix together and put a little on a cotton ball and inhale three times a day or diffuse.

ECK: Basil, Clary sage, geranium, lemon, lemongrass, orange, helichrysum.

CHRONIC PAIN—PanAway. Apply to base of big toe.

SUPPLEMENTS—BLM

NEGATIVE IONS: When dispersed into the air through a cool-air nebulizing diffuser, the following oils ionize negatively: Bergamot, cedarwood, citronella, *Eucalyptus citriodora*, grapefruit, lavandin, lavender, lemon, lemongrass, mandarin, orange, patchouli, sandalwood.

> **Negative ions** are produced naturally by wind and rain. They help stimulate the parasympathetic nervous system which controls rest, relaxation, digestion, and sleep. However, if you live in an environment with an over-abundance of negative ions, such as in the country or by the ocean, you may benefit greatly by diffusing the oils listed under POSITIVE IONS. The production of more positive ions can help bring greater balance to the area and provide a more healthy environment.

NEGATIVITY: Sandalwood (removes negative programming from the cells), Transformation.

BREAKS UP—Dream Catcher, Forgiveness.

DROWNING IN OWN—Grapefruit (aromatic).

NERVOUS SYSTEM: [F]Basil (stimulant and for nervous breakdown), bergamot, Brain Power, calamus, cedarwood (nervous tension), cinnamon bark, cumin (stimulant), Di-Tone, frankincense, geranium (regenerates nerves), ginger, Idaho balsam fir, jasmine (nervous exhaustion), juniper (better nerve function), lavender, lemon, lemongrass (for nerve damage; activates), marjoram (soothing), *Melaleuca ericifolia* (nervous tension), nutmeg (supports), orange, palmarosa (supports), Peace & Calming, pepper (stimulant), **peppermint** (soothes and strengthens; place on wrists or location of nerve damage), petitgrain (re-establishes nerve equilibrium), pine (stimulant), ravensara, Roman chamomile, rosemary, [F]sage, sandalwood, spearmint, spruce (fatigue), valerian (central nervous system depressant), vetiver.

PERSONAL CARE—NeuroGen or Regenolone (both help nerve regeneration).

SUPPLEMENTS—Coral Sea (highly bio-available calcium, contains 58 trace minerals), Mineral Essence, Sulfurzyme, Super B.

TINCTURES—Nerv-Cal (supplies nerve tissues with calcium), Nerv-Us (helps heal nerve damage and relax nervous conditions). *Both tinctures are available through Creer Labs 801-465-5423.*

NERVOUSNESS—Cypress, goldenrod, orange, Surrender, tangerine.

PARASYMPATHETIC NERVES—See PARASYMPATHETIC NERVES. [F]Marjoram (increases tone of).

VIRUS OF NERVES—Clove and frankincense.

NEURALGIA (severe pain along nerve): Cajeput, cedarwood, eucalyptus, helichrysum, junipe lavender, [F]marjoram, nutmeg, pine, [F]Roman chamomile, sage lavender.

NEURITIS: Cedarwood, clove, eucalyptus, juniper, lavender, [F]Roman chamomile, yarrow.

UROLOGICAL PROBLEMS: Limit the use of oils with high *ketone* content.

******COMMENTS—A 4 year old child was in a car accident where she suffered severe brain damage. The surgeon removed part of her brain which sent her into a coma. After being in a coma for two months, Dr. Friedmann was asked to help her. He used oils that are commonly used for neurological problems. He put Valor on the back of her neck, skull, and feet. He also used Present Time and Awaken. She came out of the coma and started doing physical therapy.***

UROMUSCULAR: Roman chamomile, tarragon.

UROPATHY: Brain Power, cedarwood, cypress, eucalyptus, geranium, helichrysum, juniper, JuvaFlex, lavender, lemongrass, peppermint, Roman chamomile, Valor.

PERSONAL CARE—NeuroGen, PD 80/20, Prenolone/Prenolone+, Progessence, Regenolone.

SUPPLEMENTS—Bodygize, Essential Manna, Mineral Essence, Sulfurzyme, Super B.

****COMMENTS—Refer to The chapter entitled "How to Use - The Personal Usage Reference" in the Essential Oils Desk Reference under "Nerve Disorders" subcategory "Neuropathy" for some excellent blends.*

PAIN—Relieve It, helichrysum (best with cold compresses), PanAway. Massage with peppermint, juniper, and geranium and reapply cold compresses.

EUROTONIC: Melaleuca, [F]ravensara, thyme.

IGHT SWEATS: See HOT FLASHES and HORMONAL IMBALANCE. EndoFlex, [F]Sage.

OSE: Melaleuca, rosemary.

BLEEDING—Cypress, frankincense, lavender, lemon.

BLEND—2 cypress, 1 helichrysum, and 2 lemon in 8 oz. ice water. Soak cloth and apply to nose and back of neck.

NASAL MUCUS MEMBRANE—Eucalyptus may help reduce inflammation.

NASAL NASOPHARYNX—Eucalyptus.

POLYPS—See POLYPS. Basil, citronella, frankincense, oregano, peppermint, Purification, RC (can be applied to inside of nose with cotton swab). Apply to exterior of nose (use caution because of close proximity to eyes) or breathe in diffused mist. A colon and liver cleanse may be helpful. Birch/wintergreen or Valor may also be applied to bridge of nose for possible structural realignment.

****COMMENTS—Nasal polyps are caused by an overproduction of fluid in the mucous membranes. They are seen with asthma, hay fever, chronic sinus infections, and cystic fibrosis. In fact, one source stated that one out of four people with cystic fibrosis have nasal polyps. They may also be a result of*

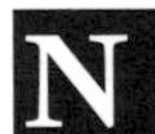

blockages in the brain or some trauma to the nose in which structural integ has been compromised. Diet may also be a factor.

NURSING: Clary sage (brings in milk production), [F]fennel or basil (increases milk production), geranium. Apply above breasts on lymph area and on spine at breast level.

INCREASE MILK PRODUCTION—

BLEND—7 to 15 drops fennel and either 7 to 15 drops geranium or 5 to 10 drops Clary sage. Dilute 1-2 drops of blend in 2 Tbs. V-6 Mixing Oil.

SUPPLEMENTS—Body Balancing Trio Hers (Bodygize, Master Formula Hers, VitaGreen).

DECREASE MILK PRODUCTION—Peppermint. Apply with cold compress over breas *Refer to Methods of Application under the Science and Application section t Reference Guide for Essential Oils for instructions on using cold compresse*

OBESITY: See DIET, WEIGHT. Fennel, grapefruit, juniper, Juva Cleanse, orange, rosemary tangerine.

SUPPLEMENTS—Berrygize Nutrition Bars, JuvaPower/JuvaSpice, Power Meal (e for breakfast as a meal replacement).

REDUCE—Juva Cleanse, Orange, tangerine.

OBSESSIVENESS: Acceptance, Awaken, Clary sage, cypress, Forgiveness, geranium, helichrysum, Humility, Inner Child, Joy, lavender, marjoram, Motivation, Present Time, rose, Sacred Mountain, sandalwood, Valor, ylang ylang.

ODORS: See DEODORANT. Bergamot, lavender, Purification (neutralizes and eliminates).

PERSONAL CARE—AromaGuard Deodorants.

BODY—Purification (obnoxious odors).

CONTROLLIING—Cedarwood.

OPENING (to receive): Fir (aromatic), Transformation.

OPPOSITION: Valor.

ORAL INFECTIONS: [F]Rosewood.

OSTEOPOROSIS: See HORMONAL IMBALANCE. Aroma Siez, birch, chamomile (Roman and German), clove, cypress, fennel, fir

Studies and clinical experience by Dr. John R. Lee indicate that bone mass can be reversed (regained) by as much as 41% with the use of Natural Progesterone. For information on Dr. Lee's book, see HORMONAL IMBALANCE.

(cortisone-like action), geranium, ginger, hyssop, lemon, nutmeg, oregano, PanAway, Peace & Calming, peppermint, pine, Relieve It, rosemary, spruce, thyme, wintergreen.

SUPPLEMENTS—BLM, Coral Sea (highly bio-available calcium, contains 58 trace minerals), PD 80/20, Prenolone/Prenolone+, Progessence, Super Cal.

'ARIES: See HORMONAL IMBALANCE. Di-Tone, geranium, Gratitude, [F]myrtle, and/or [F]rosemary (regulates).

OVARIAN CYSTS—Basil.

BLEND—5 frankincense and 5 Melrose. Mix and apply to lower back and abdomen. May also consider adding this blend to 2 tsp. of olive oil and before going to bed, while lying down, insert blend into vagina and retain with a tampon throughout the night.

PERSONAL CARE—PD 80/20, Prenolone/Prenolone+, Progessence, Protec.

SUPPLEMENTS—FemiGen (helps feed the body), Master Formula Hers.

'ERCOME AND RELEASE UNPLEASANT, DIFFICULT ISSUES IN LIFE: Acceptance, Release, Roman chamomile, SARA, Transformation, Trauma Life.

'EREATING: See EATING DISORDERS.

'ERWEIGHT: See OBESITY and WEIGHT.

'ERWHELMED: Acceptance, Hope, Release, Valor.

'YGEN:

All essential oils increase the ability of the body to take oxygen to the cells and to push toxins out. The oils pick up more oxygen and take it to the site of discomfort.

OXYGENATING—Fennel, fir, frankincense, oregano, sandalwood (increases oxygen around pineal and pituitary glands).

PERSONAL CARE—Satin Facial Scrub - Mint (deep cleansing that dispenses nutrients and oxygen).

OXYGEN EXCHANGE—Tsuga (increases by opening and dilating respiratory tract).

'IN: See ACHES AND PAINS.

'INTING: Add one 15 ml. bottle of your favorite essential oil (or oil blend) to any five gallon bucket of paint. Stir vigorously, mixing well, and then either spray paint or paint by hand. This should eliminate the paint fumes and after-smell.

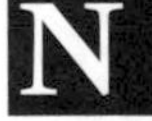
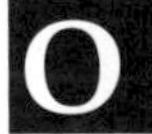
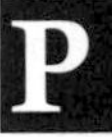

PALPITATIONS: See HEART.

PANCREAS: Coriander, [F]cypress (for insufficiencies), dill, fleabane, lemon, Raven, RC, rosemary, Thieves.
STIMULANT FOR—Fleabane, [F]helichrysum.
SUPPORT—Cinnamon bark, coriander, EndoFlex, fennel, geranium.
SUPPLEMENTS—Essentialzyme, Stevia, Thyromin, VitaGreen.

PANCREATITIS:
WEAKNESS—Lemon, marjoram.

PANIC: Awaken, bergamot, birch, fir, frankincense, Gathering, Harmony, Idaho balsam fir, lavender, marjoram, myrrh, Roman chamomile, rosemary, sandalwood, spruc thyme, Valor, White Angelica, wintergreen, ylang ylang.

PARALYSIS: Awaken, cypress, geranium, ginger, helichrysum, juniper, lemongrass, nutmeg, peppermint, Purification, Valor.
BLEND—Combine 6 cypress, 15 geranium, 10 helichrysum, 5 juniper, 2 peppermi and V-6 Mixing Oil. May rejuvenate nerve damage up to 60%. Put on locat and on feet.
SUPPLEMENTS—Support the body with Bodygize, VitaGreen, Super B, Master Formula His/Hers, Mineral Essence. When it starts to reverse there will be pa apply PanAway on location and on feet.

PARASITES: See ANTI-PARASITIC and INTESTINAL PROBLEMS. Anise, clove, Di-Tone, [F]fennel, hyssop, melaleuca, Mountain savory, mugwort (blend with thyme), [F]oregano, tangerine, [F]tarragon, [F]thyme. Apply oil on stomach and feet to help pass parasites.

ParaFree was specifically designed to help the body rid itself of parasites. The essential oils contained in this supplement are: Black cumin, anise, fennel, laurel, vetiver, nutmeg, melaleuca alternifolia, Idaho tansy, clove, and thyme.

Since this product is to be used orally and contraindications do exist, one would be well advised to review the book, Essential Oil Safety—A Guide for Health Care Professionals by Robert Tisserand and Tony Balacs or Aromatherapy for Health Professionals by Shirley and Len Price.

ANTI-PARASITIC—[F]Nutmeg.
INTESTINAL—[F]Lemon, ravensara, [F]Roman chamomile.
SUPPLEMENTS—Cleansing Trio (ComforTone, Essentialzyme, and ICP), ParaFr
****COMMENTS—Individuals have passed parasites within 12 hours using Di-To on stomach.*

ARASYMPATHETIC NERVOUS SYSTEM: [F]Lemongrass (regulates), [F]marjoram (increases tone of), Peace & Calming, Valor.

DIFFUSION—See NEGATIVE IONS for a list of oils that ionize negatively when diffused to help stimulate the parasympathetic nervous system.

The Parasympathetic Nervous System is responsible for preparing us for feeding, digestion, and rest by slowing the heart, contracting the bronchi, dilating the arteries, and stimulating the digestive system.

****COMMENTS—See the Autonomic Nervous System chart in the Science and Application section of the Reference Guide for Essential Oils.*

ARATHYROID: EndoFlex. Apply over the thyroid gland at the bottom of the throat or on the parathyroid Vita Flex point on feet.

*The **parathyroid gland** is responsible for secreting a hormone necessary for the metabolism of calcium and phosphorus. It is located near or within the posterior surface of the thyroid gland.*

ARKINSON'S DISEASE: See BRAIN, PINEAL GLAND, PITUITARY GLAND, and ALZHEIMER'S DISEASE. Acceptance, basil, bergamot, Clarity (brain function), cypress (circulation), frankincense, Gathering (high in sesquiterpenes and in frequency), geranium, helichrysum, juniper, Juva Cleanse, lavender, lemon, marjoram, nutmeg, orange, Peace & Calming, peppermint, rosemary, sandalwood, thyme, Valor, vitex.

Cedarwood, vetiver, sandalwood, Black pepper, myrrh, patchouli, ginger, German chamomile, spikenard, galbanum, and frankincense all contain sesquiterpenes which have the ability to go beyond the blood-brain barrier. See PINEAL GLAND and PITUITARY GLAND.

SUPPLEMENTS—BLM, Cleansing Trio (ComforTone, Essentialzyme, and ICP), JuvaPower/JuvaSpice, JuvaTone, Power Meal (contains Choline which is beneficial for Parkinson's disease), Sulfurzyme.

TINCTURES—Chelex.

The following recipe has been used by Dr. Terry Friedmann of Paradise Valley, Arizona:

RECIPE #1—Use the Cleansing Trio (ComforTone, Essentialzyme, and ICP) for one week, then add JuvaTone and 10 VitaGreen along with it. Drink 10 glasses of distilled water daily. Take one dropper full of Chelex tincture two times a day and diffuse the oil of helichrysum and frankincense together one hour at night.

TO PREVENT—Keep liver and blood clean with Juva Cleanse, JuvaTone and the Cleansing Trio (ComforTone, Essentialzyme, and ICP). Massage with helichrysum and sandalwood to help chelate metallics out of the body.

PAST: Present Time (helps to bring you into the present so you can go forward), Transformatio

PEACE: Juniper (aromatic), lavender (aromatic), marjoram, Peace & Calming, Release, Traum Life, ylang ylang.

FINDING—Tangerine (aromatic).

PROMOTE—Roman chamomile.

SUPPLEMENTS—Cleansing Trio (ComforTone, Essentialzyme, and ICP) and JuvaTone.

PELVIC PAIN SYNDROME: Bergamot, clove, geranium, ginger, nutmeg, thyme.

PERIODONTAL DISEASE: See GUM DISEASE.

PERSONAL GROWTH: Transformation.

ELIMINATING BLOCKED—Helichrysum, frankincense.

PERSONALITY (MULTIPLE)—Inner Child, SARA, and Sensation.

PERSPIRATION: Petitgrain, Purification.

SUPPLEMENTS—Cleansing Trio (ComforTone, Essentialzyme, and ICP).

PEST TROUBLES: See INSECT. Ravensara.

pH BALANCE: See ACIDOSIS and ALKALOSIS.

SUPPLEMENTS—AlkaLime (combats yeast and fungus overgrowth and preserves the body's proper pH balance), ComforTone (to help clean out the colon), Essentialzyme, JuvaTone (to clean the liver) and Mineral Essence (if body is too alkaline), VitaGreen (brings blood back to an alkaline pH).

PERSONAL CARE—Genesis Hand & Body Lotion (balances pH on skin).

According to Dr. Robert O. Young in his book, One Sickness, One Disease, One Treatment, "disease is an expression of pH." He believes that there is only one disease which is "the constant over-acidification of the blood and tissues which disturbs the central regulation of the human body, all of which is mainly the result of an inverted way of living and eating." All sickness and disease that leads to death begins with an over-acidification of the blood and tissues and culminates with yeast and fungus. A normal healthy body should have a pH of about 7.2. (The use of saliva and urine test strips will show a much lower pH level due to the protein present in the solution. Saliva and urine tests from a healthy body should be about 6.6 to 6.8.) To maintain this pH, our diet should consist of 80% alkaline foods to 20% acid foods. "In the healing of disease, when the individual is acidic, the higher the ratio of alkaline elements in the diet, the faster will be the recovery."

HARYNGITIS: See also RHINOPHARYNGITIS. Goldenrod.

HLEBITIS: Cypress, geranium, grapefruit, [F]helichrysum (prevents), [F]lavender, Roman chamomile, or Valor. Massage toward heart and wear support hose until healed, possibly two to three months. Use Aroma Life every morning and night. Do the Raindrop Technique on leg.

IMPLES: Clary sage, frankincense, Gentle Baby, ImmuPower (pimples in ears), lavender, lemongrass, melaleuca, Melrose, Purification, Raven, ravensara, RC.

PERSONAL CARE—Rose Ointment (apply over top of other oil(s) used to enhance and extend their effectiveness).

INEAL GLAND:

OPENS AND INCREASES OXYGEN—Acceptance, Brain Power, Canadian Red cedar cedarwood, Forgiveness, frankincense, Gathering, Harmony, Inspiration, Into the Future, Release, sandalwood (increases oxygen), spruce, Transformation, Trauma Life, 3 Wise Men (same frequency as pineal).

****COMMENTS— Just smelling the essential oils will increase the oxygen production, particularly around the pineal and pituitary glands, and will help increase the secretion of anti-bodies, endorphins, and neuro-transmitters.*

*The **pineal gland** synthesizes a hormone called melatonin in periods of darkness. The pineal gland and melatonin are being studied for their roles in aging, sleep, and reproduction. The pineal gland is also involved in the process of creativity and planning things to do. If the pineal gland is not open, negative emotions will be attracted back to the aura.*

***Oils containing sesquiterpenes are especially effective in oxygenating the pineal and pituitary glands.** These include cedarwood, vetiver, sandalwood, Black pepper, myrrh, patchouli, ginger, German chamomile, spikenard, galbanum, and frankincense in order of sesquiterpene content. Blends include 3 Wise Men, Acceptance, Brain Power, Forgiveness, Gathering, Harmony, Inspiration, Into the Future, and Trauma Life.*

ITUITARY: See ENDOCRINE SYSTEM.

SUPPLEMENTS—Ultra Young (a new spray neutriceutical which contains ingredients that are necessary for stimulating the pituitary gland into producing the human growth hormone (hGH) and allowing the body to utilize it).

BALANCES—Geranium, ylang ylang. Apply to forehead, back of neck, and Vita Flex points on big toes.

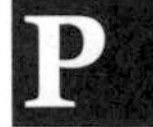

INCREASES OXYGEN— 3 Wise Men, Acceptance, Brain Power, frankincense, Forgiveness, Gathering, Harmony, Inspiration, Into the Future, sandalwood, Trauma Life. Apply to the forehead, back of neck, and Vita Flex points on big toes. Can also rub a couple drops of oil between hands, cup over nose and mouth, and breathe deeply (see COMMENT under PINEAL above).

*The **pituitary gland** is located at the base of the brain and is considered to be the master gland because its secretions stimulate the other endocrine glands. The pituitary has an anterior and a posterior lobe. The anterior lobe secretes the human growth hormone (stimulates overall body growth), adrenocorticotropic hormone (controls steroid hormone secretion by the adrenal cortex), thyrotropic hormone (stimulates the activity of the thyroid gland), and three gonadotropic hormones (control growth and reproductive activity of the ovaries and testes). The posterior lobe secretes antidiuretic hormone and oxytocin. The antidiuretic hormone causes water retention by the kidneys. Oxytocin stimulates the mammary glands to release milk and also causes uterine contractions. An overactive pituitary during childhood can cause a child to be extremely tall while an underactive pituitary can result in the opposite. (Refer to the text box for Pineal Gland above for a list of oils that are high in sesquiterpenes.)*

PLAGUE: Abundance, [F]clove, Thieves (annihilates bacteria).

PLEURISY: See LUNGS or ANTI-BACTERIAL. [F]Cypress, [F]thyme.

PMS: See HORMONAL IMBALANCE. Angelica, anise, bergamot, [F]Clary sage, Exodus II, fennel, geranium, grapefruit, jasmine, lavender (aromatic), nutmeg, Peace & Calming, Roman chamomile, [F]tarragon.

APATHETIC-TIRED-LISTLESS PMS—Bergamot, fennel, geranium, grapefruit, Roman chamomile.

BATH & SHOWER GELS—Dragon Time Bath & Shower Gel.

BLEND—10 drops Dragon Time and 4 drops basil. Rub blend around ankles, lower back, and lower stomach. Use before and during cycle.

IRRITABLE PMS—Bergamot, Clary sage, nutmeg, Roman chamomile.

MASSAGE OILS—Before and during cycle, combine 10 drops Dragon Time with 4 basil and rub around ankles, lower back and lower stomach.

SUPPLEMENTS—Berrygize Nutrition Bars, Essential Omegas, Exodus, PD 80/20, Prenolone/Prenolone+, Progessence. Three times a day one week before cycle starts, take 2 droppers full of F.H.S. (available through Creer Labs 801-465-5423) in water. One week after the cycle, take Master Formula Hers four time a day and 6 VitaGreen a day. Also FemiGen (for PMS)—take 2 FemiGen thre times a day before period, start again two days after cycle.

VIOLENT AGGRESSIVE PMS—Bergamot, geranium, nutmeg.

SUPPLEMENTS—Essential Omegas.

WEEPING-DEPRESSION PMS—Bergamot, Clary sage, geranium, nutmeg.
SUPPLEMENTS—Essential Omegas.

EUMONIA: See RESPIRATORY SYSTEM (comments and recipe #1). Cajeput, eucalyptus, Exodus II, frankincense, ImmuPower (on spine), lavender, lemon, melaleuca, *Melaleuca ericifolia*, oregano, Raven (on back and feet), ravensara, Thieves (on feet) and thyme are good to use as compresses.
SUPPLEMENTS—Exodus, Master Formula His/Hers, Ultra Young.
One or more of the following can be used with great effect:

1. RC on chest.
2. Put 15 drops of RC in 2 cups of hot water in a bowl, wet towel, ring out, and put on chest with a dry towel on top.
3. Put 4 drops of RC or eucalyptus in ½ cup hot water, inhale steam deeply.
4. Raven in rectum, RC on chest and back (reverse each night).

****COMMENTS—Refer to The chapter entitled "How to Use - The Personal Usage Reference" in the Essential Oils Desk Reference under "Pneumonia - Emphysema" for some excellent blend recipes and supplement recommendations.*

ISON OAK-IVY: Harmony, Joy, Lavender, Melrose, Roman chamomile, rose, rosewood, palmarosa.
PERSONAL CARE—Rose Ointment.

LLUTION: See PURIFICATION. Purification.
AIR—Lemon, peppermint, Purification.
CIGARETTE SMOKE—Purification.
WATER—Lemon, peppermint, Purification.

*Recently I got **Poison Ivy/Oak** for the first time. I looked in my "Reference Guide for Essential Oils" and decided to use Melrose on my poison ivy. The itching would stop for about 5 minutes and start up again. I decided to put Purification on, which stopped the itching for maybe an hour or two and then would start up again. Getting desperate I used Joy and sometimes Harmony (since I had more Harmony) on the poison ivy. The itching would stop for most of the day and I would forget about having poison ivy. I didn't start the Harmony and Joy until about 3 or 4 days into the poison ivy flare up, but it's now the 6th day and I'm not itching unless I take a shower or sweat profusely. From my experience with my poison ivy, I'm convinced that the presence of Rose, Rosewood, and Palmarosa in Joy and Harmony, have all helped in the healing of our "skin conditions". I plan to stock up on Harmony and Joy for future needs.*

-Submitted by Christie Krajewski
Batesville, Arkansas (July 2004)

LYPS: See also NOSE:POLYPS. Di-Tone, Exodus II, peppermint, spikenard, and others with strong anti-bacterial properties (See ANTI-BACTERIAL).
SUPPLEMENTS—ComforTone, Coral Sea (highly bio-available calcium, contains 58 trace minerals), Essentialzyme, Exodus, Master Formula His/Hers, Super Cal.
****COMMENTS—In two separate articles published in 1998, bacterial infection was found to exist when polyps were present. In the case of colorectal (intestinal)*

polyps, E. coli and similar bacteria were found to be adhering to the walls o the large intestine, and even partially penetrating the intestinal mucosa (Gastroenterology 1998; 115: 281-286). In the case of gastric polyps (sma growths in the stomach lining), the Helicobacter pylori bacteria was found, and when eradicated, the polyps disappeared in 71% of the patients within a 12 to 15 month period (Annals of Internal Medicine 1998; 129: 712-715).

POSITIVE FEELINGS: Acceptance, Abundance, Envision, Forgiveness, Idaho tansy, Joy, Motivation, Live with Passion, 3 Wise Men (releases negative memory/traum and reinforces positive feelings which creates greater spiritual awareness).

POSITIVE IONS: When dispersed into the air through a cool-air nebulizing diffuser, the following oils ionize positively: Cajeput, clove, cypress, eucalyptus, frankincense, helichrysum, juniper, marjoram, *Melaleuca quinquenervia*, palmarosa, pine, ravensara, rosemary, thyme, ylang ylang.

> ***Positive ions*** *are produced by electronic equipment and are typically found in man-made environments. They help stimulate the sympathetic nervous system, necessary for recovering, strengthening, and energizing. However, an over-abundance of positive ions can lead to stress and agitation. The diffusion of the oils listed under NEGATIVE IONS can help balance the ions and help produce a more stress free environment.*

POTASSIUM DEFICIENCY:
SUPPLEMENTS—Essential Manna, Master Formula His/Hers, Mineral Essence, Thyromin.

> ***Potassium*** *is important for a healthy nervous system and a regular heart rhythm. It works with sodium to control the body's water balance and regulates the transfer of nutrients to the cells.*

POTENTIAL: Acceptance, Awaken (realize our highest potential), Believe (release our unlimi potential), Gathering, Transformation, White Angelica (greater awareness of one's potential).

POWER: Sacred Mountain, Surrender (calming and relaxing to dominant personalities), Valor

POWER SURGES: See HOT FLASHES.

PRAYER: Frankincense, Inspiration, Sacred Mountain.

PREGNANCY: Elemi, Gentle Baby (relieves stress during pregnancy; can also be used by fathers to relieve stress during delivery), geranium, grapefruit, jasmine, lavender, Roman chamomile, tangerine, ylang ylang.

SUPPLEMENTS—PD 80/20, Prenolone/Prenolone+, Progessence, Thyromin (use before, during, and after).

PERSONAL CARE—ClaraDerm (Essential oil spray - apply topically to stressed skin before and after childbirth).

ANXIETY/TENSION—<u>Into the Future</u> (help let go of fear and trauma), <u>Present Time</u> (help mother focus on giving birth).

BLEND—Add 10 drops lavender, 10 orange, 2 marjoram, 2 cedarwood, 1 Roman chamomile to 4 oz. sweet almond oil or V-6 Mixing Oil. Use as a massage oil or in bath water.

SUPPLEMENTS—PD 80/20, Prenolone/Prenolone+, Progessence.

BABY (Newborn)—Frankincense (1 drop on crown for protection), myrrh (on remaining umbilical cord and around navel to protect from infection), <u>Valor</u> (1 drop - divide between both feet & 1-2 drops rubbed up spine to help ensure proper alignment).

BREASTS—Fennel (tone), Roman chamomile (sore nipples).

CONCEPTION—Do a proper cleansing for one year before. May want to start with the Master Cleanser (See CLEANSING for more information).

SUPPLEMENTS—Cleansing Trio (especially ComforTone for the colon and ICP for the intestines), JuvaTone (cleanses liver).

CONSTIPATION—ComforTone can be taken during pregnancy as long as you don't get diarrhea. Diarrhea can cause cramping which could bring on labor.

PREGNANCY SAFETY DATA

<u>Avoid During Pregnancy</u>

Single Oils: *Basil, birch, calamus, cassia, cinnamon bark, hyssop, Idaho tansy, lavandin, rosemary, sage, tarragon.*

Blends: *Di-Tone, Dragon Time, Exodus II, Grounding, Mister.*

Other: *Estro, Exodus, FemiGen, ParaFree, Protec,*

<u>Use Cautiously During Pregnancy</u>

Single Oils: *Angelica, cedarwood, chamomile (German/Blue), cistus, citronella, Clary sage, clove bud, cumin (Black), cypress, davana, fennel, laurel, marjoram, Mountain savory, myrrh, nutmeg, peppermint, rose, spearmint, vetiver, yarrow.*

Blends: *Aroma Siez, Clarity, Harmony, ImmuPower, Relieve It, Thieves.*

Other: *Prenolone/Prenolone+, ComforTone, Essentialzyme, ArthroTune, Dragon Time Massage Oil.*

It was very difficult to compile a list of oils and products to be avoided during pregnancy. Each aromatologist has a different opinion. We feel that an oil that is unsafe is an oil that has been adulterated or one that is used improperly. Oils that are diluted, applied externally and in moderation should not create a problem. This list is a compilation of the safety data contained in aromatherapy books written by the following authors: Ann Berwick, Julia Lawless, Shirley & Len Price, Jeanne Rose, Robert Tisserand, and Tony Balacs.

SUPPLEMENTS—Essentialzyme, JuvaTone (helps change genetics in the colon an purge the liver).

DELIVERY—Clary sage, Forgiveness, Gentle Baby, Harmony, lavender (stimulates circulation, calming, antibiotic, anti-inflammatory, antiseptic), nutmeg (balan hormones, calms the central nervous system, alleviates anxiety, increases circulation, and good for blood supply), Valor (align mother's hips; apply alo inside and bottom of each foot, then have someone hold feet–right palm to rig foot and left palm to left foot–to balance energy flows; rub a couple drops alo newborn's spine for alignment).

****CAUTION—Nutmeg is generally non-toxic, non-irritant, and non-sensitizing. However, large doses may cause nausea, stupor, and tachycardia. Use in moderation and with great care during pregnancy. See the safety data abou nutmeg in the APPENDIX of this book.*

AVOID EPISIOTOMY—ClaraDerm Spray (spray onto and massage into perineum three times daily), Gentle Baby or geranium (neat or added to olive oil; massa perineum).

BLEND—8 drops geranium, 5 drops lavender, 1 oz. V-6 Mixing Oil. Prepare three weeks before delivery and rub on perineum three times a day. One week befo delivery, prepare same blend and add 5 drops fennel. Continue applying three times daily.

DIFFUSE—Hope, Joy, Motivation, Live with Passion, Peace & Calming.

UTERUS—Tone uterus with 1-3 drops of Clary sage around ankles (one woman dilated and had her baby in 1 ½ hours), Dragon Time, fennel, Gathering, sage

TRANSITION—Basil.

EARLY LABOR—Lavender (rub on tummy to stop).

ENERGY—Put equal portions of Roman chamomile, geranium, and lavender in V-6 Mixi Oil.

HEMORRHAGING—Helichrysum and Gentle Baby together on lower back (prevent).

HIGH BLOOD PRESSURE—Aroma Life (heart). Avoid using hyssop, rosemary, sage, thyme, and possibly peppermint.

KEEP BABY IN BIRTH CANAL—Gentle Baby.

****COMMENTS—One mother would rub Gentle Baby on her little fingers and lit toes when contracting. The she would squeeze the sides of her little fingers while someone else squeezed her little toes. This was repeated during contractions until the baby decided to stay in the birth canal.*

LABOR (during)—Clary sage (kick labor into gear; some have combined with fennel), Gentle Baby (apply to ankles and hands when labor starts), Into the Future (tc help move past fear and trauma), jasmine (speed up contractions), Present Tir (to help mother focus).

BLEND—**(Use only when ready to deliver)**. 2 oz. V-6 Mixing Oil, 8 drops Clary sage, 8 drops lavender, 8 drops jasmine. May be useful when trying to induce labor or augment a slow, lazy labor.

PAIN—<u>PanAway</u> (apply to lower back and tummy area).

****COMMENTS—Refer to The chapter entitled "How to Use - The Personal Usage Reference" in the <u>Essential Oils Desk Reference</u> under "Pregnancy" for a wonderful blend to use during labor.*

LABOR (post)—Geranium, lavender.

****COMMENTS—Lavender is calming and has a slight analgesic effect. It also stimulates circulation, which is great for both mother and baby, and has anti-inflammatory and antiseptic properties. Geranium is one of the best oils to stimulate circulation, which in turn facilitates easy breathing. It has a contractive effect and helps pull together dilated tissues, so it is healing for the uterus and endometrium after the birth. Geranium is also an anti-depressant and is known for its uplifting effect (<u>Alternative Medicine—A Definitive Guide</u>, pp. 806-7).*

LACTATION—See MILK PRODUCTION.

MASTITIS (breast infection)—<u>Citrus Fresh</u> (with lavender), <u>Exodus II</u>, lavender, tangerine.

BLEND—Equal amounts of lavender and tangerine. Dilute with some V-6 Mixing Oil and apply to breasts and under arms twice a day.

SUPPLEMENTS—Exodus, ImmuGel.

MILK PRODUCTION—Clary sage (bring in milk), fennel or basil (increase), peppermint with cold compress (decrease). ***Caution: Fennel should not be used for more than 10 days as it will excessively increase flow through the urinary tract.***

SUPPLEMENTS—Essential Manna, Power Meal, VitaGreen.

MISCARRIAGE (after)—Frankincense, geranium, grapefruit, lavender (may help prevent), Roman chamomile, spruce (2 drops on solar plexus).

SUPPLEMENTS—JuvaTone, Cleansing Trio (ComforTone, Essentialzyme, and ICP).

MORNING SICKNESS—Calamus, <u>Di-Tone</u> (1-2 drops in water and sip or 1-2 drops around the navel), ginger, <u>M-Grain</u>, peppermint. Apply on or behind ears, down jaw bone, over stomach as a compress, on Vita Flex points on feet, on hands (rub together and smell), or put a drop on your pillow. Can also put 4 to 6 drops of spearmint in a bowl of boiled and cooled water and place on floor beside the bed overnight to keep stomach calm.

> ***Caution:*** *Although <u>Di-Tone</u> is recommended for morning sickness, it contains some oils which some aromatologists strongly discourage using. It may have a lot to do with purity. Use at your own risk. I did and it worked for me!*

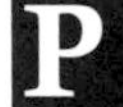

SUPPLEMENTS—ComforTone, Essentialzyme.

ON CHAKRAS—<u>Awaken</u> (after pregnancy).

PLACENTA—Basil (has been use to help retain), jasmine (helps expulsion).

POSTPARTUM DEPRESSION (Baby Blues)—See FEMALE PROBLEMS. Bergamot, Clary sage, fennel, frankincense, geranium, Gentle Baby, grapefruit, Harmony Hope, jasmine, Joy, lavender, myrrh, nutmeg (use in moderation), orange, and patchouli, Valor, vetiver, White Angelica.

SUPPLEMENTS—Essential Manna, Essential Omegas, ImmuPro.

SELF LOVE—Joy.

SKIN ELASTICITY—Aroma Life, Clarity, Dragon Time, Gentle Baby, Mister, M-Grain, Relieve It. *Again, many of these blends contain oils that many aromatologist feel should be avoided or used with caution during pregnancy.*

PERSONAL CARE—ClaraDerm (Essential oil spray - apply topically to stressed ski before and after childbirth).

STRETCH MARKS—Gentle Baby (every day on tummy).

PERSONAL CARE—ClaraDerm (Essential oil spray - apply topically to stressed ski before and after childbirth).

TOXEMIA (extremely high protein in urine)—Aroma Life.

PRIDE: Peppermint (dispels).

PROCRASTINATION: Acceptance, Envision (emotional support), Magnify Your Purpose (empowering and uplifting), Motivation (easier to take action, gets you out of the mood of procrastination).

PROGESTERONE: EndoFlex, Grounding. *Progesterone is made from cholesterol and helps to protect against cancer.*

PERSONAL CARE—PD 80/20, Prenolone/Prenolone+, Progessence.

PROSPERITY: Abundance, bergamot, cinnamon bark (aromatic), cypress.

PROSTATE: Australian Blue, Blue cypress, EndoFlex, Gratitude, helichrysum, juniper, Juva Cleanse, Mister, yarrow.

PERSONAL CARE—PD 80/20, Prenolone/Prenolone+, Protec (designed to accompany the nightlong retention enema, it helps buffer the prostate from inflammation, enlargement, and tumor activity).

SUPPLEMENTS—CortiStop (Men's), Master Formula HIS, ProGen (an herbal support for the male glandular system; it may prevent prostate atrophy and malfunction and protect men from prostate cancer).

DECONGESTANT—[F]Cypress, Di-Tone, Dragon Time, Mister (decongests prostate and balances hormones), myrrh, [F]myrtle, sage, [F]spruce, yarrow. Apply oils to insid ankle and heel. ImmuPower on lower spine and in rectum.

BLEND #1—Combine 15 frankincense and 5 Mister with 2 tsp. V-6 Mixing Oil. Insert blend into rectum with bulb syringe or pipet and retain throughout night.

BLEND #2—Combine 10 frankincense and 10 lavender with 2 tsp. V-6 Mixing Oil. Insert blend into rectum with bulb syringe and retain throughout night.

BLEND #3—Combine 10 frankincense, 5 myrrh, and 3 sage with 2 tsp. V-6 Mixing Oil. Insert blend into rectum with bulb syringe or pipet and retain through night.

ENLARGEMENT—Mix 10 drops of Mister with 1 Tbs. of V-6 Mixing oil and insert in rectum and retain overnight. May also apply either sage, fennel, or yarrow to posterior, scrotum, ankles, lower back, and bottom of feet.

INFLAMED—Cypress, lavender, thyme (Alternative Medicine—A Definitive Guide, p. 742).

STRENGTHEN—PD 80/20, Prenolone/Prenolone+, ProGen, Protec.

THOUGHT PATTERNS AND EMOTIONS—The prostate represents the masculine principle. Men's PROSTATE problems have a lot to do with self-worth and also believing that as they get older they become less of a man. Ideas may be in conflict about sex, refusing to let go of the past, fear of aging, feeling like throwing in the towel. May be feeling inadequate in sexual role, may be holding onto unpleasant memories of previous relationships, or feeling unfulfilled in love.

ROSTATE CANCER: See CANCER.

> ***Prostate Cancer** may be from repressed anger. Visualize the prostate healing, don't put energy into the cancer.*

ROTECTION: (from negative influence) Clove (aromatic), cypress, fennel (protection from psychic attack), fir (aromatic), frankincense, Harmony, Joy, Sacred Mountain, Valor, White Angelica.

ROTEIN: Carbonated water prevents absorption of protein. Protein deficiency causes Hypoglycemia.

SUPPLEMENTS—Bodygize, Essentialzyme, Polyzyme (provides enzymes necessary for proper breakdown and digestion of protein), Power Meal (pre-digested protein), Sulfurzyme (helps digest protein), VitaGreen.

> *A **protein deficiency**, either from the lack of protein intake or from the inability to digest it, creates an acidic pH in the blood. A high acidity level in the blood creates an environment for cell mutation and disease. See ACIDOSIS.*

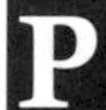

ORIASIS: Bergamot, cajeput, cedarwood, [F]helichrysum, lavender, melaleuca, patchouli, Roman chamomile, [F]thyme.

BLEND—Combine 2-3 drops each of Roman chamomile and lavender for use as ointment for pH Balance.

PERSONAL CARE—Rose Ointment (helps soften cracking skin), Lavender Volume Shampoo and Lavender Volume Conditioner for psoriasis of the scalp.

SUPPLEMENTS—Alkalime, Cleansing Trio (ComforTone, Essentialzyme, and ICP Essential Omegas, JuvaPower/JuvaSpice, JuvaTone, Sulfurzyme.

PSYCHIC: Cinnamon bark (awareness), fennel (protect from attack), lemongrass. Diffuse.

CENTERS—Elemi (balances, strengthens, fortifies).

PUBERTY: Fleabane (stimulates retarded puberty).

PULMONARY: See LUNGS.

PURGE: See CLEANSING.

PURIFICATION: Abundance, Acceptance, cedarwood, En-R-Gee, eucalyptus (aromatic), fenn (aromatic), lemon (aromatic), lemongrass (aromatic), melaleuca (aromatic), orange (aromatic), Purification, sage.

AIR—Lemon (diffuse or add to spray bottle of water to deodorize and sterilize the air).

CIGARETTE SMOKE—Purification.

DISHES—2 drops of Melrose or lemon in the dish water for sparkling dishes and a great smelling kitchen.

WATER—[F]Lemon, peppermint.

CLOTHING—Adding oils to washer or dryer decreases bacteria, improves hygiene, and clothes have a fresh, clean smell.

FURNITURE—A few drops of fir, lemon, or spruce oil on a dust cloth or 10 drops in a spray bottle work well for polishing, cleaning and disinfecting furniture, kitche and bathrooms. You may also consider adding Abundance to increase your abundance. Lemon oil for dissolving gum and grease. Purification for mold a fungus. If you don't have a diffuser, you may want to add 10-12 drops of Purification to 8 oz of distilled water in a spray bottle and spray into the air.

PUS: See INFECTION and ANTI-INFECTIOUS. Melaleuca is useful in healing pus-filled wounds.

RADIATION: See CANCER. *Melaleuca quinquenervia*, Melrose, patchouli. May apply on location, bottom of feet, kidneys, thyroid, and diffuse.

COMPUTER, T.V., MICROWAVE—Fill a wooden bowl half full of peat moss and half full of hazel nuts and 30 drops of Melrose then set on the appliance. Using an equipment diode may also help.

****COMMENTS—*Melrose* may help protect the body during radiation treatments if used 10 days before, during, and 10 days after. ***Do not use on the day of radiation treatment***. According to Dr. Pénoël, massage with Melaleuca quinquenervia helps to prevent radiation side effects. Remember to keep all massage light and away from trauma area.*

Valerie Woorwood suggests Recipe #1 below to be used at least two to three weeks before the radiation treatments begin. Don't use it during the treatment, but use it between treatments and for at least a month after your last treatment.

***RECIPE #1**—10 lavender, 5 German chamomile, 5 Roman chamomile, 5 tagetes, 5 yarrow, and 2 tsp. of vinca infused oil. Massage the entire torso, including the back and abdomen and the trauma area. This treatment will not conflict with the doctor's treatment. Note: Vinca is made from periwinkle which is known to contain alkaloids that in some cases can suppress the cancerous cells. (The Complete Book of Essential Oils & Aromatherapy, pp. 249-50).*

RADIATION BURNS—Recipe #1.

SIDE-EFFECTS–Recipe #2.

TREATMENTS—Radiation treatments can produce tremendous toxicity within the liver. Cut down on the use of oils with high *phenol* content to prevent increasing the liver toxicity.

CHEMOTHERAPY— Because of the greater amounts of toxicity produced, even greater care should be taken to limit the use of oils with high *phenol* content.

The following Dr. Westlake formula utilizes Bach Flower Remedies to counteract the side-effects of cancer patients who have received radiation therapy.

***RECIPE #2**—"Mix 3.5 grams of sea salt with 100 mils of distilled water. Put into a 10 ml dropper bottle 2 drops of each of the following Bach Flower Remedies: Cherry Plum, Gentian, Rock Rose, Star of Bethlehem, Vine, Walnut and Wild Oat, and top up the bottle with the sea salt solution. Take 2 drops, three or four times a day, or add 10 to 15 drops to a bath. People who have been exposed to radiation sources, such as X-rays, cobalt therapy or other medical radiation therapies, or have been contaminated in an escape from a nuclear power station or who regularly use office or domestic equipment that gives out low-level radiation, such as color television sets, microwaves, and visual display units, would do well to use this formula in a bath once or twice a week." (Aromatherapy—An A to Z by Patricia Davis, p. 269)*

WEEPING WOUNDS FROM—Melaleuca, oregano, thyme.

SUPPLEMENTS—The apple pectin that is contained in ICP helps remove unwanted metals and toxins. It is also valuable in radiation therapy.

ASHES: Elemi (allergic), lavender, [F]melaleuca, Melrose, palmarosa, Release (on Vita Flex points of feet), Roman chamomile. Red spots on body may indicate a Biotin deficiency; take Super C or Super C Chewable.

PERSONAL CARE—KidScents Tender Tush, Rose Ointment.

****COMMENTS—Dr. Friedmann had a patient who had a rash for three years on the side of the face and arms and the eyes were weeping. They had gone to five physicians for treatments and had no success. Dr. Friedmann did the following: 1) Did a culture of the eye and face and determined that the patient had staphylococcus. 2) Had the patient apply Melrose and lavender alternately morning and night. 3) Had the patient take Mineral Essence and Colloidal Essence (a colloidal silver product). After a short period of time, the patient's face and eyes totally cleared up and their arms were healing.*

If the rash occurs from application of oils to the skin, it may be due to the oils reacting with accumulated synthetic chemicals (toxins) that are trapped in the fatty layers of the skin. Take the following steps: 1) Try diluting the oils first (1-3 drops of oil to ½ tsp. V-6 Mixing Oil), 2) reduce the number of oils used with each application (use oils one at a time), 3) reduce the amount of oils (number of drops) used, 4) reduce the frequency of application (more time between applications). Drinking pure (steam distilled) water helps promote the elimination of accumulated toxins from the body. Initiating programs to cleanse the bowels and blood will also help remove accumulated toxins and reduce the possible recurrences of the rash. If the rashes persist, discontinue use of the oils and consult your health care professional.

RAYNAUD'S DISEASE (feel cold; hands and feet turn blue): Aroma Life, clove, cypress, fennel, geranium, helichrysum, lavender, nutmeg, rosemary.

REFRESHING:

ESSENTIAL WATERS (HYDROSOLS)—Canadian Red Cedar (exhilarating), Peppermint, Spearmint. Spray into air or directly on face (don't spray directly in eyes or ears) diffuse using the Essential Mist Diffuser.

REGENERATING: Helichrysum, lavender, Melrose, or equal parts of Thieves and V-6 Mixing Oil.

SUPPLEMENTS—Bodygize, ImmuneTune, Power Meal.

REJECTION: Acceptance, Joy.

RELATIONSHIPS:

BATH & SHOWER GELS—Sensation Bath & Shower Gel contains oils used by Cleopatra to enhance love and increase the desire to be close to that someone special.

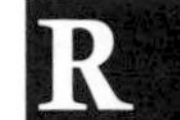

MASSAGE OILS—Sensation creates an exotic arousal; increases sexual desire. The fragrance creates a peaceful and harmonious feeling that is helpful in easing relationship stress.

PERSONAL CARE—Sensation Hand & Body Lotion.

ENHANCING—Lady Sclareol (especially for the woman - best if applied by male partner), Ylang ylang.

ENDING RELATIONSHIPS—Basil.

RELAXATION: Citrus Fresh, Clary sage, frankincense, Gentle Baby, geranium, jasmine, lavender, Peace & Calming, Roman chamomile, sandalwood, Trauma Life (calming), ylang ylang.

BATH & SHOWER GELS—Evening Peace Bath & Shower Gel.

ESSENTIAL WATERS (HYDROSOLS)—Basil (relaxing to muscles), Lavender (soothing and calming), Melissa, Western Red Cedar. Spray into air or directly on face (don't spray directly in eyes or ears) or diffuse using the Essential Mist Diffuser.

DIFFUSION—See NEGATIVE IONS for oils that produce negative ions when diffused to help promote relaxation. Lavender, Peace & Calming.

MASSAGE OILS—Relaxation Massage Oil.

SENSE OF—Ylang ylang.

BLEND—1 bergamot, 2 lavender, 2 marjoram, and 4 rosewood.

RELEASE NEGATIVE TRAUMA: Inspiration, Release, Transformation.

RESENTMENT: Forgiveness, Harmony, Humility, Idaho tansy, jasmine, Release, rose, White Angelica.

RESPIRATORY SYSTEM: Abundance, anise, basil (restorative), bergamot (infections), cajeput (infections), Canadian Red cedar, Clary sage (strengthens), clove, Di-Tone, EndoFlex, [F]eucalyptus (general stimulant and strengthens), *Eucalyptus radiata*, fennel (stimulant), [F]fir (opens respiratory tract, increases oxygenation, decongests and balances), frankincense, goldenrod (discharges mucus), helichrysum (relieves), hyssop (opens respiratory system and discharges toxins and mucus), JuvaFlex, ledum (supports), lemon, marjoram (calming), melaleuca, *Melaleuca ericifolia*, Melrose, [F]myrtle, oregano

> *Vita Flex points for the bronchial tubes are located between the bones on the tops of the feet. The sinuses are located at the base of the middle three toes on the bottom of the feet. One of the most effective ways of handling a respiratory problem is by doing rectal implants. There is a nerve that goes from the rectum to the lungs. The oils will travel in this manner in 3 seconds. The next best method is through inhalation.*

(antiseptic), [F]peppermint (aid), pine (dilates and opens bronchial tract), RC, Raven (all respiratory problems), ravensara, rosemary verbenon, Sacred Mountain (soothing), [F]spearmint, spruce, Thieves, tsuga (dilates and opens tract).

RECIPE #1—Dr. Young alternates the oils of Raven and RC in rectal implants. He uses 20 drops of the oil in 1 Tbs. of V-6 Mixing Oil and implants it rectally using a pipet (or glass dropper).

BLEND #1—3 birch/wintergreen, 8 eucalyptus, 6 fir, 6 frankincense, 1 peppermint, 10 ravensara and 1 oz. V-6 Mixing Oil.

BLEND #2—3 German chamomile, 10 fir, and 5 lemon.

ESSENTIAL WATERS (HYDROSOLS)—Canadian Red Cedar (supportive), Eucalyptus (soothing), Mountain Essence (enhanced respiratory action). Diffuse into air using the Essential Mist Diffuser.

SUPPLEMENTS—ImmuGel, Super C / Super C Chewable.

ACUTE—RC and Raven, Thieves.

BLEND #3—5 eucalyptus, 8 frankincense, 6 lemon, and 1 oz. V-6 Mixing Oil. Do a hot compress on chest and rub neat on bottom of feet under toes.

BLEND #4—3 tsp. *Eucalyptus radiata* (or any oil from the Myrtaceae botanical family), 1 tsp. Canadian Balsam fir (or any conifer oil). Apply to Vita Flex points on the feet, add to V-6 Mixing Oil and apply to chest area, or diffuse.

> *My 18 year old daughter has had **respiratory problems** for years and finally the doctors put her on inhalers. These helped, but she did not like the way they made her feel. Soon after I started using therapeutic grade essential oils we began using them on her. After a few weeks she was off her inhalers and has never needed them since. She has, however, had the occasional upper respiratory infection, which in the past has always led to a bout with bronchitis and several months of coughing. Now, we apply oils and the infection goes away without bronchitis ever showing up. This has saved vacations and more! We apply the oils to her chest, back and feet twice a day. The oils we use are hyssop, myrrh, and two Young Living blends - RC and Raven.*
>
> ***-Submitted by Lauren Martin (July 2004)***

RESTLESSNESS: Acceptance, angelica, basil, bergamot, cedarwood, frankincense, Gathering, geranium, Harmony, Inspiration, Joy, lavender, orange, Peace & Calming, rose rosewood, Sacred Mountain, spruce, Trauma Life, valerian, Valor, ylang ylang

RHEUMATIC FEVER: Ginger, [F]tarragon. Both help with pain.

RHEUMATISM: See ARTHRITIS.

RHINITIS: Basil, sage lavender.

> ***Rhinitis** is an inflammation of the nasal mucus membrane.*

IINOPHARYNGITIS: [F]Ravensara.

NGWORM: See ANTI-FUNGAL. Geranium, lavender, melaleuca (Tea Tree), Melrose, myrrh, peppermint, Purification, RC, Raven, rosemary verbenon, thyme.

BLEND #1—2 lavender, 2 melaleuca, and 2 thyme, OR

BLEND #2—3 melaleuca, 2 peppermint, and 3 spearmint.

Apply 1-2 drops of blend (#'s 1 or 2 above) or Melrose on ringworm three times a day for ten days. Then mix 30 drops of melaleuca (Tea Tree) or Melrose with 2 Tbs. V-6 Mixing Oil and use daily until ringworm is gone.

MASSAGE OILS—Ortho Ease or Ortho Sport.

PERSONAL CARE—Rose Ointment.

> *My friend's eight month old little boy had a ringworm the size of a quarter on his head. After putting lavender neat on it several times it started to go away and after a few more times it was gone altogether. Shortly after that he got a tick in his head and by putting peppermint right on the back of the tick that nasty thing backed right out. I guess he could not breath--whatever it was, it got the tick out without us trying to pull it out and perhaps getting only part of the critter out.*
>
> ***-Submitted by V. Frierdich***
> ***Overland Park, Kansas (July 2004)***

)MANTIC TOUCHES: Jasmine, Lady Sclareol, patchouli, Sensation, ylang ylang; use these in small amounts.

BATH & SHOWER GELS— Sensation Bath & Shower Gel.

MASSAGE OILS—Sensation Massage Oil.

PERSONAL CARE—Sensation Hand & Body Lotion.

)SACEA (Acne Rosacea): Lavender. Dilute with V-6 Mixing Oil and apply daily after washing face with Orange Blossom Facial Wash and before applying Sandalwood Moisture Creme or Sandalwood Toner. Can also add extra lavender oil to Sandalwood Moisture Creme or Sandalwood Toner

PERSONAL CARE—Orange Blossom Facial Wash, Sandalwood Moisture Creme, Sandalwood Toner.

> ***Rosacea*** *is a chronic, acne-like condition of the facial skin which typically first appears as a flushing or subtle redness on the cheeks, nose, chin or forehead that comes and goes. Left untreated, the condition progresses and the redness becomes more persistent, bumps and pimples appear, and small dilated blood vessels may become visible. In some cases the eyes may be affected, causing them to be irritated and bloodshot and, according to some doctors, can even cause blindness. In the more advanced cases, the nose becomes red and swollen from excess tissue. Currently, this condition can only be controlled.*

SACREDNESS: Sacred Mountain (sacred place of protection within self).

SADNESS: Acceptance, helichrysum, Inspiration, Joy (over heart), onycha (combine with rose Massage Oil Base for calming/uplifting massage), orange (overcome), 3 Wise Men, Transformation, Valor. Wear as cologne or diffuse.

SAINT VITUS DANCE (Chorea):
BLEND—5 Aroma Siez, 3 basil, 6 juniper, and 8 peppermint.

SANITATION: Citronella, lemongrass, Purification.

SCABIES: Bergamot, laurel, lavender and peppermint, pine, Thieves (needs to be diluted).

SCARRING: Frankincense (prevents), Gentle Baby, geranium, helichrysum (reduces), hyssop (prevents), [F]lavender (burns), Melrose, rose (prevents), rosehip (reduces).
PERSONAL CARE—Satin Hand & Body Lotion (moisturizes skin and promotes healing).
BLEND #1—Equal parts helichrysum and lavender mixed with liquid lecithin.
BLEND #2—3 rosemary, 15 rosewood, and 1 ¾ oz. Hazel Nut Oil.
BLEND #3—6 lavender, 3 patchouli, 4 rosewood, and Vitamin E Oil.
PREVENT FORMATION—Frankincense, helichrysum, hyssop, myrrh, rose, rosehip seed
BLEND #4—5 helichrysum, 2 patchouli, 4 lemongrass, 3 lavender in ¼ to ½ oz. V-6 Mixing Oil or Massage Oil Base.
BLEND #5—Equal parts lavender, lemongrass, and geranium.

SCHMIDT'S SYNDROME: See ADDISON'S DISEASE. En-R-Gee, EndoFlex, Joy, nutmeg (increases energy; supports adrenal glands), sage (combine with nutmeg).

> ***Schmidt's Syndrome** is the same as Addison's Disease with the additional problem of low thyroid hormone production.*

SUPPLEMENTS—ImmuPro, Master Formula His/Hers (3 times a day), Mineral Essence (help supplement mineral loss), **Sulfurzyme** (shown to slow or reverse autoimmune diseases), Super B (after each meal), Thyromin (first thing in morning), VitaGreen.

SCIATICA: Aroma Life, cardamom, **cistus (followed by peppermint)**, fir, [F]helichrysum, Gentle Baby, hyssop, M-Grain, PanAway, peppermint, Relieve It, sandalwood, spruce (alleviates pain), [F]tarragon, [F]thyme, Valor. Apply a cold compress and lightly

S

massage with Roman chamomile or lavender, and birch/wintergreen. Relief can also be obtained by applying Joy and lavender to the bottoms of the feet.

MASSAGE OIL—Ortho Ease.

:COLIOSIS: May be caused by a virus. DO THE RAINDROP TECHNIQUE!

****COMMENT—The video, listed in the Bibliography, is highly recommended for a professional visual presentation of this technique!*

BLEND—8 basil, 12 birch/wintergreen, 5 cypress, 10 marjoram, and 2 peppermint.

CORRECT—Do the following (a variation of the Raindrop Technique) every seven to ten days for a minimum of eight times to help get rid of SCOLIOSIS:

1. Rub Valor on feet.
2. Apply oregano and thyme using the Raindrop Technique up the spine.
3. Apply BLEND along the spine. Push or pull in the direction that the spine needs to be strengthened. Knead fingers clockwise three times. Then work two fingers up the spine with the other hand on top of the hand that is doing the kneading (do this three times).
4. Apply Aroma Siez and marjoram on the muscles on each side of the spine. Apply warm wet towel to back and have individual lay on their back.
5. Work the Vita Flex areas down the leg to the feet with basil, birch/wintergreen, cypress, and peppermint in V-6 Mixing Oil.
6. Work the spine Vita Flex areas on the feet then give feet a mild pull.
7. Put one hand under their chin and the other hand at the back of their neck. Have them breathe in and out as you gently rock and pull the neck in time with their breathing.
8. Take towel off. If the back gets too hot during massage apply V-6 Mixing Oil.
9. Measure the spine to see how much it has changed.

:CRAPES: Lavender, ravensara.

:CURVY: [F]Ginger. Apply over kidneys, liver, and on corresponding Vita Flex points on the feet.

SUPPLEMENTS—Super C / Super C Chewable.

ECURITY: Christmas Spirit, Sacred Mountain.

CREATING—Acceptance, Roman chamomile.

FEELING OF—Cypress (aromatic).

IN THE HOME—Bergamot.

SELF SECURE—Oregano.

EDATIVE: Among the most effective sedatives are: Bergamot, Citrus Fresh, lavender, neroli, and Peace & Calming. Other oils that may also help are: Angelica, cedarwood,

Personal Guide

Clary sage, coriander, cypress, elemi, frankincense, geranium, hyssop, jasmin juniper, lavender, lemongrass, melissa, marjoram, onycha (benzoin), orange, patchouli, Roman chamomile, rose, sandalwood, tangerine, Trauma Life, valerian, vetiver (nervous system), ylang ylang. Use intuition as to which one may be best for the given situation. In addition, check the safety data for each of the oils in the APPENDIX of this book.

SEIZURE: See EPILEPSY.

GRAND MAL—Need to support the body. Aroma Siez (apply using the Raindrop Technique up the spine), Brain Power and Peace & Calming (diffuse and put around naval), Joy (over the heart), Sacred Mountain (back of neck and crown and Valor (on feet).

SUPPLEMENTS—Cleansing Trio (ComforTone, Essentialzyme, and ICP), Essential Omegas, JuvaPower.

****COMMENTS—Grand Mal seizures can sometimes be caused by zinc and copp imbalance. Mineral Essence provides zinc and copper in both ionic and colloidal form for optimal assimilation.*

SELF ADJUSTMENT: Awaken.

SELF ESTEEM: Acceptance, Forgiveness, Joy, Valor.

BUILD—Joy, Transformation, Valor.

SELF LOVE—Joy, Valor.

SELF HYPNOSIS: Clary sage, geranium, patchouli.

SELF PITY: Acceptance, Motivation, Transformation, Valor.

SENSORY SYSTEM (Senses): See AWARENESS. Birch/wintergreen.

SEXUAL ABUSE: SARA has a fragrance that when inhaled may enable one to relax into a mental state whereby one may be able to release and let go of the memory trauma of sexual and or ritual abuse.

SEX STIMULANT: Chivalry, [F]cinnamon bark (general), ginger, goldenrod, rose, SclarEssence Sensation, [F]ylang ylang (sex drive problems).

BATH & SHOWER GELS—Sensation Bath & Shower Gel contains oils used by Cleopatra to enhance love and increase the desire to be close to that someone special.

MASSAGE OILS—Sensation creates an exotic arousal and increases sexual desire. The fragrance creates a peaceful and harmonious feeling that helps to ease relationship stress. Also Chivalry.

PERSONAL CARE—PD 80/20, Prenolone/Prenolone+ (for both males and females), Progessence (for females only), Sensation Hand & Body Lotion.

SUPPLEMENTS—Master Formula His/Hers, Mineral Essence, VitaGreen.

OTHER—SE6 Tincture (available through Creer Labs 801-465-5423). Use 10-50 drops of SE6 Tincture three times a day plus 2 droppers at bedtime for three to five days.

AROUSING DESIRE—Clary sage, Lady Sclareol.

FRIGIDITY—See FRIGIDITY. Lady Sclareol, nutmeg (overcome).

IMPOTENCE—Goldenrod, SclarEssence.

INFLUENCES—Lady Sclareol, patchouli (aromatic).

SHINGLES: Australian Blue, Bergamot, Blue cypress, eucalyptus, geranium, lavender, lemon, melaleuca (Tea Tree), [F]ravensara, Roman chamomile.

BLEND—10 drops lavender, 10 melaleuca (Tea Tree), and 10 drops thyme mixed in Genesis Hand & Body Lotion. Rub on feet.

MASSAGE OILS—Ortho Sport.

PERSONAL CARE—PD 80/20, Prenolone/ Prenolone+, Progessence.

SUPPLEMENTS—Cleansing Trio (ComforTone, Essentialzyme, and ICP), ImmuGel.

HERPES ZOSTER—Australian Blue, Bergamot, Blue cypress, *Eucalyptus radiata*, geranium, lavender, melaleuca (Alternative Medicine—The Definitive Guide, p. 972), Roman chamomile.

> ***Shingles** is an acute viral infection with inflammation of certain spinal or cranial nerves and the eruption of vesicles along the affected nerve path. It usually strikes only one side of the body is often accompanied by severe neuralgia. Also called herpes zoster. Some say it is necessary to cleanse the liver.*
>
> *Dr. Schnaubelt says that his greatest success in helping individuals with shingles came from applying a blend of 50 percent Ravensara aromatica and 50 percent Calophyllum inophyllum (Tamanu). "Drastic improvements and complete remission occur within seven days." (Alternative Medicine—The Definitive Guide, p. 56).*

SHOCK: See FAINTING. Aroma Life, Australian Blue, basil, Clarity (to keep from going into shock), Gathering, Grounding, helichrysum, Highest Potential, Inspiration, Joy, melaleuca, melissa, myrrh, neroli, [F]peppermint, [F]Roman chamomile, rosemary, Valor, ylang ylang.

SHOULDER (Frozen): Basil, birch/wintergreen, lemongrass, oregano, peppermint, White fir. Begin by applying White fir to shoulder Vita Flex point on foot (same side of body as frozen shoulder) to deal with any inflammation. Work it in with Vita Flex technique. Then check for improvement in pain reduction and/or range of motion (check after each oil to help determine what problem really was). In a similar manner apply lemongrass (for torn or pulled ligaments), basil (for muscle spasms), and birch/wintergreen (for bone problems) on the same Vita Flex point on the foot. After applying the oils to the foot and determining which oil(s) get the best results, apply same oil(s) on the shoulder and work it into the area with Vita Flex. Then apply peppermint (for nerves) and oregano (create thermal reaction to enhance elasticity of muscle and help it to stretch) on the shoulder and work each one into the area with Vita Flex. Finally, apply White fir to the other shoulder to create balance as the opposite shoulder will compensate for the sore one. Drink lots of water.

PERSONAL CARE—Regenolone.

SUPPLEMENTS—Sulfurzyme.

SINUS: Cedarwood, eucalyptus, [F]helichrysum, [F]myrtle, PanAway, RC, or Thieves on feet.

****COMMENTS—Eucalyptus and other sinus oils work really well when rubbed on each side of the nose. It seems to clear the sinuses almost immediately.*

SINUSITIS: See RESPIRATORY SYSTEM. Cajeput, elemi, [F]eucalyptus, *Eucalyptus radiata*, fir, ginger, *Melaleuca ericifolia*, myrtle, [F]pine, ravensara, RC, [F]rosemary, sage lavender.

SUPPLEMENTS— ImmuneTune.

SKELETAL SYSTEM: See SCOLIOSIS. Valor ("chiropractor in a bottle"). Also try the RAINDROP TECHNIQUE.

SKIN: See ACNE, ALLERGIES, BRUISES, CUTS, DERMATITIS, ECZEMA, FACIAL OILS, PSORIASIS, WRINKLES. Acceptance, Aroma Life, cajeput, cedarwood, Roman and German chamomile (inflamed skin), Clarity, cypress, Dragon Time, frankincense, Gentle Baby (youthful skin), geranium,

> ***Contact-sensitization*** *is a type of allergic reaction which can occur when a substance comes into contact with the body. A few essential oils applied to the skin may cause sensitization, perhaps only after repeated application (the amount used is not significant). The skin reaction appears as redness, irritation, or vesiculation. A rule of thumb when applying oils to someone is that people with darker hair usually have less sensitive skin while those with blond or red hair are generally more sensitive.*
>
> ***Single oils:*** *Bergamot, cassia, cinnamon bark, citronella, clove, fennel, Laurus nobilis, ylang ylang.*
>
> *For a list of possible skin irritants, please see the APPENDIX of this book.*

helichrysum, Inner Child, jasmine (irritated skin), juniper, lavender, ledum (all types of problems), lemon, marjoram, [F]melaleuca (healing), Melrose, Mister, M-Grain, myrrh (chapped and cracked), [F]myrtle (antiseptic), orange, palmarosa (rashes, scaly, and flaky skin), patchouli (chapped; tightens loose skin and prevents wrinkles), [F]peppermint (itching skin), Relieve It, rosehip, rosemary, rosewood (elasticity and candida), sage, sandalwood (regenerates), Sensation, Valor, vetiver, Western Red cedar (nourishing), and ylang ylang.

AFTERSHAVE—Awaken can be used instead of aftershave lotion. Try adding Awaken to Sandalwood Moisture Creme, Satin Hand & Body Lotion, Sensation Hand & Body Lotion, or Genesis Hand & Body Lotion as an aftershave. KidScents Lotion makes a great aftershave as it soothes and rehydrates the skin (and smells good too).

BAR SOAPS—Lavender Rosewood Moisturizing Soap, Lemon Sandalwood Cleansing Soap, Peppermint Cedarwood Moisturizing Soap, Sacred Mountain Moisturizing Soap for Oily Skin, Thieves Cleansing Soap.

BATH & SHOWER GELS—Dragon Time (for women who have lower back pain, stress and sleeping problems due to menstruation), Evening Peace (relaxes tired, fatigued muscles and helps to alleviate tension), Morning Start (dissolves oil and grease), and Sensation (aphrodisiac).

ESSENTIAL WATERS (HYDROSOLS)—Clary Sage, German Chamomile (soothes irritation and swelling), Eucalyptus (helps cleanse oily skin), Juniper (helps detoxify and cleanse), Lavender (soothing), Spearmint (helps cleanse blemished and oily skin). Spray directly onto the skin (don't spray directly into the eyes of ears).

PERSONAL CARE—Boswellia Wrinkle Creme, Genesis Hand & Body Lotion (hydrates, heals, and nurtures the skin), Satin Facial Scrub - Mint (eliminates layers of dead skin cells and slows down premature aging of the skin), NeuroGen (provide nutrients and moisturizers to deeper layers of the skin), Orange Blossom Facial Wash combined with Sandalwood Toner and Sandalwood Moisture Creme (cleans, tones, and moisturizes dry or prematurely aging skin), Prenolone , Progessence, Regenolone (helps moisturize and regenerate tissues), Rose Ointment (for skin conditions and chapped skin), Satin Hand & Body Lotion (moisturizes skin leaving it feeling soft, silky, and smooth), Sensation Hand & Body Lotion (moisturizes, softens, and protects the skin from weather, chemicals, and household cleaners).

SUPPLEMENTS FOR SKIN—JuvaTone, Sulfurzyme, Ultra Young (helps firm and tighten skin by activating the production of skin proteins, collagen, and elastin).

TINCTURES—AD&E

AGING/WRINKLES—Carrot, frankincense, patchouli (prevents wrinkles), rose, rosehip (retards), rosewood (slows).

BATH & SHOWER GELS—Bath Gel Base (cleanses the pores of the skin) plus use your own choice of oils or blends to create the fragrance or therapeutic action you desire.

PERSONAL CARE—Boswellia Wrinkle Creme, Genesis Hand & Body Lotion, Satin Facial Scrub - Mint, PD 80/20, Prenolone/Prenolone+, Progessence, Rose Ointment, Sandalwood Moisture Creme and Sandalwood Toner.

SUPPLEMENTS—Ultra Young (helps firm and tighten skin by activating the production of skin proteins, collagen, and elastin).

CHAPPED/CRACKED—Davana, elemi, myrrh, onycha (benzoin), patchouli.

BLEND #1—1 geranium, 1 patchouli, and 1 rosemary in Genesis Hand & Body Lotion or Satin Hand & Body Lotion.

BLEND #2—1-3 drops of both onycha (benzoin) and rose in Genesis Hand & Body Lotion, Satin Hand & Body Lotion (makes a wonderful hand cream), or Rose Ointment. May also add lemon and/or lavender for their additional healing properties.

PERSONAL CARE—Cinnamint Lip Balm.

DISEASE—Rose, Melrose.

DRY—Davana, Gentle Baby, geranium, jasmine, lavender, lemon, neroli, patchouli, Roman chamomile, [F]rosewood, sandalwood.

ESSENTIAL WATERS (HYDROSOLS)—Clary Sage (supports cells). Spray directly onto the skin (don't spray directly into eyes or ears).

MASSAGE OILS—Sensation Massage Oil (silky and youthful skin).

> *For years, I had been troubled with an* ***actinic keratosis*** *on the back of my hand. It had been caused by excessive sun exposure when I was younger. Farmers often get them on their foreheads. My dermatologist said there was no way to get rid of it - unless I wanted to freeze it off with liquid nitrogen. He didn't want to do that because it was over 1/2 inch in diameter and would have made a hole in my hand. The growth continued to bother me. It was red, scaly, and itchy. One day, in desperation, I put some "Thieves" blend on it. The Thieves seemed to make it feel better so I continued to apply it once a day. It is now several months later and the growth has almost disappeared. I intend to continue using Thieves on it until it is gone. It doesn't bother me anymore and the redness and itching have disappeared.*
>
> ***-Submitted by Judy Brown***
> ***Geneva, New York*** **(July 2004)**

PERSONAL CARE—Genesis Hand & Body Lotion (hydrates, heals, and nurtures), NeuroGen, Orange Blossom Facial Wash (gently cleanses the skin), PD 80/20, Prenolone/Prenolone+, Progessence, Sandalwood Toner, Sandalwood Moisture Creme (hydrates), Satin Hand & Body Lotion (nourishes and moisturizes)

FACIAL MASK—Orange Blossom Facial Wash, Satin Facial Scrub - Mint.

FEEDS SKIN AND SUPPLIES NUTRIENTS—All applicable Essential Oils, Boswellia Wrinkle Creme, NeuroGen (deeper layers of the skin), Rose Ointment.

ITCHING—Peppermint.

PERSONAL CARE— ClaraDerm (essential oil spray), Satin Hand & Body Lotion.

OILY (greasy) COMPLEXION— Bergamot, cajeput, Clary sage, cypress, jasmine, lavender, lemon, nutmeg, orange, ylang ylang.

ESSENTIAL WATERS (HYDROSOLS)— Eucalyptus (helps cleanse), Spearmint. Spray directly onto the skin (don't spray into eyes or ears).

SAGGY SKIN—Combine 8 drops each of sage, pine, lemongrass, and 1 oz. V-6 Mixing Oil. Rub on areas.

SENSITIVE—Geranium, German chamomile, jasmine, lavender, neroli.

PERSONAL CARE—Satin Hand & Body Lotion.

SUNBURN—Add a little lavender or tamanu oil to some Satin Hand & Body Lotion. Australian Blue.

PERSONAL CARE—LavaDerm Cooling Mist (use as often as necessary to keep skin cool and moist). May also use Satin Hand & Body Lotion later to help maintain moisture.

SUNTAN—Sunsation Suntan Oil filters out the ultraviolet rays without blocking the absorption of vitamin D. It may also accelerate tanning.

TONES—Patchouli.

MASSAGE OILS—Cel-Lite Magic.

PERSONAL CARE—Satin Facial Scrub - Mint, Sandalwood Toner with Sandalwood Moisture Creme.

SUPPLEMENTS—Ultra Young (helps firm and tighten skin by activating the production of skin proteins, collagen, and elastin).

WRINKLES—(see WRINKLES for recipes/blends) Carrot, cistus, Clary sage, cypress, elemi, fennel, frankincense, galbanum, geranium, helichrysum, lavender, lemon, lime, myrrh, neroli, orange, oregano, patchouli, rose, rosemary, rosewood, sandalwood, spikenard, thyme, ylang ylang.

PERSONAL CARE—Boswellia Wrinkle Creme (collagen builder), NeuroGen (helps moisturize deep tissues), Rose Ointment, Sandalwood Moisture Creme, Satin Hand & Body Lotion, Satin Facial Scrub - Mint, Wolfberry Eye Creme. The following three items can be used together to help tone the skin and prevent wrinkles: Orange Blossom Facial Wash, Sandalwood Toner, Sandalwood Moisture Creme.

SUPPLEMENTS—Essentialzyme, PD 80/20, Prenolone/Prenolone+, Progessence, Thyromin (thyroid function affects the skin), Ultra Young.

LEEP: Lavender (on spine), marjoram (aromatic), Peace & Calming, Roman chamomile (aromatic), valerian (disturbances).

DIFFUSION—See NEGATIVE IONS for oils that produce negative ions when diffused to help promote sleep. Lavender, Peace & Calming.

ESSENTIAL WATERS (HYDROSOLS)—Lavender (promotes). Spray into the air, on face (don't spray directly into eyes or ears) or diffuse using the Essential Mist diffuser).

SUPPLEMENTS—Ultra Young (restores deep sleep).

ANIMALS—Oils can be used on the paws of animals to help them relax and sleep when i pain. Peace & Calming, Trauma Life.

GOOD NIGHT SLEEP—1/4 cup bath salts, 10 drops geranium or lavender in bath and soak. Bath with Evening Peace Bath Gel.

RESTLESS—Lavender and Gathering.

SLEEPING SICKNESS—Geranium, juniper, Peace & Calming (on big toes, back of neck and navel), peppermint, or Valor (on feet).

SLIMMING AND TONING OILS: Basil, grapefruit, lavender, lemongrass, orange, rosemar sage, thyme.

SLIVERS (SPLINTERS): Mix 10 drops Thieves with 4 Tbs. V-6 Mixing Oil and massage bottom of feet, arm pits, throat, and lower stomach. Put 30 drops of Thieves Bath Gel Base and use in shower each day (this helps pull the slivers to gently massage them out) .

SMELL-LOSS OF: Basil (helps when loss of smell is due to chronic nasal catarrh), peppermint.

STIMULATE SENSORY CORTEX—Brain Power. Place under the tongue, behind the ears, and on the forehead. Can also place a couple drops of oil in the hands, rub them together in a clockwise motion, cup over nose and mouth, and breathe deeply.

****COMMENTS—According to the Essential Oils Desk Reference, "Massage 1 or drops [of Brain Power] with a finger on the insides of cheeks in the mouth. Doing this 1 or 2 times a day will immediately improve the smell sensory cortex." (EDR-June 2002; Ch. 8; Brain Power; Application)*

> *Just smelling the oils helps stimulate the sense of smell. **To smell the oils**, first close the eyes, hold the left nostril closed, breathe in the smell of the oil through the right nostril, then breathe out through the mouth. Breathing in the fragrance of the oils in this manner stimulates every endocrine gland in the brain. Next hold the right nostril closed and repeat the process.*

SMOKING: Purification.

CIGARETTE—Purification.

STOP SMOKING—See ADDICTIONS. Clove (removes desire), Present Time (helps wi insecurity), Thieves (on tongue before lighting up helps remove desire).

SUPPLEMENTS—JuvaTone, Super C / Super C Chewable.

****COMMENTS—One individual used JuvaTone to break a habit of smoking 2½ packs of cigarettes a day for 20 years. Another individual who used JuvaTo went from smoking a pack a day to 1 cigarette in 1½ weeks.*

S

)OTHING: Gentle Baby, myrrh, onycha (benzoin), Release, Roman chamomile, .

)RES: Melaleuca, pine, Thieves.

)RE THROAT: See THROAT.

'ACING OUT: Grounding, Acceptance, Present Time, Sacred Mountain.

'ASMS: See MUSCLES, ANTISPASMODIC. Aroma Siez, **basil**, calamus, [F]cypress, jasmine (muscle), lavender (antispasmodic), marjoram (relieves), oregano, Peace & Calming, peppermint, Roman chamomile, spikenard, tarragon, and thyme.

SPASTICITY—Cypress, ginger, juniper, lavender, lemon, rosemary, sandalwood.

'INA BIFIDA: Work on the nervous system with eucalyptus, lavender, lemon, nutmeg, orange, Roman chamomile, rosemary, 3 Wise Men. Apply oil(s) to bottom of feet, along spine, forehead, back of neck, and diffuse. Do the Raindrop Technique.

> ***Spina Bifida** is a congenital defect of the back bone, usually the lower vertebrae varies from a small area of numbness to paralysis from the waist down. A mental handicap can occur.*

'INE: See BACK. Oils can be applied along the Vita Flex spine points on the feet as an alternative to working directly on the spine.

SUPPLEMENTS—BLM

CALCIFIED—Geranium, PanAway (on spine), rosemary.

MASSAGE OILS—Ortho Ease for body massage.

SUPPLEMENTS—ArthroTune, and Super C / Super C Chewable.

DETERIORATING—PanAway.

MASSAGE OILS—Ortho Ease.

SUPPLEMENTS—ArthroTune, BLM, Super C / Super C Chewable.

PAIN—Valor and PanAway may relieve pain along the spine when applied to spine and Vita Flex points on feet.

MASSAGE OILS—Ortho Sport.

STIFFNESS—Marjoram, Valor. Do the Raindrop Technique.

MASSAGE OILS—Ortho Sport.

VIRUS—*Eucalyptus radiata*, ImmuPower, oregano, and Ortho Ease on Spine. Viruses tend to hibernate along the spine.

PIRITUAL: Awaken, Believe, Dream Catcher, Gathering, Gratitude, Humility, Inspiration.

AWARENESS—Acceptance, Canadian Red cedar, cedarwood, juniper, myrrh, Sacred Mountain, spruce, Transformation, White Angelica (Aromatic), White lotus.

BALANCING—Joy, Into the Future, spruce.

INCREASE—Believe, cedarwood (enhances), frankincense (opening and enhancing spirit receptivity; aromatic), Gratitude, Transformation.

INNER AWARENESS—Believe, Gratitude, Inner Child, Inspiration.

MEDITATION—Believe, Canadian Red cedar, frankincense, Inspiration, tsuga, White Angelica.

PRAYER—Gratitude, Inspiration, White Angelica.

PROTECTION—3 Wise Men (on crown and shoulders).

PURITY OF SPIRIT—Myrrh.

SPIRITUALLY UPLIFTING—Believe, Gratitude, Sacred Mountain, Transformation.

SPLEEN: is a major receptor for infections. Laurel, marjoram.

SPORTS: See ACHES AND PAINS, BONES, INJURY, MUSCLES, TISSUE.

EXCEL IN—Clarity (on forehead), Peace & Calming (back of neck), PanAway (injuries), Valor (on feet for courage and confidence).

INJURIES—Helichrysum, lemongrass, Melrose, PanAway, Peace & Calming.

SUPPLEMENTS—BLM

TRACK COMPETITION—

BLEND—5 basil, 5 bergamot, and 2 tsp. V-6 Mixing Oil.

MASSAGE OILS—Ortho Ease, Ortho Sport. Massage into the muscles to increase oxygen and elasticity in the tissues to prevent the muscles and ligaments from tearing during strenuous exercise. It may also be used after to prevent the muscle from cramping.

SUPPLEMENTS—VitaGreen.

SPRAINS: Aroma Siez, ginger, jasmine, lavender, [F]marjoram, PanAway, Peace & Calming, ro sage. Make a cold compress with eucalyptus, lavender, Roman chamomile, or rosemary.

SPURS-BONE: See BONES. Lavender, RC (dissolves). Apply directly on location.

STAINS: Lemon (removes).

STAPH INFECTION: Black pepper or peppermint will make it more painful. Use oregano an hyssop; alternate with oregano and thyme to relieve the pain. Helichrysum, lavender, Purification.

ERILITY: Clary sage, [F]geranium, rose (wonderful for both men and women). Can also try jasmine, neroli, sage lavender, sandalwood, SclarEssence (taken internally, helps increase estradiol and testosterone levels), rosewood, and vetiver. Apply several together (or alternate individually) by massage or aromatic baths.

PERSONAL CARE—Prenolone/Prenolone+, Progessence.

SUPPLEMENTS—Bodygize, Power Meal.

IMULATING: Basil, Black pepper, En-R-Gee, eucalyptus, fir, ginger, grapefruit, orange, patchouli, [F]peppermint, rose, rosemary, [F]sage, Transformation. Dilute with Massage Oil for stimulating massage. Adding a little Black pepper to an oil like rosemary can give it a little more power. Can also add a few drops of an oil or a couple oils to Bath Gel Base then add to bath water as the tub is filling.

ESSENTIAL WATERS (HYDROSOLS)—Basil, Juniper (to the nervous system), Thyme (to the scalp). Spray into air or directly on face (don't spray directly into eyes or ears) or diffuse using the Essential Mist Diffuser.

INGS: See BITES.

OMACH: [F]Basil, calamus (supports), ginger, peppermint. Apply to stomach Vita Flex points on feet or use with a hot compress over the stomach area.

ACHE—Di-Tone (behind ears and down jaw bone), eucalyptus, geranium, lavender, peppermint, or rosemary.

ACID—Peppermint (put drop on finger and place on tongue). Put several drops of fresh lemon juice in warm water and sip slowly.

SUPPLEMENTS—AlkaLime (acid-neutralizing mineral formula).

BACTERIA or GERMS—Peppermint.

BLOATING—Fennel (1-2 drops in liquid as dietary supplement).

CRAMPS—Blue cypress, ginger, [F]helichrysum, lavender, onycha (benzoin), rosemary cineol, [F]thyme (general tonic for), or flavor water with 5 drops of Di-Tone and drink for stomach pains.

TONIC—Tangerine.

UPSET—Di-Tone. Apply over stomach and colon, behind the ears, on Vita Flex points on the feet, and/or add 1 drop to 8 oz. rice or almond milk and drink. Can also place a couple of drops on the palms of the hands, rub together clockwise, then cup over nose and mouth and breathe deeply.

RENGTH: Cypress (aromatic), Hope, oregano, patchouli, [F]peppermint, Raven, Roman chamomile (strengthens positive imprinting in DNA), Sacred Mountain, White Angelica.

S

Personal Guide

SUPPLEMENTS—Be-Fit (enhances strength by promoting muscle formation), Pow Meal, WheyFit (provides three high-quality sources of protein for enhanced strength), Wolfberry Bar.

STREP THROAT: See THROAT.

STRESS: Aroma Life, basil, Believe, [F]bergamot, Clarity, Clary sage, cypress, elemi, Evergreen Essence, frankincense, geranium, grapefruit, Harmony, Inspiration, Joy, lavender (aromatic), Lazarus (available through Creer Labs 801-465-5423), marjoram, neroli, onycha (benzoin), Peace & Calming, pine, Roman chamomile (relieves stress), rosewood, Sacred Mountain, spruce, Surrender, tangerine, 3 Wise Men, Valor, White Angelica and ylang ylang.

BATH & SHOWER GELS—Evening Peace, Relaxation, or Sensation Shower Gel.

MASSAGE OILS—Relaxation or Sensation Massage Oil.

PERSONAL CARE—Sensation Hand & Body Lotion.

SUPPLEMENTS—Coral Sea (highly bio-available, contains 58 trace minerals), ImmuPro, Master Formula His/Hers (Multi-Vitamin), Thyromin, Super B, an Super Cal.

CHEMICAL—Clary sage, geranium, grapefruit, lavender, lemon, patchouli, rosemary.

EMOTIONAL STRESS—Bergamot, Clary sage, Evergreen Essence, Forgiveness, Gathering, geranium, Joy, ravensara, sandalwood (layer on navel and chest), Surrender, Transformation, Trauma Life.

ENVIRONMENTAL STRESS—Basil, bergamot, cedarwood, cypress, geranium, Roman chamomile.

MENTAL STRESS—Basil, bergamot, Evergreen Essence, geranium, grapefruit, lavende patchouli, pine, sandalwood, Surrender.

PERFORMANCE STRESS—Bergamot, ginger, grapefruit, rosemary.

PHYSICAL STRESS—Believe, bergamot, fennel, Gentle Baby, geranium, Harmony, lavender, marjoram, Peace & Calming, Roman chamomile, rosemary, thyme, Trauma Life (calming).

SUPPLEMENTS—ImmuPro.

RELATIONSHIP STRESS—See SEX STIMULANT.

BATH & SHOWER GELS—Sensation Bath & Shower Gel.

MASSAGE OILS—Sensation Massage Oil creates an exotic arousal, increasing sex desire. The fragrance creates a peaceful and harmonious feeling that helps ea relationship stress. Relaxation Massage Oil also creates a peaceful and harmonious feeling. You may want to add jasmine and ylang ylang.

PERSONAL CARE—Sensation Hand & Body Lotion.

STRESS THAT STARTS WITH TIREDNESS, IRRITABILITY, OR INSOMNIA—

BLEND—15 Clary sage, 10 lemon, 5 lavender, and 1 oz. V-6 Mixing Oil.

SUPPLEMENTS—ImmuPro, Super B.

S

RETCH MARKS: Gentle Baby, [F]lavender, mandarin, [F]myrrh, neroli.

BLEND #1—3 rosemary, 15 rosewood, and 1 ¾ oz. Hazel Nut Oil.

BLEND #2—6 lavender, 4 rosewood, 3 patchouli, and Vitamin E Oil.

****COMMENTS—Patricia Davis recommends adding mandarin and neroli to either rosehip seed oil or Almond oil to massage over tummy and hips.*

ROKE: See BLOOD: CLOTS and BROKEN BLOOD VESSELS. Aroma Life, calamus, cypress, helichrysum. Breathe deeply and apply to neck and forehead.

SUPPLEMENTS—Master Formula Hers/His, Power Meal, Sulfurzyme, Ultra Young, Wolfberry Power Bars.

HEAT—Lavender or peppermint (rub on neck and forehead).

MUSCULAR PARALYSIS—Lavender.

BLEND—Mix together equal parts of basil, lavender, and rosemary. Rub spinal column and paralyzed area (Alternative Medicine—The Definitive Guide, p. 978).

RUCTURAL ALIGNMENT: Aroma Siez, basil, birch, cypress, peppermint, Valor, wintergreen (apply on feet to reduce time and effort necessary for alignments and to increase amount of time the alignment remains effective). Do the Raindrop Technique.

Valor is considered a "chiropractor in a bottle." It may help to realign the spine and keep the body in balance.

MASSAGE OILS—Ortho Ease.

BCONSCIOUS: Believe, Gratitude, helichrysum (uplifts when diffused), Idaho balsam fir, Transformation, Western Red cedar.

ESSENTIAL WATERS (HYDROSOLS)—Western Red Cedar.

DORIFIC: Hyssop, juniper, lavender, Roman chamomile, rosemary, thyme.

*A **sudorific** is an agent that causes sweating. It may be helpful in times of fever or when toxins need to be released through the skin.*

GAR:

SUPPLEMENTS—Allerzyme (aids the digestion of sugars, starches, fats, and proteins).

REMOVE ADDICTIONS TO SUGAR—Dill (on wrists).

Honey goes into the blood stream faster than sugar and can be harder on the system than sugar. Maple syrup is one of the most perfect sugars because it has equal proportions of positive and negative ions. It also has the same pH as the blood and it doesn't go into the blood as fast as honey or sugar. Diabetics and pre-diabetics should use black strap molasses instead of maple syrup.

STOP EATING—Peace & Calming, Purification.
SUPPLEMENTS—JuvaTone.
SUBSTITUTE—Stevia (liquid) or Stevia Select (powder). *Stevia Select can even be use on cereals and in other recipes as a sugar replacement. Experimentation m be necessary for proper amounts as Stevia Select tends to be more sweet th regular sugar.*

SUICIDE: See DEPRESSION and EMOTIONS.

SUNBURN: See BURNS. Australian Blue, [F]melaleuca, peppermint. Spray or rub with Roman chamomile and lavender. 5-6 drops of Roman chamomile added to lukewarm bath water helps reduce the burning sensation.

> *My niece came to me in a panic. She had been at the beach all day and acquired a nasty sunburn on her face, chest, and arms. She was planning to go to a fancy party the next day and decided that she absolutely could not go to the party unless the sunburn was gone. I immediately applied a layer of lavender oil, followed a few minutes later by a layer of peppermint oil. The next day to her amazement the sunburn had vanished and she was able to enjoy her party.*
>
> ***-Submitted by J.S., Florida (July 2004***

SUPPLEMENTS—Mineral Essence (can apply directly on affected area).
PERSONAL CARE—LavaDerm Cooling Mist (use as often as needed to keep skin cool and moist), Satin Hand & Body Lotion.
PREVENT BLISTERING—Apply 2-3 drops of lavender with Satin Hand & Body Lotio

SUN SCREEN: [F]Helichrysum, Tamanu (used by the natives as a natural sunscreen for centuri
PERSONAL CARE—Sunsation Suntan Oil helps filter out the ultraviolet rays with blocking the absorption of vitamin D, which is important to skin and bone development. It also ACCELERATES TANNING.

SUPPORTIVE: Myrrh.

SWELLING: See EDEMA (for swelling from water retention). Helichrysum, lemongrass, **tangerine**.

SYMPATHETIC NERVOUS SYSTEM: Black pepper, Brain Power, Clarity, *Eucalyptus radiata*, ginger, peppermint.

> ***The Sympathetic Nervous System*** *is responsible for preparing our bodies for action by stimulating the heart, dilating the bronchi, contracting the arteries, and inhibiting the digestive system.*

Stimulation of certain areas of the Sympathetic Nervous System can be achie by application of any of the above oils at the appropriate places along the spi column (*refer to the Autonomic Nervous System chart in the Science and Application section of the Reference Guide for Essential Oils*).

SUPPLEMENTS—Coral Sea (highly bio-available, contains 58 trace minerals), Mineral Essence, Power Meal, Sulfurzyme, Super Cal, Ultra Young.

YMPATHY: Acceptance, Awaken, Present Time.

ACHYCARDIA (Rapid Heartbeat): See ANXIETY, HEART, SHOCK, or STRESS. Aroma Life (combine with ylang ylang), Australian Blue, goldenrod, Idaho tansy, lavender, neroli, orange, PanAway, Relieve It, Roman chamomile, rose, [F]rosemary, [F]ylang ylang (smell on tissue or straight from bottle in emergency). Apply over heart and to heart Vita Flex points on the left hand and elbow (see illustration under HEART) and on the left foot. Add oils to V-6 Mixing Oil or Massage Oil for massage, or add them to Bath Gel Base for an aromatic bath. Continue to use regularly to help prevent recurrence.

TINCTURES—HRT.

SUPPLEMENTS—CardiaCare, Sulfurzyme.

ALKATIVE: Cypress (for over-talkative).

ASTE: Helichrysum (1 drop on tongue), peppermint (for impaired taste).

SUPPLEMENTS—Mineral Essence, Super B, Super C / Super C Chewable (enhances flavor).

EETH: See DENTAL INFECTION.

CAVITIES—Brush teeth with Thieves. *Put a drop on your toothpaste if you can't handle it straight.*

PERSONAL CARE—Dentarome/Dentarome Plus Toothpaste (contains Thieves), Fresh Essence Mouthwash (contains Thieves), KidScents Toothpaste (for children).

****COMMENTS—People have had regeneration of their teeth in as little as four months by brushing their teeth with Thieves.*

FILLINGS—(to help eliminate toxins from mercury in the system) Idaho balsam fir (22 drops in a capsule, once in morning, once at night). Can also combine Idaho balsam fir with helichrysum and/or frankincense.

SUPPLEMENTS—Super C / Super C Chewable, Cleansing Trio (ComforTone, Essentialzyme, and ICP), Detoxzyme (5 in morning and 5 at night until body says stop! Then back off to 1 or 2 per day).

GUM SURGERY—Helichrysum every 15 minutes for the pain.

TEETHING PAIN—German chamomile, Thieves.

TOOTHACHE—Cajeput, [F]**clove**, melaleuca, Purification (anti-bacterial), Roman chamomile. Apply on location (on gums) and along jawbone.

PERSONAL CARE— Dentarome/Dentarome Plus Toothpaste (contains Thieves), Fresh Essence Mouthwash (contains Thieves).

TOOTHPASTE—Thieves.

****COMMENTS—You may want to put 10-12 drops of Thieves in 2 oz. of water in a small spray bottle. Mist in mouth or on toothbrush and brush.*

PERSONAL CARE— Dentarome/Dentarome Plus/Dentarome Ultra Toothpaste (contains Thieves), Fresh Essence Mouthwash (contains Thieves), KidScents Toothpaste (for children).

*RECIPE—*Combine 4 tsp. green or White clay, 1 tsp. salt, 1 to 2 drops peppermint, to 2 drops lemon, mix clockwise.

NERVE PAIN—Melaleuca (put 1 drop in small amount of water and hold in mouth for on to two minutes to help calm nerves).

My husband has very cavity prone teeth that have needed much dental work in the past 5 years. He has been going in for cleanings every 3 months. His dentist had once prescribed a special mouth wash that was supposed to help his decaying teeth. He didn't use the mouthwash regularly enough to see any improvement. About a year ago, he started using Dentarome Plus toothpaste instead of the brand he had been using from the local grocer. That was the only change he made to his dental hygiene routine. At his cleaning in March, his dentist wanted to know what he was doing differently, because his x-rays showed no dental work needed to be done and they didn't have to work as hard to polish his teeth. He told them that all he changed was the toothpaste he was using. They wanted to know if it had fluoride in it, because to be any good (in their eyes) it must have fluoride in it; he brushed them off not wanting to get into the dangers of fluoride with them that day. Then at his cleaning just last week, the dentist had to look at his x-rays twice as well as call on two other colleagues to look at his x-rays to be sure that nothing was being missed because they could not find anything that needed to be fixed. They also told him to come back in six months (instead of 3) for his next cleaning. Now, if I could only get him to use the Fresh Essence Plus mouthwash...

-Submitted by A. Corn
Machesney Park, Illinois (July 2004)

TEMPERATURE: See FEVER or THYROID.

*SUPPLEMENTS—*Thyromin (balances the temperature in the body).

LOWER—Bergamot, eucalyptus, lavender, melissa, peppermint. Cypress and rosemary induce sweating to lower temperature indirectly. Use oils in baths or mix with cool water and sponge over body or area.

*ESSENTIAL WATERS (HYDROSOLS)—*Lavender, Melissa, Peppermint. Spray directly on body or diffuse with Essential Mist Diffuser.

RAISE—Marjoram, onycha (benzoin), thyme. Add to V-6 Mixing Oil or Massage Oil for brisk massage. Locally warming (rubefacient) oils like Black pepper, juniper, and rosemary help raise temperature in cold extremities.

TENDONITIS: Basil, [F]birch, cypress, ginger, Idaho Balsam fir, lavender, PanAway, peppermint, Relieve It, rosemary, wintergreen. Apply oils in Raindrop fashion on location and ice pack.

SUPPLEMENTS—BLM

PAIN RELIEF—Birch/wintergreen and peppermint. If pain and inflammation is a result of torn or infected ligaments or tendons, then lemongrass and helichrysum can be helpful when added to any of these oils.

Tendonitis Blend
This has worked for my tendonitis and for several other people I have given it to. In a 15 ml amber glass bottle I mix the following essential oils: 3 drops each of helichrysum, pepper, bergamot, and geranium, 5 drops each of Idaho Balsam fir and lemongrass, then 3 drops each of hyssop, Blue tansy, pine, and myrtle. Then I fill the bottle with V-6 Mixing Oil. This is applied to the area where the pain is and followed with a layer of peppermint oil. This can be done several times per day. If a sensitivity develops, stop using it for a few weeks.
-Submitted by J.S.
West Saint Paul, Minnesota (July 2004)

TENNIS ELBOW: Birch, eucalyptus, helichrysum, PanAway, peppermint, rosemary, wintergreen.

Tennis Elbow *is the painful inflammation of the tendon on the outer side of the elbow that usually results from excessive strain on and twisting of the forearm.*

BLEND #1—10 eucalyptus, 10 peppermint, 10 rosemary, and 1 Tbs. V-6 Mixing Oil. Mix and apply, then ice pack. Can also try alternating cold and hot packs.

BLEND #2—Equal parts lemongrass, helichrysum, marjoram, and peppermint. Mix and apply, then ice pack.

TENSION: Basil (nervous), bergamot (nervous), [F]cedarwood, frankincense, Harmony, lavender, *Melaleuca ericifolia* (nervous), Peace & Calming, Trauma Life (balances and calms), valerian, ylang ylang. Apply on hands, cup over nose and mouth and breathe deeply or diffuse. Mix a few drops of oil, or oils of choice, in ½ cup Epsom salts and add to bath water.

AQUA ESSENCE BATH PACKS—Finally, some of the most popular essential oil blends have been combines with the latest hydro-diffusion technology to create the perfect solution for adding oils to your bath water. Just place a packet in the tub while hot water is being added and the oils are perfectly dispersed into the water. The packets contain 10 ml of oil and are reusable. Try either Valor or Peace & Calming.

RELIEVE—Grapefruit, Roman chamomile, Transformation.

MASSAGE OILS—Ortho Ease, Relaxation.

PERSONAL CARE—Prenolone/Prenolone+, Progessence.

TESTICLES: [F]Rosemary.

REGULATION—Aroma Siez (combine with Mister), Clary sage, geranium, sandalwood, yarrow.

PERSONAL CARE—Prenolone+.

SUPPLEMENTS—Mineral Essence, ProGen, Ultra Young+.

THOUGHTS: Inspiration (relieves negative), ravensara (lifts emotions).

THROAT: Calamus (helps remove phlegm), [F]cypress, oregano. Myrrh and peppermint are also very effective for removing phlegm and mucus from the throat area.

DRY—Grapefruit, lemon.

INFECTION IN—Clary sage, [F]lemon, oregano, [F]peppermint.

LARYNGITIS—See LARYNGITIS.

SORE—Rub one of the following on the throat: Bergamot, cajeput, geranium, ginger, ImmuPower, [F]melaleuca, myrrh, oregano, RC, sandalwood, Thieves, or put 1 drop of Thieves in 32 oz. water and drink. Inhalations with Clary sage, eucalyptus, lavender, sandalwood, thyme.

PERSONAL CARE—Gargle with Fresh Essence or Fresh Essence Plus Mouthwash.

SUPPLEMENTS—Thieves Lozenges.

STREP—Geranium, ginger, or Thieves (rub on throat every time it feels sore; dilute well!) Also hyssop, laurel, melaleuca (combine with Thieves and dilute), oregano, ravensara (combine with Melrose).

PERSONAL CARE—Gargle with Fresh Essence or Fresh Essence Plus Mouthwash (every hour).

SUPPLEMENTS—ImmuneTune, ImmuPro, Super C / Super C Chewable, Thieves Lozenges.

THRUSH: Bergamot, eucalyptus, [F]lavender, marjoram, rose, thyme.

VAGINAL—Geranium, [F]melaleuca, [F]myrrh, patchouli, rosemary.

THYMUS: Elemi, ImmuPower (apply on throat and chest), ravensara, Thieves (dilute with V-6 Mixing Oil and apply over thymus or apply neat on bottom of feet).

STIMULATES—ImmuPower, [F]spruce.

SUPPLEMENTS—Ultra Young (reverses aging of the thymus gland).

THYROID:

DYSFUNCTION—Clove.

NORMALIZES HORMONAL IMBALANCE OF—Myrtle.

HYPERTHYROIDISM—EndoFlex, [F]myrrh, myrtle, [F]spruce.

SUPPLEMENTS— Sulfurzyme.

BLEND #1—Equal parts lemongrass and myrrh. Can apply undiluted on thyroid and parathyroid Vita Flex points under big toes or dilute with small amount of V-6 Mixing Oil and apply on throat just under the Adam's apple.

BLEND #2—Equal parts myrrh and spruce. Apply as directed in Blend #1 above.

T

HYPOTHYROIDISM—Clove, EndoFlex (apply on top of big toes), [F]myrtle, peppermint, spearmint. Combine lemongrass with any or all of these oils and apply as directed in BLEND #1 above.

> *The **thyroid gland** is situated in the neck and regulates the body's metabolic rate.*
>
> *To determine whether or not the thyroid needs help, you must monitor your basal cell temperature. Place a thermometer under your arm pit before getting out of bed in the morning and rest quietly for 10 minutes. A temperature below 97.6º F (36.5º C) may indicate hypothyroidism (low thyroid function) and a temperature above 98º F (36.7º C) may indicate hyperthyroidism.*

SUPPLEMENTS—Thyromin (regulates metabolism, balances body temperature, prevents fatigue; *follow directions for use as specified in the Supplements section under Thyromin*).

****COMMENTS—One of the signs of thyroid deficiency is rough, dry skin on the bottoms of the feet.*

REGULATION—Ledum.

SUPPORTS—EndoFlex, myrrh (rub on hands and feet), myrtle.

SUPPLEMENTS—Cleansing Trio (ComforTone, Essentialzyme, and ICP), Power Meal, VitaGreen (enhances effect of Thyromin), Thyromin (regulates metabolism, balances body temperature, prevents fatigue; *follow directions for use as specified in the Supplements section of the Reference Guide for Essential Oils under Thyromin*).

NNITUS: (Ringing in the ears.) See EAR. Juniper, helichrysum. Apply to mastoid bone behind ear.

RED: See ENERGY, EXHAUSTION, and FATIGUE.

SSUE: Basil, elemi (rejuvenates), helichrysum, lavender, lemongrass, lime (tightens connective tissue), marjoram, Melrose, Roman chamomile, sandalwood.

SUPPLEMENTS—Be-Fit (builds muscle tissue), Bodygize (for elasticity in tissues), AminoTech (builds lean muscle tissue), Power Meal (pre-digested protein), WheyFit. Biotin (found in Bodygize) is important for damaged tissue.

ANTI-INFLAMMATORY—Myrrh.

BONE AND JOINT REGENERATION—(See Blend on following page)

BLEND—5 drops birch/wintergreen, 2 German chamomile, 1 Blue tansy, 7 fir, 5 helichrysum, 5 hyssop, 4 lemongrass, 8 sandalwood, 8 spruce, and 1 oz. V-6 Mixing Oil.

CLEANSES TOXINS FROM—Fennel.

CONNECTIVE TISSUE, WEAK—Aroma Siez, helichrysum, lavender, lemongrass, patchouli.

MASSAGE OILS—Ortho Ease.

DEEP TISSUE PAIN—Helichrysum, PanAway, Relieve It.

MASSAGE OILS—Ortho Ease and Ortho Sport.

REPAIR—Elemi (builds), helichrysum (scar tissue and reduces tissue pain), hyssop (scar lemongrass (repairs connective tissue), orange, rosewood, sage (firms tissue) Relieve It (deep tissue damage).

PERSONAL CARE—Rose Ointment (to help maintain, protect, and keep the scab soft), Satin Hand & Body Lotion (to moisturize and promote healing).

REGENERATE—Geranium, helichrysum, lemongrass, Melrose, [F]patchouli, rosehip.

****COMMENTS—Use helichrysum and Melrose together for traumatized tissue (cuts, wounds, and abrasions).*

TMJ (Temporomandibular Joint Disorder or TMD): 3 Wise Men. Apply on temple and si of face, in front of ear and down to the jaw. Cover with ice packs for 10 minutes at a time, 3-4 times a day. May be best to seek advise from a healthcare professional, especially a dentist.

TONIC:

DIGESTIVE—[F]German chamomile, *Melaleuca quinquenervia*.

GENERAL—Angelica, basil, cajeput, cardamom, cinnamon bark, cistus, Clary sage, cu galbanum, geranium, ginger, grapefruit, juniper, lemon, lemongrass, lime, mandarin, marjoram, melissa, Mixta chamomile, Mountain savory, myrrh, neroli, nutmeg, orange, palmarosa, patchouli, sandalwood, spruce, ylang yla Best way to restore tone in a body that is run-down is to apply oils by massa when possible. Baths are next in effectiveness to massage is not possible or between massages.

HEART—Lavender, thyme.

NERVE—Carrot, Clary sage, melaleuca, [F]ravensara, thyme.

SKIN—lemon, lime, spearmint, spikenard.

STOMACH—Tangerine.

UTERINE—Jasmine, thyme.

TONSILLITIS: (Inflamed tonsils, most often due to streptococcal infection.) See STREP THROAT. Bergamot, clove, goldenrod, [F]ginger, lavender, lemon (gargle),

[F]melaleuca, Roman chamomile, Thieves. Apply on throat, lungs, and Vita Flex points.

DIFFUSE—Bergamot, clove, geranium, lavender, lemon, melaleuca (Tea Tree), onycha (benzoin), Thieves, thyme. Breathe deeply through mouth.

PERSONAL CARE—Fresh Essence Mouthwash.

SUPPLEMENTS—Thieves Lozenges.

****COMMENTS—Use caution when considering surgery (tonsillectomy) for recurring tonsillitis as doctors have discovered that the only area of the body that can synthesize the antibody to poliomyelitis (polio) is the tonsils.*

***Toxemia**—poisoned condition of the blood caused by the presence of toxic materials, usually bacterial but occasionally chemical or hormonal in nature. When bacteria themselves find entrance into the bloodstream, the condition is known as bacteremia. The term toxemia is also sometimes applied to preeclampsia, a condition that occasionally occurs in late pregnancy and is characterized by high blood pressure and kidney malfunction.* *(Microsoft® Encarta® Online Encyclopedia 2000)*

OTHACHE: See TEETH.

XEMIA: Aroma Life, cypress.

SUPPLEMENTS—Essential Manna, Exodus.

TINCTURES—Rehemogen.

XINS: Fennel, fir, hyssop (opens respiratory system and discharges toxins and mucus), lemongrass (helps increase lymphatic circulation for enhanced toxin removal), patchouli (digests toxic wastes).

SUPPLEMENTS—Cleansing Trio (ComforTone, Essentialzyme, and ICP). These cleansing products may help remove toxic by-products from the body.

****COMMENTS—Another way to help remove toxins through the skin is to add 2 cups of Apple Cider Vinegar to warm bath water and soak for 25 minutes.*

ANSITION IN LIFE: Acceptance, Awaken (into achieving success), basil, cypress, **Transformation**. May also want to concentrate on the emotional blends of Valor, Motivation, Grounding, Release, Hope, and Joy (*refer to the pages on "Auricular Emotional Therapy" and "Emotional Release" in the Science and Application section of the Reference Guide for Essential Oils*).

AUMA: See SHOCK. Release (feet and liver), Joy (heart), 3 Wise Men (crown); use all three blends in succession. May also diffuse. Australian Blue, Envision, Forgiveness, Hope, and Release can also aid in releasing emotional trauma (*Refer to each blend separately in the Blends section of the Reference Guide for Essential Oils for possible applications*). Trauma Life is an excellent blend for helping to cope with shock or emotional trauma. Apply on forehead and on palms then rub palms together, cup over nose and mouth, and inhale deeply. Others that may help are Valor (on the feet), SARA (on temples), Peace & Calming (on palms; place hands together over heart in prayer position).

****COMMENTS—Concentrate on relaxing to help release the trauma. Also, if after an emotional or physical trauma you find you don't like the smell of a particula oil, it may be the one you need most to help unlock the trauma. Try exposin yourself to it a little at a time until the healing is finished.*

SUPPLEMENTS—ImmuPro, Mineral Essence, Super C / Super C Chewable.

TRAVEL SICKNESS: See MOTION SICKNESS.

TUBERCULOSIS (T.B.): Cajeput, [F]cedarwood, [F]cypress, [F]*Eucalyptus radiata*, lemon, [F]myrtle peppermint, rosemary verbenon, sandalwood, or [F]thyme linalol. Exodus II (on spine and Raven on back with a hot compress), ImmuPower (on spine daily), Raven (1-2 drops in V-6 Mixing Oil as a rectal implant), RC (on chest and back– reverse each night with Raven), rose, rosemary, Thieves (on feet). A h compress can be used when applying oils to the chest or back. DO THE RAINDROP TECHNIQUE.

SUPPLEMENTS—Exodus, ImmuGel, ImmuneTune, ImmuPro, Super C / Super C Chewable, VitaGreen. Do a colon and liver cleanse with the Cleansing Trio (ComforTone, Essentialzyme, and ICP), and JuvaTone.

TINCTURES—Rehemogen.

BLEND—1-2 drops each of *Eucalyptus radiata*, myrtle, Mountain savory, and ravensara in 1 Tbsp. V-6 Mixing Oil. Apply as a rectal implant.

****COMMENTS—Refer to The chapter entitled "How to Use - The Personal Usage Reference" in the* Essential Oils Desk Reference *under "Tuberculosis" for a specific regimen using the blends and supplements.*

AIRBORNE BACTERIA—Purification, Raven, RC, Sacred Mountain, Thieves. Alterna diffusing different oils to help control spread of bacteria like *Mycobacterium tuberculosis*.

BLEND—Equal amounts of cypress and Sacred Mountain. Diffuse.

PULMONARY—Cypress, eucalyptus, Inspiration, [F]oregano, ravensara.

BLEND—Equal amounts of frankincense and ImmuPower. Diffuse or dilute with V Mixing Oil and massage on chest or back. Can also apply to Vita Flex lung points on hands and feet.

TUMORS: See CANCER.

ANTI-TUMORAL—Clove, [F]frankincense, ledum (may be more powerful than frankincense). Apply directly on tumor.

LIPOMA–Frankincense and clove, grapefruit, ginger, ledum.

PERSONAL CARE—Prenolone/Prenolone+, Progessence.

****COMMENTS—Avoid the use of elemi as the oxidation of d-limonene (a principle constituent of elemi) has been known to cause tumor growth!*

YPHOID: (Fever from contamination of the Salmonella typhosa bacteria) See ANTI-BACTERIAL. [F]Cinnamon bark, lemon, Melrose, Mountain savory, peppermint, Purification, Raven, ravensara, RC. Diffuse or dilute with V-6 Mixing Oil or Massage Oil Base and apply over intestines and on Vita Flex points on the feet.

T

U

LCERS: Bergamot, cinnamon bark, clove, elemi, [F]frankincense, geranium, [F]German chamomile, lemon, [F]myrrh, oregano, rose, thyme, vetiver. Add one drop of oil to rice or almond milk and take as dietary supplement. May also be applied over stomach by hot compress.

> *While some sources claim that sixty percent of all* ***ulcers*** *are caused by bacteria, F. Batmanghelidj, M.D. maintains that the majority of ulcers are only dehydration of the stomach lining. In his book, Your Body's Many Cries for Water, Dr. Batmanghelidj shows that rehydration is the simplest cure for this and many other adverse health conditions.*

SUPPLEMENTS—Use ComforTone to help destroy the bacteria, then use Essentialzyme, Master Formula His/Hers.

DUODENAL—(Damaged mucous membrane in a portion of the small intestine). Same oils as listed above.

SUPPLEMENTS—AlkaLime.

GASTRIC—See GASTRITIS. [F]Geranium.

LEG—(From lack of circulation in lower extremities and possible bacterial, fungal, or viral infection). Gentle Baby, geranium, German chamomile, lavender, Melrose, patchouli, Purification, Roman chamomile, rosewood, Sensation.

****COMMENTS—Dilute oils with V-6 Mixing Oil or Massage Oil Base and massage lower extremities to stimulate circulation. Thyromin may be needed to help with overall circulation.*

MASSAGE OILS—Sensation.

PERSONAL CARE—Rose Ointment.

BLEND—Equal drops of lavender and either Melrose or Purification applied to location. Can cover with Rose Ointment.

MOUTH—See CANKERS. Basil (mouthwash), myrrh, orange.

BLEND #1—1 drop each of sage and clove and 1-3 drops lavender. Apply directly on location.

PEPTIC—Flavor a quart of water with 1 drop of cinnamon bark oil and sip all day.

SUPPLEMENTS—AlkaLime.

STOMACH—Bergamot, frankincense, geranium, orange, peppermint. Use as food flavoring, apply to stomach, and Vita Flex points.

SUPPLEMENTS—AlkaLime, Cleansing Trio (ComforTone, Essentialzyme, and ICP), Master Formula His/Hers, Royaldophilus (can help coat stomach and protect sensitive tissues while rebuilding).

ULCERATIONS—Cleanse liver and colon (See CLEANSING). Lavender, Melrose, rose.

Personal Guide

PERSONAL CARE—Rose Ointment.

VARICOSE ULCERS—See VARICOSE ULCERS.

ULTRAVIOLET RAYS: Sunsation Suntan Oil blocks ultraviolet rays without blocking the absorption of Vitamin D.

UNWIND: See MASSAGE. Lavender, Peace & Calming. Diffuse, rub between hands and inhale deeply, or combine with V-6 Mixing Oil or Massage Oil for massage.

MASSAGE OILS—Relaxation.

BATH & SHOWER GELS—Evening Peace.

UPLIFTING: Believe, bergamot, birch, Brain Power, fir (emotionally uplifting), grapefruit, helichrysum, Idaho balsam fir, Idaho tansy, jasmine, lavender, myrrh, orange, Live with Passion, ravensara, Sacred Mountain, Sensation, spruce, 3 Wise Me Transformation, tsuga, wintergreen. Diffuse or wear as perfume or cologne.

BLEND—3 birch/wintergreen, 3 lavender, 3 orange, 3 spruce and 1 oz. V-6 Mixing Oil. Wear a few drops of this blend as a perfume or cologne or apply over the heart, on the chest, neck, and/or shoulders, and behind the ears. Can also appl a few drops on both hands, rub together, cup over nose and mouth and breathe deeply.

BATH & SHOWER GELS—Morning Start, Sensation.

ESSENTIAL WATERS (HYDROSOLS)—Basil, Melissa, Mountain Essence, Peppermint, Idaho Tansy (mentally). Spray into air directly on face (don't spray directly into eyes or ears) or diffuse using the Essential Mist Diffuser.

URETER:

*The **ureter** is the duct that carries the urine away from the kidneys to the bladder.*

INFECTION IN—See BLADDER: INFECTION or KIDNEYS: INFECTION. [F]Lemon, [F]myrtle. Apply as specified below in Urinary Tract Infection.

URINARY TRACT: Bergamot, ImmuPower, lavender, ledum, melaleuca (Tea Tree), pine (antiseptic), [F]sage, [F]sandalwood, rosemary, tarragon, [F]thyme (infection).

GENERAL—Bergamot, [F]eucalyptus (general stimulant).

INFECTION—See BLADDER INFECTION. Bergamot, cajeput, [F]cedarwood, Di-Tone, EndoFlex, geranium, hyssop, ImmuPower, Inspiration (effective by itself), juniper, lemongrass, Melrose, onycha, Purification (effective by itself), tarrago Apply 2-3 drops of oil directly over bladder. May also apply a hot compress.

BLEND #1—Equal parts sage and Purification.

BLEND #2—Equal parts thyme and Melrose.

BLEND #3—Equal parts oregano and Thieves.

BLEND #4—Equal parts juniper and EndoFlex.

SUPPLEMENTS—AlkaLime.

TINCTURES—K&B.

RECIPE #1—Add 1 drop of Mountain savory to 3 droppers of K&B tincture in distilled water and drink every few hours.

With any of these blends, dilute with V-6 Mixing Oil and massage over lower back and pubic area or apply with hot compress.

****COMMENTS—Refer to The chapter entitled "How to Use - The Personal Usage Reference" in the Essential Oils Desk Reference under "Urinary Tract/Bladder Infection" for a unique blend of 14 different oils to specifically help with infection.*

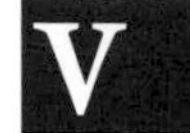

STONES IN—[F]Fennel, [F]geranium. Apply oils over pubic area and lower back with hot compress. *See Master Cleanser under CLEANSING.*

SUPPORT—Cypress, geranium, goldenrod, juniper, laurel, melaleuca.

TINCTURES—K&B.

ERUS: Cedarwood, frankincense, geranium, jasmine, lemon, myrrh.

INFLAMMATION—Elemi.

REGENERATION OF TISSUE—Frankincense, sage, tarragon. Add 1-3 drops of each to 1 tsp. V-6 Mixing Oil, insert into vagina, and retain overnight.

PERSONAL CARE—PD 80/20, Prenolone/Prenolone +, Progessence.

SUPPLEMENTS—Bodygize, FemiGen.

UTEROTONIC—Thyme.

UTERINE CANCER—See CANCER. Cedarwood, frankincense, geranium, Gratitude, ImmuPower, lemon, myrrh. Oils can be applied to the reproductive Vita Flex points on the feet, mostly around the front of the ankle, on either side of the ankle under the ankle bone, and up the Achilles tendon. The most effective application of oils is by vaginal retention implant. Add 2-5 drops of any of these single oils or a combination of any of them to 1 tsp. V-6 Mixing Oil, insert into vagina and retain overnight. A tampon may be used if necessary to help retain the oil.

UTERINE CYSTS—See OVARIAN CYSTS under OVARIES.

GINAL:

APPLICATION METHODS—Mix desired oil(s) with water and either use in a douche or sitz bath. After a douche, a capsule of Royaldophilus can be inserted in the vagina to help repopulate friendly bacteria and flora. Desired oil(s) may also be mixed with V-6 Mixing Oil and either applied directly or by soaking a tampon in mixture, inserting, and leaving in all day or night.

CANDIDA (thrush)—[F]Bergamot, lavender, laurel, [F]melaleuca, [F]myrrh, rosemary, spikenard, [F]thyme. *See Application Methods above.*

SUPPLEMENTS—AlkaLime, Royaldophilus, and/or Stevia Select with FOS (important to re-establish the intestinal flora). Yogurt or Royaldophilus mixe with a little bit of water may be applied directly to relieve the pain associated with candida.

****COMMENTS—Focus on the underlying problem of system-wide yeast infectio See CANDIDA. Also, refer to The chapter entitled "How to Use - The Personal Usage Reference" in the Essential Oils Desk Reference under "Fungal Infections" for some excellent blend recipes for dealing with vagin yeast infections.*

INFECTION—[F]Cinnamon bark (be extremely careful; dilute well), Clary sage, cypress, eucalyptus, hyssop, Inspiration, juniper, lavender, laurel, melaleuca, Melrose, myrrh, Mountain savory, oregano, [F]rosemary, [F]rosewood, sage, 3 Wise Men, thyme. Apply oregano and thyme along the spine using the Raindrop Technique. *See also Application Methods above.*

BLEND #1—Equal parts oregano, thyme, and Melrose. Dilute with V-6 Mixing Oi or Massage Oil and apply as described in Application Methods above.

BLEND #2—3 drops rosemary, 2 drops *Melaleuca quinquenervia*, 2 drops oreganc and 1 drop thyme. Dilute with V-6 Mixing Oil or Massage Oil and apply as described in Application Methods above. Can also apply as hot compress ove lower abdominal area.

BLEND #3—5 drops Melrose, 2 drops oregano, and 1 drop thyme in 1 Tbsp. V-6 Mixing Oil or Massage Oil. Use as douche or vaginal retention implant as described in Application Methods above.

INFLAMMATION OF VAGINA—Eucalyptus, lavender, melaleuca, yarrow.

RETENTION IMPLANT—Used to cleanse and nourish the female reproductive system c as a support when taking products like the FemiGen supplement. Best when done after a colon and liver cleanse using the Cleansing Trio (ComforTone, Essentialzyme, ICP).

BLEND #4—Dilute 2 drops *Melaleuca quinquenervia*, 1 drop lavender, and 1 drop bergamot in 1 Tbsp. V-6 Mixing Oil. Insert and retain overnight.

BLEND #5—Dilute 2 drops frankincense and 7 drops Purification in 1 Tbsp. V-6 Mixing Oil. Insert and retain overnight.

VAGINITIS—[F]Cinnamon bark (be extremely careful; dilute well), *Eucalyptus radiata*, [F]rosemary, [F]rosewood. Valerie Woorwood suggests the following douche reci that should be used daily for three days a week only.

RECIPE #1—1 lavender, 1 melaleuca (Tea Tree), 1 tsp. of vinegar, ½ tsp. lemon juice, and 2 ½ cups of warm water. Mix thoroughly.

VARICOSE ULCERS: Eucalyptus, geranium, lavender, melaleuca (Tea Tree), thyme, yarrov

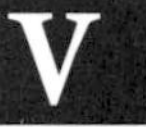

ARICOSE VEINS: Aroma Life, Aroma Siez, basil, bergamot, Citrus Fresh, [F]cypress (as bath oil), geranium, helichrysum (especially during pregnancy), Idaho tansy (helps weak veins), juniper, lavender, [F]lemon (tonic for circulatory system), [F]lemongrass, orange, [F]peppermint, rosemary, spikenard, tangerine, yarrow.

Varicose veins are abnormal swelling of the veins in the legs. It is most often a symptom of poor circulation and a loss of elasticity of the vascular walls and particularly their valves. If the valves do not work properly, blood accumulates in the veins instead of flowing back to the heart. This accumulation of blood causes the vein to become swollen and twisted. ***Hemorrhoids*** *are varicose veins of the anus or rectum usually resulting from constipation. Cleanse the colon.*

Helichrysum dissolves the coagulated blood inside and outside of the veins. Cypress strengthens the veins. Massage ***above*** *the affected vein toward the heart with helichrysum and cypress every morning and night; wear support hose until healed; it may take from three months to a year to heal completely. It is important to vary the essential oils being used. Try using lavender, juniper or rosemary instead of cypress and helichrysum. See DIET, CIRCULATORY SYSTEM.*

Caution: *Do not rub below the affected area as it may increase the pressure on the vein*

MASSAGE OILS—Cel-Lite Magic (strengthens vascular walls).

SUPPLEMENTS—Super B, Thyromin, VitaGreen.

TINCTURES—Rehemogen.

BLEND #1—1-3 drops each of lemongrass and Aroma Life with Cel-Lite Magic.

BLEND #2—1-3 drops each of basil and Aroma Siez. Massage above the affected vein toward the heart.

****COMMENTS—Refer to The chapter entitled "How to Use - The Personal Usage Reference" in the Essential Oils Desk Reference under "Varicose Veins" for more specific blend recipes and instructions regarding treatment.*

ASCULAR SYSTEM: Aroma Life, cypress, frankincense, helichrysum, [F]lemongrass (strengthens vascular walls). Apply as a full body massage, over heart, and on bottom of the feet.

The ***vascular system*** *refers to the vessels or veins that carry and circulate fluids (blood and lymph) throughout the body.*

MASSAGE OILS—Cel-Lite Magic (strengthens vascular walls).

CLEANSING—See CHELATION and METALS. Juva Cleanse.

SUPPLEMENTS—JuvaTone, and VitaGreen work very well together. Other supplements include AD&E, Essentialzyme, ImmuGel, ImmuneTune, and Super C / Super C Chewable.

TINCTURES—HRT, K&B, Rehemogen.

BLEND—1-3 drops each of helichrysum and Aroma Life with Cel-Lite Magic Massage Oil. Massage on the body to help dilate the blood vessels and enhance the chelation of metallics.

VASODILATOR: See BLOOD. Lemongrass, marjoram.

VEINS: See VASCULAR SYSTEM above.

CIRCULATION IN VASCULAR WALLS OF VEINS—Aroma Life, cypress, lemon.

BLOOD CLOT IN VEIN—Cypress and helichrysum (rub neat on location to dissolve).

VERTIGO: See EARS, EQUILIBRIUM and DIZZINESS. Ginger.

VIRAL DISEASE: Cinnamon bark.

SUPPLEMENTS—ParaFree, Super C / Super C Chewable, ImmuneTune, ImmuPro, ImmuGel.

ANTI-VIRAL—Oregano.

INFECTION—Cajeput, melaleuca, oregano, ravensara, thyme. Apply along spine, bottom of feet, and diffuse.

BLEND—Mix one drop each of lavender, orange, and spruce and apply to chest. Then put 10 drops of frankincense in a cap full of Evening Peace Bath Gel and add to bath as a bubble bath and soak.

VIRUSES: (often hibernate along the spine) Massage ImmuPower and oregano along the spine. Also use bergamot, Blue cypress (especially for HPV), cypress, *Eucalyptus radiata*, lavender, *Melaleuca quinquenervia* (viral and fungal infection), ravensara (viral infection), [F]rosemary, Thieves. DO THE RAINDROP TECHNIQUE!

SUPPLEMENTS—ImmuPro, Royaldophilus (up to 4 a day, 30 minutes before eating), Thieves Lozenges.

*When my friend contracted the **West Nile virus** from a mosquito bite last summer, her neck became stiff, and she had swelling in her ears and behind her ears at the base of her brain. She was in great pain and her ears felt "full" all of the time. We applied an oil blend from Young Living Oils called Thieves. She placed the oil at the base of her head and down both sides of her neck and jaw area. This gave her relief from the intense pain in her neck and reduced the swelling in her ears and head. She also drank a couple of drops of the Thieves oil blend in fluids several times a day. She continued doing this for at least a month while she fought this disease. We both agree this probably kept her from more serious complications due to the severity of the illness. We also believe it kept her out of the hospital.*

-Submitted by C. Ness
Rapid City, South Dakota (July 2004)

AIRBORNE VIRUSES—ImmuPower on throat and chest, Thieves on feet. Diffuse.

ASTHMA—See ASTHMA.

EBOLA VIRUS—This virus cannot live in the presence of cinnamon bark or oregano.

EPSTEIN BARR VIRUS—See EPSTEIN BARR. Strengthen immune system, ensure proper thyroid function, and work on hypoglycemia. ImmuPower, Thieves.

SUPPLEMENTS—Exodus, ImmuneTune, ImmuGel, ImmuPro, Wolfberry Bars.
RESPIRATORY—*Eucalyptus radiata*.
SPINE—5 oregano and 5 thyme. Put on bottom of the feet and up the spine using the Raindrop Technique.

ISUALIZATION: Awaken, Dream Catcher, helichrysum, PanAway. Diffuse or wear as perfume or cologne.

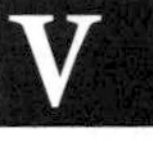

V

ITAL CENTERS: Oregano and sage may strengthen the vital centers of the body.

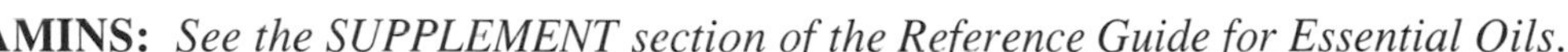

ITAMINS: *See the SUPPLEMENT section of the Reference Guide for Essential Oils.*
SUPPLEMENTS—Bodygize, Coral Sea (highly bio-available, contains 58 trace minerals), Power Meal, Sulfurzyme (sulfur necessary for proper assimilation of Vitamin C), Super B, Super C / Super C Chewable, Super Cal.
TINCTURES—AD&E.
CHILDREN—
SUPPLEMENTS—KidScents Mighty Mist (vitamin spray), KidScents Mighty Vites (chewable vitamin tablets), KidScents MightyZyme (chewable enzymes).

ITILIGO: Frankincense, Melrose, myrrh, Purification, sage, sandalwood, vetiver. Apply behind ears and to back of neck. Then rub hands together, cup over nose and mouth, and breathe deeply. Can also be applied to Vita Flex points relating to the pineal and pituitary glands on the feet and hands.

> ***Vitiligo*** *is a disease in which the skin pigmentation is absent in certain areas of the body. It looks as if patches of skin have been bleached white. This may be due to a malfunction of the pineal gland and possibly the pituitary gland as well. See PINEAL and PITUITARY for oils and products that can help oxygenate these glands. Another possible remedy includes daily exposure of the eyes to full-spectrum light without contacts or eyeglasses.*

OICE (hoarse): Bergamot, jasmine.
BLEND—Add one drop each of Melrose and lemon to 1 tsp. honey. Swish around in mouth for a couple of minutes to liquify then swallow.

OID: 3 Wise Men (replaces the void; place on crown).

OMITING: See NAUSEA. [F]Fennel, nutmeg, [F]peppermint (aromatic).
MASSAGE OR COMPRESS (over stomach)—Black pepper, fennel, lavender, peppermint, Roman chamomile, rose.

WARMING: Cinnamon bark, onycha (benzoin), oregano, thyme.

WARTS: Cinnamon bark, colloidal silver, clove, cypress, frankincense (excellent for more stubborn warts), jasmine, lavender, lemon (may dilute in 2 tsp. apple cider vinegar), Melrose, oregano, Thieves. Dilute 1 to 2 drops of oil in a few drops of V-6 Mixing Oil and apply on location.

My son had a really big wart on his hand and I started using Lavender and Melrose and it seemed to help. Then I decided to try something new. I used Melrose, Purification, Thieves, and Clove–one drop each–and rubbed them in one by one and within a few days the wart was gone. I was so impressed and happy!

-Submitted by Caroline Rood
Toledo, Ohio (July 2004)

BLEND—5 cypress, 10 lemon, 2 Tbs. apple cider vinegar, AD&E tincture. Apply twice daily and bandage. Keep a bandage on it until wart is gone.

TINCTURES—AD&E.

GENITAL—Frankincense (excellent for more stubborn warts), hyssop, melaleuca, oregano, Thieves, thyme. Dilute 1-2 drops of oil in a few drops of V-6 Mixing Oil and apply on location.

PLANTAR—Oregano.

In late October of last year, Cathy brought her 15 year old daughter to see me for massage therapy. Amanda was dealing with a huge plantar's wart grown deep into the ball of her foot. She was dealing with a great deal of pain with every step, and Cathy was planning to make an appointment for her to see a medical doctor. Cathy also suffered from these warts and had undergone months of treatment at her doctor's office having them repeatedly cut and burned with liquid nitrogen. She was also told you could never get rid of them. I suggested that Amanda rub essential oil of oregano on the infected area which Amanda did diligently each day, covering it with a bandage. They were amazed that the wart had completely disappeared in 6 weeks and has had no recurrence of the virus. Amanda's only complaint was she got tired of going to school every day smelling like a pizza.

-Submitted by Ellie Ayers (July 2004)

WASTE: *Refer to the chapter entitled, "Cleansing and Diets" in the Essential Oils Desk Reference for lots of information on cleansing.*

ELIMINATING—[F]Lavender (through lymphatic system).

SUPPLEMENTS—Cleansing Trio (ComforTone, Essentialzyme, and ICP). These cleansing products help eliminate toxic waste from the body.

WATER DISTILLATION: Add 3-5 drops of your favorite oil to the post-filter on your distille The oils will help increase the oxygen and frequency of the water. Try lemon, and peppermint.

WATER PURIFICATION: [F]Lemon, orange. H2Oils packets are wonderful for purifying and flavoring drinking water at the same time. Packets can be left in a container of water overnight to allow the oils to be effectively dispersed throughout the water. Try lemon, lemon/grapefruit, or lemon/orange.

REMOVE NITRATES—Peppermint.

ATER RETENTION: See EDEMA, DIURETIC, and HORMONAL IMBALANCE.

EAKNESS:

AFTER ILLNESS—Thyme (physical).

EALTH: Abundance, bergamot.

ATTRACTS—Cinnamon bark (aromatic).

MONEY—Ginger, patchouli.

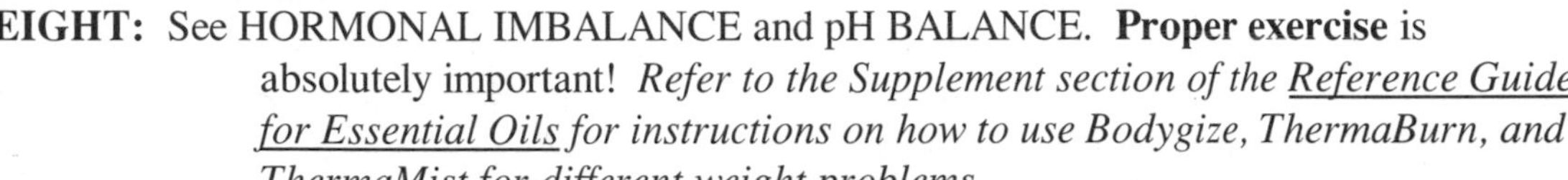

EIGHT: See HORMONAL IMBALANCE and pH BALANCE. **Proper exercise** is absolutely important! *Refer to the Supplement section of the Reference Guide for Essential Oils for instructions on how to use Bodygize, ThermaBurn, and ThermaMist for different weight problems.*

SUPPLEMENTS—Enzyme products: Allerzyme (aids the digestion of sugars, starches, fats, and proteins), Carbozyme (aids the digestion of carbohydrates), Detoxzyme (helps maintain and support a healthy intestinal environment), Fiberzyme (aids the digestion of fiber and enhances the absorption of nutrients), JuvaPower/JuvaSpice, Polyzyme (aids the digestion of protein and helps reduce swelling and discomfort), and Lipozyme (aids the digestion of fats). Body Balancing Trio (BodyBalance Mater Formula His/Her, VitaGreen), Cleansing Trio (ComforTone, Essentialzyme, and ICP).

> ***Weight gain** is often attributed to slow metabolism, lack of exercise, low fiber, poor diet, stress, enzyme deficiency, hormonal imbalance, low thyroid function, and poor digestion and assimilation. It can also result from too much insulin being produced by the body.*

CONTROL—EndoFlex (while taking Thyromin, a drop of EndoFlex under the tongue two or three times a day can help).

SUPPLEMENTS—Berrygize Nutrition Bars, Thyromin.

EMOTIONS—Excessive weight may be due to unresolved childhood emotions. Any or all of the following may help: Acceptance, Forgiveness, Inner Child, SARA (*Refer to the "Emotional Release" part of the Science and Application section or to the Blend section of the Reference Guide for Essential Oils for more information on each of these blends*).

WEIGHT LOSS—EndoFlex (on throat, under big toes), Joy, and Motivation.

BLEND #1—Put 5 lemon and 5 grapefruit in 1 gallon of water and drink during the day. Add more grapefruit to dissolve fat faster. This same thing can now be done easier and more effectively by using the H2Oils packet with lemon/grapefruit. Just leave the packet in a gallon of purified drinking water overnight and the oils will disperse throughout the water.

BLEND #2—4 lavender, 4 basil, 3 juniper, 8 grapefruit, 5 cypress. Mix and apply t feet, on location, as a body massage, or use in bath. Blend is used to emulsify fat.

MASSAGE OILS—Massage whole body with Cel-Lite Magic after showering.

PERSONAL CARE—If the weight problem is related to a hormonal imbalance, Prenolone/Prenolone+ / Progessence combined with Thyromin and EndoFlex may help.

SUPPLEMENTS—Use Bodygize (helps to be at ideal weight) to replace breakfast a dinner, ComforTone, ICP, and Essentialzyme to promote proper elimination o waste material from the bowels, ThermaBurn or ThermaMist to naturally suppress the appetite and regulate the metabolism, and Thyromin to ensure proper thyroid function. Eat a normal meal at lunch, but watch fat intake. Other products that may help are AlkaLime (improves digestion), Berrygize Nutrition Bars, JuvaPower/JuvaSpice, Power Meal, Sulfurzyme, Ultra Young (may help improve fat-to-lean ratios), and WheyFit (high quality, lactose-free proteins from three different sources). Master Formula His/Hers is also important to use.

UNDERWEIGHT—Drink Bodygize with meals. Feed cells with Mineral Essence.

WELL BEING: Citrus Fresh, Idaho tansy, Release (emotional), rose, Transformation.

FEELING OF—Harmony, spearmint.

PROMOTES—Eucalyptus, geranium, lavender, lemon, lime.

SUPPLEMENTS—Cleansing Trio (ComforTone, Essentialzyme, and ICP).

WHIPLASH: See TRAUMA or SHOCK. Aroma Siez, basil, birch (bones), helichrysum (bruising), hyssop (inflammation), juniper, lemongrass (strained ligaments), marjoram (muscles), PanAway, Relieve It, Roman chamomile, spruce, wintergreen (bones).

SUPPLEMENTS—ArthroTune, Sulfurzyme, Super C / Super C Chewable.

****COMMENTS—Remember to think through every physical aspect of the injury (ie. muscle damage, nerve damage, inflammation, ligament strain, bone injury, fever, and emotions). Select oils for each area of concern.*

WHOLENESS: Ones own spirituality and oneness with the Creator. Apply each of the follow blends, one right after the other: Awaken over the heart and on the forehead, Sacred Mountain on the crown of the head and over the thymus, and White Angelica on the shoulders. Then rub hands together, cup over nose and mouth and breathe deeply to inhale the aroma of all three blends together.

'HOOPING COUGH: See CHILDHOOD DISEASES. Cinnamon bark, Clary cage, cypress, grapefruit, hyssop, lavender, [F]oregano. Apply on chest, throat, and Vita Flex points. Use a hot compress for deeper penetration.

DIFFUSE—Basil, eucalyptus, lavender, melaleuca, peppermint, Roman chamomile, rose, thyme.

'ITHDRAWAL: See ADDICTIONS.

'ORKAHOLIC: Basil, geranium, lavender, marjoram. Rub a couple drops between hands, cup over nose and mouth and breathe deeply. Can also be diffused.

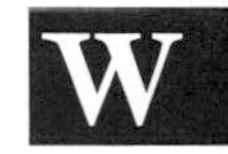

'ORMS: See RINGWORM or PARASITES. Bergamot, Di-Tone (helps expel intestinal worms), lavender, melaleuca, peppermint, Roman chamomile, rosemary verbenon, thyme. For intestinal worms, apply a few drops over abdomen with a hot compress or add to V-6 Mixing Oil (½ to 1 oz.) and use as a retention enema for 15 minutes or more. Can also apply on intestine and colon Vita Flex points on the feet.

BLEND—Mix 6 drops Roman chamomile, 6 eucalyptus, 6 lavender, and 6 lemon with 2 Tbs. V-6 Mixing Oil. Apply 10-15 drops of blend over abdomen with a hot compress and on intestine and colon Vita Flex points on the feet.

SUPPLEMENTS—Cleansing Trio (ComforTone, Essentialzyme, and ICP), ParaFree.

'ORRY: Bergamot. Diffuse.

'OUNDS: Bergamot, cajeput, [F]clove (infected wounds), cypress, elemi (infected), eucalyptus, frankincense, galbanum, geranium, juniper, lavender (combine with any of these other oils), melaleuca (Tea Tree), myrrh, onycha (benzoin), peppermint (when wound has closed, will soothe, cool, and reduce inflammation), Roman chamomile (add to Rose Ointment for an excellent first aid salve), rose, rosemary, rosewood, thyme, tsuga.

One Sunday morning I tripped and rammed my foot into a dirty pair of grass clippers, cutting my 4th toe at the base where it joins my foot. I washed it out as best I could with hydrogen peroxide, and then applied lavender oil and a bandage, and went on to church. When I came home, I kept my foot elevated and applied more lavender oil throughout the day. My friend looked at my wound and commented that it wasn't just a gash, it was punctured. That evening I also applied clove oil, along with the lavender oil. I slept with it unbandaged, and then bandaged it during the day while I was at work. I applied the oils morning and night. I had no infection, and by the following Sunday evening, it was almost totally healed. My friend who looked at it again was amazed, and she's an EMT!

-Submitted by C. Ness
Rapid City, South Dakota (July 2004)

BLEND #1—Lavender with Purification or Melrose.

RECIPE #1—First, 1-3 drops of helichrysum on the fresh wound will help stop the bleeding and a drop of clove will help with pain. Once bleeding is stopped, a drop of lavender (to help start the healing), a drop of Melrose (to help fight infection), and a drop of lemongrass (for possible ligament damage) can be applied. Other oils such birch/wintergreen, thyme, or sage may also be applie depending on the extent of the injury. Rose Ointment can then be applied to he seal the wound and extend the effectiveness of the applied oils, and then cover all with a bandage. When changing the bandage, myrrh, onycha, or patchouli can be applied to help promote further healing. Thieves or Purification may b necessary to help fight any occurrence of infection.

PERSONAL CARE—Rose Ointment (seals and protects).

SUPPLEMENTS—Stevia extract (apply on closed wound to help reduce scarring).

CHILDREN (and INFANTS)—Lavender and/or Roman chamomile. Helichrysum and peppermint are best diluted with lavender or Rose Ointment first to help minimize stinging effect on open wounds.

BLEND #2—(for Bruises or Wounds) 1-3 drops each of helichrysum and lavender diluted in 1/8 oz. V-6 Mixing Oil or Massage Oil Base.

BLEEDING—Rose, helichrysum, lemon, lavender.

BLEND #3—Equal amounts of Roman chamomile, geranium, and lemon. Can alternate with cypress, hyssop, palmarosa, and rose. Apply directly with a compress 2-3 times a day for 3-4 days then reduce to once a day until healed.

DISINFECT—Hyssop, Idaho tansy, lavender, melaleuca, Mountain savory, thyme (thymol and linalol). Apply 1-2 drops directly on wound.

HEALING—See SCARRING. Helichrysum, Idaho tansy, lavender, melaleuca (pus-filled wounds), myrrh, neroli, onycha (benzoin),

My husband, Tom, was taking apart a rabbit cage and the roof with the nails poking through fell on his hand and punctured it. Blood was dripping everywhere and he was becoming sick with pain and weakness. He applied pressure to the wounds but it still bled until I applied lavender and Pan Away. Before our very eyes it immediately stopped bleeding. It did swell up, but he kept applying lavender and Pan Away and it would take away the pain and bring the swelling down. It was healed in a matter of three days without a trip to the doctor. We feel so blessed to have oils on hand to treat emergencies like this one.

-Submitted by Diana Wolford
Olive Branch, Mississippi (July 2004)

*Dr. Marcy Foley maintains that "Each person will have a unique picture which created their healing challenges, and will require that each of these areas be addressed for a complete healing to take place." This is especially true for surface **wounds** where each aspect of the trauma must be considered. For example, there may also be damage to muscles, nerves, ligaments, or bones; there may be infection or inflammation; and there may be an emotion or even fever to deal with. Oils should be considered for each of these different areas as well.*

patchouli, ravensara, sandalwood, tsuga, yarrow. Apply directly on wound followed by Rose Ointment.

INFLAMMATION—German chamomile (helps reduce).

SURGICAL—Melrose, peppermint (cooling and soothing), Purification, Thieves.

BLEND #4—3 helichrysum, 3 frankincense, 4 lavender in 2 tsp. V-6 Mixing Oil. Reapply a few drops of blend when changing bandages.

WEEPING—Juniper, myrrh, patchouli, tarragon.

BLEND #5—5 drops Roman chamomile, 10 lavender, 3 tarragon, and 2 oz. V-6 Mixing Oil. Apply as a hot compress.

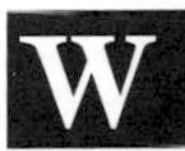
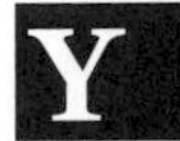
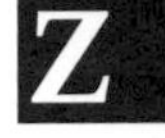

WRINKLES: Carrot, cistus, Clary sage, cypress, elemi, fennel, frankincense, galbanum, geranium, helichrysum, lavender, lemon, myrrh, neroli, orange, oregano, patchouli, rose, rosemary, rosewood, sandalwood, spikenard, thyme, ylang ylang.

> ***Wrinkles*** *occur as we mature and as we lose oxygen to the tissues. Essential oils oxygenate the tissues and thereby slow down the premature aging of the skin.*

AFTERSHAVE—Awaken can be used instead of aftershave lotion. KidScents Lotion works well to rehydrate the skin after shaving.

BLEND #1—3 lavender, 4 geranium, 2 patchouli, 6 rosewood, and 1 oz. V-6 Mixing Oil. Rub on wrinkles in an upward, lifting motion.

BLEND #2—1 frankincense, 1 lavender, and 1 lemon. It's like magic for wrinkles. Rub on morning and night around the eyes.

BLEND #3—5-10 drops frankincense added to Sandalwood Moisture Creme.

BLEND #4—Equal amounts of sandalwood, helichrysum, geranium, lavender, and frankincense. Combine with either Genesis Hand & Body Lotion or Satin Hand & Body Lotion and apply.

PERSONAL CARE—Rose Ointment, Sandalwood Moisture Creme, Satin Hand & Body Lotion.

SUPPLEMENTS—Essentialzyme, PD 80/20, Prenolone/Prenolone+, Progessence, Thyromin (thyroid function affects the skin), Ultra Young.

PREVENT—Gentle Baby and patchouli (prevents and retards).

PERSONAL CARE—Boswellia Wrinkle Creme (collagen builder), Satin Facial Scrub - Mint, NeuroGen (helps moisturize deep tissues), Wolfberry Eye Creme. The following three items can be used together to help tone the skin and prevent wrinkles: Orange Blossom Facial Wash, Sandalwood Toner, Sandalwood Moisture Creme.

SMOOTH—Add 2 drops frankincense to a little Genesis Hand & Body Lotion or Satin Hand & Body Lotion and apply.

PERSONAL CARE—Boswellia Wrinkle Creme (collagen builder).

YEAST: See CANDIDA.

YIN and YANG: Ylang ylang (balances)

YOGA: Cedarwood, sandalwood, spruce, tsuga.

ZEST (for life): En-R-Gee, Motivation, nutmeg, Legacy, Live with Passion. Diffuse.

Peace & Calming Saves the Day

My husband works at an elementary school as a LAN technician. Last spring the secretaries union went on strike for 2 weeks. All the other unions in the school district, in a show of support for the secretaries, forbade any of their members helping out with the secretarial duties. That left 3 people in my husband's school (my husband included) who were not union and able to attempt to keep the school running normally. After his first day of secretarial duties he took in a travel diffuser soaked in Peace & Calming, to help calm the kids who were sent to the office because they were trouble makers in their classes as well as to keep himself calm. He still is not sure who the Peace & Calming helped more (him or the kids), but the rest of the 2 weeks were less stressful thanks to the Peace & Calming.

-Submitted by A. Cornn, Machesney Park, Illinois (July 2004)

Appendix

Body System Chart

The following chart lists all of the products discussed within this book and indicates which body systems they primarily affect. While this chart does not include every system that could possibly be affected by each product, it attempts to list the primary systems that are most often affected. It is provided to give the beginning aromatherapy student a starting point for personal use and analysis.

Essential Oil	Cardiovascular System	Digestive System	Emotional Balance	Hormonal System	Immune System	Muscles and Bones	Nervous System	Respiratory System	Skin and Hair
Wise Men			X						
Abundance			X		X			X	
Acceptance			X				X		
AD&E					X		X		X
Agave				X		X			
AlkaLime	X	X				X			
Allerzyme		X						X	
AminoTech						X			
Angelica			X				X		
Animal Scents Products									X
Anise	X	X		X				X	
Aroma Life	X								
Aroma Siez						X		X	
AromaGuard Deodorants									X
ArthroTune						X			
Australian Blue			X						
Awaken			X						
Basil	X					X			
Be-Fit						X			
Believe			X						
Bergamot		X	X						X
Berry Young Juice					X				

Essential Oil	Cardiovascular System	Digestive System	Emotional Balance	Hormonal System	Immune System	Muscles and Bones	Nervous System	Respiratory System	Skin an Hair
Berrygize Bars		X			X	X			
Birch						X			
BLM						X			
Bodygize		X			X	X			
Boswellia Wrinkle Creme									X
Brain Power			X				X		
Cajeput	X							X	
Carbozyme		X							
Cardamom		X							
CardiaCare	X								
Carrot	X						X		X
Cedar, Canadian Red			X					X	X
Cedar, Western Red									X
Cedarwood							X	X	
Cel-Lite Magic									X
Celery Seed		X				X	X		
Chamomile, German			X				X		X
Chamomile, Roman			X				X		X
Chelex					X				
Chivalry			x						
Christmas Spirit	X		X				X		
Cinnamint Lip Balm									X
Cinnamon Bark					X				
Cistus					X				X
Citronella						X			X
Citrus Fresh			X		X				
ClaraDerm									X
Clarity			X				X		
Clary Sage				X					
Clove	X	X			X			X	
ComforTone		X			X				
Coral Sea						X			
Coriander		X		X					
CortiStop				X					
Cumin		X			X				

ssential Oil	Cardiovascular System	Digestive System	Emotional Balance	Hormonal System	Immune System	Muscles and Bones	Nervous System	Respiratory System	Skin and Hair
ress	X					X			
ress, Blue		X			X				
vana				X					
oxzyme		X			X				
Tone		X							
		X							
agon Time			X	X					
eam Catcher			X						
mi									X
R-Gee			X				X		
doFlex				X					
vision			X						
ential nna		X			X	X			
ential egas	X						X		X
entialzyme		X							
ro				X					
calyptus						X		X	
calyptus iodora								X	
calyptus iata								X	X
ening Peace									X
ergreen ence			X						
odus					X				
odus II					X				
niGen				X					
nnel		X		X					
erzyme		X							
								X	
, Balsam						X	X		
, Douglas						X		X	
, White			X			X		X	
abane onyza)	X			X					
rgiveness			X						
ankincense			X		X		X		X
lbanum					X				
thering			X						

Essential Oil	Cardiovascular System	Digestive System	Emotional Balance	Hormonal System	Immune System	Muscles and Bones	Nervous System	Respiratory System	Skin Ha
Genesis Lotion									X
Gentle Baby			X						X
Geranium			X						X
Ginger		X					X		
Goldenrod	X			X					
Grapefruit	X								
Gratitude			X						
Grounding			X						
Harmony			X						
Helichrysum	X					X			
Highest Potential			X						
Hope			X						
HRT	X								
Humility			X						
Hyssop	X						X	X	
ICP	X	X							
ImmuGel					X			X	
ImmuneTune					X				
ImmuPower					X				
ImmuPro					X				
Inner Child			X						
Inspiration			X						
Into the Future			X						
Jasmine			X	X					
Joy			X						
Juniper		X	X				X		X
Juva Cleanse		X							
JuvaFlex		X							
JuvaPower		X							
JuvaSpice		X							
JuvaTone		X			X				
K&B		X							
KidScents MightyZyme		X							
Lady Sclareol			X						X
Laurel		X			X			X	
LavaDerm Cooling Mist			X						X
Lavandin	X					X		X	
Lavender	X		X				X		X

Essential Oil	Cardiovascular System	Digestive System	Emotional Balance	Hormonal System	Immune System	Muscles and Bones	Nervous System	Respiratory System	Skin and Hair
edum		X			X				X
egacy			X						
emon		X			X			X	
emongrass					X	X			
ime		X			X			X	
ipozyme		X							
ive with assion			X				X		
ongevity	X		X						
ongevity apsules	X								
-Grain						X	X		
agnify Your urpose			X				X		
andarin		X							X
arjoram	X					X			
aster ormula	X		X		X		X		
egaCal	X					X	X		
elaleuca					X	X		X	X
elaleuca ricifolia								X	X
elaleuca uinquenrvia						X		X	
elissa			X						X
elrose								X	X
ineral ssence	X		X	X	X	X	X		
ister				X					
orning Start			X						X
otivation			X				X		
ountain avory					X				
yrrh				X	X		X		X
yrtle		X		X		X		X	
eroli		X							X
euroGen				X		X	X		
utmeg				X	X		X		
nycha	X		X						X
range		X	X		X				X
range lossom Facial Vash									X

Essential Oil	Cardiovascular System	Digestive System	Emotional Balance	Hormonal System	Immune System	Muscles and Bones	Nervous System	Respiratory System	Skin a Hai
Oregano					X	X		X	
Ortho Ease						X			
Ortho Sport						X			
Palmarosa	X		X						X
PanAway						X	X		
ParaFree		X			X				
Patchouli									X
PD 80/20			X	X		X			
Peace & Calming			X				X		
Pepper, Black		X					X		
Peppermint		X				X	X	X	X
Petitgrain			X						
Pine			X					X	
Polyzyme		X				X			
Power Meal	X	X			X	X			
Prenolone			X	X		X	X		X
Present Time			X						
ProGen				X					
Progessence			X	X		X	X		X
Protec				X					
Purification		X	X						X
Raven								X	X
Ravensara					X			X	
RC								X	
Regenolone				X		X	X		X
Rehemogen	X	X							
Relaxation			X			X			X
Release			X						
Relieve It						X			
Rose			X						X
Rose Ointment									X
Rosemary camphor	X	X				X			
Rosemary cineol					X		X	X	
Rosemary verbanon		X		X					X
Rosewood									X
Royaldophilus		X			X				

sential Oil	Cardiovascular System	Digestive System	Emotional Balance	Hormonal System	Immune System	Muscles and Bones	Nervous System	Respiratory System	Skin and Hair
red untain			X						
e				X	X				
e Lavender			X	X		X	X	X	X
dalwood			X			X	X		X
dalwood isture me									X
dalwood ter									X
RA			X						
n Hand & y Lotion									X
n Facial ubs									X
rEssence		X		X					
sation ion									X
sation Oil nd			X	X					
armint		X	X						
kenard			X						X
uce			X				X	X	
via & Stevia ect	X	X			X				
furzyme					X	X	X		X
sation tan Oil									X
er B	X					X	X		
er C					X			X	
er C ewable					X	X			
er Cal	X		X			X	X		
render			X				X		
gerine			X		X				X
sy, Blue							X		
sy, Idaho					X				
ragon		X					X		
rmaBurn						X			
rmaMist		X				X			
eves					X				
eves aning Prod					X				

Essential Oil	Cardiovascular System	Digestive System	Emotional Balance	Hormonal System	Immune System	Muscles and Bones	Nervous System	Respiratory System	Skin Ha
Thieves Lozenges					X				
Thyme					X	X			
Thyme linalol								X	X
Thyromin				X					
Transformation			X						
Trauma Life			X						
Tsuga	X							X	
Ultra Young				X	X				
Valerian							X		
Valor			X			X	X		X
Vetiver			X	X			X		X
VitaGreen	X	X			X	X	X		
WheyFit						X			
White Angelica			X						
White Lotus					X				
Wintergreen						X			
Wolfberry Bar		X			X	X			
Wolfberry Crisp Bars		X			X	X			
Wolfberry Eye Creme									X
Yarrow				X	X				X
Ylang Ylang	X		X	X					

Single Oil Property Chart

The following chart presents some of the properties of each of the single oils. An attempt ; been made to indicate the effectiveness of the oils for each property, where supporting ɔrmation existed. However, this information should not be considered conclusive. It is provided give the beginning aromatherapy student a starting point for personal use and analysis. Also, ·p in mind the applicable safety data when applying an oil for its property. For example, namon bark is one of the best known antiseptics, but it is also extremely irritating to the skin. It y work well to sanitize the bathroom with, but should be used with extreme caution on the skin.

ssential Oil	A-Bac	A-Cat	A-Dep	A-Fun	A-Inf	A-Infl	A-Mic	A-Par	A-Rhe	A-Sep	A-Spa	A-Vir	Analg	Imm
gelica		+										+		
sil	++	+	+		+	+++				+	+	+		
·gamot					+	+++		+		+	+		+	
ch						++			++	+	+++		++	
ieput	+	+			+					+	+		+	
·rdamom										+	+			
dar, nadian Red	+		+							+				
darwood				+	+					+				
amomile, rman	+		+		+	+++				+	+		++	
amomile, man	+					++		+++			+++		+	
namon ·k	+		+	+	+	+	++	+		++++	+	+		
tus							+			+				+
ronella	+			+		+				+++	+			
ry Sage	+		+		+					+	+			
ve	+++	+		++	+			++	+	+		+++		
riander	++		++		++			+			+		+	
min	+							+		+	++	+		+
press	+				+			+	+	+	+			
vana					++									
l	+	+									+			
mi		++	++		+					+				
calyptus	++	++++			+	+		+	++	+	++	+++	++	
calyptus, ·iodora	++	++		+	++					+		++		
calyptus, liata	++	++			+	+						+++	++	+
nnel	+	++				+	+	+		+	+			
		+								++			+	

Essential Oil	A-Bac	A-Cat	A-Dep	A-Fun	A-Inf	A-Infl	A-Mic	A-Par	A-Rhe	A-Sep	A-Spa	A-Vir	Analg	I
Frankincense		++	++				+				+			+
Galbanum		+			+	+	+			+	+	++	++	
Geranium	+++		++	++	+	+				+				
Ginger		++								++			++	
Grapefruit	++									++				
Helichrysum	++	+++		+		++	++			+	+++			
Hyssop	++	++++			+	++		+	+	+	+	+++		
Jasmine		+	++				++				+	+	+	
Juniper					+			+	++	+	+			
Laurel				+						+				
Lavender			++		+	++	+	+	+	+	++		++	
Lavandin	+			+		++				+++	++		++	
Lemon	++				+		++		+	+++	+			+
Lemongrass	+		+	+		++	+			+			++	
Lime	++									++		+		
Mandarin				+						++	+			
Marjoram	+	+		+	+					++	++	+	++	
Melaleuca	+++			++++	+	+		+		+		+++		+
Melaleuca Ericifolia	+			+	+		+++							
Melaleuca Quinquenrvia	+++			++++		+				+		+++		
Melissa	+		++				+				++	++		
Mountain Savory	+++	+		+	++		+++	++		+	+	++	++	+
Myrrh		+		+	+	+++	++	+		+		+++		
Myrtle	+	+++			+					+				
Neroli	+		++		+			+		++	++	+		
Nutmeg						+		+		+				
Orange	++		++	+		+				++				
Oregano	+++	+		+++	+++			+++	++	+	+	++	++	+
Palmarosa	+			+			+			+		+		
Patchouli	+		+	+	+	+	+			+		+		
Pepper, Black	+						+			+	+		++	
Peppermint	+	+		+	+	++	+			+	+	+	++	
Petitgrain	+				++	++				+	++			
Pine	+	+		+	++		+			+		+	+	
Ravensara	+	+++		+	+					++		++++		
Rose			++		++	+								
Rosemary	+	+++		+	+		++	+	++	+	+	+	++	
Rosewood	+++		+	++	+		+	+		+	+	++	+	+

ssential Oil	A-Bac	A-Cat	A-Dep	A-Fun	A-Inf	A-Infl	A-Mic	A-Par	A-Rhe	A-Sep	A-Spa	A-Vir	Analg	Imm
ge	+	+	+	++	+	+	++			+	+	+++		
udalwood	+	+++	++	+						++	+			
earmint	+			++		++				+	+			
ikenard	+			+	++	++		++			++			
ruce		+			+	+++	+		+	+				+
ngerine														
rragon	++				++	++		+		+	++	++		
yme	+	+		+++			++	+	++		+	+		++
lerian	+										++			
tiver					+					+	+			+
aho Tansy	++				++	++					+	++		+
arrow						++				++				
ang Ylang			+		+					+	+			

ossary

Bac (Anti-bacterial): an agent which prevents the growth of, or destroys, bacteria.

Cat (Anti-catarrhal): an agent which helps remove excess catarrh from the body. Expectorants help promote the removal of mucus from the respiratory system.

Dep (Anti-depressant): an agent which helps alleviate depression.

Fun (Anti-fungal): an agent which prevents and combats fungal infection.

Inf (Anti-infectious): an agent which prevents and combats the spread of germs.

Infl (Anti-inflammatory): an agent which alleviates inflammation.

Mic (Antimicrobial): an agent which resists or destroys pathogenic micro-organisms.

Par (Anti-parasitic): an agent which prevents and destroys parasites.

Rhe (Anti-rheumatic): helps prevent and relievé rheumatism.

Sep (Antiseptic): destroys and prevents the development of microbes.

Spa (Antispasmodic): prevents and eases spasms or convulsions.

Vir (Antiviral): a substance which inhibits the growth of a virus.

alg (Analgesic): a substance which relieves pain.

m (Immune-stimulant): an agent which stimulates the natural defense mechanism of the body.

Single Oil Summary Information

The following chart displays summary information about each of the single oils, including botanical name, safety data, and the products (blends, personal care products, bath and shower gels, tinctures, massage oils, and supplements) that contain the single oil. The safety data includ possible skin reactions and conditions during which use of that particular oil should be limited o completely avoided (refer to the legend following the Blend Summary Information). **Note:** This safety data is provided for **EXTERNAL USE ONLY! Essential oils should never be taken internally** unless specifically instructed by a professional aromatherapist.

Single Oil Name	Botanical Name	Safety Data	Products containing Single Oi
Angelica	*Angelica archangelica* (Umbelliferae)	(GRAS), D, P, PH Dilute 1:1	Awaken, Forgiveness, Grounding, Harmony, Legacy, Live with Passion, Surrender
Anise	*Pimpinella anisum* (Umbelliferae)	(GRAS), CS Dilute 1:1	Awaken, Di-Tone, Dream Catcher, Allerzyme, Carbozyme, ComforTone, Detoxzyme, Essentialzyme, Fiberzyme, ICP, JuvaPower, JuvaSpice, Lipozyme, ParaFree, Polyzyme, Power Meal
Basil	*Ocimum basilicum* (Labiatae)	(GRAS), E*, P*, SI, Dilute 1:1	Aroma Siez, Clarity, Legacy, M-Grain, ArthroTune
Bergamot	*Citrus bergamia* (Rutaceae)	(GRAS), CS*, PH* Dilute 1:1	Awaken, Chivalry, Clarity, Dream Catcher, Forgiveness, Gentle Baby, Harmony, Joy, Joy Aqua Essence, Legac White Angelica, Genesis Hand and Bod Lotion, Prenolone, Prenolone+, Progessence, Rosewood Moisturizing Shampoo, Rosewood Moisturizing Conditioner, Sandalwood Moisture Creme, Sandalwood Toner, Dragon Tim Bath Gel, Evening Peace Bath Gel
Birch	*Betula alleghaniensis* (Betulaceae)	E*, P* Dilute 1:1	
Black Cumin	*Nigella sativa*		ParaFree
Buplevere	*Bupleurum fruticosum*		Legacy
Cajeput	*Melaleuca leucadendra* (Myrtaceae)	(FA/FL), SI Dilute 1:1	Legacy
Calamus	*Acorus calamus (Araceae)*	Dilute 1:4	Exodus II
Cardamom	*Elettaria cardamomum* (Zingiberaceae)	(GRAS) Dilute 1:1	Clarity, Legacy, Transformation

Single Oil Name	Botanical Name	Safety Data	Products containing Single Oil
rrot	*Daucus carota* (Umbelliferae)	(GRAS) Dilute 1:1	Legacy, Animal Scents Pet Ointment, Rose Ointment
ssia	*Cinnamomum cassia* (Lauraceae)	(GRAS), CS*, SI*, Dilute 1:4	Exodus II
dar	*Cedrus canadensis* (Cupressaceae)		Evergreen Essence
dar, Canadian Red	*Thuja plicata* (Cupressaceae)	CS Dilute 1:1	Legacy
dar, Western Red	*Thuja plicata* (Cupressaceae)	Dilute 1:1	Red Cedar Essential Water, KidScents Lotion
dar Leaf	*Thuja occidentalis* (Cupressaceae)	Dilute 1:1	Legacy
darwood	*Cedrus atlantica* (Pinaceae)	P	Australian Blue, Brain Power, Grounding, Inspiration, Into the Future, Legacy, Live with Passion, Sacred Mountain, SARA, AromaGuard Deodorants, KidScents Bath Gel, KidScents Lotion, Sacred Mountain Aqua Essence, Sacred Mountain Bar Soap, Peppermint Cedarwood Bar Soap, Cel-Lite Magic Massage Oil
lery Seed	*Apium graveolens* (Umbeliferae)	(GRAS), CS, SI, P, Dilute 1:1	Juva Cleanse
amomile erman/Blue)	*Matricaria chamomilla/recutita* (Compositae)	(GRAS), P, SI	EndoFlex, Legacy, Surrender, K&B Tincture, JuvaTone, ComforTone
amomile lixta)	*Chamaemelum mixtum* (Compositae)		
amomile oman)	*Chamaemelum nobile* (Compositae)	(GRAS), SI	Clarity, Forgiveness, Gentle Baby, Harmony, Joy, Joy Aqua Essence, JuvaFlex, Legacy, M-Grain, Motivation, Surrender, ClaraDerm, Genesis Hand and Body Lotion, KidScents Tender Tush, Lemon Sage Clarifying Shampoo, Lemon Sage Clarifying Conditioner, Sandalwood Toner, Satin Hand & Body Lotion, Wolfberry Eye Creme, Dragon Time Bath Gel, Evening Peace Bath Gel, Chelex Tincture, K&B Tincture, Rehemogen Tincture

Single Oil Name	Botanical Name	Safety Data	Products containing Single Oi
Cinnamon Bark	*Cinnamomum verum* (Lauraceae)	CS*, P*, SI* Dilute 1:4	Christmas Spirit, Exodus II, Gathering, Legacy, Magnify Your Purpose, Thieves Cinnamint Lip Balm, Thieves Bar Soap ImmuGel, Mineral Essence, Wolfberry Bar
Cistus	*Cistus ladanifer* (Cistaceae)	(FA/FL), P	ImmuPower, Legacy, ImmuneTune, KidScents Tender Tush
Citronella	*Cymbopogon nardus* (Gramineae)	(GRAS), CS*, P, SI, Dilute 1:1	Legacy, Purification, Sunsation Suntan Oil, Animal Scents Pet Shampoo
Citrus Hystrix (Combava)	*Citrus hystrix* (Rutacae)	PH*, Dilute 1:1	Trauma Life
Clary Sage	*Salvia sclarea* (Labiatae)	(GRAS), A, P Dilute 1:1	Dragon Time, Into the Future, Lady Sclareol, Legacy, Live with Passion, SclarEssence, Transformation, Lavende Volume Shampoo, Lavender Volume Conditioner, Prenolone, Prenolone+, Progessence Cream, Rosewood Moisturizing Shampoo, Rosewood Moisturizing Conditioner, Dragon Time Bath Gel, Evening Peace Bath Gel, Estr Tincture, Cel-Lite Magic Massage Oil, Dragon Time Massage Oil, CortiStop (Women's), FemiGen
Clove	*Syzygium aromaticum* (Myrtaceae)	(GRAS), CS*, P, SI Dilute 1:4	Abundance, En-R-Gee, ImmuPower, Legacy, Longevity, Melrose, PanAway, Thieves, AromaGuard Deodorants, Dentarome Plus Toothpaste, KidScents Toothpaste, Thieves Bar Soap, K&B Tincture, BLM, Essential Omegas, ImmuGel, Longevity Capsules, Essentialzyme, ParaFree
Coriander	*Coriandrum sativum* L. (Umbelliferae)	(GRAS), ST Dilute 1:1	Legacy
Cumin	*Cuminus cyminum* (Umbelliferae)	(GRAS), P, PH* Dilute 1:1	ImmuPower, Legacy, Detoxzyme, Prote
Cypress	*Cupressus sempervirens* (Cupressaceae)	P Dilute 1:1	Aroma Life, Aroma Siez, Legacy, RC, HRT Tincture, Cel-Lite Magic Massage Oil, ArthroTune, Bodygize, Power Meal Super Cal
Cypress, Blue	*Callitris intratropica* (Cupressaceae)		Australian Blue, Brain Power, AromaGuard Deodorants
Davana	*Artemisia pallens* (Compositae)	(FA/FL), P Dilute 1:1	Trauma Life

ingle Oil Name	Botanical Name	Safety Data	Products containing Single Oil
	Anethum graveolens (Umbellifcrac)	(GRAS), E Dilute 1:1	Legacy
mi	*Canarium luzonicum* (Burseraceae)	(FA/FL)	Legacy, Ortho Sport Massage Oil
calyptus	*Eucalyptus globulus* (Myrtaceae)	(FA/FL) Dilute 1:1	Legacy, RC, Fresh Essence Mouthwash, Chelex Tincture, Ortho Sport Massage Oil
calyptus riodora	*Eucalyptus citriodora* (Myrtaceae)	CS Dilute 1:1	Legacy, RC
calyptus Dives	*Eucalyptus dives* (Myrtaceae)	Dilute 1:1	Legacy
calyptus Polybractea	*Eucalyptus polybractea* (Myrtaceae)	Dilute 1:1	Legacy
calyptus Radiata	*Eucalyptus radiata* (Myrtaceae)	Dilute 1:1	Legacy, Raven, RC, Thieves, Thieves Bar Soap
nel	*Foeniculum vulgare* (Umbelliferae)	(GRAS), CS, E, P Dilute 1:1	Di-Tone, Dragon Time, JuvaFlex, Legacy, Mister, SclarEssence, Allerzyme, Carbozyme, Detoxzyme, Essentialzyme, Fiberzyme, JuvaPower, JuvaSpice, Lipozyme, Prenolone, Prenolone+, Progessence Cream, Dragon Time Bath Gel, Estro Tincture, K&B Tincture, Dragon Time Massage Oil, CortiStop (Women's), FemiGen, ICP, ParaFree, Power Meal, ProGen
	Abies alba (Pinaceae)	(FA/FL), SI Dilute 1:1	En-R-Gee, Grounding, Into the Future, ArthroTune, ImmuneTune
, Balsam aho Balsam Fir)	*Abies balsamea* (Pinaceae)	(FA/FL), SI Dilute 1:1	Legacy, Sacred Mountain, Transformation, Sacred Mountain Aqua Essence, Animal Scents Pet Ointment, Sacred Mountain Bar Soap, BLM
, Douglas	*Pseudotsuga menziesii* (Pinaceae)	SI Dilute 1:1	Legacy, Regenolone
, Red	*Abies magnifica* (Pinaceae)	SI Dilute 1:1	Evergreen Essence, Legacy
, White	*Abies grandis* (Pinaceae)	SI Dilute 1:1	Australian Blue, Believe, Evergreen Essence, Gratitude, Legacy, Mountain Essence Essential Water
abane	*Conyza canadensis* (Compositae)	Dilute 1:1	Legacy, CortiStop (Men's and Women's), Progessence Cream, ThermaBurn, Ultra Young, Ultra Young Plus

Single Oil Name	Botanical Name	Safety Data	Products containing Single O
Frankincense	*Boswellia carteri* (Burseraceae)	(FA/FL)	Abundance, Acceptance, Believe, Brai Power, Exodus II, Forgiveness, Gatheri Gratitude, Harmony, Humility, ImmuPower, Inspiration, Into the Futur Legacy, Longevity, 3 Wise Men, Transformation, Trauma Life, Valor, Boswellia Wrinkle Creme, ClaraDerm, KidScents Tender Tush, Protec, Wolfb Eye Creme, Valor Bar Soap, Valor Aq Essence, CortiStop (Men's and Women's), Exodus, ThermaBurn
Galbanum	*Ferula gummosa* (Umbelliferae)	(FA/FL)	Exodus II, Gathering, Gratitude, Legac
Geranium	*Pelargonium graveolens* (Geraniaceae)	(GRAS), CS	Acceptance, Clarity, EndoFlex, Envisi Forgiveness, Gathering, Harmony, Humility, Joy, Joy Aqua Essence, JuvaFlex, Lady Sclareol, Legacy, Relea SARA, Trauma Life, White Angelica, Animal Scents Pet Ointment, AromaGuard Deodorants, Boswellia Wrinkle Creme, Genesis Hand and Bo Lotion, Lemon Sage Clarifying Shamp Lemon Sage Clarifying Conditioner, Prenolone, Prenolone+, Progessence Cream, Rosewood Moisturizing Shamp Rosewood Moisturizing Conditioner, Satin Hand & Body Lotion, Wolfberry Creme, Animal Scents Pet Shampoo, Dragon Time Bath Gel, Evening Peace Bath Gel, KidScents Bath Gel, KidSce Lotion, Melaleuca Geranium Bar Soap, K&B Tincture, JuvaTone
Geranium, Rose	*Pelargonium x asperum* (Geraniaceae)		Gentle Baby
Ginger	*Zingiber officinale* (Zingiberaceae)	(GRAS), CS, PH Dilute 1:1	Abundance, Di-Tone, Legacy, Live wit Passion, Magnify Your Purpose, Allerzyme, Carbozyme, ComforTone, Fiberzyme, ICP, Lipozyme
Goldenrod	*Solidago canadensis* (Asteraceae)	Dilute 1:1	Legacy
Grapefruit	*Citrus x paradisi* (Rutaceae)	(GRAS) Dilute 1:1	Citrus Fresh, Legacy, Cel-Lite Magic Massage Oil, Bodygize, Power Meal, Super C, ThermaMist

Single Oil Name	Botanical Name	Safety Data	Products containing Single Oil
lichrysum	*Helichrysum italicum* (Compositae)	(GRAS)	Aroma Life, Brain Power, Forgiveness, Juva Cleanse, JuvaFlex, Legacy, Live with Passion, M-Grain, PanAway, Trauma Life, ClaraDerm, Chelex Tincture, ArthroTune, CardiaCare
ssop	*Hyssopus officinalis* (Labiatae)	(GRAS), E*, HBP*, P*, D-1:1	Exodus II, Harmony, ImmuPower, Legacy, Relieve It, White Angelica, Exodus
mine	*Jasminum officinale* (Oleaceae)	(GRAS)	Clarity, Dragon Time, Forgiveness, Gentle Baby, Harmony, Highest Potential, Inner Child, Into the Future, Joy, Joy Aqua Essence, Lady Sclareol, Legacy, Live with Passion, Sensation, Genesis Hand & Body Lotion, Lavender Volume Shampoo, Lavender Volume Conditioner, Satin Hand & Body Lotion, Sensation Hand & Body Lotion, Dragon Time Bath Gel, Evening Peace Bath Gel, Sensation Bath Gel, Dragon Time Massage Oil, Sensation Massage Oil
iper	*Juniperus osteosperma* and/or *J. scopulorum* (Cupressaceae)	Dilute 1:1	Di-Tone, Dream Catcher, En-R-Gee, Grounding, Hope, Into the Future, Legacy, 3 Wise Men, Allerzyme, Carbozyme, Fiberzyme, Lipozyme, NeuroGen, Morning Start Bath Gel, Morning Start Bar Soap, K&B Tincture, Cel-Lite Magic Massage Oil, Ortho Ease Massage Oil, ArthroTune
urel	*Laurus nobilis* (Lauraceae)	(GRAS), CS, P* Dilute 1:1	Legacy, Exodus, ParaFree
vandin	*Lavandula x hybrida* (Labiatae)	(GRAS), E, P*	Purification, Release, Animal Scents Pet Shampoo
vender	*Lavandula angustifolia* CT linalol (Labiatae)		Aroma Siez, Brain Power, Dragon Time, Envision, Forgiveness, Gathering, Gentle Baby, Harmony, Legacy, M-Grain, Mister, Motivation, RC, SARA, Surrender, Trauma Life, AromaGuard Deodorants, ClaraDerm, LavaDerm Cooling Mist, Lavender Essential Water, Lavender Volume Shampoo, Lavender Volume Conditioner, KidScents Tender Tush, Orange Blossom Facial Wash, Sandalwood Moisture Creme, Sunsation Suntan Oil, Wolfberry Eye Creme, Dragon Time Bath Gel, Lavender Rosewood Bar Soap, Estro Tincture, Dragon Time Massage Oil, Relaxation Massage Oil, ProGen

Single Oil Name	Botanical Name	Safety Data	Products containing Single O
Ledum	*Ledum groenlandicum* (Ericaceae)		Juva Cleanse, Legacy
Lemon	*Citrus limon* (Rutaceae)	(GRAS), PH*, SI* Dilute 1:1	Citrus Fresh, Clarity, Forgiveness, Ger Baby, Harmony, Joy, Joy Aqua Essence Legacy, Raven, Surrender, Thieves, Transformation, AromaGuard Deodora Genesis Hand and Body Lotion, Anima Scents Pet Shampoo, KidScents Shamp Lavender Volume Shampoo, Lavender Volume Conditioner, Lemon Sage Clarifying Shampoo, Lemon Sage Clarifying Conditioner, Orange Blosso Facial Wash, Dragon Time Bath Gel, Evening Peace Bath Gel, Thieves Bar Soap, Lemon Sandalwood Bar Soap, H Tincture, AlkaLime, AminoTech, Berr Young Juice, Bodygize, CardiaCare, ImmuGel, ImmuneTune, JuvaTone, MegaCal, Mineral Essence, Power Me Super C, Super C Chewable, VitaGree WheyFit
Lemongrass	*Cymbopogon flexuosus* (Gramineae)	(GRAS), SI* Dilute 1:4	Di-Tone, En-R-Gee, Inner Child, Legac Purification, Allerzyme, Carbozyme, Fiberzyme, Lipozyme, NeuroGen, Sunsation Suntan Oil, Morning Start B Gel, Morning Start Bar Soap, Ortho Ea Massage Oil, Ortho Sport Massage Oil Be-Fit, Bodygize, ICP, VitaGreen
Lime	*Citrus aurantifolia* (Rutaceae)	(GRAS), PH* Dilute 1:1	Legacy, Lemon Sage Clarifying Shamp Lemon Sage Clarifying Conditioner, AlkaLime, AminoTech, KidScents Mig Vites, Super C
Mandarin	*Citrus reticulata* (Rutaceae)	(GRAS), PH Dilute 1:1	Citrus Fresh, Joy, Joy Aqua Essence, Legacy, Dragon Time Bath Gel, KidScents Mighty Vites, Super C
Marjoram	*Origanum majorana* (Labiatae)	(GRAS), P Dilute 1:1	Aroma Life, Aroma Siez, Legacy, M-Grain, RC, Ortho Ease Massage Oil, Ortho Sport Massage Oil, ArthroTune, CardiaCare, Super Cal
Melaleuca (Tea Tree)	*Melaleuca alternifolia* (Myrtaceae)	(FA/FL), CS Dilute 1:1	Legacy, Melrose, Purification, Animal Scents Pet Ointment, AromaGuard Deodorants, ClaraDerm, Rose Ointmen Sunsation Suntan Oil, Melaleuca Geranium Bar Soap, Rehemogen Tinct ParaFree

Single Oil Name	Botanical Name	Safety Data	Products containing Single Oil
Ielaleuca ericifolia Rosalina)	*Melaleuca ericifolia* (Myrtaceae)	(FA/FL) Dilute 1:1	Legacy, Melaleuca Geranium Bar Soap
Ielaleuca uinquenervia Niaouli)	*Melaleuca quinquenervia* (Myrtaceae)	(FA/FL), CS Dilute 1:1	Melrose, AromaGuard Deodorants
Ielissa	*Melissa officinalis* (Labiatae)	(GRAS)	Brain Power, Forgiveness, Hope, Humility, Legacy, Live with Passion, Melissa Essential Water, White Angelica, VitaGreen
Iountain Savory	*Satureja montana* (Labiatae)	(GRAS), P*, SI* Dilute 1:4	ImmuPower, Legacy, Surrender
Iugwort	*Artemisia vulgaris* (Asteraceae)	P* Dilute 1:1	
Iyrrh	*Commiphora myrrha* (Burseraceae)	(FA/FL), P	Abundance, Exodus II, Gratitude, Hope, Humility, Legacy, 3 Wise Men, White Angelica, Animal Scents Pet Ointment, Boswellia Wrinkle Creme, ClaraDerm, Protec, Rose Ointment, Sandalwood Moisture Creme, Sandalwood Toner, Thyromin
Iyrtle	*Myrtus communis* (Myrtaceae)	Dilute 1:1	EndoFlex, Inspiration, Legacy, Mister, Purification, RC, JuvaTone, ProGen, ThermaBurn, Thyromin
Iyrtle, Lemon	*Backhousia citriodora* (Myrtaceae)	CS, SI Dilute 1:4	
eroli	*Citrus aurantium bigaradia* (Rutaceae)	(GRAS) Dilute 1:1	Acceptance, Humility, Inner Child, Legacy, Live with Passion, Present Time
utmeg	*Myristica fragrans* (Myristicaceae)	(GRAS), E*, P Dilute 1:2	EndoFlex, En-R-Gee, Legacy, Magnify Your Purpose, Be-Fit, ParaFree, Power Meal, ThermaBurn
nycha	*Styrax benzoin* (Styracaceae)	(FA/FL)	
range	*Citrus sinensis* (Rutaceae)	(GRAS), PH* Dilute 1:1	Abundance, Christmas Spirit, Citrus Fresh, Envision, Harmony, Inner Child, Lady Sclareol, Legacy, Longevity, Peace & Calming, Peace & Calming Aqua Essence, SARA, Berry Young Juice, Bodygize, Essential Omegas, ImmuneTune, ImmuPro, Longevity Capsules, KidScents Mighty Vites, Power Meal, Super C, Wolfberry Bar

Single Oil Name	Botanical Name	Safety Data	Products containing Single Oil
Oregano	*Origanum compactum* (Labiatae)	(GRAS), SI* Dilute 1:4	ImmuPower, Legacy, Regenolone, Ortho Sport Massage Oil, ImmuGel
Palmarosa	*Cymbopogon martinii* (Gramineae)	(GRAS) Dilute 1:1	Clarity, Forgiveness, Gentle Baby, Harmony, Joy, Joy Aqua Essence, Legacy, Animal Scents Pet Ointment, Genesis Hand & Body Lotion, Rose Ointment, Dragon Time Bath Gel, Evening Peace Bath Gel
Patchouli	*Pogostemon cablin* (Labiatae)	(FA/FL)	Abundance, Di-Tone, Legacy, Live with Passion, Peace & Calming, Allerzyme, Carbozyme, Fiberzyme, Lipozyme, Peace & Calming Aqua Essence, Animal Scents Pet Ointment, Orange Blossom Facial Wash, Rose Ointment
Pepper, Black	*Piper nigrum* (Piperaceae)	(GRAS), SI* Dilute 1:1	Dream Catcher, En-R-Gee, Legacy, Relieve It, Cel-Lite Magic Massage Oil, ArthroTune
Peppermint	*Mentha piperita* (Labiatae)	(GRAS), CS, HBP, P Dilute 1:2	Aroma Siez, Clarity, Di-Tone, Legacy, M Grain, Mister, PanAway, Raven, RC, Relieve It, SclarEssence, Transformation, Allerzyme, Carbozyme, Cinnamint Lip Balm, Dentarome/ Dentarome Plus Toothpaste, Fiberzyme, Fresh Essence ar Fresh Essence Plus, Lipozyme, Mint Sat Facial Scrub, NeuroGen, Polyzyme, Regenolone, Satin Hand & Body Lotion, Morning Start Bath Gel, Peppermint Cedarwood Bar Soap, Peppermint Essential Water, Morning Start Bar Soap Ortho Ease Massage Oil, Ortho Sport Massage Oil, Relaxation Massage Oil, ComforTone, CortiStop (Men's and Women's), Essential Manna (Carob Min Flavor), Essentialzyme, Mineral Essence ProGen, ThermaMist, Thyromin
Petitgrain	*Citrus aurantium* (Rutaceae)	(GRAS) Dilute 1:1	Legacy
Pine	*Pinus sylvestris* (Pinaceae)	(FA/FL), SI Dilute 1:1	Evergreen Essence, Grounding, Legacy, RC, Lemon Sage Clarifying Shampoo, Lemon Sage Clarifying Conditioner, ImmuneTune
Pine, Black	*Pinus nigra* (Pinaceae)	SI	Evergreen Essence
Pine, Lodge Pole	*Pinus contorta* (Pinaceae)	SI	Evergreen Essence

Single Oil Name	Botanical Name	Safety Data	Products containing Single Oil
ne, Piñon	*Pinus edulis* (Pinaceae)	SI	Evergreen Essence
ne, Ponderosa 'ellow Pine)	*Pinus ponderosa* (Pinaceae)	SI	Evergreen Essence, Legacy
ıvensara	*Ravensara aromatica* (Lauraceae)		ImmuPower, Legacy, Raven, ImmuneTune
ɔse (Bulgarian)	*Rosa damascena* (Rosaceae)	(GRAS), P	Envision, Forgiveness, Gathering, Gentle Baby, Harmony, Humility, Joy, Joy Aqua Essence, Legacy, SARA, Trauma Life, White Angelica, Rose Ointment
ɔsehip	*Rosa canina* (Rosaceae)	(GRAS)	Legacy, Animal Scents Pet Ointment, Rose Ointment, Sandalwood Moisture Creme, Wolfberry Eye Creme
ɔsemary Cineol	*Rosmarinus officinalis* CT 1,8 cineol (Labiatae)	(GRAS), E*, HBP*, P* Dilute 1:1	En-R-Gee, JuvaFlex, Legacy, Melrose, Purification, Thieves, Transformation, AromaGuard Deodorants, Morning Start Bath Gel, Thieves Bar Soap, Morning Start Bar Soap, Chelex, Rehemogen, Be-Fit, ComforTone, ICP, ImmuGel, JuvaTone, Polyzyme, VitaGreen
ɔsemary Verbenon	*Rosmarinus officinalis* CT verbenon (Labiatae)	(GRAS), E*, HBP, P Dilute 1:1	Clarity, Orange Blossom Facial Wash, Sandalwood Moisture Creme
ɔsewood	*Aniba rosaeodora* (Lauraceae)	(GRAS)	Acceptance, Believe, Clarity, Forgiveness, Gentle Baby, Gratitude, Harmony, Humility, Inspiration, Joy, Joy Aqua Essence, Lady Sclareol, Legacy, Magnify Your Purpose, Sensation, Valor, Valor Aqua Essence, White Angelica, Animal Scents Pet Ointment, AromaGuard Deodorants, Genesis Hand & Body Lotion, KidScents Lotion, KidScents Tender Tush, Rose Ointment, Rosewood Moisturizing Shampoo, Rosewood Moisturizing Conditioner, Sandalwood Moisture Cream, Sandalwood Toner, Satin Hand & Body Lotion, Sensation Hand & Body Lotion, Wolfberry Eye Creme, Dragon Time Bath Gel, Evening Peace Bath Gel, Sensation Bath Gel, Lavender Rosewood Bar Soap, Valor Bar Soap, HRT Tincture, Relaxation Massage Oil, Sensation Massage Oil

Single Oil Name	Botanical Name	Safety Data	Products containing Single Oil
Sage	*Salvia officinalis* (Labiatae)	(GRAS), E*, HBP*, P* Dilute 1:1	EndoFlex, Envision, Legacy, Magnify Your Purpose, Mister, Progessence Cream, Protec, Lemon Sage Clarifying Shampoo, Lemon Sage Clarifying Conditioner, Dragon Time Bath Gel, K& Tincture, Dragon Time Massage Oil, FemiGen, ProGen
Sage, Spanish (Sage Lavender)	*Salvia lavandulifolia* (Labiatae)	(GRAS) Dilute 1:1	Harmony, Lady Sclareol, SclarEssence
Sandalwood	*Santalum album* (Santalaceae)	(FA/FL)	Acceptance, Brain Power, Dream Catch Forgiveness, Gathering, Harmony, Inner Child, Inspiration, Lady Sclareol, Legac Live with Passion, Magnify Your Purpo Release, 3 Wise Men, Transformation, Trauma Life, White Angelica, Boswelli Wrinkle Creme, KidScents Tender Tush Rosewood Moisturizing Shampoo, Rosewood Moisturizing Conditioner, Sandalwood Moisture Creme, Sandalwc Toner, Satin Hand & Body Lotion, Evening Peace Bath Gel, Lemon Sandalwood Bar Soap, Ultra Young, Ul Young Plus
Spearmint	*Mentha spicata* (Labiatae)	(GRAS), P Dilute 1:2	Citrus Fresh, EndoFlex, Legacy, Cinnamint Lip Balm, Fresh Essence Plu Mouthwash, Relaxation Massage Oil, ThermaBurn, ThermaMist, Thyromin
Spikenard	*Nardostachys jatamansi* (Valerianaceae)		Exodus II, Humility, Legacy, Exodus, Animal Scents Pet Shampoo
Spruce	*Picea mariana* (Pinaceae)	(FA/FL) Dilute 1:1	Abundance, Christmas Spirit, Envision, Gathering, Grounding, Harmony, Hope, Inner Child, Inspiration, Legacy, Motivation, Present Time, RC, Relieve Sacred Mountain, Sacred Mountain Aqu Essence, Surrender, 3 Wise Men, Traur Life, Valor, Valor Aqua Essence, White Angelica, Sacred Mountain Bar Soap, Valor Bar Soap, ArthroTune
Spruce, Colorado Blue	*Picea pungens* (Pinaceae)		Evergreen Essence
Tangerine	*Citrus nobilis* (Rutaceae)	(GRAS) Dilute 1:1	Citrus Fresh, Dream Catcher, Inner Chi Legacy, Peace & Calming, KidScents Shampoo, Peace & Calming Aqua Essence, Relaxation Massage Oil, ComforTone

Single Oil Name	Botanical Name	Safety Data	Products containing Single Oil
ansy, Blue	*Tanacetum annum* (Compositae)	Dilute 1:1	Acceptance, Australian Blue, Dream Catcher, JuvaFlex, Legacy, Peace & Calming, Release, SARA, Valor, KidScents Shampoo, KidScents Tender Tush, Peace & Calming Aqua Essence, Valor Aqua Essence, Dragon Time Bath Gel, Evening Peace Bath Gel, Valor Bar Soap, JuvaTone
ansy, Idaho	*Tanacetum vulgare* (Compositae)	Dilute 1:1	ImmuPower, Into the Future, Lady Sclareol, Legacy, ParaFree
arragon	*Artemisia dracunculus* (Compositae)	(GRAS), E*, P* Dilute 1:1	Di-Tone, Legacy, Allerzyme, Carbozyme, ComforTone, Fiberzyme, ICP, Lipozyme, Essentialzyme
hyme	*Thymus vulgaris* (Labiatae)	(GRAS), HBP Dilute 1:4	Longevity, Dentarome Plus Toothpaste, Fresh Essence Mouthwash, KidScents Toothpaste, Rehemogen, ImmuGel, Longevity Capsules, ParaFree
hyme linalol	*Thymus vulgaris* CT Linalol (Labiatae)	(GRAS) Dilute 1:2	Legacy
hyme, Red	*Thymus serpyllum* (Labiatae)	(GRAS)	Ortho Ease
suga	*Tsuga canadensis* (Pinaceae)	(FA/FL), SI* Dilute 1:1	Legacy
alerian	*Valeriana officinalis* (Valerianaceae)	(FA/FL), CS	Legacy, Trauma Life
etiver	*Vetiveria zizanoides* (Gramineae)	P	Lady Sclareol, Legacy, Fresh Essence Plus Mouthwash, Melaleuca Geranium Bar Soap, Ortho Ease Massage Oil, Ortho Sport Massage Oil, ParaFree
hite Lotus	*Nymphaea lotus* (Nymphaeaceae)		SARA
intergreen	*Gaultheria procumbens* (Ericaceae)	E*, P* Dilute 1:2	Legacy, PanAway, Raven, Dentarome/ Dentarome Plus Toothpaste, Fresh Essence Mouthwash, Regenolone, Rosewood Moisturizing Shampoo, Rosewood Moisturizing Conditioner, Ortho Ease Massage Oil, Ortho Sport Massage Oil, ArthroTune, Be-Fit, BLM, Super Cal
arrow	*Achillea millefolium* (Compositae)	CS, P Dilute 1:1	Dragon Time, Legacy, Mister, Prenolone/ Prenolone+, Progessence Cream, Dragon Time Massage Oil, ProGen

Single Oil Name	Botanical Name	Safety Data	Products containing Single Oi
Ylang Ylang	*Cananga odorata* (Annonaceae)	(GRAS), CS Dilute 1:1	Aroma Life, Australian Blue, Clarity, Dream Catcher, Forgiveness, Gathering, Gentle Baby, Gratitude, Grounding, Harmony, Highest Potential, Humility, Inner Child, Into the Future, Joy, Joy Ac Essence, Lady Sclareol, Legacy, Motivation, Peace & Calming, Peace & Calming Aqua Essence, Present Time, Release, Sacred Mountain, Sacred Mountain Aqua Essence, SARA, Sensation, White Angelica, Boswellia Wrinkle Creme, Genesis Hand & Body Lotion, Lemon Sage Clarifying Shampo Lemon Sage Clarifying Conditioner, Prenolone/Prenolone+, Progessence Cream, Satin Hand & Body Lotion, Sensation Hand & Body Lotion, Dragon Time Bath Gel, Evening Peace Bath Ge Sensation Bath Gel, Sacred Mountain B Soap, HRT Tincture, Dragon Time Massage Oil, Relaxation Massage Oil, Sensation Massage Oil, CardiaCare, FemiGen

Safety Data Legend:

A **Avoid** during and after consumption of **alcohol**

CS Could possibly result in **contact sensitization** (redness or irritation of the skin due to repeated application of a substance) (rotate or use different oils)

CS* Repeated use can result in **extreme contact sensitization** (rotate between different oils)

D **Avoid** if **diabetic**

E Use with **caution** if susceptible to **epilepsy** (small amounts or in dilution)

E* **Avoid** if susceptible to **epilepsy** (can trigger a seizure)

HBP Use with **caution** if dealing with **high blood pressure** (small amounts)

HBP* **Avoid** if dealing with **high blood pressure**

P Use with **caution** during **pregnancy** (small amounts or in dilution)

P* **Avoid** during **pregnancy**

PH **Photosensitivity**–direct exposure to sunlight after use could cause dermatitis (test first)

PH* **Extreme Photosensitivity**–direct exposure to sunlight after use can cause severe dermatiti (avoid exposing affected area of skin to direct sunlight for 12 hours)

SI Could possibly result in **skin irritation** (dilution may be necessary)

SI* Can cause **extreme skin irritation** (dilution highly recommended)

ST Can cause **stupification** in high doses (use only small amounts or in dilution)

Dilute - Dilution ratios shown equal Essential Oil:Vegetable Oil

Blend Summary Information

The following chart displays summary information about each of the oil blends, including: ıgle oils contained in the blend, possible uses or areas of application, and safety data. The safety ta includes possible skin reactions and conditions during which use of that particular blend ould be limited or completely avoided (refer to the legend following the chart). **Note:** This safety ta is provided for **EXTERNAL USE ONLY!**

Blend Name	Single Oil Contents	Uses/Application Areas	Safety Data
bundance	Myrrh, frankincense, patchouli, orange, clove, ginger, spruce	Diffuse; Wrists, ears, neck, face; Wallet/Purse; Painting; Perfume	CS*, SI Dilute 1:1
cceptance	Geranium, Blue tansy, frankincense, sandalwood, neroli, rosewood (Carrier: Almond oil)	Diffuse; *Liver*, heart, *chest*, face, ears, neck, thymus, wrists; Sacral chakra; Perfume	
roma Life	Cypress, marjoram, helichrysum, ylang ylang (Carrier: Sesame seed oil)	Heart; Vita Flex heart points—under left ring finger, under left ring toe, above left elbow, arteries; Spine	
roma Siez	Basil, marjoram, lavender, peppermint, cypress	Muscles; Neck; Heart; Vita Flex points; Full body massage; Bath	Dilute 1:1
ustralian Blue	Blue cypress, ylang ylang, cedarwood, Blue tansy, White fir	Diffuse; Perfume; Forehead	CS, SI
waken	Oil Blends of Joy, Forgiveness, Dream Catcher, Present Time, Harmony	Diffuse; Chest, heart, *forehead*, neck, temples, wrists; Perfume; Full body massage; Bath	
elieve	Idaho balsam fir, rosewood, frankincense	Diffuse; *Heart, forehead, temples*; Perfume	Dilute 1:1
rain Power	Cedarwood, sandalwood, frankincense, melissa, Blue cypress, lavender, helichrysum	Diffuse; Neck, throat, nose; Inside of cheeks; Perfume	
hivalry	Oil Blends of Valor, Joy, Harmony, Gratitude	Diffuse; *Heart, forehead, temples*; Perfume	Dilute 1:1
hristmas Spirit	Orange, cinnamon bark, spruce	Diffuse; Crown; Perfume; Place on pine boughs or fireplace logs; Add to potpourri	CS*, SI* Dilute 1:1
itrus Fresh	Orange, tangerine, mandarin, grapefruit, lemon, spearmint	Diffuse; Ears, heart wrists; Perfume; Full body massage; Bath; Purify drinking water	SI*, PH* Dilute 1:1
larity	Basil, cardamom, rosemary verbenon, peppermint, rosewood, geranium, lemon, palmarosa, ylang ylang, bergamot, Roman chamomile, jasmine	Diffuse; Forehead, neck, temples, wrists; Perfume; Bath	SI, P, PH*

Blend Name	Single Oil Contents	Uses/Application Areas	Safety Dat
Di-Tone	Tarragon, ginger, peppermint, juniper, anise, fennel, lemongrass, patchouli	Vita Flex points—feet and ankles; stomach; abdomen, bottom of throat; Compress	P, E
Dragon Time	Clary sage, fennel, lavender, jasmine, yarrow	Vita Flex points; Diffuse; Abdomen, lower back, location	P
Dream Catcher	Sandalwood, bergamot, ylang ylang, juniper, Blue tansy, tangerine, Black pepper, anise	Diffuse; Forehead, eye brows, *temples*, ears, throat chakra; Perfume; Pillow; Bath or sauna	PH
En-R-Gee	Rosemary cineol, juniper, nutmeg, fir, Black pepper, lemongrass, clove	Diffuse; Wrists, ears, neck, temples, feet; Full body massage; Perfume	SI*, E Dilute 1:1
EndoFlex	Spearmint, sage, geranium, myrtle, nutmeg, German chamomile (Carrier: Sesame seed oil)	Thyroid, kidneys, liver, pancreas, glands; Vita Flex points	SI, E
Envision	Spruce, sage, rose, geranium, orange, lavender	Vita Flex points; Diffuse; Wrists, *temples*; Bath; Massage	HBP, E, P
Evergreen Essence	Colorado Blue spruce (*Picea pungens*), Ponderosa pine (*Pinus ponderosa*), pine, Red fir (*Abies magnifica*), cedar (*Cedrus canadensis*), White fir, Black pine (*Pinus nigra*), Piñon pine (*Pinus edulis*), Lodge Pole pine (*Pinus contorta*)	*Diffuse*; Hands, bottoms of feet	CS, SI Dilute 1:1
Exodus II	Cinnamon bark, cassia, calamus, myrrh, hyssop, frankincense, spikenard, galbanum (Carrier: Olive oil)	Vita Flex points; Spine (dilute well)	CS*, SI*, P* Dilute 1:1
Forgiveness	Frankincense, sandalwood, lavender, melissa, angelica, helichrysum, rose, rosewood, geranium, lemon, palmarosa, ylang ylang, bergamot, Roman chamomile, jasmine (Carrier: Sesame seed oil)	Diffuse; *Navel*, heart, ears, wrists; Perfume	
Gathering	Galbanum, frankincense, sandalwood, lavender, cinnamon bark, rose, spruce, geranium, ylang ylang	Diffuse; *Forehead, heart, temples*, neck, thymus, face, chest; Perfume	
Gentle Baby	Rose geranium, rosewood, palmarosa, lavender, Roman chamomile, ylang ylang, rose, lemon, bergamot, jasmine	Diffuse; Ankles, lower back, abdomen, feet, face, neck; Massage; Perfume; Bath	

Blend Name	Single Oil Contents	Uses/Application Areas	Safety Data
ratitude	Idaho balsam fir, frankincense, rosewood, myrrh, galbanum, ylang ylang	Diffuse; *Heart, forehead, temples*; Perfume	Dilute 1:1
rounding	Juniper, angelica, ylang ylang, cedarwood, pine, spruce, fir	Diffuse; *Brain stem, back of neck, sternum*, temples	SI
armony	Hyssop, spruce, lavender, frankincense, geranium, ylang ylang, orange, sandalwood, angelica, sage lavender, rose, rosewood, lemon, palmarosa, bergamot, Roman chamomile, jasmine	Diffuse; Each chakra; Ears, feet, heart; *Energy meridians*, crown; Perfume	P, E*, HBP, PH
ighest Potential	Oil Blends of Australian Blue, Gathering, and Single Oils of ylang ylang and jasmine	Diffuse; *Heart, forehead, temples*; Perfume	Dilute 1:1
ope	Melissa, myrrh, juniper, spruce (Carrier: Almond oil)	Diffuse; *Ears*; Chest, heart, temples, solar plexus, neck, feet, wrists; Perfume	
umility	Geranium, ylang ylang, frankincense, spikenard, myrrh, rose, rosewood, melissa, neroli (Carrier: Sesame seed oil)	Diffuse; *Heart, neck, temples*	
nmuPower	Cistus, frankincense, hyssop, ravensara, Mountain savory, oregano, clove, cumin, Idaho tansy	Diffuse; Throat, chest, spine, feet; Thymus; Veins in neck, under arm pits	SI, P, E Dilute 1:1
nner Child	Orange, tangerine, jasmine, ylang ylang, spruce, sandalwood, lemongrass, neroli	Diffuse; *Navel, chest, temples, nose*	SI
nspiration	Cedarwood, spruce, rosewood, sandalwood, frankincense, myrtle, mugwort	Diffuse; *Horns*, crown, shoulders, back of neck	
nto the Future	Frankincense, jasmine, Clary sage, juniper, Idaho tansy, fir, ylang ylang (Carrier: Almond oil)	Diffuse; Bath; Heart, wrists, neck; Compress; Full body massage	
oy	Lemon, mandarin, bergamot, ylang ylang, rose, rosewood, geranium, palmarosa, Roman chamomile, jasmine	Diffuse; *Heart*, ears, neck, thymus, temples, forehead, wrists; Bath; Compress; Massage; Perfume	PH*
uva Cleanse	Helichrysum, celery seed, ledum	Liver; Vita Flex points on feet	SI
uvaFlex	Fennel, geranium, rosemary cineol, Roman chamomile, Blue tansy, helichrysum (Carrier: Sesame seed oil)	Vita Flex points; Feet, spine, LIVER; Full body massage	SI Dilute 1:1

Blend Name	Single Oil Contents	Uses/Application Areas	Safety Dat
Lady Sclareol	Rosewood, vetiver, geranium, orange, Clary sage, ylang ylang, sandalwood, sage lavender, jasmine, Idaho tansy	On Location (by male partner); Massage; Bath; Compress over abdomen; Diffuse, *Perfume*	
Legacy	(See LEGACY in Blend section for complete list of 90 single oils)	Diffuse; Forehead, wrists, sternum, feet; Perfume	CS, SI Dilute 1:4
Live with Passion	Melissa, helichrysum, Clary sage, cedarwood, angelica, ginger, neroli, sandalwood, patchouli, jasmine	Wrists, *temples, chest, forehead*; Bath; Perfume or cologne	
Longevity	Thyme, orange, clove, frankincense	Internally as Dietary Supplement;	CS, SI, PH Dilute 1:4
M-Grain	Basil, marjoram, lavender, peppermint, Roman chamomile, helichrysum	DIFFUSE; Forehead, crown, shoulders, neck, temples; Vita Flex points; Massage	Dilute 1:1
Magnify Your Purpose	Sandalwood, nutmeg, rosewood, cinnamon bark, ginger, sage	Vita Flex points; Feet, wrists, *temples*; Diffuse; Bath; Massage	E, P, CS, SI
Melrose	Melaleuca (*alternifolia* & *quinquenervia*), rosemary cineol, clove	Diffuse; Forehead, liver; Topically on location	CS, SI Dilute 1:1
Mister	Sage, fennel, lavender, myrtle, yarrow, peppermint (Carrier: Sesame seed oil)	Vita Flex points; Ankles, lower pelvis, prostate (dilute); Compress	P*, E
Motivation	Roman chamomile, ylang ylang, spruce, lavender	Diffuse; Chest, neck; *Solar plexus*, sternum, feet, navel, ears; wrists, palms; Perfume	
PanAway	Wintergreen, helichrysum, clove, peppermint	Compress on spine; Vita Flex on feet; Topically on location	Dilute 1:1
Peace & Calming	Tangerine, orange, ylang ylang, patchouli, Blue tansy	Diffuse; Navel, nose, neck, feet; Bath; Perfume	PH
Present Time	Neroli, spruce, ylang ylang (Carrier: Almond oil)	*Thymus*; Neck, forehead	
Purification	Citronella, lemongrass, rosemary cineol, melaleuca, lavandin, myrtle	Diffuse; Vita Flex points; Ears, feet, temples; Topically on location	CS, SI
Raven	Ravensara, *Eucalyptus radiata*, peppermint, wintergreen, lemon	Diffuse; Vita Flex points; Lungs, throat; Pillow; Suppository (diluted)	SI Dilute 1:1
RC	4 eucalyptuses (E. globulus, E. radiata, E. australiana, E. citriodora), myrtle, marjoram, pine, cypress, lavender, spruce, peppermint	DIFFUSE; Chest, back, feet; Sinuses, nasal passages; Ears, neck, throat; Compress; Massage	

Blend Name	Single Oil Contents	Uses/Application Areas	Safety Data
lease	Ylang ylang, lavandin, geranium, sandalwood, Blue tansy (Carrier: Olive oil)	*Compress on liver*; Ears, feet, Vita Flex points; Perfume	Dilute 1:1
lieve It	Spruce, Black pepper, hyssop, peppermint	Apply on location of pain	SI, P, E, HBP Dilute 1:1
cred Mountain	Spruce, ylang ylang, Idaho balsam fir, cedarwood	Diffuse; *Solar plexus, brain stem*, crown, neck, ears, thymus, wrists; Perfume	SI
RA	Blue tansy, rose, lavender, geranium, orange, cedarwood, ylang ylang, White lotus (Carrier: Almond oil)	*Energy centers*; Vita Flex points; *Temples, nose*; Places of abuse	
larEssence	Clary sage, peppermint, sage lavender, fennel	Internally as Dietary Supplement	
nsation	Rosewood, ylang ylang, jasmine	Diffuse; Apply on location; Massage; Bath	
rrender	Lavender, Roman chamomile, German chamomile, angelica, Mountain savory, lemon, spruce	*Forehead, rim of ears, nape of neck, chest, solar plexus*; Bath	P, SI
hieves	Clove, lemon, cinnamon bark, *Eucalyptus radiata*, rosemary cineol	Diffuse; Feet, throat, stomach, intestines; Thymus, arm pits (Dilute well for topical uses!)	CS*, SI*, P Dilute 1:4
Wise Men	Sandalwood, juniper, frankincense, spruce, myrrh (Carrier: Almond oil)	Diffuse; *Crown of head*; Neck, forehead, solar plexus, thymus; Perfume	
ransformation	Lemon, peppermint, sandalwood, frankincense, Clary sage, Balsam fir, rosemary cineol, cardamom	Diffuse; *Forehead, heart*	
rauma Life	*Citrus hystrix* (Leech Lime), davana, geranium, spruce, helichrysum, rose, sandalwood, frankincense, lavender, valerian	Diffuse; Spine; Feet, chest, ears, neck, forehead	
alor	Spruce, rosewood, Blue tansy, frankincense (Carrier: Almond oil)	*FEET*; Diffuse; Heart, wrists, solar plexus, neck to thymus, spine; Perfume	
/hite Angelica	Geranium, spruce, myrrh, ylang ylang, hyssop, bergamot, melissa, sandalwood, rose, rosewood (Carrier: Almond oil)	Diffuse; *Shoulders*, crown, chest, ears, neck, forehead, wrists; Bath; Perfume	PH*

ote: Italicized application areas represent the most effective areas for **emotional applications**. Refer the safety data legend shown previously (following the Single Oil Summary Information chart).

Glossary of Terms

Topic	Definition
Acne	Acne is a blockage of a skin pore by dead skin cells, tiny hairs, and oil secreted by the sebaceous glands locate near hair follicles in the face, neck, and back. This blockage occurs deep within the skin. Acne is not caused b dirt on the face or by eating certain foods. Over scrubbing the face may actually make acne worse. For more information, visit the website of the American Academy of Dermatologists at www.aad.org, or the National Institute of Arthritis and Musculoskeletal and Skin Diseases at http://www.niams.nih.gov/hi/topics/acne/acne.htm.
ADD/ADHD	Attention Deficit Disorder or Attention Deficit/Hyperactive Disorder is a psychological condition characterize by inattentiveness, restlessness, and difficulty concentrating. For more information, visit www.help4adhd.org/
Alcoholism	Alcoholism is an increasing dependency on alcohol that interferes with health, career, or family and social interactions. This problem affects between 5-10% of all people who use alcohol. Alcoholism has also been defined as any irresponsible drinking (such as binge drinking, or drunk driving).
Allergies	An allergy is an immune response to a harmless substance that most people donít react to. Allergies can cause sneezing, stuffy or runny noses, hives, itching, red eyes, breathing problems, stomach cramps, or vomiting.
Alopecia Areata	Alopecia Areata is an autoimmune disease where the bodyís immune system attacks fast-growing cells in the hair follicles, causing patches of hair, or all of the hair to fall out. For more information, visit the National Institute of Arthritis and Musculoskeletal and Skin Diseases: http://www.niams.nih.gov/hi/topics/alopecia/alopecia.htm
Analgesic	A substance that acts as a pain reliever
Anemia	Anemia is a lack of red blood cells in the body resulting in weakness and impaired motor and mental development. It is most common in infants and small children and is often (although not always) caused by a deficiency of iron in the diet. For more information, visit www.cdc.gov.
Aneurysm	A swelling or dilation of a blood vessel in the area of a weakened blood vessel wall.
Anorexia	A psychological disorder where an individual is addicted to depriving themselves of food.
Arteriosclerosis	A thickening or hardening of the artery walls due to high blood pressure, calcification, or fatty deposits.
Arthritis	Arthritis is any painful swelling of a joint.
Asthma	Asthma is a disease that causes the lungís airways to narrow, making it difficult to breath. Episodes (or attacks of asthma can be triggered by any number of things, including smoke, pollution, dust mites, and other allergen For more information, visit www.cdc.gov/nceh/airpollution/asthma/faqs.htm
Autism	Autism is a disorder caused by an abnormality in the brain which makes it difficult for an individual to communicate or interact with other people. For more information, visit www.cdc.gov/ncbddd/dd/ddautism.htm
Baldness	Baldness is usually caused by the hair follicles in the scalp failing to replace the hair when it falls out. This failure to replace the hairs is typically attributed to either aging, hormone imbalance, or an increase in the male hormone testosterone.
Boils	Boils (furuncles) are infections of the upper layers of the skin by staphylococcus or streptococcus bacteria. The infections often become filled with pus and dead cells, causing painful pea to golf ball sized swellings
Bronchitis	Inflammation of the bronchi (the tubes that lead from the trachea to the lungs).
Bruises	A bruise is an injury to tissue that results in blood capillaries breaking and spilling blood into the tissue.
Bulimia	Bulimia is a chronic psychological desire to purge the body of recently eaten foods either through vomiting or through the abuse of laxatives.
Calluses	A callus is a thickening of the outer layer of skin in a small area caused by friction or rubbing. Calluses can sometimes lead to serious infections.
Cancer	Cancer is when damaged or abnormal DNA causes a cell to divide out of control, resulting in clumps of rapidl dividing cells, or tumors, within healthy tissue.
Cataracts	A cataract is a clouding of the lens of an eye, causing blurriness, double-vision, or blindness. Cataracts can be caused by medications, injury, disease, or the natural aging process.
Catarrh	Chronic inflammation of the mucus membranes in the nose and throat.

ellulite	Fat deposits.
harley Horse	A Charley horse, or painful muscle spasm in the calf, is often caused by overuse, dehydration, or a lack of potassium, sodium, calcium, or magnesium in the body. Stretching the muscle and applying an initial hot compress, followed by a cold compress or ice pack once the pain starts to subside can often alleviate the pain associated with a muscle spasm.
higgers	Chiggers are the parasitic larvae of certain types of mites found in wooded areas, or areas of high grass. When chiggers bite, they cause red, severely itching bumps to appear.
holera	Cholera is a bacterial illness that can cause severe diarrhea, vomiting, and leg cramps. The most important treatment for cholera is to re-hydrate the body by drinking large amounts of an oral rehydration solution. (In an emergency when no commercially prepared re-hydration solution is available, mix 6 tsp. sugar, ½ tsp. salt, and 1 liter of water and drink.)
horea	Involuntary twisting, jumping, dancing, or other coordinated body movements that interfere with normal movement. Often caused by a previous strep (streptococcus) infection. A sign of rheumatic fever.
olic	Periods of loud crying in young infants that seem to be caused by pain in the abdomen.
olitis	Inflammation of the large intestine.
onjunctivitis	Also called "pinkeye" or "red eye", conjunctivitis is an inflammation of the membrane that covers the whites of the eyes and the inside of the eyelid due to infection, allergies, or irritation.
onvulsions	Uncontrolled rapid contracting and relaxing of muscles, usually caused by a seizure (sudden random electrical activity in the brain).
orns	A small, sometimes painful, callus caused by the friction between a bone and an outside pressure (such as a shoe) on the intermediate tissues.
ortisone	A natural hormone created in the outer layers of the adrenal gland that has anti-inflammatory and anti-arthritic properties. Cortisone has also been synthetically developed as a drug for rheumatoid arthritis.
rohn's Disease	A disease that causes chronic ulceration (either mild or severe) of the large and sometimes the small intestine.
ushing's Disease	(or Cushing Syndrome) describes many different symptoms (including weight gain, weakness, bruising, & osteoporosis) caused by an overabundance of the cortisol hormone. This disease is often caused by taking artificial cortisone or cortisone-like substances
ystic Fibrosis	Cystic fibrosis is a potentially deadly genetic disease that causes an excess of mucus to build up, inhibiting pancreas function and slowly clogging the airways.
ermatitis	Dermatitis is redness, itching or soreness of the skin caused either by an allergic reaction or contact with a skin irritant.
iaper Rash	Irritation of the skin in the area covered by the diaper caused by infection, sweat, friction, or allergic reactions.
iphtheria	Diphtheria is a rare bacterial infection that causes sore throat, low fevers, and swelling of the neck and throat that can possibly lead to airway obstruction and other complications.
iuretic	Any substance that causes an increase in the amount of urine created by the body.
own Syndrome	Down Syndrome is a genetic condition characterized by an extra chromosome 21. This extra chromosome causes the formation of various distinguishing physical attributes, and slight to severe mental disabilities or retardation.
ysentery	Dysentery is a painful intestinal inflammation due to an infection of the intestine by an ameba, causing severe cramping, diarrhea, vomiting, and bloody stools. Rehydration is critical to anyone suffering from dysentery.
czema	Itchy or painful patches of inflamed skin caused by allergic reactions, irritating substances, infection, or disease.
dema	A swelling in the body caused by the accumulation of water, blood, or other fluids.
lectrolytes	Any substance that acquires the ability to conduct electricity when it is dissolved in a solution. Sodium, calcium, and potassium are three electrolytic substances that play an important role in the body. Low levels of any of these substances in the blood can lead to muscle cramps and other problems.
mphysema	Damaged or burst air sacs in the lungs caused by smoking or a long-lasting lung infection.
nzymes	An enzyme is any biological agent that mediates the speed or frequency of chemical reactions.
atigue	Being unable to work or think at full capacity.
iber	Complex carbohydrates that cannot be digested by the body. Fiber serves to help clean the colon and regulate bowel movements. Fiber can be found in fruits, vegetables, whole grain breads and cereals.

Fibroids	A benign tumor found in the uterus that can cause pain, reproductive problems, or heavy menstrual bleeding.
Fever	A fever is defined as any body temperature above 98.6 degrees F. A fever is the body's natural way of fighting disease (many pathogens cannot survive, or are weakened in these elevated temperatures). High fevers (over 1 degrees F.), however, can cause convulsions and other undesired effects.
Fibrositis	(See Fibromyalgia)
Flu	(See also Influenza) Any of several viral diseases that cause fever, nausea, fatigue, soreness, impaired breathin and other cold-like symptoms.
Gangrene	Localized decay of body tissue caused by a loss of blood to that area. Gas gangrene is caused by bacteria invading a deep wound that has lessened the blood supply, or cut it off entirely. The bacteria create gases and pus in the infected area, causing severe pain and accelerating decay of t tissue.
Gingivitis	A gum disease that results in sore gums that bleed easily. This condition can sometimes be corrected with more frequent/longer brushing and flossing.
Glaucoma	Glaucoma is an increasing eye pressure caused by a slowing in fluid drainage from the eye. Glaucoma can cau damage to the optical nerve or loss of sight over time.
Goiter	An enlarged thyroid gland. Goiter is often attributed to a deficiency of iodine in the body (found in iodized salts). While this is one possible cause, goiter is often a symptom of any of several diseases or conditions.
Gout	Gout is a painful inflammation of a joint caused by a buildup of uric acid crystals deposited in the joint. Uric acid is formed during the natural breakdown of dead tissues in the body. An excess of uric acid in the bloodstream can lead to the formation of crystals in the joints or kidneys (kidney stones). Some good ways to prevent the formation of uric acid crystals include maintaining a healthy body weight (which leaves less body tissue to be broken down), exercise, and drinking plenty of water.
Grave's Disease	Toxicity of the thyroid gland which leads to goiter, an autoimmune skin disease, and an eye disease that often causes bulging of the eyes.
Hashimoto's Disease	An autoimmune disease of the thyroid gland, leading to goiter and a decreased ability of the thyroid to produce essential hormones.
Heartburn	A burning pain in the chest caused by stomach acid rising up into the esophagus.
Hemorrhaging	Any internal or external bleeding.
Hepatitis	Hepatitis is a liver disease caused by one of five different Hepatitis viruses. The symptoms and seriousness of t disease depend on the type of virus causing the disease. www.cdc.gov/ncidod/diseases/hepatitis/
Hernia	A hernia is the protrusion of any tissue or organ outside of the cavity in which it is normally contained.
High Blood Pressure	Blood pressure that is consistently higher than 140 over 90. Chronic high blood pressure can cause severe heal problems. High blood pressure can often be reduced by losing weight if overweight, cutting back on salty food and regular exercise.
Hodgkin's Disease	Hodgkin disease is a cancer that develops in the lymph system, causing enlarged lymph nodes, fever, sweating, fatigue, and loss of weight.
Inflammation	Inflammation is the body's response to infection, irritation, or injury in a localized area. The tissue becomes inflamed due to dilation of the blood vessels (which allows greater blood flow into the affected area).
Insomnia	Lack of adequate sleep. Insomnia is caused by a variety of factors, including stress, disease, the environment, overuse of caffeine and other stimulants, and changes in sleeping times or behaviors.
Irritable Bowel Syndrome	Chronically irregular bowel movements that result in frequent bouts of constipation and diarrhea.
Jet Lag	Jet lag is caused by the hypothalamus (the body's internal clock) trying to re-adjust the body's schedule to differing environmental cues (such as when the sun rises) after a person has traveled rapidly across different tin zones.
Laryngitis	Inflammation of the larynx due to viral or bacterial infection. Often causes hoarseness, or voice loss.
Lice	Lice are any of three varieties of small, parasitic insects that are found either on the head, body, or pubic hair. Lice can be passed to another person through personal contact or by sharing bed linens, clothing, hats, hair ribbons, scarves, combs or brushes.

ou Gehrig's sease — Lou Gehrig's disease (or ALS) is caused by the atrophy of certain nerve cells in the body that control voluntary movement. This atrophy leads to weakness in the muscles controlled by these nerve cells. Lou Gehrig's disease usually leads to death within several years due to opportunistic infections overcoming an already weakened body.

yme Disease — Lyme disease is a disease caused by an infection of B. Burgdorferi bacteria transmitted by the bite of a deer tick. Symptoms of Lyme disease include a red circular rash, arthritis, neurological problems, and possible heart irregularities.
For more information on Lyme disease, visit: www.niaid.nih.gov/publications/lyme/contents.htm

alaria — Malaria is a disease caused by one of four types of parasites transmitted to humans from several species of mosquitoes. Symptoms can include muscle pains, headaches, fevers, sweating, and chills. More serious cases involve anemia and kidney failure that can lead to death.
www.cdc.gov/malaria/

elanoma — A type of malignant skin cancer that presents itself as a rapidly growing/spreading, irregularly shaped mole. This type of cancer can be very dangerous if not detected and treated early.

enopause — The natural cessation of menstruation in women associated with a decline in the ovary hormones estrogen and progesterone.

etabolism — The entire range of chemical processes that build up and break down substances within the body.

igraine eadaches — A throbbing headache caused by spasms in the brain's blood vessels. Sometimes accompanied by an "aura"—perception of lights, or sounds that do not exist.

old — Mold is a type of fungus that grows in damp, warm conditions. The CDC recommends using a weak bleach solution (1 part bleach, 10 parts water) to remove any mold growths within the house.
www.cdc.gov/nceh/airpollution/mold/moldfacts.htm

ononucleosis — Mononucleosis—an illness characterized by fever, sore throat, fatigue, and swollen lymph nodes—is caused by an infection of the Epstein-Barr virus during adolescence or early adulthood. The Epstein-Barr virus is very common in humans (it can be found in 95% of people over the age of 40), and many people acquire the virus with few or no symptoms during infancy and early childhood. When an individual acquires the virus during adolescence and early adulthood, it can sometimes develop into mononucleosis (about 35-50% of the time).
www.cdc.gov/ncidod/diseases/ebv.htm

umps — Mumps is a viral disease that causes fever, sore muscles, headache, and swelling of the lymph nodes by the jaw.
www.cdc.gov/nip/diseases/mumps/default.htm

uscular ystrophy — Any of several genetic diseases that cause gradual weakening of the skeletal muscles.

yelin Sheath — The myelin sheath is the fatty protective layer that surrounds the nerve fibers allowing nerve cells to transmit their signals properly. It is composed of lipids (70%), and proteins (30%). It is produced by oligodendrocyte cells surrounding the nerve fibers.

euritis — Inflammation of the nerve cells.

europathy — Any nerve malfunction or disease.

ncreatitis — Inflammation of the pancreas, often associated with alcohol or gallstones.

rkinson's isease — A neurological disease that over time causes progressively worse shaking, muscle weakness, and other symptoms.

aryngitis — (See also Sore Throat) Inflammation of the Pharynx (throat).

lebitis — Inflammation or swelling of a vein, usually caused by a blood clot.

ague — Plague is a potentially deadly bacterial disease that is caused by the *Yersinia pestus* bacteria transmitted to humans and animals through close contact or bites from fleas that have previously bitten infected animals. Symptoms include fever, headaches, and extremely swollen and hot lymph nodes. If left untreated, plague can quickly invade the lungs causing severe pneumonia, high fever, bloody coughing, and death.
www.cdc.gov/ncidod/dvbid/plague/index.htm

eurisy — Pleurisy is the inflammation of one or both of the two protective layers that surround the lungs. This inflammation causes sharp pains that are intensified by breathing. Pleurisy can be caused by infection, injury, blood clots, or disease.

ison Oak/Ivy — These two plants create a chemical that is caustic to the skin, causing inflammation, redness, itching, and pain in the areas it comes in contact with.

lyps — An outgrowth of tissue on the inside of hollow organs.

Progesterone	A female hormone produced by the ovaries responsible for regulating the lining of the uterus.
Psoriasis	Psoriasis is a chronic skin disease that causes skin cells to be rotated to the surface before they are mature, resulting in inflamed patches of scaly, red skin that either itch or are sore. About 20% of the time, psoriasis als causes arthritis in adjoining joints. Psoriasis occurs when T cells (white blood cells that help fight infections) become unnecessarily active, triggering inflammation and causing skin cells to rotate to the surface before they are mature. One possible treatment for the itching and soreness is to soak for 15 minutes in a bath with Epsom dead sea salts, oiled oatmeal, or oil, followed by application of a moisturizer on the affected areas. www.niams.nih.gov/hi/topics/psoriasis/psoriafs.htm
Radiation	Radiation is any of several different forms of energy that may or may not be harmful to the human body. Common forms of radiation include light, radio waves, and x-rays. The three types of radiation considered mo dangerous to humans include alpha particles (large, slow moving particles that typically bounce off the skin, a are not dangerous unless the source of these particles is ingested into the body), beta particles (tiny, fast movin particles that can penetrate deep within the body when emitted within several thousand feet), and gamma rays (bursts of energy that can penetrate deep within the body). Each of these types of radiation can change the chemical state or break chemical bonds of molecules they collide with, potentially damaging vital life processe within a cell. www.epa.gov/radiation/
Rheumatic Fever	An illness that causes pain in the joints, fever, nausea, and vomiting. This disease follows an infection by the streptococcus bacteria or scarlet fever. Rheumatic fever can cause severe damage to the heart, joints, and brain Rheumatic fever often returns once a person develops it.
Ringworm	Ringworm is a skin disease cause by a fungus that can result in ring-shaped red rashes that can be itchy, crusty or scaly.
Scabies	Scabies is an infestation of a microscopic mite (*Sarcoptes scabei*) that burrows into your skin, leaving pimple like burrows that itch. www.cdc.gov/ncidod/dpd/parasites/scabies/default.htm
Sciatica	Lower-back/upper-leg pain caused by irritation of the sciatic nerve (a large nerve that extends from the lower back down into the legs). The cause of this irritation is often a herniated disk pressing on the nerve, but it can also be caused by inflammation or other irritants.
Scoliosis	Scoliosis is a sideways curving of the spine. www.niams.nih.gov/hi/topics/scoliosis/scochild.htm
Scurvy	A disorder caused by a lack of vitamin C that causes bleeding in the gums, anemia, and bumpy skin.
Shingles	(Already in book) www.cdc.gov/nip/diseases/varicella/faqs-gen-shingles.htm
Spurs, Bone	Outgrowths of bone (typically in the heel or sole of the feet) that cause inflammation of the surrounding tendon making movement painful. Ice packs on the inflamed tendons can help reduce pain and swelling.
Staph Infections	Staph infections are any type of infection caused by the *Staphylococcus* bacteria. While skin infections caused by the *staphylococcus* bacteria are very common, and usually require no treatment, they can become very serious—especially when they occur in surgical wounds, or open bed sores. www.cdc.gov/ncidod/hip/ARESIST/mrsafaq.htm
Strep Throat	Strep throat is an infection caused by the streptococcal bacteria in the throat that causes a sore throat and fever www.cdc.gov/ncidod/dbmd/diseaseinfo/groupastreptococcal_g.htm
Tendonitis	Tendonitis is the painful inflammation of the tendons (the tissue that connects muscles to bones) due to injury, overuse, or disease.
Thrush	Thrush is an overgrowth of the fungus *Candida* (found normally on the skin and mucus membranes) caused b an imbalance in the environment in the mouth or throat that results in white patches in the mouth and potential painful swallowing. www.cdc.gov/ncidod/dbmd/diseaseinfo/candidiasis_opc_g.htm
Tinnitus	Tinnitus, or a ringing in the ears, is caused by many different things, including: ear damage from loud noises, excess ear fluid, infections, diseases, and some medications.
TMJ	TMJ (temporomandibular joint) disorder or syndrome is characterized by chronic pain in the joint connecting the jawbone to the skull and in the surrounding area. This pain is often caused by clenching or grinding the jaw due to stress or habit. It can also be caused by an injury to the joint or arthritis.
Tonsillitis	Inflammation of the tonsils due to infection or disease.
Tuberculosis	Tuberculosis is a disease caused by bacteria that can attack the lungs, resulting in a severe, bloody cough, ches pains, fever, chills, and loss of appetite. www.cdc.gov/nchstp/tb/faqs/qa.htm

umors	An abnormal growth of tissue. A tumor may be either cancerous (malignant) or non-cancerous (benign).
yphoid	Typhoid is a bacterial disease that causes a high, sustained fever, weakness, stomach pains, headache, and loss of appetite. If untreated, the fever may last for weeks, or even months, and could result in death. www.cdc.gov/ncidod/diseases/submenus/sub_typhoid.htm
asodilator	Any agent that causes the blood vessel walls to relax, increasing the diameter of the blood vessel and allowing more blood to flow through.
ertigo	A feeling that the environment is spinning around you, or that you are spinning. Typically caused by a problem in the inner ear.
'arts	A small outgrowth of skin caused by a virus.
'hiplash	Over stretching or tearing the muscles and tendons in the neck and head due to a collision pushing the body in one direction, while the head's tendency is to remain in the same place, causing the head to quickly rock in the opposite direction the body is going.
'hooping Cough	Whooping cough (or pertussis) is caused by *Bordetella pertussis* bacteria. This highly contagious disease causes severe bouts of coughing, whooping, and vomiting; and in small children and infants can lead to seizure, apnea (closure of airways), pneumonia, malnutrition, and other serious complications. www.cdc.gov/health/pertussis.htm

rces (besides those listed above):
v.MedTerms.com
ter for Disease Control (www.cdc.gov)
ironmental Protection Agency (www.epa.gov)
line Plus Medical Encyclopedia (www.nlm.nih.gov/medlineplus/ency)

Taxonomical Information

following chart is the taxonomical breakdown of the plant families for each of the essential oils found in this book. On the pages owing this division chart, there is further information for each family, including the plants within that family that essential oils are ved from, the body systems affected by these essential oils, the properties of these oils, and general uses for these oils.

ision: Embryophyte Siphonogama (plants with seeds)
- Subdivision: Gymnosperm (plants with concentric rings, exposed seeds, & resinous wood)
  - Class: Coniferae (cone-bearing plants) & Taxaceae (yew-like plants)
    - Family: **Pinaceae** (Trees or shrubs with cones and numerous "scales")
      - Genus: Abies (firs, balsam trees), Cedrus (cedars), Pinus (pines), Picea (spruces), Pseudotsuga (false hemlock), Tsuga (hemlocks)
    - Family: **Cupressaceae**
      - Genus: Callitris (blue cypress), Cupressus (cypresses), Juniperus (junipers), Thuja (Arbor vitae or cedars)
- Subdivision: Angiosperm (highly evolved plants with seeds enclosed by fruits)
  - Class: Monocotyledons (plants with one-leaf embryos)
    - Family: **Gramineae**, **Zingiberaceae**
  - Class: Dicotyledons (plants with multiple-leaf embryos)
    - Family: **Annonaceae, Betulaceae, Burseraceae, Cistaceae, Compositae, Ericaceae, Geraniaceae, Guttiferae, Labiatae, Lauraceae, Myristicaceae, Myrtaceae, Oleaceae, Piperaceae, Rosaceae, Rutaceae, Santalaceae, Styracaceae, Umbelliferae, Valerianaceae**

NONACEAE (shrubs, trees, climbers; fragrant flowers; 128 genera, 2000 species; mostly tropical, found in Old World & rain forest)
dy Systems: Cardiovascular System, Nervous System (calming), Hormonal System (aphrodesiac)
perties: extreme fire and water; nervous sedative, balancing
neral Uses: depression, frigidity, impotence, palpitations, skincare
ianga odorata; two forms exist:
- var. odorata (var. genuina., *Unona odorantissimum*): ylang-ylang
- var. macrophylla: cananga

BETULACEAE (shrubs, trees; fruit is one-seeded nut, often winged; includes birches, alders, hornbeams and hazels; 6 genera, 150 species; from northern hemisphere to tropical mountains)
Body Systems: Digestive and Respiratory Systems, Muscles and Bones
Properties: analgesic, draining (lymph), purifying
General Uses: auto intoxication, muscle pain
Betula alleghaniensis: yellow birch
Betula lenta: sweet birch

BURSERACEAE (means "dry fire"; resinous tropical timber trees; drupe or capsule fruit; 21 genera, 540 species)
Body Systems: Respiratory System (secretions), Emotional Balance (psychic centers), Skin
Properties: cooling, drying, fortifying
General Uses: anti-inflammatory, expectorant, scar tissue (reducing), ulcers, wounds (healing)
Boswellia carterii: frankincense
Canarium luzonicum: elemi
Commiphora myrrha: myrrh

CISTACEAE (low shrubs, few herbs; capsule fruit; Cistus species have large flowers; 7 genera, 175 species; Mediterranean, Europe, central Asia and America)
Body Systems: Emotional Balance, Skin (care)
Properties: calming, fortifying, healing
General Uses: anxiety, depression, stress-related disorders, wound healing
Cistus ladanifer: labdanum, cistus

COMPOSITAE (ASTERACEAE) (largest family of flowering plants; inflorescence, small flowers; 1317 genera, 21,000 species; fou everywhere, especially around Mediterranean)
Body Systems: Digestive System, Skin
Properties: "perfect balance of etheric and astral forces, promoting realization, reorganization, structure" [Lavabre, *Aromatherapy Workbook*]; adaptive, calming, regeneration (note: because of the large variety of plants withing this family, the therapeutic activity is very diversified; some plants are neurotoxic)
General Uses: infections, inflammation, regeneration
Achillea millefolium: yarrow
Artemisia dracunculus: tarragon
Artemisia pallens: davana
Artemisia vulgaris: mugwort
Chamaemelum mixtum (*mixta*): chamomile
Chamaemelum nobile: Roman chamomile
Conyza canadensis: Canadian fleabane
Helichrysum angustifolium (var. *Italicum*): helichrysum
Matricaria recutita: German chamomile
Solidago odora (*Solidago canadensis*): goldenrod
Tanacetum annum: blue tansy
Tanacetum vulgare: wild tansy

CUPRESSACEAE (conifer cypress family, needle-like leaves and cones; 17 genera, 113 species, most in northern temperate zones)
Body Systems: Hormonal, Respiratory, and Nervous Systems
Properties: appeasing, reviving, tonic, warming
General Uses: anti-rheumatic, astringent, cellulite (reduces), insomnia, nervous tension (reduces), respiration (when taken through inhalation), stress-related conditions
Callitris intratropica: blue cypress
Cupressus sempervirens: cypress
Juniperus communis: juniper
Juniperus scopulorum (*J. osteosperma*): Rocky Mountain juniper
Thuja occidentalis: cedarleaf
Thuja plicata: Western red cedar (leaf), Canadian red cedar (bark)

ICACEAE (shrubs and small trees with leathery evergreen leaves, fruit berry, drupe or capsule; 103 genera, 3350 species; cosmopolitan centered in northern hemisphere)

y Systems: Cardiovascular and Digestive Systems

perties: detoxifying

eral Uses: hypertension, kidney and liver stimulant

um groenlandicum: Labrador tea

ltheria procumbens: wintergreen

RANIACEAE (herbs or low shrubs, 14 genera, 730 species; temperate and tropical zones)

y Systems: Hormonal System, Digestive System (kidneys - excretion, liver & pancreas - metabolism), Nervous System, Emotional Balance

perties: balancing (nervous system)

eral Uses: burns, depression, diabetes, hemorrhage, nervous tension, skin, sore throat, ulcers, wounds

rgonium graveolens: geranium, rose geranium (*P. x asperum*)

AMINEAE (or POACEAE) (nutritious grass family; used for ground covering and food (wheat, rice, corn, barley); large root systems; 737 genera, 7950 species; distributed throughout the world)

y Systems: Cardiovascular System, Digestive System (stimulant), Respiratory System, Skin

perties: air purifier, calming, refreshing, sedative

eral Uses: air deodorizer, calm digestion, cleanse and balance skin (acne)

ibopogon flexuosus: lemongrass

ibopogon martinii: palmarosa

ibopogon nardus: citronella

veria zizanoides: vetiver

TTIFERAE (or HYPERICACEAE) (trees and shrubs; many useful for timber and edible fruits; 47 genera, 1350 species; mainly in tropics)

y Systems: Muscles and Bones, Skin

perties: anti-inflammatory, analgesic

eral Uses: infections, muscle pain, wounds

ophyllum inophyllum: tamanu

BIATE (LAMIACEAE) (herbs or low shrubs with quadrangular stems; largest of all essential oil producing plant families; oils are mostly non-toxic and non-hazardous; some antiseptic oils; some oils used for flavoring; most oils helpful for headaches, congestion, muscular problems (analgesic, anti-inflammatory), and stimulate one or more body systems; 224 genera, about 5600 species; main distribution in tropical and warmer temperate regions)

y Systems: Digestive and Respiratory Systems

perties: appeases overactive astral body [Lavabre, *Aromatherapy Workbook*], curative, stimulates, warms

eral Uses: anemia, diabetes, digestion (poor), headaches, respiratory problems; "good for people with intense psychic activity to prevent exhaustion and loss of self" [Lavabre, *Aromatherapy Workbook*]

sopus officinalis: hyssop

ndula angustifolia: lavender

ndula x hybrida: lavandin

ssa officinalis: melissa

tha piperita: peppermint

tha spicata: spearmint

num basilicum: basil

anum majorana: marjoram

anum vulgare: oregano

ostemon cablin: patchouli

narinus officinalis: rosemary several varieties

var. *officinalis*: common rosemary; numerous cultivars and forms;

chemotypes: CT I: camphor; CT II: cineole; CT III: verbenone

ia lavendulifolia: Spanish sage

ia officinalis: sage

Salvia sclarea: clary sage
Satureja montana: winter savory
Thymus vulgaris: thyme
chemotypes: linalool; thymol (or geraniol)
Vitex negundo: vitex

LAURACEAE (trees and shrubs with evergreen leaves and aromatic oils; some valued for timber, as ornamentals, or for oils or spices genera, 200-2500 species; found in tropics and sub-tropics in Amazona and South-east Asia)
Body Systems: Cardiovascular System (cardiac-stimulates, pulmonary-stimulates), Nervous System (regulates), Hormonal System (aphrodisiac), Skin (cellular-regenerates)
Properties: anti-fungal, anti-viral, anti-bacterial, stimulant, tonic (some oils in this family are irritant)
General Uses: depression, headache, hypotension, scars, sexual debility
Aniba roseodora var. amazonica: Brazilian rosewood, bois de rose
Cinnamomum cassia: cassia
Cinnamomum zeylanicum (C. *verum*): cinnamon bark
Laurus nobilis: laurel
Ravensara aromatica: ravensara

MYRISTICACEAE (plants whose bark produces watery, blood-like exudate; fruit is fleshy with one large seed; 19 genera, about 40(species; found throughout tropics, centered in Malaysia lowland rain forest)
Body Systems: Digestive, Hormonal, and Nervous Systems, Emotional Balance
Properties: analgesic, aphrodisiac, circulation, nervous system stimulant
General Uses: digestion, fatigue (mental and physical), impotence, nervousness, rheumatism
Myristica fragrans: nutmeg

MYRTACEAE (mainly tropical and sub-tropical plants with dotted leaves and oil glands; fruit is woody capsule or berry with one or many seeds; some have ornamental or showy flowers; many produce valuable timber; 121 genera, 3850 species; found in tropical and warm regions, especially Australia)
Body Systems: Respiratory and Immune Systems
Properties: "balances interaction of four elements (earth, air, fire, water)" [Lavabre, *Aromatherapy Workbook*], antiseptic, stimulant, tonic
General Uses: antiseptic, energy (balances), respiratory (infections), stimulant, tonic
Backhousia citriodora: lemon myrtle
Eucalyptus citriodora: lemon-scented eucalyptus
Eucalyptus dives: peppermint eucalyptus
Eucalyptus globulus: eucalyptus
Eucalyptus polybractea: blue leaved mallee
chemotype: cineole
Eugenia caryophyllata (*Syzygium aromaticum*): clove bud
Melaleuca alternifolia: tea tree
Melaleuca ericifolia: rosalina
Melaleuca leucadendra: cajeput
Melaleuca quinquenervia: niaouli
Myrtus communis: Myrtle (two sub-species exist: green and red)

OLEACEAE (trees or shrubs; including olive and ash; used for timber; 24 genera, 900 species; widely distributed, centered on Asia)
Body Systems: Emotional Balance, Hormonal System (aphrodisiac)
Properties: calming, soothing, uplifting
General Uses: anxiety, depression, frigidity, impotence, stress
Jasminum officinale: jasmine

PINACEAE (ABIETACEAE) (conifers with male and female cones; 9 genera, 194 species; found in northern hemisphere, temperate climates)
Body Systems: Hormonal, Nervous, and Respiratory Systems; signifies air element
Properties: antiseptic, appeasing, reviving, tonic, warming

eneral Uses: arthritis, congestion (inhaled), oxygen deficiency, respiratory disorders, rheumatism, stress

ies alba: fir, silver fir

ies balsamea: balsam fir

ies grandis: white fir, giant fir

drus atlantica: Atlas cedarwood

cea mariana: black spruce

nus ponderosa: ponderosa pine

nus sylvestris: Scotch pine

eudotsuga menziesii: Douglas fir

uga canadensis: hemlock spruce (or tsuga)

PERACEAE (pepper family; small trees, shrubs and climbers; small fleshy drupe with single seed; some widely cultivated for condiments; 4 genera, over 2000 species; found throughout tropics, mostly in rainforests)

dy Systems: Cardiovascular, Digestive, and Nervous Systems; root chakra

operties: drying, heating, stimulant, tonic

eneral Uses: fevers, indigestion, pain (muscle, tooth), grounding

per nigrum: black pepper

OSACEAE (trees, shrubs, and herbs; some edible fruits; many cultivated for fruits (almond) or flowers (rose); 107 genera, 3100 species; found in temperate climates throughout the world)

dy Systems: Hormonal System (female reproductive); heart chakra

operties: aphrodisiac, harmonizing, tonic, uplifting

eneral Uses: emotional shock, frigidity, grief, impotence

sa canina: rosehip

sa damascena: Bulgarian rose

UTACEAE (aromatic trees and shrubs; sometimes thorny; dotted, compound leaves with aromatic glands; includes citrus fruits; 161 genera, about 1650 species; found in tropical and warm temperate regions, especially Australia and South Africa)

dy Systems: Digestive (kidneys, liver) and Nervous Systems, Skin

operties: cooling, refreshing, secretion (fruits), sedative (flowers)

eneral Uses: inflammation, over-sensitivity, water balance

trus aurantifolia: lime

trus aurantium: neroli (var. *bigaradia*), petitgrain

trus bergamia: bergamot

trus hystrix: leech-lime

trus limon: lemon

trus nobilis: tangerine

trus x paradisi: grapefruit

trus reticulate: mandarin

trus sinensis: orange

NTALACEAE (herbs, shrubs and trees which are semi-parasitic on roots and stems of other plants; 36 genera, about 500 species; found in tropical and temperate regions)

dy Systems: Digestive System (excretory-balances, genito-urinary-disinfects), Nervous System (balances), and Respiratory System (balances)

operties: balancing, calming, constriction, grounding

neral Uses: genito-urinary tract infections, impotence, lung congestion, stress-related disorders

ntalum album: East Indian sandalwood, Mysore sandalwood, sandalwood

YRACACEAE (trees and shrubs with resinous bark used medicinally; used for incense, obtained by wounding tree; 12 genera, 165 species; found in tropical and warm temperate climates in Americas, Malaysia, Mediterranean, and South-east Asia)

dy Systems: Cardiovascular and Nervous Systems; first chakra

operties: calming, grounding, soothing

eneral Uses: hyper-activity

rax benzoin: benzoin, onycha

UMBELLIFERAE (APIACEAE) (herbs and a few shrubs, flowers borne in umbels (flowers radiating from a central point, like an umbrella); some important as food (carrot, celery), while others are very poisonous; some have medicinal actions; 420 genera 3100 species; found throughout the world, mainly in norther temperate regions)

Body Systems: Digestive System (balances), Hormonal System (stimulates uterus), Respiratory System, Skin (regenerates)

Properties: air element; accumulation (elimination, excretion), secretion

General Uses: gas, glandular problems, spasms

Anethum graveolens: dill

Angelica archangelica: angelica

Apium graveolens: celery

Coriandrum sativum: coriander

Cuminum cyminum: cumin

Daucus carota: carrot seed oil

Ferula galbaniflua: galbanum

Foeniculum vulgare: fennel

Pimpinella anisum: aniseed

VALERIANACEAE (herb family; fruit is dry; roots often used medicinally (valium); 17 genera, 14 species; found throughout the worl (except Australia))

Body Systems: Nervous System (calming)

Properties: grounding, sedative; balances upper and lower body

General Uses: anxiety, insomnia, nervous headaches, palpitations, stomach; living in one's head

Nardostachys jatamansi: spikenard

Valeriana officinalis: valerian

ZINGIBERACEAE (ginger family comprising rhizomatous herbs; 53 genera, 1200 species; found mostly in rain forests throughout the tropics, but mainly in Indo-Malaysia)

Body Systems: Digestive and Hormonal Systems, Muscles and Bones

Properties: analgesic, fever reducing, scurvy (prevents), stimulant, tonic, warming

General Uses: digestive (stimulant), rheumatism, sexual tonic

Elettaria cardamomum: cardamom

Zingiber officinale: ginger

Index

The following index has been manually verified and adjusted to increase its effectiveness ıd reduce its length. Due to the extent that the single oils are listed throughout this reference ıide, we thought it best to list only the most relevant page numbers for each single oil listing. The ngle oils are all listed in bold print to make it easy to identify them. All other page numbers that e listed in bold print, are the most relevant for their respective listing.

Bibliography

ch, M.D., James, and Phyllis Balch, C.N.C. *Prescription for Nutritional Healing*. Garden City Park, NY: Avery Publishing Group, 1990.

ker, M.D., Robert O. *The Body Electric*. New York, NY: Wm. Morrow, 1985.

roughs, Stanley. *Healing for the Age of Enlightenment*. Auburn, CA: Burroughs Books, 1993.

ton Goldberg Group, The. *Alternative Medicine: The Definitive Guide*. Fife, WA: Future Medicine Publishing, Inc., 1994.

Vita, Sabina M. *Electromagnetic Pollution. A Hidden Stress to Your System.* Marble Hill, MO: Stewart Publishing Company, 2000.

----------. *Essential Oils Desk Reference*. Essential Science Publishing. Third Edition, First Printing March 2004.

cher-Rizzi, Suzanne. *Complete Aromatherapy Handbook*. New York, NY: Sterling Publishing, 1990.

ey, Marcy. *Embraced by the Essence! Your Journey into Wellness Using Pure Quality Essential Oils*. Boulder, Colorado: Holistic Wellness Foundation I, April 2000.

tefosse, Ph.D., Rene-Maurice. *Gattefosse's Aromatherapy*. Essex, England: The C.W. Daniel Company Ltd., 1937 English translation.

en, Mindy. *Natural Perfumes: Simple Aromatherapy Recipes.* Loveland CO: Interweave Press Inc., 1999.

----------. *Integrated Aromatic Medicine*. Proceedings from the First International Symposium, Grasse, France. Essential Science Publishing, March 2000.

vless, Julia. *The Encyclopaedia of Essential Oils*. Rockport, MA: Element, Inc., 1992.

, M.D., John R. *Natural Progesterone: The Multiple Roles of a Remarkable Hormone*. Sebastopol, CA: BLL Publishing, 1995.

ury, Marguerite. *Marguerite Maury's Guide to Aromatherapy*. C.W. Daniel, 1989.

oël, M.D., Daniel and Pierre Franchomme. L'aromatherapie exactement. Limoges, France: Jollois, 1990.

ce, Shirley, and Len Price. *Aromatherapy for Health Professionals*. New York, NY: Churchill Livingstone Inc., 1995.

ce, Shirley, and Penny Price Parr. *Aromatherapy for Babies and Children*. San Francisco, CA: Thorsons, 1996.

se, Jeanne. *The Aromatherapy Book: Applications and Inhalations*. Berkeley, CA: North Atlantic Books, 1992.

man, Danièle. *Aromatherapy: The Complete Guide to Plant & Flower Essences for Health and Beauty*. New York: Bantam Books, 1993.

ppard-Hanger, Sylla. *The Aromatherapy Practitioner Reference Manual*. Tampa, FL: Atlantic Institute of Aromatherapy, Twelfth Printing February 2000.

Stewart, Ph.D., R.A., David. *A Statistical Validation of Raindrop Technique*. Marble Hill, MO: Care Publications, 2003.

Tisserand, Maggie. *Aromatherapy for Women: a Practical Guide to Essential Oils for Health and Beauty*. Rochester, VT: Healing Press, 1996.

Tisserand, Robert. *Aromatherapy: to Heal and Tend the Body*. Wilmot, WI: Lotus Press, 1988.

Tisserand, Robert. *The Art of Aromatherapy*. Rochester, VT: Healing Arts Press, 1977.

Tisserand, Robert, and Tony Balacs. *Essential Oil Safety: A Guide for Health Care Professionals*. New York, NY: Churchill Livingstone, 1995.

Valnet, M.D., Jean. *The Practice of Aromatherapy: a Classic Compendium of Plant Medicines and their Healing Properties*. Rochester, VT: Healing Arts Press, 1980.

Watson, Franzesca. *Aromatherapy Blends & Remedies*. San Francisco, CA: Thorsons, 1995.

Wilson, Roberta. *Aromatherapy for Vibrant Health and Beauty: a practical A-to-Z reference to aromatherapy treatments for healt skin, and hair problems*. Honesdale, PA: Paragon Press, 1995.

Worwood, Valerie Ann. *The Complete Book of Essential Oils & Aromatherapy*. San Rafael, CA: New World Library, 1991.

Young, N.D., D. Gary. *An Introduction to Young Living Essential Oils*. Payson, UT: Young Living Essential Oils, 2000.

Young, N.D., D. Gary. *Aromatherapy: The Essential Beginning*. Salt Lake City, UT: Essential Press Publishing, 1995.

Young, Ph.D., Robert O. *One Sickness, One Disease, One Treatment*. Alpine, UT: Self-published, 1995.

Video Listing

---------------. *Essential Tips for Happy, Healthy Pets*. The Vision Firm, LLC, 2000.

Eaton, Cathy. *Raindrop Therapy*. Health is Your Wealth Enterprises, 1997.

Woloshyn, Tom. *Vita Flex Instruction*. Vita-Gem Enterprises, 1998.

Young, ND, D. Gary. *Raindrop Technique*. Young Living Essential Oils, 2000.

Products Available from Abundant Health

de	Wt‡	Product Description	Price
		HEALTH RELATED BOOKS	
00	50	**COIL BOUND - REFERENCE GUIDE BUNDLE** (1001 & 1002)	$31.95
01	34	**COIL BOUND - Reference Guide for Essential Oils**	24.95
02	12	**COIL BOUND - Quick Reference Guide for Using Essential Oils**	10.95
48	64	**Essential Oils Desk Reference** (3rd Edition)	38.00
47	16	**Essential Oils Pocket Reference**	14.75
49	80	**Essential Oils Desk Reference/Pocket Reference Bundle**	49.00
16	4	**Pregnenolone**	3.50
12	7	**A Stastical Validation of Raindrop Technique**	9.50
03	48	**Essential Oils Integrative Medical Guide**	34.00
19	17	**Healing with Aromatherapy**	12.00
35	12	**Releasing Emotional Patterns with Essential Oils**	14.00
74	16	**Holistic Aromatherapy for Animals**	16.50
36	19	**What To Do When Antibiotics Don't Work**	19.50
62	12	**Making Aromatherapy Creams & Lotions**	16.95
46	18	**Healing Oils of the Bible**	16.85
04	20	**Healing Oils, Healing Hands**	22.50
66	13	**Saving Face**	16.95
73	17	**Aromatherapy for the Healthy Child**	16.95
14	17	**Advanced Aromatherapy - The Science of Essential Oil Therapy**	16.50
15	20	**Medical Aromatherapy - Healing with Essential Oils**	16.50
07	9	**Natural Perfumes**	12.50
06	16	**500 Formulas for Aromatherapy**	12.50
02	22	**Clinical Aromatherapy**	34.95
30	20	**Feelings Buried Alive Never Die...**	14.00
31	17	**Healing Feelings... From Your Heart**	14.00
52	12	**Electromagnetic Pollution**	8.50
43	12	**Alkalize or Die**	14.45
77	28	**Prozac, Panacea or Pandora?**	23.95
65	10	**Li ver Cleansing Handbook**	9.50
41	6	**The Master Cleanser** (Booklet)	5.95
61	1	**Rub a Dub, Dub... Is Cancer in your Tub?** (Booklet)	1.00
38	1	**How's Your pH?** (Booklet)	1.50
		VIDEOS (Volume Discounts Available)	
02	11	**Raindrop Technique** by D. Gary Young, ND	19.50
14	11	**Healing Oils of the Bible** by David Stewart, Ph.D.	29.50
27	11	**Essential Tips for Happy, Healthy Pets**	14.00

SHIPPING CHARGES

Total Weight	UPS Ground	UPS 2nd Day Air	Priority Mail
0-16 oz.	$5.90	$12.00	$3.85
17-32 oz.	6.42	13.60	5.40
33-48 oz.	6.78	15.20	7.85
49-64 oz.	7.08	16.80	9.45
65-80 oz.	7.37	18.60	11.00
81-96 oz.	7.61	20.80	11.30
97-112 oz.	7.84	22.90	12.55
113-128 oz.	8.13	25.10	13.80
129-144 oz.	8.48	27.20	15.05
145-160 oz.	8.95	29.30	16.30
161-176 oz.	9.47	31.40	17.55
177-192 oz.	9.99	33.20	18.80
193-208 oz.	10.51	34.70	20.05
209-224 oz.	11.03	36.40	21.25
225-240 oz.	11.55	38.20	22.50
241-256 oz.	12.04	39.90	23.75
257-272 oz.	12.54	41.70	25.00
273-288 oz.	13.04	43.60	26.25
289-304 oz.	13.54	45.70	27.50
305-320 oz.	14.04	47.60	28.75
321-336 oz.	14.53	49.40	30.00
337-352 oz.	15.02	51.20	31.20
353-368 oz.	15.51	53.20	32.45
369-384 oz.	16.02	55.00	33.70
385-400 oz.	16.53	56.70	34.95
401-416 oz.	16.99	58.40	36.20
417-432 oz.	17.46	60.00	37.45
433-448 oz.	17.93	61.70	38.70
449-464 oz.	18.45	63.40	39.95
465-480 oz.	18.97	65.00	41.20
481-496 oz.	19.49	66.80	42.40
497-512 oz.	20.01	68.50	43.65
513-528 oz.	20.54	70.30	44.90
529-544 oz.	21.06	72.30	46.15
545-560 oz.	21.58	74.30	47.40
561-576 oz.	22.10	76.10	48.65
577-592 oz.	22.62	77.90	49.90
593-608 oz.	23.14	79.70	51.15
609-624 oz.	23.66	81.40	52.40
625-640 oz.	24.18	83.20	53.60
641-656 oz.	24.70	84.90	54.85
657-672 oz.	25.22	86.60	56.15
673-688 oz.	25.73	88.60	57.40
689-704 oz.	26.24	90.50	58.70
705-720 oz.	26.75	92.30	59.95
721-736 oz.	27.20	94.10	61.20
737 oz. +	Call	Call	Call

This is only a partial list of products available from Abundant Health. For a complete list or to order, call 1-888-718-3068 / 801-798-0642 or visit our web site at www.abundant-health4u.com.

		VITA FLEX PRODUCTS (Volume Discounts Available)	
9302	11	**VIDEO: Vita Flex Instruction**	25.00
9301	20	**Vita Flex Roller** (Also known as **"Relax-a-Roller"**)	20.00
9040	11	**Healing for the Age of Enlightenment** (book)	11.00
		GLASS and PLASTIC PRODUCTS	
9100	3	**5/8 Dram Amber Glass Vials** (w/ orifice reducers) - 1 doz.	3.75
9155	4	**5 ml Amber Glass Vials** (w/ orifice reducer & white cap) - ½ doz.	3.50
9156	4	**10 ml Amber Glass Vials** (w/ orifice reducer & white cap) - ½ doz.	3.75
9157	4	**15 ml Amber Glass Vials** (w/ orifice reducer & white cap) - ½ doz.	4.00
9158	3	**10 ml Roll-On Bottles** (clear glass w/ white cap) - ½ doz.	4.00
9150	2	**1/6 Dram Clear Sample Vials** (w/ dabber cap or clip) - 1 doz.	2.00
9160	4	**2 Dram (7.4 ml) Amber Glass Vials** (w/ dropper cap) - ½ doz.	3.75
9180	12	**1 oz. Amber Glass Vials** (w/ dropper cap) - ½ doz.	4.00
9123	.5	**Spray Top for 1 oz. Amber Glass Vial**	.40
9190	4	**2 oz. Plastic Bottles** (w/ snap top cap) - ½ doz.	2.00
9251	1	**1 ml Syringe** (w/ drop markings - perfect for blending - other sizes avail.)	0.38
9259	1	**5 ml Vaginal Syringe** (rounded tip - ideal for vaginal insertion of oils)	1.10
9260	1	**20 ml Rectal Syringe** (w/ special rectal insertion tip)	1.47
9271	1	**Adapt-A-Cap Bottle Adapters (Size A - fits 5, 10, & 15 ml bottles)** Use these with the syringes to easily transfer oils from larger to smaller bottles or to accurately blend single oils.	1.21
		DIFFUSERS (Volume Discounts Available)	
9310	18	**Battery Operated Diffuser w/ Power Adapter & 5 Pads**	35.00
9320	19	**Economy Model Diffuser**	32.00
9346	32	**Tranquility Deluxe Diffuser**	62.00
9348	48	**Tubeless, Top-Loading Diffuser**	68.00
9315	48	**The "FanFuser™"** (Ultra quiet fan diffuser with replaceable pad)	34.95
9360	12	**Diffuser Timer** with on/off switch and 96 possible settings (programmable in 15 minute increments over a 24 hour period!)	12.00
		VIAL CARRYING CASES and OIL STORAGE/DISPLAY RACKS	
9550	6	**Essential Bags**–Carrying Case for 30 - 15 ml vials (Qty Disc. Avail.)	31.95
9559	4	**Essential Bags**–Carrying Case for 16 - 5/8 dram vials (Qty Disc. Avail.)	14.95
9530	30	**Essential Portfolios**–Professional Case for 64 vials (Qty Discounts Avail.)	39.95
9535	18	**Essential Portfolios**–Professional Case for 32 vials (Qty Discounts Avail.)	29.95
9570	192	**PREMIUM 3-Shelf Solid Oak Storage/Display Rack** (Holds 144 vials) It is 15" high x 21.75" wide x 8.5" deep; has two removable shelves with routed holes to keep your oils in place.	119.95
		ELECTROMAGNETIC FIELD (EMF) PROTECTION	
9700	1	**Cellular Phone Diode** provides excellent protection against EMF from cellular or cordless phones, blow dryers, or any appliance.	19.95

‡ Weight is all shown in ounces.

Call or visit our web site for Wholesale Prices & Volume Discounts!!!

Prices subject to change without notice!

Orders: 1-888-718-3068 (toll-free) / 801-798-0642 (

Fax: 1-877-568-1988 (toll-free) / 801-798-0644 (

E-Mail: orders@abundant-health4u

Web Site: www.abundant-health4u

(Check out our monthly Internet Spe

LING INFORMATION (as it appears on the credit card statement)

:____

ess:____

State/Zip:____________________________________

#:____

l Address:____________________________________

P-TO INFORMATION (to which order will be sent)

:____

ess:____

State/Zip:____________________________________

#:____

Mail to:
Abundant Health
1460 N. Main St., #9
Spanish Fork, UT 84660

Orders: 1-888-718-3068 / 801-798-0642
Fax: 1-877-568-1988 / 801-798-0644
E-Mail: orders@abundant-health4u.com
Web Site: www.abundant-health4u.com

Return Policy:
Any damaged or defective products must be reported within 10 days of receipt and will be replaced with an exact product replacement only. An RMA number must first be obtained from Abundant Health for all returns. Purchase price of returned items will be refunded less a 10% restocking fee. No refunds will be issued for any outdated, used, or damaged items.

International Shipping:
Global Priority Mail envelopes are $9.00 and hold one Reference Guide and one Quick Reference Guide. Call for all other shipping costs.

YMENT INFORMATION

sa ☐ MC
neck/Money Order
nclude with order form)

Credit Card Number:______________________________

Exp. Date:__________________________________

Signature:__________________________________

Code	Wt. (oz)	Qty	Unit Price	Discount	Total
				-	=
				-	=
				-	=
				-	=
				-	=
				-	=
				-	=
				-	=
				-	=
				-	=
				-	=
				-	=
				SUBTOTAL:	=
				Sales Tax (Utah residents only) x 0.0625:	+
(Add Ounces & See Chart on Products Page)				**Shipping/Handling:**	+
				TOTAL COST:	=

LING INFORMATION (as it appears on the credit card statement)

:____

ss:____

tate/Zip:______________________________________

#:____

Address:______________________________________

P-TO INFORMATION (to which order will be sent)

:____

ss:____

tate/Zip:______________________________________

#:____

Mail to:
Abundant Health
1460 N. Main St., #9
Spanish Fork, UT 84660

Orders: 1-888-718-3068 / 801-798-0642
Fax: 1-877-568-1988 / 801-798-0644
E-Mail: orders@abundant-health4u.com
Web Site: www.abundant-health4u.com

Return Policy:
Any damaged or defective products must be reported within 10 days of receipt and will be replaced with an exact product replacement only. An RMA number must first be obtained from Abundant Health for all returns. Purchase price of returned items will be refunded less a 10% restocking fee. No refunds will be issued for any outdated, used, or damaged items.

International Shipping:
Global Priority Mail envelopes are $9.00 and hold one Reference Guide and one Quick Reference Guide. Call for all other shipping costs.

'MENT INFORMATION

sa ☐ MC
eck/Money Order
clude with order form)

Credit Card Number:______________________________________

Exp. Date:____

Signature:____

Code	Wt. (oz)	Qty	Unit Price	Discount	Total
				-	=
				-	=
				-	=
				-	=
				-	=
				-	=
				-	=
				-	=
				-	=
				-	=
				-	=
				-	=
				SUBTOTAL:	=
				Sales Tax (Utah residents only) x 0.0625:	+
(Add Ounces & See Chart on Products Page)				**Shipping/Handling:**	+
				TOTAL COST:	=

About the Cover Painting and the Artist

n you identify the plants in this painting?
The answers are at the bottom of the page.

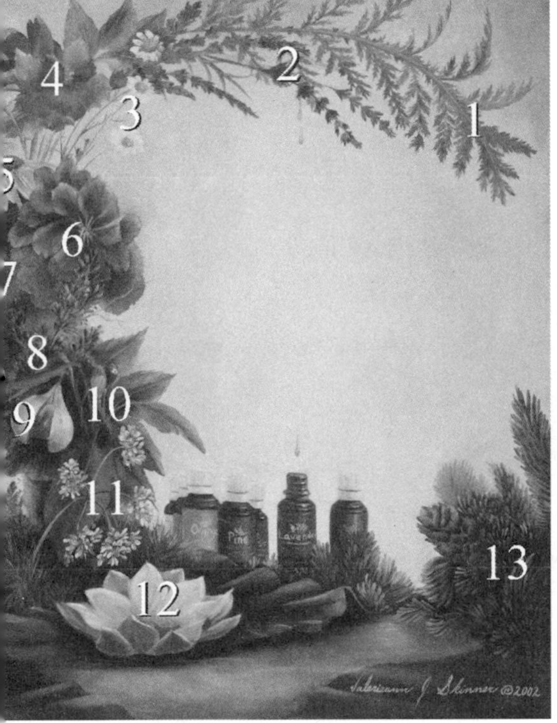

This painting was created by

Valerieann J. Skinner,

artist and author from Georgetown, Idaho. For nineteen years, Valerieann has taught others how to heal, better know themselves and express their uniqueness through art. This and painting professionally for over twenty years, has taught her much—especially about color and its affect on people. She has discovered the importance of using color *consciously*. You can learn how to use it more effectively in your own life by reading her book, *Cashing in on the "Simple Magic" of Color*. Get a FREE copy by visiting her website.

Her newest book, *The World of Mirrors—A Bridge to Knowing and Being Your "True" Self*, is a self-empowering book that gives the reader a life changing perspective on everything happening in their life and the world. Read this book and your orld will come alive with the answers, guidance and healing you are seeking. **Valerieann's oks, handmade "essential oil" greeting cards, and art prints are available through undant Health.**

Do you need a cover for your book, CD or creation?
Contact Valerieann and discuss your ideas with her.
Inner Light Creations
P.O. Box 32, Georgetown, Idaho 83239
Phone: 208-847-3129 Website: www.valerieann.com
E-mail: valerieann@valerieann.com Website: www.valerieann.com

1.Tansy 2. Lavender 3. Chamomile 4. Rose 5. Echinacea 6. Geranium
7. Goldenseal 8. Hyssop 9. Nutmeg 10. Clove 11. Coriander 12. Lotus 13. Pine